Skull Base Reconstruction

Edward C. Kuan • Bobby A. Tajudeen
Hamid R. Djalilian • Harrison W. Lin

Editors

Skull Base Reconstruction

Management of Cerebrospinal Fluid Leaks
and Skull Base Defects

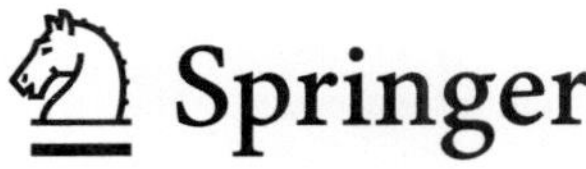 Springer

Editors
Edward C. Kuan
Otolaryngology-Head and Neck Surgery
and Neurological Surgery
University of California, Irvine
Irvine, CA, USA

Hamid R. Djalilian
Otolaryngology-Head and Neck Surgery
and Neurological Surgery
University of California, Irvine
Irvine, CA, USA

Bobby A. Tajudeen
Otorhinolaryngology-Head and
Neck Surgery
Rush University Medical Center
Chicago, IL, USA

Harrison W. Lin
Otolaryngology-Head and Neck Surgery
and Neurological Surgery
University of California, Irvine
Irvine, CA, USA

ISBN 978-3-031-27939-3   ISBN 978-3-031-27937-9   (eBook)
https://doi.org/10.1007/978-3-031-27937-9

This Springer imprint is published by the registered company Springer Nature Switzerland AG
The registered company address is: Gewerbestrasse 11, 6330 Cham, Switzerland

To my family, mentors, mentees, and, above all, patients, from whom we have the privilege of caring for and their generosity for helping us learn more about how to treat others.

Foreword

Before I reviewed the book, I could not help wondering whether the scope was too narrow for a book of this size. I was completely and totally wrong. Firstly, the authors have done a magnificent job of bringing together the disciplines of both neurosurgery and otolaryngology with the leading authors that they chose. The book will be an important reference for surgeons in both specialties. Secondly, the work is particularly relevant, because the appropriate diagnosis and management of CSF leaks has changed dramatically, has major potential complications, and at least from the otolaryngological standpoint, has become a significant issue medicolegally.

The endoscopic closure of CSF leaks was first formally described in 1989, although Wigand had made a reference to it well prior to that point in time [1–3]. Since the first formal descriptions of endoscopic closure, the appropriate management of anterior, middle, and posterior fossa CSF leaks has been radically transformed, in terms of diagnosis, when to operate, and in terms of the preferred surgical approach. Accordingly, this book is very timely in terms of bringing every otolaryngologist and neurosurgeon up to date. Whereas previously the morbidity from CSF leak closure performed from above was high, with endoscopic techniques the morbidity from the closure itself is now typically minimal. This morbidity reduction has called into question the appropriateness of conservative or medical management in the absence of associated intracranial injuries, and this is one of the most important evolutions. Additionally, with the epidemic of obesity, the frequency of spontaneous CSF leaks appears to likely be on the rise, making the importance of dealing with this issue and skull base meningoencephaloceles ever more important. Finally, the ever-increasing opportunity to manage skull base lesions extracranially has created increasingly large skull base defects.

The text starts with an overview of the anatomy of both the anterior and lateral skull base, and then discusses CSF physiology and leak diagnosis, anterior and lateral skull base pathologies, repair materials and anesthesia. There are separate sections for anterior and for lateral base reconstruction. In addition to free grafts and vascularized flaps, there are chapters on free flaps and the management of posterior fossa defects. I was also delighted to see that the authors have included chapters on both anterior and lateral skull base approaches, as well as anesthesia during skull base reconstruction and CSF diversion. In terms of reconstructive techniques, in addition to free grafts and vascularized flaps, the work also contains chapters on extracranial and microvascular repairs. One of the most difficult areas to repair, clival and craniocervical junction defects, has an excellent chapter for the management of such frequently high flow defects. This chapter carefully elucidates the options for multilayer reconstruction, the importance of judicious packing in the region, and additional options when a vascularized posterior septal flap is not available. Overall, the book is comprehensive in its approach and truly a multidisciplinary work.

The dramatically reduced morbidity and higher closure success rates associated with extracranial repair have tipped the scales in favor of surgical closure of leaks, and at an earlier point in time than had previously been considered appropriate. It is important that all specialists in both otolaryngology and neurosurgery are aware of this significant shift, as well as of the most applicable approaches for CSF leak closure. Failure to manage this issue appropriately can be devastating to the patient and raise questions of appropriate standard of care. During my career as a rhinologist/skull base surgeon, I have been asked to get involved in a number of medico-legal cases, where the creation, diagnosis, or management of a CSF leak has been the major focus. Inaccurately believing that the success rate for closure is higher with an intracranial approach, utilizing outdated diagnostic tests, and inappropriately managing an iatrogenic CSF leak have all been issues that can be difficult to defend. However, more importantly, with the increasing use of extracranial approaches to skull base lesions, the defects created have become significantly more sizeable and it is important to be familiar with different closure options available today.

I am delighted with the way that the authors have utilized a comprehensive multidisciplinary approach in putting this text together. I believe that it will be the definitive text on this issue for years to come and I hope that it is read by all otolaryngologists and neurosurgeons. It is an important book even among those not performing skull base surgery, as traumatic and iatrogenic CSF leaks can present unexpectedly and it is critical for our patients that they are managed appropriately and with some confidence on the part of the treating surgeon.

University of Pennsylvania David W. Kennedy
Philadelphia, PA, USA

References

1. Wigand ME (1981). Transnasal Ethmoidectomy Under Endoscopic Control. Rhinology, 19:7–15, 1981
2. Papay FA, Benninger MS, Levine HL, Lavertu P (1989). Transnasal transseptal endoscopic repair of sphenoidal cerebral spinal fluid fistula. Head and Neck Surg 101(5):595–7.
3. Mattox DE, Kennedy DW (1990). Endoscopic management of cerebrospinal fluid leaks and cephaloceles. Laryngoscope, 100:857–862.

Preface

The skull base poses a unique challenge to the medical community, as it is a highly anatomically sensitive area at the intersection of multiple disciplines. The traditional problem of accessing or approaching the skull base has largely been circumvented with the advent of multiportal techniques, including open, endoscopic, other minimally invasive, and combined means, and our ability to deliver appropriate treatment has also improved with advances in surgical and nonsurgical modalities. However, a longstanding problem in skull base surgery is reconstruction, which may challenge even the most experienced of surgeons, for which there is currently no dedicated text. The importance of skull base reconstruction cannot be understated to prevent patient morbidity and to restore normal physiologic function surrounding the brain and meninges, sinonasal cavity, temporal bone, and aerodigestive tract.

To fill this gap, we pooled our academic interests and expertise and proposed the first edition of this text. There is currently no updated book uniquely dedicated to the topic of skull base reconstruction. We hoped to create a centralized, multidisciplinary, comprehensive, and balanced text that would allow readers to access all queries on this developing topic. We were fortunate to have been able to invite a truly stellar group of multidisciplinary authors, all of whom have academic and clinical focus areas in skull base reconstruction, to share their expertise and experiences on various topics. The first section is dedicated to basic principles, anatomy, physiology, imaging, and anesthetic considerations. The second and third sections discuss pathological processes which lead to cerebrospinal fluid leaks and the need for skull base reconstruction within the anterior and lateral skull base, respectively. The fourth and fifth sections focus on anterior and lateral skull base reconstruction, respectively, with attention to reconstruction techniques and strategies for managing each defect type. The sixth section comprehensively reviews postoperative care and management strategies, where there is high variability and limited evidence, and is intended to present multiple perspectives and provide experiential guidance on this topic. The final section highlights developments, research, and emerging ideas.

The intended audience of the book includes skull base surgeons, otolaryngologists, neurosurgeons, medical and radiation oncologists, radiologists, pathologists, ophthalmologists, endocrinologists, neurologists, trauma physicians, and emergency physicians, and trainees and students in all of those areas. We hope that our efforts will provide a user-friendly and informative resource for this exciting area, and further stimulate curiosity in how we can improve the status quo.

Irvine, CA, USA   Edward C. Kuan
Chicago, IL, USA   Bobby A. Tajudeen
Irvine, CA, USA   Hamid R. Djalilian
Irvine, CA, USA   Harrison W. Lin

Contents

Part I
Anatomy, Physiology, and General Principles

Chapter 1
Anterior Skull Base Anatomy

Sarah Khalife, Rickul Varshney, and Rohit Garg

Introduction

An increasing shift from open approaches to less invasive endoscopic techniques for surgical treatment of sinonasal and skull base pathology has taken precedence over the last 30 years. It was in the 1990s that the first endoscopic surgery team of otolaryngologists and neurosurgeons was created [1]. Subsequently, endoscopic access gained popularity and has now become the mainstay of treatment for many sinonasal and anterior skull base pathologies with fewer complications and good outcomes [2]. For the endoscopic surgical team, knowledge of the complex anatomy of the nasal cavity, orbit, and anterior skull base and its many variations is essential to ensure proper surgical resection while avoiding devastating complications of surrounding structures [3]. In this chapter, we discuss their important anatomical features and key surgical landmarks to remain safe during endoscopic surgery.

S. Khalife (✉)
Department of Otolaryngology—Head and Neck Surgery, McGill University Health Centre, Montreal, QC, Canada
e-mail: Sarah.khalife@mcmaster.ca

R. Varshney
Department of Otolaryngology—Head and Neck Surgery, CIUSSS Ouest-de-l'Ile de Montréal & McGill University, Montreal, QC, Canada
e-mail: rickul.varshney@mcgill.ca

R. Garg
Department of Head and Neck Surgery, Kaiser Permanente Orange County Anaheim Medical Center, Anaheim, CA, USA
e-mail: Rohit.X.Garg@kp.org

E. C. Kuan et al. (eds.), *Skull Base Reconstruction*,
https://doi.org/10.1007/978-3-031-27937-9_1

Nasal Cavity

Nasal septum: The nasal septum is separated into an anterior cartilaginous part and a posterior bony portion formed by the maxilla, vomer, and perpendicular plate of the ethmoid bone [4]. It is important to assess the anatomy of the nasal septum both on physical exam and on preoperative imaging in order to identify a septal deviation, a septal spur, or, rarely, pneumatization of the posterior septum [3]. These anatomic abnormalities can hinder proper access and visualization during surgery, thus increasing the risks of complications. A 26–97% prevalence of septal anomalies has previously been reported [3]. In the latter cases, one would proceed with a septoplasty to optimize endoscopic visualization and maximize space for the surgical instruments.

Lateral nasal wall (Fig. 1.1): The lateral nasal wall is formed by the uncinate process; the inferior, middle, and superior turbinates; and occasionally supreme turbinate. The embryological origin of these structures is from the ethmoturbinals that appear by the tenth week of gestation and develop over time into ridges with ascending and descending portions [5]. Each ethmoturbinal and its final anatomical structure are listed in Table 1.1. However, there is much debate on the accuracy of each of these embryological associations which varies from one source to another [5].

The uncinate process is an extension of the ethmoid bone that is sickle-shaped in a sagittal plane [5]. It is attached anteriorly to the lacrimal bone and inferior-posteriorly to the inferior turbinate and palatine bone, and superiorly, six alternative attachment points have been reported [5]. The most common superior attachment is to the lamina papyracea which shifts the frontal drainage pathway lateral to the uncinate and into the middle meatus [4, 5]. Attachments to the skull

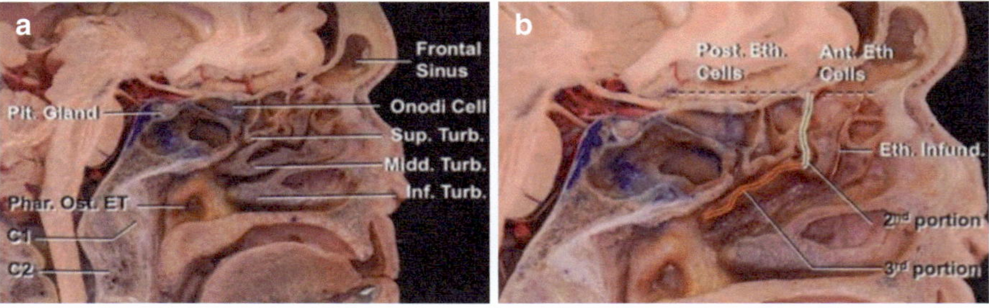

Fig. 1.1 Lateral nasal wall cadaveric image in sagittal view. (**a**) The inferior, middle, and superior turbinates can be seen protruding from the lateral nasal wall. Posteriorly, above the sphenoid, an Onodi cell can also be seen. (**b**) The second portion of the middle turbinate (white double-line) in coronal plane separates the anterior and posterior ethmoid air cells. The third portion in axial orientation is shown as an orange double-line. (With permissions from Peris-Celda et al. 2019)

Table 1.1 Embryology of the lateral nasal wall and their ethmoturbinal origin

Ethmoturbinal	Final anatomical structure
First	Agger nasi/uncinate process
Second	Ethmoid bulla
Third	Middle turbinate basal lamella
Fourth	Superior turbinate (+/− supreme turbinate)

base and middle turbinate are less common, and both lead to frontal sinus drainage into the ethmoid infundibulum [4, 5]. The ethmoid infundibulum is bordered medially by a 2-D structure known as the hiatus semilunaris. The latter is formed by the uncinate process antero-inferiorly and the ethmoid bulla postero-superiorly. From a surgical standpoint, it is important to determine the uncinate's lateral distance from the lamina papyracea and to identify its superior attachment, as this may alter the frontal drainage pathway as mentioned above [5]. Anatomical variations of the uncinate process must also be identified preoperatively and can include its pneumatization, paradoxical shape, medialization, atelectasis, absence, and its different attachment points [5, 6]. Atelectasis increases the risk of orbital injury during uncinectomy, while pneumatization can lead to sinus obstruction [6].

The inferior turbinate is known to have a separate embryological origin and becomes its own separate bone that develops by endochondral ossification [7]. Beneath each turbinate lies an anatomical space known as a meatus, into which drain different components of the nasal cavity. The inferior meatus lies beneath the inferior turbinate and receives drainage from the nasolacrimal duct via Hasner's valve [5, 6]. The middle meatus is an anatomical space beneath the middle turbinate that drains the anterior compartment of the nasal cavity, notably the frontal sinus, anterior ethmoid sinuses, and the maxillary sinus [6]. The superior meatus, beneath the superior turbinate, drains the posterior component of the nasal cavity, including the sphenoid sinus and posterior ethmoids [6].

The middle turbinate merits a more detailed description of its structure, as it is subdivided into three parts [4]. Its first segment, visualized in the sagittal plane, is attached superiorly to the skull base at the cribriform plate; its second segment in the coronal plane (also known as the basal lamella) is attached laterally to the lamina papyracea; and its third segment, in the axial plane, also inserts onto the lamina papyracea. Understanding the orientations of each of these segments is essential in order to avoid destabilization of the middle turbinate during endoscopic sinus surgery and also to be able to identify the basal lamella as the landmark that separates the anterior and posterior ethmoid compartments [4]. In addition, anatomical differences of the middle concha include its size and shape [4], the presence of a concha bullosa in 15–80% of patients (Fig. 1.2a), concha bullosa mucocele or mucopyocele, or a paradoxical middle turbinate [3].

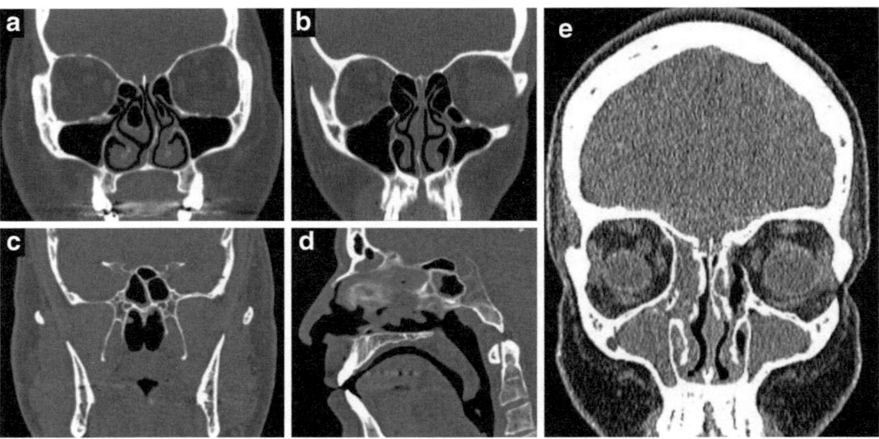

Fig. 1.2 Anatomic variations in sinus anatomy can be seen on CT scans preoperatively. (**a**) Right concha bullosa. (**b**) Left haller cell. (**c** and **d**) Coronal and sagittal views of an Onodi cell. (**e**) Dehiscence of left lamina papyracea with orbital prolapse

Paranasal Sinuses

The four pairs of paranasal sinuses are complex and have variations in pneumatization and timing of development. Embryologically, the maxillary sinus is the first to start developing at 10 weeks of gestation, followed by the ethmoids, sphenoids, and then frontals. Sinuses are fully developed during adolescence in the following order: ethmoids, maxillary, and sphenoid followed by frontals, which are not even present at birth.

The maxillary sinus in its adult form is bounded superiorly by the floor of the orbit, in which the infraorbital canal and infraorbital nerve cross and inferiorly by the maxilla's alveolar process [5]. Infraorbital nerve dehiscence has been reported in up to 14% of patients, making it a nerve structure that should be identified during sinus surgery and trans-antral surgeries to avoid its inadvertent injury [3, 6]. The maxillary sinus ostium opens within the medial wall of the sinus with a 3–10 mm opening through the lateral nasal wall behind the nasolacrimal duct and lateral to the uncinate process [5]. When performing a maxillary antrostomy, one must be cognizant of the fact that the true ostium is not visible with a 0° endoscope and is hidden by the uncinate process. The pterygopalatine fossa is an inverted pyramidal space that is located posterior to the posterior wall of the maxillary sinus. Sieur cells are found between these two structures in 34–42% of cases [3]. Septations of the maxillary sinus are also quite commonly found in 29% of patients, and other variations include sinus hypoplasia, aplasia, and hyper-pneumatization [3, 6]. The sinus surgeon must be aware of these differences, as they can increase the risk of orbital injury during surgery.

The ethmoid sinuses are divided into anterior and posterior compartments separated by the basal lamella of the middle turbinate. An important landmark to identify is the largest air cell of the anterior ethmoids, known as the ethmoid bulla [5]. The latter is the most constant anteriorly, where it forms the posterior edge of the ethmoid infundibulum and semilunar hiatus, laterally, where it attaches to the lamina papyracea and, medially, where the middle turbinate is a consistent landmark [4, 5]. However, its anatomy superiorly and posteriorly can vary depending on its pneumatization. Posteriorly, an air space known as the "retrobullar recess" can be present as an air space between the bulla and the second segment of the middle turbinate [5]. Similarly, the "supra bullar recess" is a potential space between the bulla and the skull base. However, if no air space is found, the superior border of the ethmoid bulla/ethmoid roof forms the posterior aspect of the frontal recess [5].

Other patterns of pneumatization of surgical importance include the agger nasi cell, haller cells, and sphenoethmoidal cells (Fig. 1.2). The agger nasi is known as the most anterior ethmoid air cell and serves as an important landmark for frontal sinus dissection. When an ethmoid cell pneumatized into the maxillary sinus and lies beneath the inferior orbital wall, this is known as a "haller cell" [5] (Fig. 1.2b). It can lead to maxillary sinus obstruction and can mislead the surgeon during surgery if he/she is not aware of its presence. The sphenoethmoidal cell, also known as an Onodi cell (Fig. 1.2c, d), can also increase the surgical risk, notably to the optic nerve, internal carotid artery, and skull base [5]. By definition, it consists of a posterior ethmoid air cell pneumatized into the superior-lateral sphenoid sinus [5].

The sphenoid sinuses are also paired and separated by an intersinus septum, which can occasionally insert itself onto the carotid canal in 4.7% of cases [3] or optic nerve. The pneumatization of the sphenoid sinuses varies and can be classified into conchal (Fig. 1.3), pre-sellar, and sellar, in order of least to most pneumatized [1]. Sternberg's canal is an anatomic variation of the sphenoid sinus that can be present in 4% of the adult population and results in lateral sphenoid sinus pneumatization and more specifically a defect of congenital origin [5]. A more detailed anatomy of the sphenoid bone and sinus will be discussed in the ventral skull base section.

Frontal sinus endoscopic procedures can be considered the most complex of all sinuses. The frontal sinus can be asymmetric when comparing both sides and can be aplastic in up to 33% of patients bilaterally and 7.4% unilaterally [3]. In endoscopic surgery, comfort with the use of angled endoscopes and instruments is necessary to approach the frontal sinus due to its posterior and superior location to the frontal beak [8]. In addition, the frontal sinus has a drainage pathway that can vary

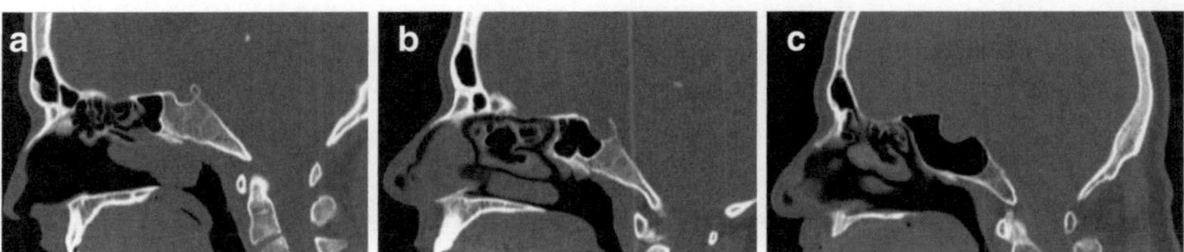

Fig. 1.3 Sphenoid sinus pneumatization variations on sagittal cut CT sinus: (**a**) conchal, (**b**) pre-sellar, and (**c**) sellar

extensively from one patient to another, notably due to the numerous air cells that can obstruct the frontal recess or the frontal sinus itself. The boundaries of the frontal recess, into which the frontal sinus ostium drains, consist of the frontal beak anteriorly, the basal lamella of the middle turbinate posteriorly, the lacrimal bone and the lamina papyracea laterally, and the first sagittal segment of the middle turbinate and the cribriform plate's lateral lamella medially [8]. Multiple classifications and their modifications over the years have been followed. The most recent classification published in 2016 by Wormald et al. is "The International Frontal Sinus Anatomy Classification (IFAC)" [8]. This new IFAC classification separates cells into anterior, posterior, and medial [8]. Anterior cells consist of cells that move the frontal drainage pathway in a medial, posterior, or posteromedial direction and include the three following cells: agger nasi cell, supra agger cell, and supra agger frontal cell [8]. Posterior cells move the frontal drainage pathway anteriorly and include the three following cells: supra bulla cell, supra bulla frontal cell, and supraorbital ethmoid cell [8]. The frontal septal cell is the only medial cell that forces the frontal drainage in a lateral direction. Understanding the anatomy and the differences between these cells is vital and will allow for appropriate and safe surgery of the frontal sinus. A more detailed description can be found in the IFAC classification article by Wormald et al. [8]. It is important to note that an associated "Classification of the Extent of Endoscopic Frontal Sinus Surgery (EFSS)" was also described in the same publication [8] but will not be discussed for the purposes of this chapter.

Orbit

The orbit is in very close proximity to all sinuses and is therefore a structure at high risk of injury during endoscopic sinus surgery and endoscopic skull base surgery. It lies in a bony compartment bounded superiorly by the orbital process of the frontal bone and the sphenoid; laterally by the frontal, sphenoid, and zygomatic bones; inferiorly by the sphenoid, palatine, and maxillary bone; and medially by the frontal process of maxilla, lamina papyracea (ethmoid bone), and lacrimal and sphenoid bones [9]. The lamina papyracea is normally 0.2–0.4 mm in thickness, decreasing in width from posterior to anterior, making it susceptible to injury and invasion [5]. Preoperatively, it is always important to note any evidence of dehiscence and orbital prolapse (Fig. 1.2e) or if the lamina is uncharacteristically medial to the maxillary sinus ostium, which all increase the risk of orbital injury [3, 5, 6]. The globe itself is surrounded by the periorbita and contains orbital fat, nerves, vessels, and extraocular muscles. The extraocular muscles include the superior and inferior oblique muscles and the superior, medial, inferior, and lateral rectus muscles [5]. Together with their fibrous attachments, the rectus muscles form a ring that is anatomically known as the annulus of Zinn [9]. During endoscopic surgery, the medial rectus muscle is at greatest risk of injury due to its close proximity to the lamina papyracea.

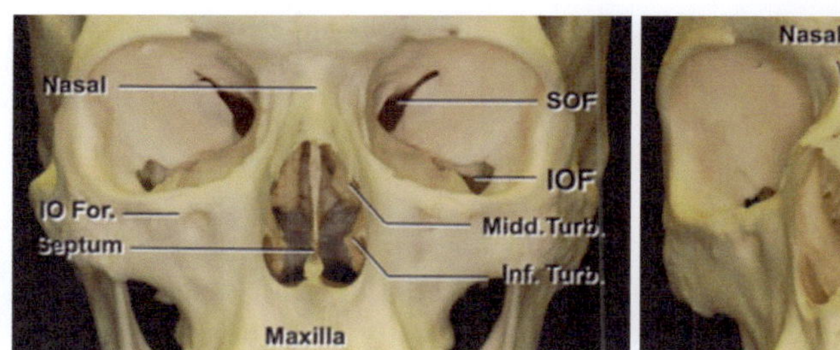

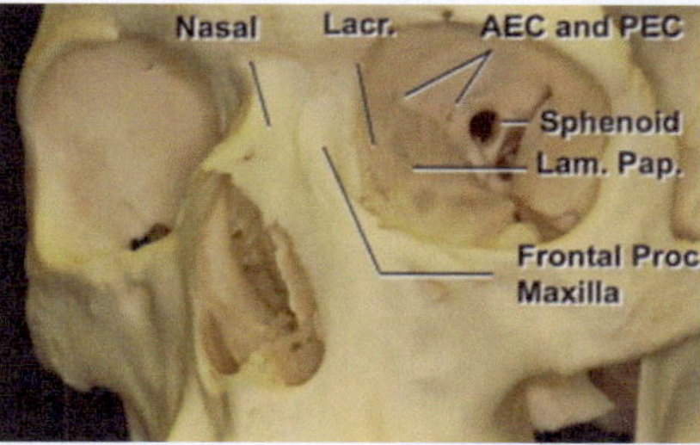

Fig. 1.4 Bony anatomy of the orbit demonstrates the superior orbital fissure (SOF) and inferior orbital fissure (IOF) within the posterior orbital wall formed by the sphenoid bone. The medial orbital wall is formed by the frontal process of maxilla (Frontal Proc. Maxilla), lamina papyracea (Lam. Pap.), lacrimal (Lacr.), and sphenoid bones. AEC, anterior ethmoid canal; PEC, posterior ethmoid canal; IO For., infraorbital foramen; Midd Turb., middle turbinate; Inf. Turb., interior turbinate (Modified from Peris-Celda et al., 2019)

Along the posterior orbital wall is the optic canal which courses the ophthalmic artery, optic nerve, and sympathetic fibers [9, 10]. Lateral to this canal are the superior and inferior orbital fissures (Fig. 1.4). The superior orbital fissure carries numerous cranial nerves and vessels including cranial nerves III (oculomotor nerve), IV (trochlear nerve), VI (abducens nerve) V1 branches of cranial nerve V (trigeminal nerve), inferior and superior ophthalmic veins [9, 10]. The inferior orbital fissure carries the infraorbital nerve, artery, and vein [9].

Ventral Skull Base

The ventral skull base can be described as a bony division that separates the anterior intracranial contents from the nasal cavity. Its boundaries can be subdivided into the lamina papyracea laterally, the planum sphenoidale posteriorly, and the posterior table of the frontal sinus anteriorly [11, 12].

If we begin anatomically from a front to back approach, the first anterior skull base structure that is encountered endoscopically is a part of the ethmoid bone known as the cribriform plate. Its boundaries consist of the frontal bone anteriorly, planum sphenoidale of the sphenoid bone posteriorly, laterally the middle and superior turbinates, and medially the nasal septum [5]. The crista galli of the ethmoid bone attaches posteriorly to the anterior edge of the falx cerebri and divides the paired cribriform plates into right and left [5, 13]. Although rare, pneumatization of the crista galli is present in approximately 13% of patients [5, 13]. Together, the crista galli, the cribriform plate, and the lateral lamella form the olfactory fossa that house the olfactory bulbs [5]. Olfactory epithelium is found in specific locations of the nasal cavity, notably the upper nasal septum, the cribriform plate, and the superior and medial portions of the superior and middle turbinates [5]. Multiple olfactory nerve fibers pass through the little foramina of the cribriform

Table 1.2 Olfactory fossa depth measurement as described by the "Keros classification" [5]

Keros type	Lateral lamella vertical height
1	1–3 mm
2	4–7 mm
3	8–16 mm

plate to reach the olfactory bulbs and allow for the sense of smell. From a surgical standpoint, the lateral lamella of the cribriform is the thinnest bone of the skull base and is at high risk of cause of a cerebrospinal fluid leak in the anterior skull base [5]. In addition, it is important to remember that increased depth and asymmetry of the olfactory fossa also increases this risk [5, 13]. The Keros classification is most commonly used to determine this depth as described in Table 1.2 (Fig. 1.5) [5, 13].

Between the lateral lamella of the cribriform plate and the lamina papyracea sits the fovea ethmoidalis (also known as the ethmoid roof) across which one can identify the anterior and posterior ethmoid arteries [5, 13]. The course of the anterior (AEA) and posterior ethmoid arteries (PEA) are important to understand as their injury can lead to significant bleeding. They both derive from the internal carotid artery's ophthalmic branch and branch off between the medial rectus and superior oblique muscles [2]. The AEA then enters the anterior ethmoid foramen, crosses the ethmoid sinuses through an ethmoid canal in a slanted anteromedial direction, and enters the lateral lamella of the cribriform plate forming the anterior ethmoid sulcus [1, 5, 13]. Here, it branches into an intracranial component and a nasal component that supplies the septum and middle turbinate [5]. During endoscopic sinus surgery, the AEA is often found posterior to the frontal recess or in the suprabullar recess [1, 5]. In more than 40% of patients [5, 6], the AEA can be found on a mesentery rather than within its bony canal; therefore it is very important to identify any dehiscence of the AEA on preoperative CT scans [5, 6] (Fig. 1.6). Its injury can lead to excessive bleeding and even retroorbital hematoma. Conversely, the PEA is not at an increased risk of injury, as it enters the posterior ethmoid foramen and crosses the posterior ethmoids skull base almost always within a bony canal between the planum sphenoidale and the cribriform plate [1, 5].

Anatomically, it is conventionally taught that the distance in order from the lacrimal crest to the AEA, PEA, and optic nerve is 24 mm, 12 mm, and 6 mm from one another [5]. Song et al. conducted a cadaver study that determined the distance from the columella to the AEA was on average 64 mm on the right and 63 mm on the left, whereas the PEA was on average 72 mm on the right and 71 mm on the left [2]. A middle ethmoid artery has also been described in the literature in 29–38% of cases, but is not always present [13]. Variations in all three arteries including their number, course, location, and absence have also been described; one should therefore be cognizant of these potential differences.

The posterior edge of the cribriform plate comes into contact with the planum sphenoidale: the superior wall of the body of the sphenoid bone and sphenoid sinus [1]. To understand this association, the sphenoid bone anatomy must be discussed.

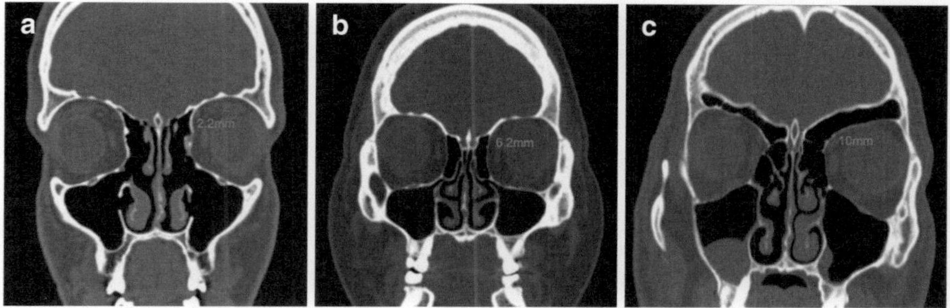

Fig. 1.5 CT sinus coronal views demonstrating examples of olfactory fossa depth measurements. (**a**) Keros type 1 (2.2 mm depth shown in orange) in a patient who had previously undergone endoscopic sinus surgery. (**b**) Keros type 2 (6.2 mm depth shown in orange) in a and (**c**) Keros Type 3 (10 mm depth shown in orange), in patients without a history of endoscopic sinus surgery

Fig. 1.6 Coronal CT scans demonstrating anterior ethmoid arteries on a mesentery

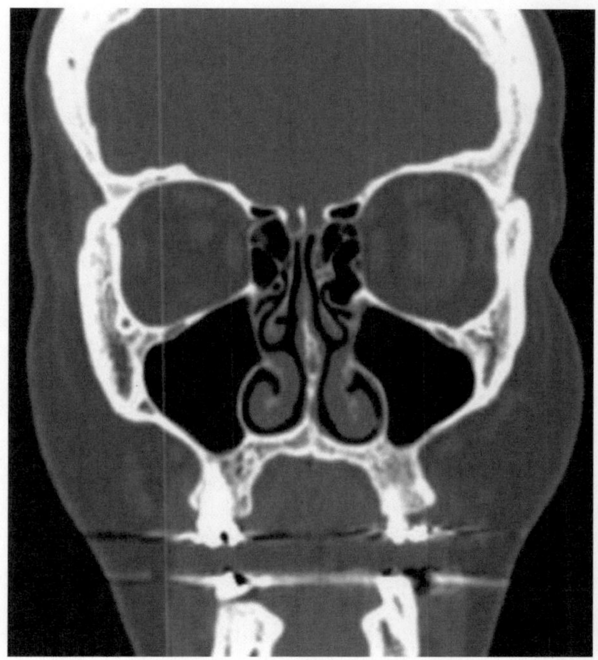

The sphenoid bone (Fig. 1.7) separates the anterior from the middle cranial fossa [5]. It is important to understand its unique shape and associations to surrounding structures. In the center is the body of the sphenoid bone in which lie the sphenoid sinuses and their variable pneumatization and septations as described above [5]. A greater wing and a lesser wing extend from the lateral aspect of the body bilaterally, and together, these wings form a space on either side named the superior orbital fissures [1]. Inferiorly, the bony structure known as the pterygoid process and medial

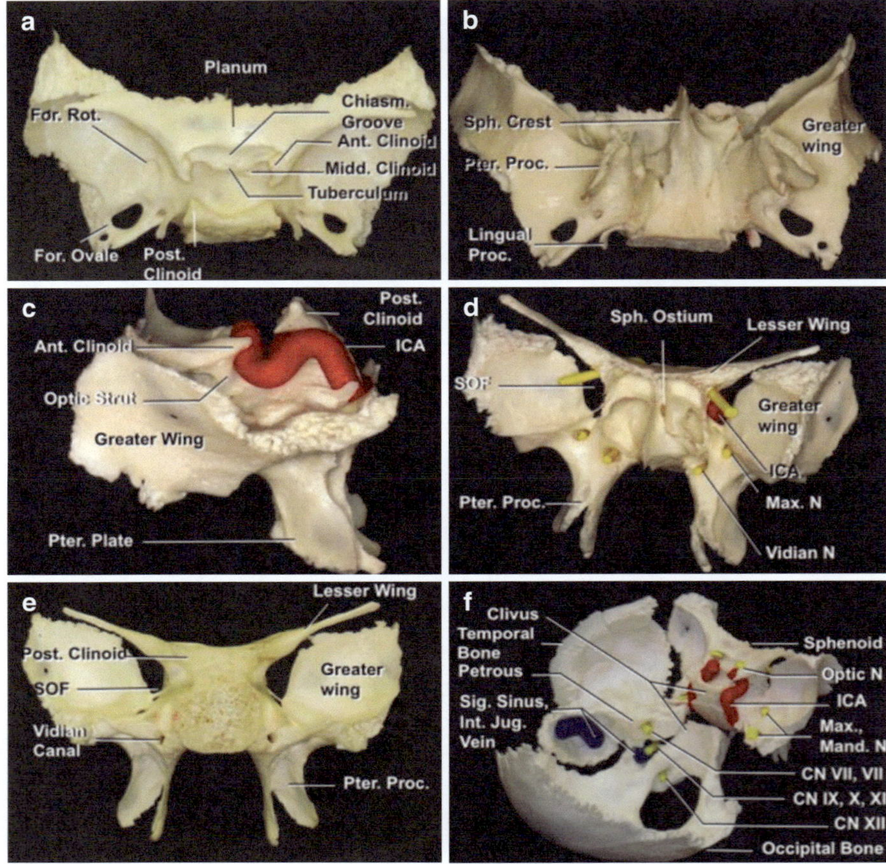

Fig. 1.7 Sphenoid bone anatomy from the following views: (**a**) superior, (**b**) inferior, (**c**) lateral, (**d**) anterior, (**e**) posterior. (**f**) Sphenoid bone location in relation to temporal and occipital bones. (With permissions from Peris-Celda et al., 2019)

and lateral pterygoid plates also branch out from both sides of the sphenoid body [1, 5].

When looking at the sphenoid bone in posterior view, one can visualize small bony projections bilaterally. These are the anterior, posterior, and occasionally medial clinoid processes that extend from the posterior-medial lesser wings of the sphenoid, superior-lateral dorsum sellae, and the superior-lateral sella turcica, respectively [1]. Medial to the anterior clinoid process projections are the optic canals, through which the optic nerve crosses and in between which the optic chiasm's prechiasmatic sulcus is found [1]. The ophthalmic artery and sympathetic nerves of the orbit also run through the optic canal [5]. Other canals to keep in mind within the sphenoid are the vomerovaginal canal, the palatovaginal canal (also known as the pharyngeal canal), and the vidian canal (also known as the pterygoid canal). A branch of the sphenopalatine artery passes through the vomerovaginal canal, but is not always present [5]. The pharyngeal branches of the maxillary artery and nerve cross through the palatovaginal canal, and the vidian nerve courses through the pterygoid canal, which is the most lateral of the three canals [5]. The pterygoid canal begins at the foramen lacerum and ends in the pterygopalatine fossa [5]. The vidian nerve, which consists of the greater and deep petrosal nerves carrying parasympathetic and autonomic fibers, respectively, can be dehiscent into the sphenoid sinus, partially bulging into it or completely covered by the bone [5].

The sella turcica is an essential anatomical space within the middle cranial fossa, in which the pituitary gland is found. It does not hold any cerebrospinal fluid since it is below the arachnoid layer [1]. It is this space that can be accessed by transsphenoidal approach to resect pituitary adenomas, for example. The boundaries of the sella turcica consist of the cavernous sinuses laterally, the tuberculum sella anteriorly, the dorsum sella posteriorly, the body of the sphenoid inferiorly, and the diaphragma sella superiorly [1]. The latter is formed by dura, separates the sella from the arachnoid space, and has a small pituitary aperture through which the pituitary stalk which attaches to the hypothalamus is found [1, 5]. Laterally, within the cavernous sinuses are found important neurovascular structures including the internal carotid artery (ICA), oculomotor nerve, trochlear nerve, abducens nerve, and V1 and V2 branches of the trigeminal nerve [5].

The sella turcica can be visualized from an endoscopic view through the sphenoid sinus (Fig. 1.8). In this view, the middle prominence consists of the sella; beneath it is the clival recess; above it is the planum sphenoidale [1]. Laterosuperiorly is the opticocarotid recess, which has variable pneumatization, but allows clear identification of the optic nerve superior to it and the ICA inferior and medial to it [1].

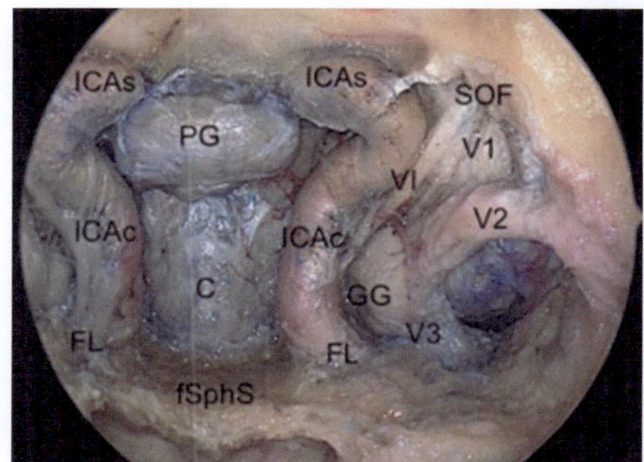

Fig. 1.8 Endoscopic image of the posterior sphenoid sinus and lateral recess. C, clivus; ICAc and ICAs, internal carotid artery paraclival and parasellar segments, respectively; FL, foramen lacerum; fSphS, sphenoid sinus floor; GG, Gasserian ganglion; PG, pituitary gland; SOF, superior orbital fissure; V1, V2, V3, nerve branches of cranial nerve V; VI, cranial nerve VI (abducens nerve). (With permissions from Cavallo et al. 2016)

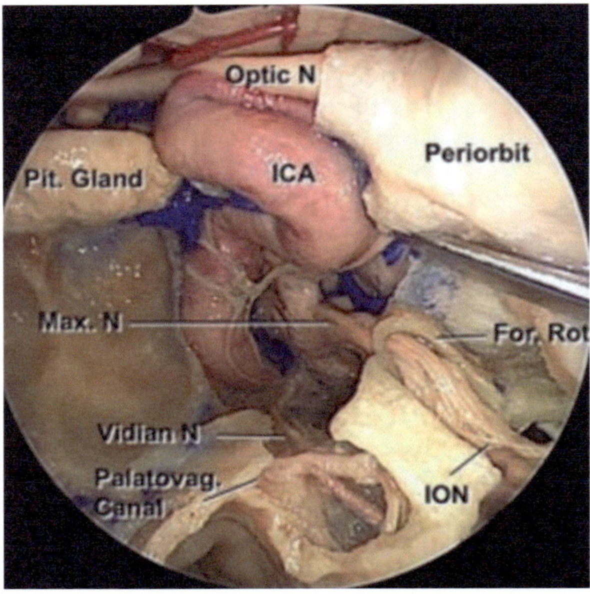

Fig. 1.9 Endoscopic view of the anatomy of the left cavernous sinus as viewed from the sphenoid sinus. ICA, internal carotid artery; For. Rot, foramen rotundum; Palatovag. Canal, palatovaginal canal; Max n., maxillary nerve; Pit Gland, pituitary gland; N, nerve. (With permissions from Peris-Celda et al. 2019)

The ICA's cavernous division has a peculiar course that must be understood prior to any endoscopic skull base surgery. It originates as the paraclival vertical carotid arteries on either side of the of the clival recess before entering the cavernous sinus as a vertical posterior segment [1]. The latter curves anteriorly forming the posterior genu, followed by a horizontal segment that eventually curves into the anterior genu and forms the paraclinoid segment anteriorly [5] (Fig. 1.9). The incidence of dehiscence of the cavernous ICA within the sphenoid sinus ranges from 2 to 25% and must be assessed on preoperative imaging [3, 5].

Another important reported finding is the presence of ICA and optic nerve projection into the sphenoid which can be, respectively, present in 5.2–67% and 7–35% of patients [3]. In addition, anterior clinoid pneumatization and its possible link to an increased incidence of optic nerve projection into the sphenoid sinus has also been reported and must be noted preoperatively due to the increased risk of injury to this nerve that can lead to blindness [3].

Conclusion

The anatomy of the nasal cavity, paranasal sinuses, orbit, and anterior skull base is complex yet essential to understand for the endoscopic skull base surgeon. With such proximity to important structures including the orbits, brain, arteries, and nerves, surgery in this area can lead to devastating and life-threatening injuries if the intricate anatomy is not well understood. To enable a better understanding, this chapter focused on the anatomical aspects most relevant to the endoscopic sinus surgeon.

Acknowledgments Reprinted/adapted by permission from [Springer nature]: [Springer nature] [2 Sinonasal and Parasellar Anatomy] by [Maria Peris-Celda, Carlos D. Pinheiro-Neto, Rowan Valentine et al [2019].

Reprinted/adapted by permission from [Springer nature]: [Springer nature] [Anatomy of the Sellar and Parasellar Region] by [Luigi Maria Cavallo, Domenico Solari, Alessandro Villa et al [2016].

References

1. Patel CR, Fernandez-Miranda JC, Wang WH, Wang EW. Skull Base Anatomy. Otolaryngol Clin N Am. 2016;49(1):9–20.
2. Song M, Zong X, Wang X, Pei A, Zhao P, Cui S, et al. Anatomic study of the anterior skull base via an endoscopic transnasal approach. Clin Neurol Neurosurg. 2011;113(4):281–4.
3. Papadopoulou AM, Chrysikos D, Samolis A, Tsakotos G, Troupis T. Anatomical variations of the nasal cavities and paranasal sinuses: a systematic review. Cureus. 2021;13(1):e12727.
4. Dalgorf DM, Harvey RJ. Chapter 1: Sinonasal anatomy and function. Am J Rhinol Allergy. 2013;27(Suppl 1):S3–6.
5. Lund VJ, Stammberger H, Fokkens WJ, Beale T, Bernal-Sprekelsen M, Eloy P, et al. European position paper on the anatomical terminology of the internal nose and paranasal sinuses. Rhinol Suppl. 2014;24:1–34.
6. Vaid S, Vaid N. Normal anatomy and anatomic variants of the paranasal sinuses on computed tomography. Neuroimaging Clin N Am. 2015 25(4):527–48.
7. Cankaya H, Egeli E, Kutluhan A, Kiris M. Pneumatization of the concha inferior as a cause of nasal obstruction. Rhinology. 2001;39(2):109–11.
8. Wormald PJ, Hoseman W, Callejas C, Weber RK, Kennedy DW, Citardi MJ, et al. The international frontal sinus anatomy classification (IFAC) and classification of the extent of endoscopic frontal sinus surgery (EFSS). Int Forum Allergy Rhinol. 2016;6(7):677–96.
9. Hu S, Colley P. Surgical Orbital Anatomy. Semin Plast Surg. 2019;33(2):85–91.
10. Gospe SM 3rd, Bhatti MT. Orbital Anatomy. Int Ophthalmol Clin. 2018;58(2):5–23.
11. Parmar H, Gujar S, Shah G, Mukherji SK. Imaging of the anterior skull base. Neuroimaging Clin N Am. 2009;19(3):427–39.
12. Solari D, Chiaramonte C, Di Somma A, Dell'Aversana Orabona G, de Notaris M, Angileri FF, et al. Endoscopic anatomy of the skull base explored through the nose. World Neurosurg. 2014;82(6 Suppl):S164–70.
13. Ferrari M, Mattavelli D, Schreiber A, Nicolai P. Macroscopic and endoscopic anatomy of the anterior Skull Base and adjacent structures. Adv Otorhinolaryngol. 2020;84:1–12.

Chapter 2
Lateral Skull Base Anatomy

Renata M. Knoll and Elliott D. Kozin

As the lateral skull base has an intricate and complex anatomy, the understanding of the anatomic interrelationships of its components and appropriate identification of its multiple anatomical landmarks are critical to accurately diagnosing and managing neurotologic disorders. Thus, this chapter presents an overview of the anatomy of the lateral skull base.

Osseous Anatomy of the Lateral Skull Base

The temporal bone is located centrally in lateral skull base and forms part of the middle and posterior cranial fossae. It articulates with the occipital, parietal, sphenoid, and zygomatic bones and is divided into five parts: squamous, petrous, mastoid, and tympanic portions and the styloid process.

The squamous portion forms part of the lateral wall of the middle fossa, the posterior part of the zygomatic arch, and the upper part of the mandibular fossa (Figs. 2.1, 2.2, and 2.3). It articulates with the sphenoid bone and zygomatic process anteriorly, with the parietal bone superiorly, and with the tympanic portion in the external auditory canal (EAC), which forms the tympanosquamous suture. The lateral surface of the squamous portion is grooved with the sulcus for the middle temporal artery and provides an anchor for the temporalis muscle. Its medial surface contains the sulcus for the middle meningeal artery.

The tympanic portion forms the inferior, anterior, and part of the posterior wall of the bony EAC, part of the wall of the tympanic cavity, the osseous portion of the

R. M. Knoll · E. D. Kozin (✉)
Department of Otolaryngology, Massachusetts Eye and Ear Infirmary, Boston, MA, USA

Department of Otolaryngology, Harvard Medical School, Boston, MA, USA
e-mail: Elliott_Kozin@meei.harvard.edu

© The Author(s), under exclusive license to Springer Nature Switzerland AG 2023
E. C. Kuan et al. (eds.), *Skull Base Reconstruction*,
https://doi.org/10.1007/978-3-031-27937-9_2

17

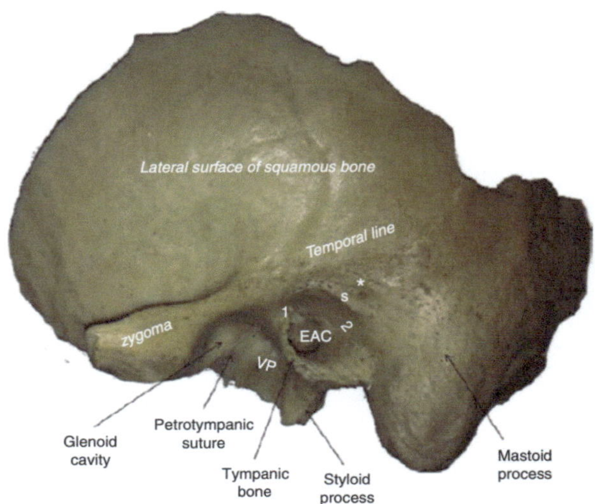

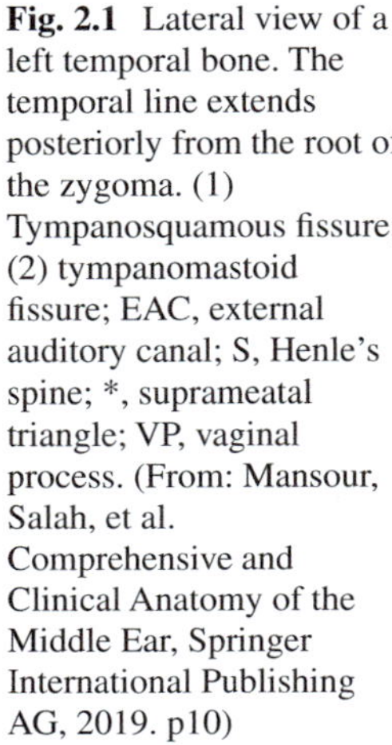

Fig. 2.1 Lateral view of a left temporal bone. The temporal line extends posteriorly from the root of the zygoma. (1) Tympanosquamous fissure; (2) tympanomastoid fissure; EAC, external auditory canal; S, Henle's spine; *, suprameatal triangle; VP, vaginal process. (From: Mansour, Salah, et al. Comprehensive and Clinical Anatomy of the Middle Ear, Springer International Publishing AG, 2019. p10)

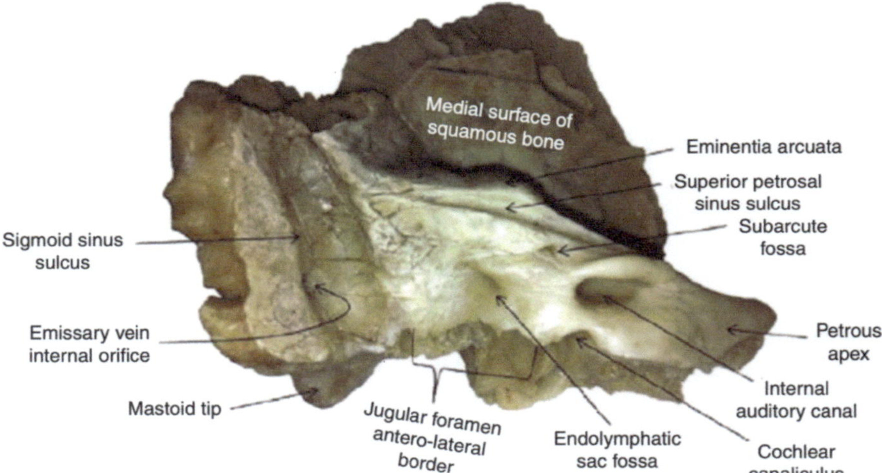

Fig. 2.2 Posterior view of a left temporal bone. (From: Mansour, Salah, et al. Comprehensive and Clinical Anatomy of the Middle Ear, Springer International Publishing AG, 2019. p 11)

eustachian tube, and the posterior wall of the glenoid fossa. Within the EAC, it interfaces with the mastoid and squamous portions forming the tympanomastoid and tympanosquamous sutures, respectively. Medially within the middle ear, it joins the petrous part at the petrotympanic fissure through which the chorda tympani and anterior tympanic artery pass. These sutures are important anatomical landmarks during ear surgery [1, 2]. Laterally, the tympanic bone ends at the cartilaginous portion of the EAC, whereas medially it ends at the tympanic (or annular) sulcus, into which the tympanic membrane attaches.

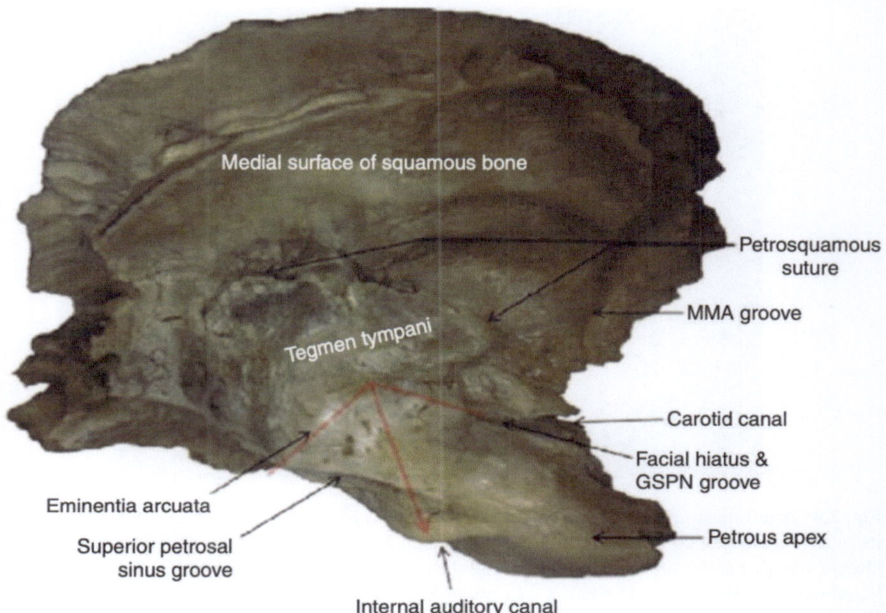

Fig. 2.3 Superior view of a left temporal bone. The red lines represent the relation of the internal auditory canal with respect to the eminencia arcuata and the greater superficial petrosal nerve (GSPN), middle meningeal artery (MMA). (From: Mansour, Salah, et al. Comprehensive and Clinical Anatomy of the Middle Ear, Springer International Publishing AG, 2019. p 13)

The mastoid portion (mastoid bone) forms the posterior part of the temporal bone and projects downwards on its lateral surface in a somewhat triangular shape to form the mastoid process (Fig. 2.1). It is composed by an extension of both the squamous and petrous portions, which are separated medially by the Körner's (petrosquamous) septum. The sternocleidomastoid muscle attaches to the inferior aspect of the mastoid, while the posterior belly of the digastric muscle attaches to the mastoid groove on the posteroinferior aspect of the mastoid process. In the lateral surface of the mastoid, the MacEwen's triangle (suprameatal triangle) can be identified, which is limited superiorly by the temporal line and anteriorly by the posterior wall of the EAC. This triangle contains numerous perforating small blood vessels (cribriform area), which are located immediately posterior to the suprameatal spine of Henle (Fig. 2.1) and serve as a landmark for mastoidectomy drilling [1–3]. The mastoid antrum is located deep to the cribriform area (Fig. 2.4). The mastoid foramen is located posteriorly on the mastoid process, through which the mastoid emissary vein and mastoid artery pass (Fig. 2.2). The medial aspect of the mastoid process is grooved by the sigmoid sinus, which represents the posterior limit of the mastoid cavity. The mastoid bone articulates posteriorly with the parietal bone superiorly and with the occipital bone inferiorly forming the parietomastoid and

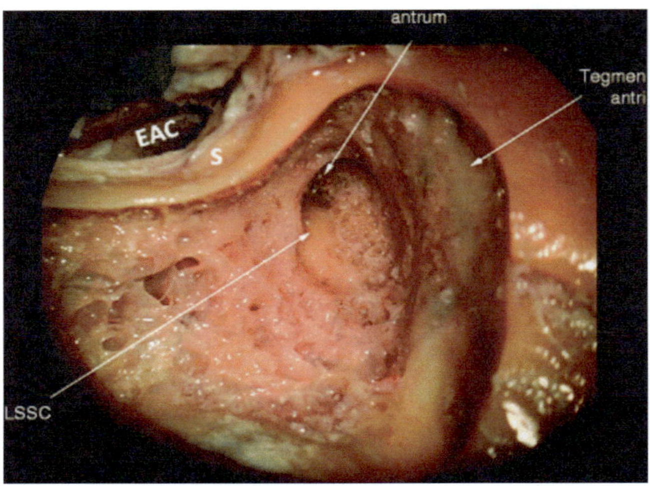

Fig. 2.4 A left mastoidectomy showing the antrum, with the lateral semicircular canal (LSSC) in its medial wall. Notice the relation between the Henle's spine (S) and the antrum: the antrum is always superior and posterior to the spine and the external auditory canal (EAC). (From: Mansour S., Magnan J., Haidar H., Nicolas K., Louryan S. (2013) The Mastoid. In: Comprehensive and Clinical Anatomy of the Middle Ear. Springer, Berlin, Heidelberg. p 105–122)

occipitoparietal suture, respectively. The union of these sutures is an important surgical landmark for craniotomies in retrosigmoid craniotomies [3].

The petrous portion has a pyramidal shape and is the densest bone of the lateral skull base, containing the sensory organs of the inner ear. The superior surface of the petrous bone contributes to the middle cranial fossa floor and contains the arcuate eminence, which corresponds to the bony prominence of the superior semicircular canal (Figs. 2.2 and 2.3). The superior surface also contains the tympanic tegmen overlying the middle ear and is grooved by the trigeminal impression of the CN V anteriorly. More medially and anteriorly to the arcuate eminence, the superficial petrosal nerve can be found exiting the facial hiatus. The foramen spinosum is found anterolaterally, through which the middle meningeal artery passes. The posteromedial surface (cerebellar surface) forms the anterolateral wall of the posterior cranial fossa, containing the opening (operculum) of the vestibular aqueduct and the subarcuate fossa through which the subarcuate artery and vein pass. The medial surface of the petrous bone (Fig. 2.2) contains the opening (porus) of the internal auditory canal (IAC).

The styloid process is located just laterally to the posterior aspect of the jugular fossa and projects down and forward from under the surface of the temporal bone (Figs. 2.1 and 2.5). The stylomastoid foramen lies just posterior to the styloid process, through which the facial nerve exits the skull. The distal part of the styloid process provides attachment to several muscles associated with the tongue and larynx.

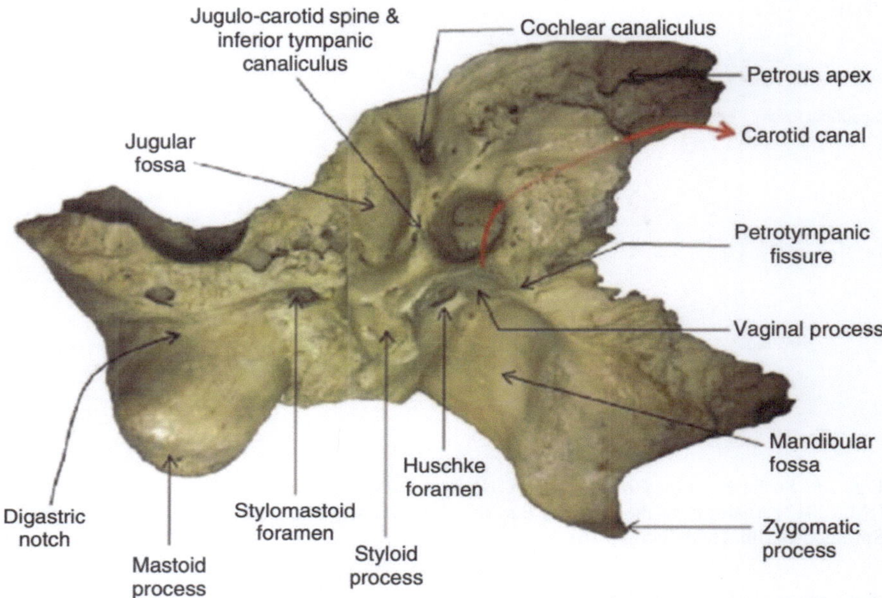

Fig. 2.5 Inferior view of a left temporal bone. The red arrow passes through the carotid canal. (From: Mansour, Salah, et al. Comprehensive and Clinical Anatomy of the Middle Ear, Springer International Publishing AG, 2019. p 16)

Anatomy of the Auricle and External Canal

The auricle (or pinna) comprises the external cartilaginous portion of the ear. Its size and shape are determined by the configuration of the cartilage frame. The major concavity of the lateral aspect of the auricle is the concha, which is contiguous with the cartilaginous portion of the EAC (Fig. 2.6). The auricle is attached to the cranium by its skin, cartilage, and a complex of and ligaments and muscles.

The EAC is approximately 3.5 cm in length and can be divided into two parts—the lateral one-third (cartilaginous) and medial two-thirds (bony). The cartilaginous part comprises a continuation of the cartilage of the auricle, and its skin has a thick subcutaneous layer, replete with hair follicles, sebaceous glands, and ceruminal glands. The osseous part of the EAC is formed by the tympanic portion of the temporal bone and contains a very thin skin with no hair follicles or sebaceous glands and is contiguous with the skin of the tympanic membrane. The sensory innervation of the EAC is supplied by branches of the CN V (V_3), CN VII, and CN X (Arnold's nerve), lesser occipital nerve (C2 and C3 via cervical plexus), and greater auricular nerve (C2 and C3 via cervical plexus). The arterial blood supply is derived from branches of the external carotid artery, and the veins accompanying the arteries drain into the internal jugular vein by either the facial or external jugular veins.

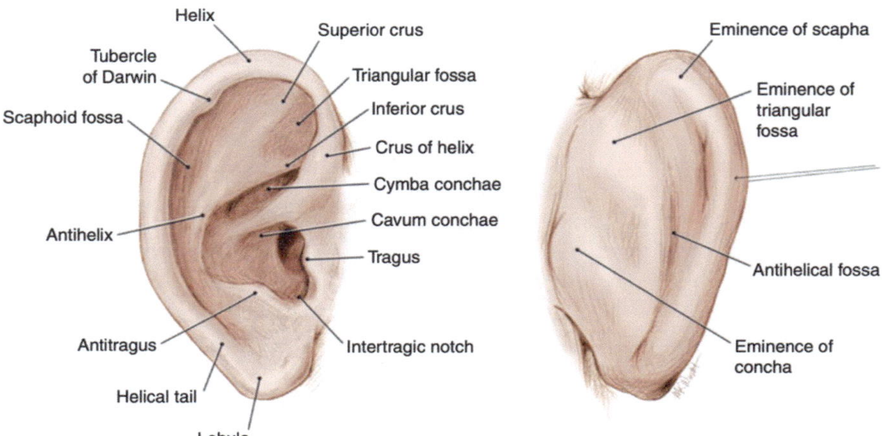

Fig. 2.6 Surface anatomy of the auricle. (Left) Anterior. (Right) Posterior. (From: Prendergast P.M. (2013) Anatomy of the External Ear. In: Shiffman M. (eds) Advanced Cosmetic Otoplasty. Springer, Berlin, Heidelberg. p 16)

Anatomy of the Middle Ear and Eustachian Tube

The middle ear is composed by the tympanic membrane and cavity, which contains the ossicular chain (malleus, incus, and stapes), two muscles, and neurovascular supply.

The tympanic membrane is a trilaminar structure with an irregular conical shape given the attachment of the manubrium of the malleus in its surface (Fig. 2.7). The adult tympanic membrane is about 9 mm in diameter, and it is separated into a superior pars flaccida (Shrapnell's membrane) and an inferior pars tensa.

The middle ear space (Fig. 2.8), or tympanic cavity, is limited by the tympanic membrane laterally, the cochlea medially, the tegmen superiorly, the mastoid posteriorly, the jugular bulb inferiorly, and the carotid artery and Eustachian tube anteriorly. The tympanic cavity is lined with a mucosal epithelium and can be divided into compartments, including the epitympanum (attic), mesotympanum, hypotympanum, and protympanum.

The ossicular chain consists of three small ossicles: the malleus, incus, and stapes. The malleus is the most lateral of the ossicles and attaches directly to the tympanic membrane. It has a head, manubrium (handle), neck, and anterior and lateral processes, and it is suspended via several ligaments. The incus is located immediately medial to the malleus, and it is the largest of the three ossicles. It has a body and a long, a short, and a lenticular process. While the body of the incus articulates with the head of the malleus in the epitympanum, the lenticular process articulates with the stapes. The stapes is the smallest and the most medial ossicle. It has a head, a footplate, and two crura. Its head articulates with the lenticular process of the incus, whereas its footplate sits in the oval window.

Fig. 2.7 Endoscopic view of a normal left tympanic membrane. Surface features of the tympanic membrane include (1) pars flaccida, (2) lateral process of malleus, (3) malleus umbo, (4) inferior central pars tensa, and (5) fibrous annulus. (From: Isaacson, B. (2018). Anatomy and Surgical Approach of the Ear and Temporal Bone. Head & Neck Pathology (Totowa, N.J.), 12 (3) p 324)

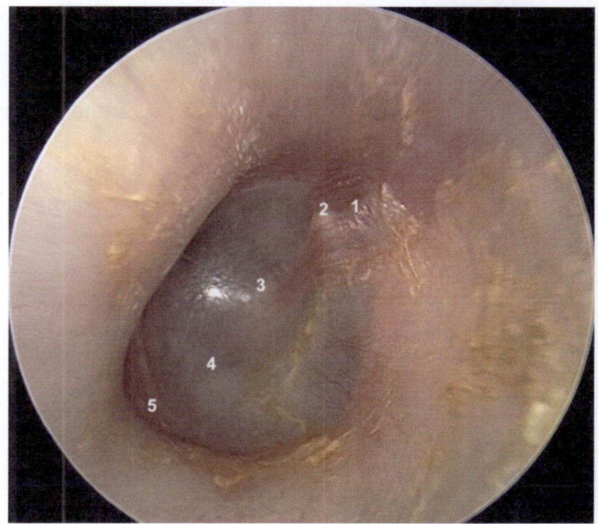

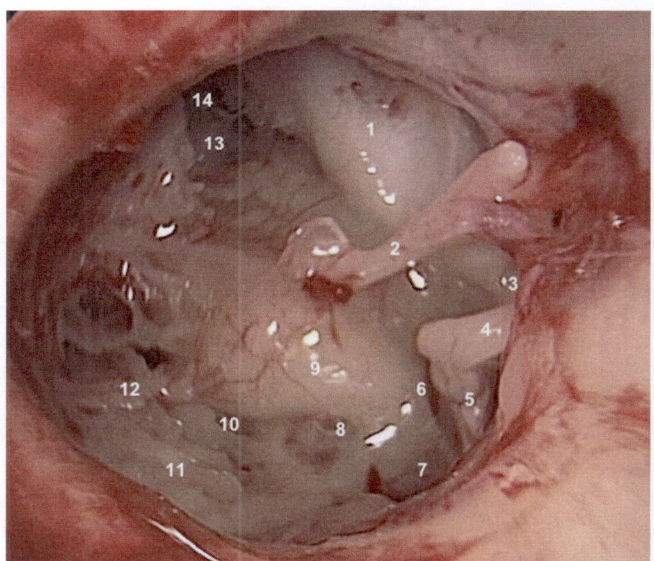

Fig. 2.8 Transcanal endoscopic view of the left middle ear after removal of the tympanic membrane: (1) semicanal of the tensor tympani muscle, (2) malleus handle, (3) tympanic facial nerve, (4) incus long process, (5) stapes capitulum and incudostapedial joint, (6) inferior margin of oval window niche, (7) sinus tympani, (8) round window niche, (9) cochlear promontory, (10) subcochlear canaliculus leading to inferior petrous apex, (11) high, non-dehiscent jugular bulb, (12) Jacobson's nerve, (13) horizontal petrous carotid artery, (14) eustachian tube. (From: Isaacson, B. (2018). Anatomy and Surgical Approach of the Ear and Temporal Bone. Head & Neck Pathology (Totowa, N.J.), 12 (3) p 325)

The tensor tympani muscle, which is innervated by the CN V, originates from the greater wing of the sphenoid and cartilage of the Eustachian tube. Its tendon inserts onto the cochleariform process and to the neck of the malleus. The stapedius muscle is innervated by the facial nerve and connects the pyramidal eminence to the posterior crus of the stapes.

The Eustachian tube connects the nasopharynx to the middle ear, traveling downward anteromedially at an angle of 45° and measuring approximately 35 mm in length in adulthood. The anteromedial two-thirds of the eustachian tube are fibrocartilaginous, whereas the posteromedial two-thirds is bony. The tympanic orifice is located in the anterior wall of the tympanic cavity, and the posterior lip of the pharyngeal orifice forms the torus tubarius in the nasopharynx. The Eustachian tube remains mostly closed, opening only during actions such as yawning and swallowing, which is accomplished by the tensor veli palatini muscle.

Anatomy of the Inner Ear

The inner ear is located within the petrous portion of the temporal bone, consisting of the cochlea, vestibule, and three semicircular canals.

The cochlea is a spiral canal with $2^{1/2}$ turns around its central axis (modiolus) that contains three main compartments with different fluids: the scala tympani and vestibuli which contain perilymph and the scala media (the cochlear duct) which contains endolymph. The latter houses the organ of Corti, which consists of inner and outer hair cells. The spiral ganglion neurons are located in the spiral canal of the cochlea (Rosenthal's canal), and the cochlear nerve fibers pass through the cribrosa area and spiral osseous lamina.

The vestibule is the central chamber, consisting of two membranous components: the utricle and saccule. Each of these organs contains a macula, which includes clusters of sensory hair cells. The utricle communicates with the endolymphatic duct through the utriculo-endolymphatic valve, whereas the saccule communicates with the scala media through the ductus reuniens. The semicircular canals (superior, lateral, and posterior canals) are situated posteriorly to the vestibule arranged in a perpendicular plane to each other. Each canal has a non-ampullated end and a large ampullated end, which contains a cluster of hair cells (crista ampullaris). The non-ampullated end of the posterior and superior canals fuse to form the common crus, whereas the non-ampullated ends of the lateral canal form an anterior and a posterior crura.

The Scarpa's ganglion neurons are located in the vestibular nerves within the IAC, projecting nerve fibers to the vestibule and semicircular canals through cribrosa

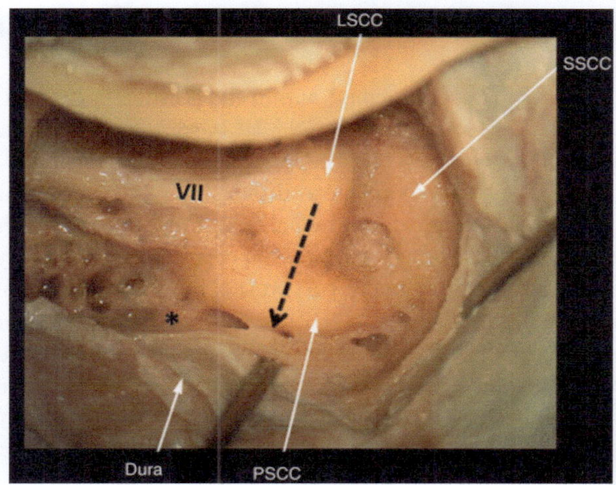

Fig. 2.9 Cadaveric left mastoidectomy showing lateral semicircular canal (LSCC), the superior semicircular canal (SSCC), and the posteriorsemicircular canal (PSCC). Notice the relationship between the PSCC and the facial nerve (VII). Notice the Donaldson's line (the black dotted line) and the endolymphatic sac (*). (From Mansour S., Magnan J., Haidar H., Nicolas K., Louryan S. (2013) The Mastoid. In: Comprehensive and Clinical Anatomy of the Middle Ear. Springer, Berlin, Heidelberg. p 105–122)

areas. The superior vestibular nerve innervates the utricle and the superior and lateral semicircular canals, while the inferior vestibular nerve innervates the saccule and the posterior semicircular canal.

The endolymphatic system includes the endolymphatic duct and sac. The endolymphatic duct is located in the posterolateral wall of the vestibule, starting at the utriculo-endolymphatic valve and ending at the aperture of the vestibular aqueduct. The endolymphatic sac has an intraosseous and an intradural portion, lying approximately 10 mm inferior and lateral to the porus of the IAC. It can be located inferiorly to the Donaldson's line (Fig. 2.9), which is an important surgical landmark derived by extending the plane of the lateral semicircular that also divides the posterior semicircular canal [1].

The cochlear aqueduct is a small opening from the scala tympani of the basal turn of the cochlea, close to the round window membrane, which runs inferiorly and medially to open at the posterior cranial fossa just at the anterior division of the jugular foramen. Surgically, the cochlear aqueduct is an important landmark during translabyrinthine craniotomy to prevent injury of the lower cranial nerves [1].

The vascular supply of the inner ear is provided by branches of the anterior inferior cerebellar artery (AICA), the labyrinthine and subarcuate arteries. The latter is not an essential vascular supply and is commonly encountered during labyrinthectomies as it courses within the arc of the superior canal [1].

Anatomy of the IAC, Jugular Foramen, and Petrous Apex

The IAC is a bony, neurovascular canal within the petrous portion of the temporal bone that houses CN VII (facial nerve), CN VIII (vestibulocochlear nerve), and the labyrinthine artery and vein. The average length and diameter of the IAC is 8 mm and 3.4 mm, respectively, although these dimensions may suffer variations. The canal ends laterally at the fundus and medially at the porus. The lateral portion of the IAC is divided into two compartments—superior and inferior—by a horizontal bony ridge called transverse (or falciform) crest. The superior compartment is further divided by a smaller vertical crest (Bill's bar), which separates the facial nerve (anteriorly) from the superior vestibular nerve (posteriorly) and is a useful landmark in translabyrinthine surgery (Fig. 2.10) [2]. As the nerves approach the cerebellopontine angle (CPA), the cochlear and vestibular fibers rotate, with the vestibular nerve fibers assuming a superior position to the cochlear fibers at the brainstem. The facial nerve also rotates from an initial anteroinferior position relative to the vestibular nerve at the pons.

The jugular foramen is located in the medial-inferior surface of the petrous pyramid, between the temporal and occipital bones. It can be divided into three compartments: (1) a sigmoid compartment posteriorly, through which the sigmoid sinus drains; (2) a petrous compartment anteromedially, through which the inferior petrosal sinus drains; and (3) a neural intrajugular compartment, which is located between the other two and is traversed by the glossopharyngeal (CN IX), vagus (CN X), and spinal accessory (CN XI) cranial nerves and meningeal branches of the ascending pharyngeal artery as they exit the skull. Within the jugular foramen, the CN IX provides a tympanic branch (i.e., Jacobson's nerve) to form the tympanic plexus of the middle ear while the CN X an auricular branch (Arnold nerve) to provide sensory

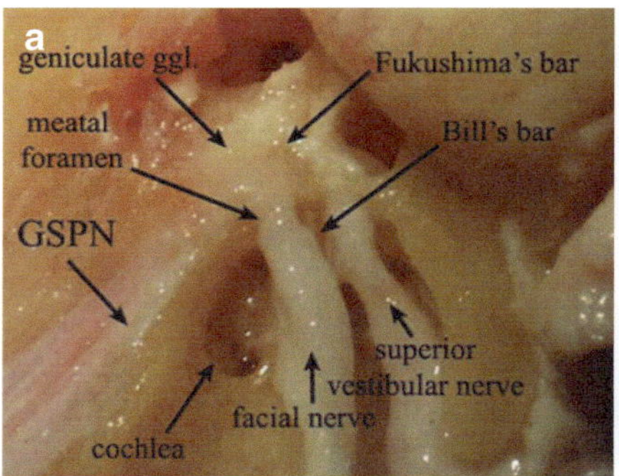

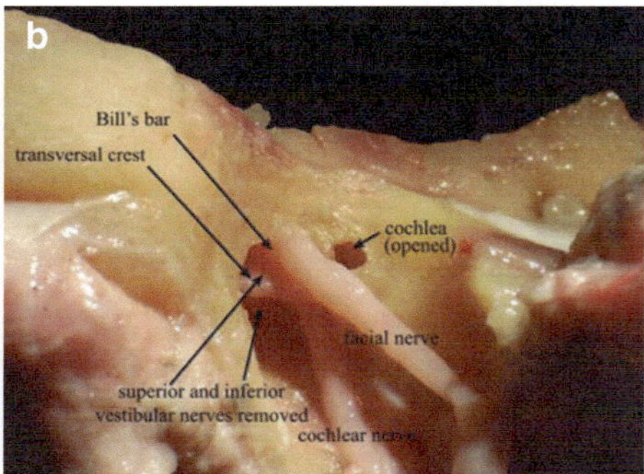

Fig. 2.10 Cadaveric Internal acoustic canal (IAC) unroofed with middle cranial fossa approach. (**a**) Superior view into the unroofed right IAC; the vertical crest (Bill's bar) separates the facial and superior vestibular nerves at the fundus of the IAC; (**b**) posterior view to the fundus of left IAC. The superior and inferior vestibular nerves are located posteriorly and the facial and cochlear nerves anteriorly in the IAC; (From: Battelino S., Bošnjak R. (2013) Surgical Approaches and Anatomy of the Lateral Skull Base. In: Kountakis S.E. (eds) Encyclopedia of Otolaryngology, Head and Neck Surgery. Springer, Berlin, Heidelberg. https://doi.org/10.1007/978-3-642-23499-6_567 p 2648)

innervation to the posterior wall of the external auditory canal. Of note, the anatomy of the jugular foramen may be highly variable, which has important implications for neurotological surgery [1]. Additionally, the right jugular foramen is generally larger than the left due to its larger venous drainage.

The petrous apex is the anteromedial limit of the petrous pyramid. Its anterosuperior portion forms the floor of the middle cranial fossa, whereas the posterosuperior portion constitutes the anterior wall of the posterior cranial fossa. The petrous apex can be divided by the IAC into an anterior (larger) and a posterior (smaller) portion. It often contains bone marrow and can be pneumatized in up to 35% of patients, which may provide a direct pathway for diseases to spread from the mastoid or middle ear cavity, in addition to being a preferred location for malignant metastasis and cholesterol granulomas [1].

Anatomy of the Middle Cranial Fossa

The middle cranial fossa comprises the area between the sphenoid ridge anteriorly and the petrous ridge posteriorly. Within its medial aspect, from medial to lateral, four foramina can be identified: (1) the superior orbital fissure, through which the ophthalmic division of the CN V (V_1) passes; (2) foramen rotundum, though which the maxillary division of the CN V (V_2) passes; (3) foramen ovale, though which the mandibular division of the CN V (V_3) passes; and (4) foramen spinosum, through which the middle meningeal artery enters the middle cranial fossa. Medially to the middle meningeal artery, the greater superficial petrosal nerve can be found, serving as an important surgical landmark for middle cranial fossa procedures (Fig. 2.11) [4]. The lateral aspect of the middle cranial fossa contains the carotid canal, the hiatus of the greater petrosal nerve, and the hiatus of the lesser petrosal nerve. The

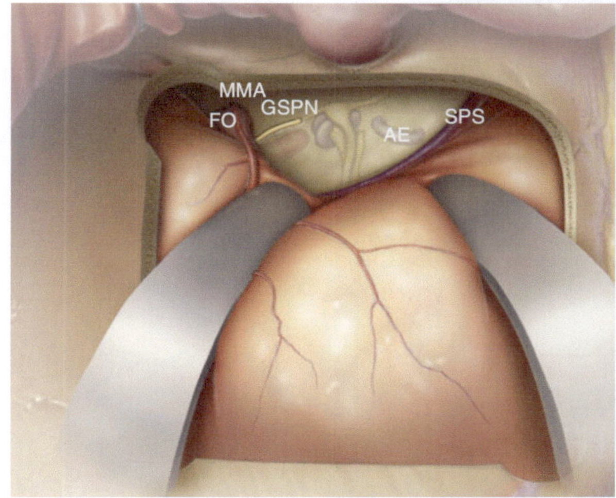

Fig. 2.11 Surgical view of the middle cranial fossa. Greater superficial petrosal nerve (GSPN), superior petrosal sinus (SPS), middle meningeal artery (MMA) from the foramen ovale (FO). (From: Oghalai, J. S., & Driscoll, C. L. W. (2015). Atlas of neurotologic and lateral skull base surgery. p 23)

horizontal portion of the carotid canal passes in an inferomedial position to the greater superficial petrosal nerve.

The greater superficial petrosal nerve ends posteriorly at the level of the geniculate ganglion, which is covered by a thin lamina of the bone. The IAC can be found at an angle of approximately 60° medially to the long axis of the superior semicircular canal. The labyrinthine segment of the facial nerve emerging from the IAC is located medially and posteriorly to the geniculate ganglion. The cochlea can be identified within an obtuse angle of approximately 120° formed between the greater superficial petrosal nerve and labyrinthine segment of CN VII.

The tegmen tympani and mastoideum can be identified lateral to the arcuate eminence and geniculate ganglion, forming the roof of the middle ear and mastoid, respectively. Just inferiorly to the tegmen, the epitympanum, the tympanic segment of the facial nerve, and the incudomalleolar joint can be accessed anteriorly, whereas the mastoid antrum and the three semicircular canals are found posteriorly.

The superior petrosal sinus creates a longitudinal groove in the petrous ridge, which is an important surgical landmark corresponding to the medial limit of the middle fossa approach [3].

Anatomy of the Posterior Cranial Fossa

The posterior cranial fossa is located between the foramen magnum and the tentorial incisura. The posterior surface of the temporal bone forms the anterior border of the posterior cranial fossa, whereas posterior and lateral walls are formed by the occipital bone.

The posterior cranial fossa contains the CPA, a space located between the superior and inferior limbs of the angular cerebellopontine fissure, from which the intracranial segments of many cranial nerves and vascular structures traverse. Both the CN VII and VIII leave the brainstem at the lateral end of the pontomedullary sulcus immediately rostral to the foramen of Luschka, with the VII assuming a position about 1 to 2 mm anteroinferior to the CN VIII. Additionally, the AICA courses between the CN VII and VIII. The CN V can be found superiorly, whereas the CN IX, X, and XI pass inferiorly within the CPA (Fig. 2.12).

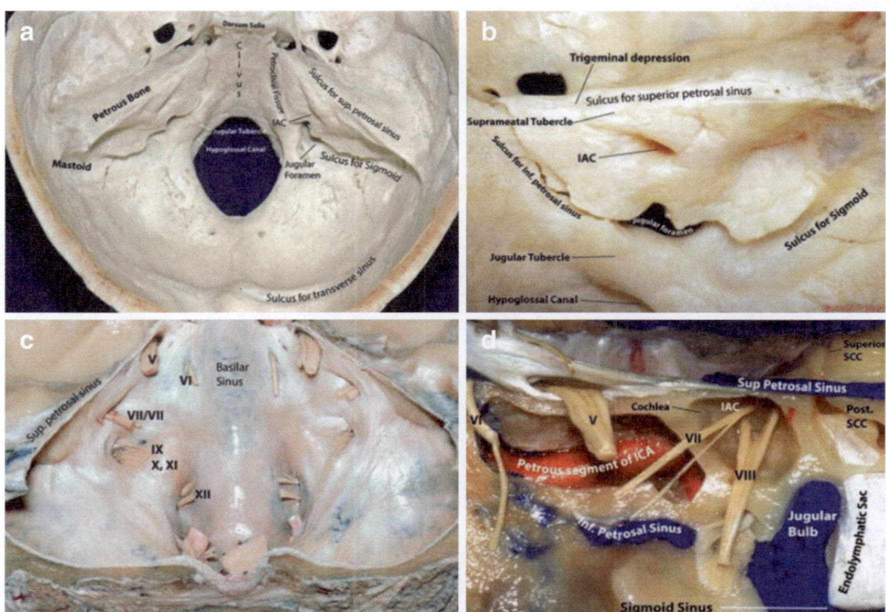

Fig. 2.12 Anatomy of the posterior cranial fossa. (**a**) Superior view; (**b**) Medial view; (**c**) Superior view with the dura lining the posterior fossa; (**d**) The posterior cranial fossa dura opened to expose the internal structures; (From: Surgical Anatomy of the Posterior Fossa Basma, Jaafar; Sorenson, Jeffrey Skull Base Surgery of the Posterior Fossa, 2017-11-12, p 3–24)

Anatomy of the Infratemporal Fossa

The infratemporal fossa is a space bounded superiorly by the infratemporal surface of the greater wing of the sphenoid bone, inferiorly by the superior limit of the posterior belly of the digastric muscle and the angle of the mandible, anteriorly by the posterolateral surface of the maxillary sinus, and posteriorly by the styloid process and the mastoid and tympanic portions of the temporal bone. The ascending ramus of the mandible forms the lateral limit, whereas the medial pterygoid and tensor veli palatini muscles form the medial border (Fig. 2.13).

The medial and lateral pterygoid muscles are located within the infratemporal fossa. The latter servers as a surgical landmark and is divided into two parts: the upper head and the lower head. The upper head originates from the infratemporal surface and the greater wing of the sphenoid bone, whereas the lower head originates from the lateral aspect of the lateral pterygoid plate. While the lower head inserts onto the pterygoid fovea under the condylar process of the mandible, the upper head inserts onto the joint capsule of the temporomandibular joint. The medial pterygoid muscle arises with two heads rising from the maxillary tuberosity and lateral pterygoid plate, which insert onto the inferior and posterior part of the medial surface of the ramus and angle of the mandible.

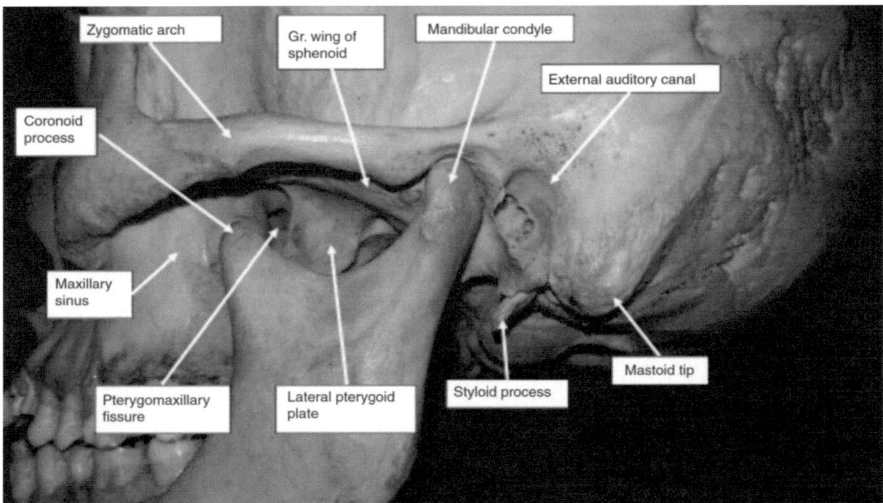

Fig. 2.13 Bone landmarks of the infratemporal fossa. (From: Infratemporal Fossa Approach Gidley, Paul W; DeMonte, Franco; Weber, Randal S, Temporal Bone Cancer, 2018-05-04, p 267–282)

The mandibular branch of the CN V (V_3) arises from the foramen ovale and transverses the infratemporal fossa to provide motor and sensory innervation to several muscles. The vasculature encountered within the infratemporal fossa includes the maxillary artery and associated branches, including the middle meningeal artery and accessory meningeal artery. The venous drainage of the infratemporal fossa occurs though the pterygoid venous plexus, which also forms anastomoses with the cavernous sinus and eventually drains into the maxillary and facial veins.

References

1. Adunka OF. Anatomy of the temporal bone and adjacent structures. In: Adunka OF, Buchman CA, eds. Otology, neurotology, and lateral Skull Base surgery. Vol 1. New York, NY: Thieme Verlagsgruppe; 2011:6-22.
2. Gulya AJ. Anatomy of the temporal bone and Skull Base. In: Glasscock ME, Gulya AJ, editors. Glasscock-Shambaugh surgery of the ear, vol. xvi. 5th ed. Hamilton, Ont: BC Decker; 2010. p. 808.
3. Blevins NH, Selesnick SH, Alyono JC. Surgical anatomy of the lateral Skull Base. In: Flint PW, Haughey BH, Lund VJ, et al., editors. Cummings otolaryngology. 7th ed. Amsterdam: Elsevier Inc; 2021. p. 2624–2633.e2621.
4. Tedeschi H, Tzu WH, Oliveira E. Anatomia microcirúrgica das fossas posterior e média relacionadas com o osso temporal. In: Cruz OLM, Costa SS, editors. Otologia Clínica e Cirúrgica. Rio de Janeiro: Editora Revinter; 2000.

Chapter 3
CSF Physiology and Intracranial Pressure

Jordan Davies, Michelle Paff, Jefferson W. Chen, Kiarash Golshani, and Frank P. K. Hsu

Introduction

Since the time of Hippocrates and Galen, the form and function of cerebrospinal fluid (CSF) has been debated and postulated. Additional knowledge has led to additional disputes. The most widely accepted dogma is that CSF is primarily secreted by the choroid plexus, tufts of highly vascular structures lined by epithelial cells in the ventricles of the brain. This fluid then circulates through the ventricular system and eventually bathes the brain and spinal cord in the subarachnoid spaces. Absorption is done via protrusions of the subarachnoid space, arachnoid granulations, into the dural venous sinuses, primarily the superior sagittal sinus, and various sources of lymphatic drainage. Of course, it isn't all that straightforward, which will be discussed further below, and there are alternative theories to even the longest accepted principles.

CSF is a clear fluid, derived primarily from ultra-selective filtration of plasma, but with about 20% derived from CNS synthesis. It has the density of water, appearing hypodense on CT imaging and bright on T2 MRI sequencing. The functions of CSF include mechanical protection, cerebral environment homeostasis, and delivery and removal of neuroactive substances—all through a tightly controlled process involving osmotic pressures, specialized receptors, and active transport to create a specialized ultra-filtrate of plasma. It's no wonder the brain requires 20% of total body oxygen and 15% of basal cardiac output despite occupying only 2% of total body weight [1].

As with all things in the cranium, this process relies on several processes being in sync to deliver function. Several different pathologies, both spontaneous and iatrogenic, can throw off this delicate balance to produce devastating side effects.

J. Davies · M. Paff · J. W. Chen · K. Golshani · F. P. K. Hsu (✉)
Department of Neurological Surgery, University of California Irvine, Irvine, CA, USA
e-mail: mpaff@hs.uci.edu; jeffewc1@hs.uci.edu; kgolshan@hs.uci.edu; fpkhsu@hs.uci.edu

E. C. Kuan et al. (eds.), *Skull Base Reconstruction*,
https://doi.org/10.1007/978-3-031-27937-9_3

Understanding the pathology requires beginning with two principles: first, the Monro-Kellie doctrine, which states the skull is of finite volume and the pressure within is a balance between the three constituents of the brain, blood, and CSF. And second, disturbance in the balance of CSF typically can be attributed to alteration of its production, circulation, or resorption.

CSF Production

The choroid plexus is considered one of the most active secretory systems in the body, producing about 0.4 ml of CSF/min or an average of 500 ml of CSF per day [2]. At any given time, there is 150 ml of CSF in the CNS, which indicates the volume of CSF undergoes turnover 3–4 times per day [3]. This turnover and renewal is an important part of maintaining neuronal homeostasis and clearing cerebral by-products in the interstitial milieu surrounding neurons and glial cells. The ventricles contain about 25 ml of CSF, and the CSF in and around the spinal cord is approximately 30 ml [4], leaving about 100 ml of CSF to circulate in the subarachnoid spaces and cisterns. This provides a mechanical protection against traumatic forces as it will cushion the brain as it propels toward the skull and the resulting reverberations. This buoyancy also decreases the weight of the brain tenfold to avoid compression of vital structures at the base of the brain against the skull.

As noted, the choroid plexus is considered the primary site of CSF production, accounting for about 60–75% of CSF production. This is supplemented by CSF production from the brain interstitial fluid (fluid transport across the blood-brain barrier to the spaces between neuronal and glial cells) and ependymal lining. The choroid plexus is contained in the temporal horns and body of the lateral ventricles, the roof of the third ventricle, and the caudal part of the fourth ventricle [3].

Overall production rate of CSF is affected by multiple factors. One is time of the day, with diurnal fluctuations increasing CSF production and turnover in the evening and during sleep. The intracranial pressure will also impact production, as well as resorption, with production decreasing during periods of elevated pressure. The autonomic nervous system also synapses on cells in the choroid plexus, with the noradrenergic-sympathetic nervous system decreasing production, while the cholinergic-parasympathetic nervous system will increase production [3].

CSF Contents

Although CSF is touted as an ultra-filtrate of plasma, significant energy and work is expended to create a fluid designed for the special functions of the neurons and supporting cells. The sodium, chloride, and magnesium concentrations are higher in CSF than plasma. The potassium and calcium concentrations are lower. In addition, the glucose and protein concentrations are lower, with protein being significantly

Table 3.1 Normal cellular and metabolic values in blood vs. cerebrospinal fluid

Content	Blood	CSF
Red blood cells	$4.2–6.1 \times 10^6/mm^3$	$0/mm^3$
White blood cells	$5–10 \times 10^3//mm^3$	$0–5/mm^3$
Glucose	90–110 mg/dL	45–80 mg/dL
Protein	$6.0–8.3 \times 10^3/mg/dL$	20–40 mg/dL
Sodium	135–145 mmol/L	135–150 mmol/L
Chloride	96–106 mmol/L	116–127 mmol/L
Magnesium	1.3–2.1 mEq/L	2.0–2.5 mEq/L
Potassium	3.5–4.5 mmol/L	2.7–3.9 mmol/L
Calcium	9–11 mg/dL	4.0–5.0 mg/dL

lower [3]. Unless disturbed, no red blood cells should enter the CSF, while only a few white blood cells will be found. A summary comparing the cellular and metabolic contents of blood and cerebrospinal fluid is shown in Table 3.1.

Diffusion of molecules across both the blood-CSF and blood-brain barriers is influenced by lipid solubility and size. The Oldendorf line was created after the observation that smaller, lipophilic molecules have greater rates of diffusion into the CNS [5]. This knowledge is used to increase cerebral bioavailability of drugs by modifying size, structure, and solubility of such medications as antibiotics to increase penetrance [6].

Also found in CSF are hormones made in the CNS to circulate to distant organs, as well as exert influences locally. Some examples include T4 (thyroxine), vasopressin, insulin growth factor (IGF), and brain-derived neurotrophic factor (BDNF). Both IGF and BDNF are upregulated in response to chronic stress. IGF has also been found to enhance clearance of beta amyloid via aquaporin channels. Regulations of electrolytes and minerals can also occur in response to intracranial pathology. For example, iron concentration is significantly decreased during viral diseases of the brain to reduce viral activity [2].

CSF Circulation

Again, tradition has largely postulated unidirectional flow of CSF from sites of production to sites of resorption. This is shown in Fig. 3.1. This was thought to be driven by the pulsations of CSF secretions, which is a mirror of the arterial pulse wave. This was a system of flow from high pressure to low pressure areas of the venous sinuses and resorption sites [3, 4]. Additional knowledge of CSF as an agent in neuronal homeostasis and drug delivery has yielded evidence of CSF as bidirectional, and at times convective, flow between subarachnoid spaces, brain interstitium, perivascular spaces, and lymphatic drainage.

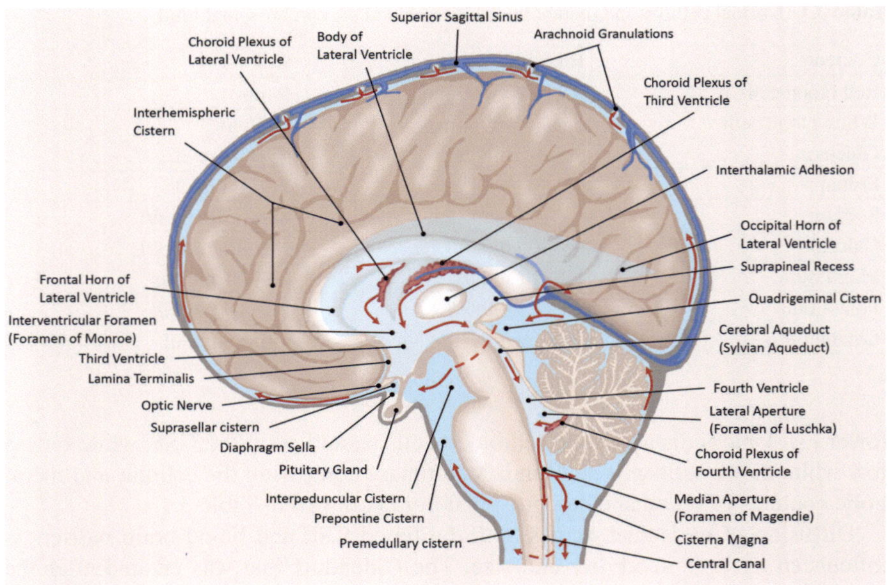

Fig. 3.1 CSF circulation. (Image courtesy of Dr. Michelle Paff, University of California Irvine, Neurosurgery Department, 2021)

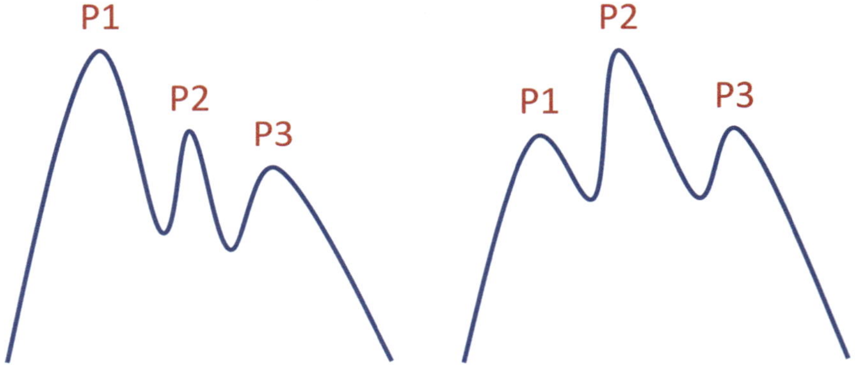

Fig. 3.2 Intracranial pressure (ICP) waveforms. Percussion wave (P1) represents arterial pulsation, tidal wave (P2) represents brain tissue compliance, and dicrotic wave (P3) is due to closure of the aortic valve. Under normal conditions, P1 > P2, indicative of normal complaint brain. In acute brain injury, brain compliance starts decreasing resulting in reversal of P1:P2 ratio (i.e., P2 > P1) which is a sensitive predictor of poor brain compliance

The arterial pulse wave and its impact in intracranial pressure (ICP) differentials are embodied in ICP pressure waves seen during invasive monitoring, shown in Fig. 3.2. There are three components to an ICP wave, the first being the largest and representing the arterial pulsation, or rush of blood through the cerebral arteries during systole. The second wave is a response of the brain pushing back, or recoiling, against the arterial wave and is a rough measurement of brain compliance. The third wave is the smallest and a representation of the pressure wave sent through the arterial system with aortic valve closure [7].

Despite this correlation, there appears to be multiple components of CSF circulation, including mechanical assistance via cilia and microvilli observed on the surface of the choroid plexus [2]. Another component is gravity and posture, which assists in decreasing venous pressure. Increased abdominal or thoracic pressure, physical activity, or Valsalva maneuvers will increase venous pressure and decrease the pressure gradient driving resorption [8].

Ventricular Anatomy

The majority of the choroid plexus and CSF production is in the lateral ventricles, which then flows through the interventricular foramen (or foramen of Monro) from each lateral ventricle into the third ventricle. From the third ventricle, CSF flows down the cerebral aqueduct (or Sylvian aqueduct) connecting the third ventricle to the fourth ventricle. CSF exits the fourth ventricle via the two lateral apertures (foramen of Luschka) and the median aperture (foramen of Magendie) and enters the subarachnoid space to then surround and bathe the brain and spinal cord. It is resorbed back into the blood circulation through a variety of means which will be explored later in this chapter. A visual reference of ventricular anatomy is provided in Fig. 3.3, as the individual components are described in the following paragraphs.

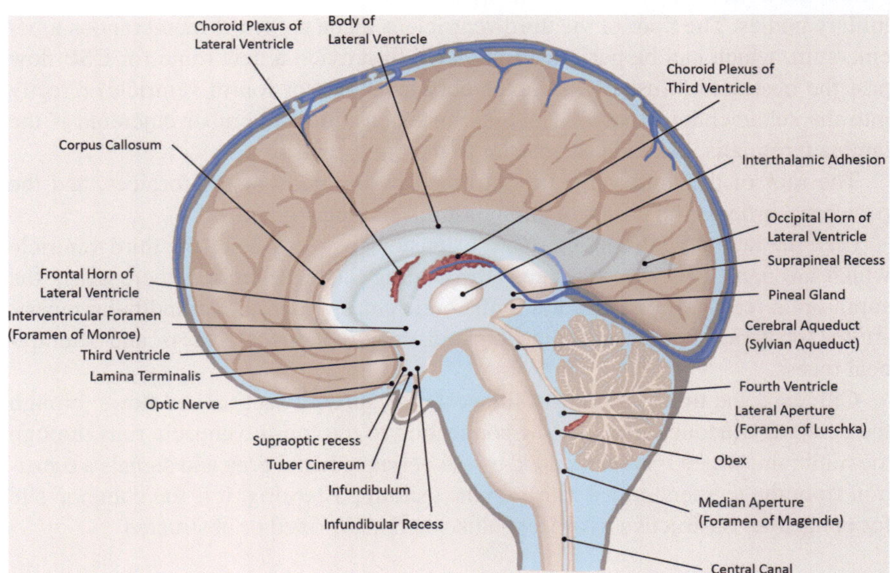

Fig. 3.3 Ventricular system anatomy. (Image courtesy of Dr. Michelle Paff, University of California Irvine, Neurosurgery Department, 2021)

Lateral Ventricles

The lateral ventricles are the largest ventricles and located near the center of the brain on either side of midline. The structure that connects both cerebral hemispheres, the corpus callosum, lies superior, and the ventricles are medial to the bilateral thalami while having projections into multiple lobes. The main part is the body with a projection, or horn, into the frontal lobe, which hugs the head of the caudate. The body becomes the atrium more posterior where the occipital horn and temporal horn diverge into their respective lobes. The choroid plexus runs along the inferomedial part of the body before it turns into the third ventricle via the foramen of Monro. Posteriorly, it wraps around the atrium of the ventricles and then runs along the roof of the temporal horn.

Third Ventricle

The third ventricle is a midline cavity between the two thalami. Occasionally, the two thalami connect forming the interthalamic adhesion in the middle of the third ventricle. Choroid plexus comes through the foramen of Monro and rides the roof of the third ventricle but stops prior to the channel to the fourth ventricle, called the cerebral aqueduct. The anterior border and floor of the third ventricle contains multiple vital structures, which are often viewed when performing an endoscopic third ventriculostomy (ETV) for obstructive hydrocephalus. These structures include the fornix, the anterior commissure, the optic chiasm, the infundibulum, and the mammillary bodies. The floor of the third ventricle is made up by the membranous tuber cinereum, which can be perforated via ETV to provide a new route for CSF flow past the obstruction (usually at the cerebral aqueduct or fourth ventricle) directly into the subarachnoid spaces. The anterior extension of the tuber cinereum is the lamina terminalis, located just anterior to the optic chiasm.

The roof of the third ventricle is formed by the body of the fornices, and the posterior border is the posterior commissure and pineal gland.

Like the lateral ventricle, there are extensions or recesses of the third ventricle which are named by the structures surrounding them. Anteriorly there exists the supra-optic recess (for its relation to the optic chiasm) and the infundibular recess. At the posterior border, the pineal gland creates a pineal recess and suprapineal recess.

CSF exits the third ventricle at the posterior, inferior section and flows through the cerebral aqueduct. This hollow connection to the fourth ventricle runs through the midbrain, where it is surrounded by the periaqueductal gray and signals a transition from the tegmentum anteriorly to the tectum posteriorly. It is the common site for congenital obstructive hydrocephalus when malformed or obstructed.

Fourth Ventricle

The fourth ventricle is a diamond-shaped structure that lies posterior to the brain stem and anterior to the cerebellum. The cerebral aqueduct lies at the superior tip with the obex at the inferior tip. The floor of the fourth ventricle is the anterior portion or the dorsal side of the pons. The floor of the fourth ventricle contains the facial colliculus, the vagal triangle, and the hypoglossal triangle. Also found is the area postrema, which is responsible for detecting toxins and inducing vomiting to assist the body in removing them [9].

The roof of the fourth ventricle is formed by the medullary velum, which is a membranous covering between the ventricle and the cerebellum, and contains choroid plexus. The peak of the roof is at the level of the pontomedullary junction and lies near the fastigial nucleus of the cerebellum. The walls, or lateral borders, are formed by extensions of the medullary velum and the cerebellar peduncles.

CSF flow down from the cerebral aqueduct continues to the spinal cord via the obex into the central canal or exits the fourth ventricle via the foramen of Magendie (medial) into the cisterna magna or via the two foramen of Luschka into the cerebellopontine cistern.

Subarachnoid Space

As noted previously, CSF enters the subarachnoid space via the foramen of Magendie into the cisterna magna and the foramina of Luschka into the cerebellopontine cistern. As CSF surrounds the brain and spinal cord, it does so in the subarachnoid space. The subarachnoid space is between the pia mater on the surface of the brain and the arachnoid mater. The subarachnoid space is made up of numerus trabeculae and channels. It also contains the major branches of the cerebral vasculature and cranial nerves. The subarachnoid space is relatively small at the gyri of the brain, but enlarge in the sulci as space is created between separate gyri. The subarachnoid space has pools or pockets of CSF as part of the drainage system mainly at the base of the brain, called subarachnoid or basal cisterns, shown in Fig. 3.4. These are located often in areas where more fluid is needed to help support the form and function of the brain and protect it from contact with the skull. This is commonly at the skull base. These cisterns have subarachnoid membranes that often form incomplete borders. Though CSF does communicate across these borders, the arachnoid does serve to blunt the communication of flow, particularly with pulsations of the brain. The basal cisterns are important aspects of intracranial surgical anatomy, as they are often accessed to aid in brain relaxation via CSF egress and thus decrease injury from brain retraction. However, this also results in increased transmission of pulsatile flow, which can impact the integrity of a surgical dural closure.

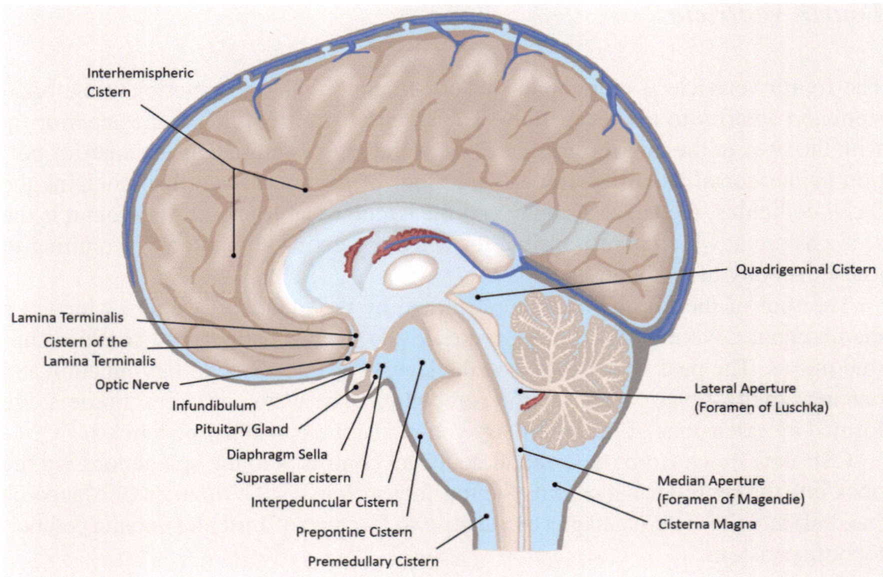

Fig. 3.4 Subarachnoid cisterns. (Image courtesy of Dr. Michelle Paff, University of California Irvine, Neurosurgery Department, 2021)

Basal Cisterns

The cisterna magna is the largest basal cistern and is the most caudal, sitting posterior to the medulla near the foramen magnum, or the opening of the skull where the spinal cord passes. It receives CSF from the fourth ventricle via the foramen of Magendie. The cisterna magna can be enlarged in a finding called mega cisterna magna. This is typically an incidental finding with no relation to pathology or symptomology. However, when noted perinatally, it can be associated with chromosomal abnormality, infection, or a result of accompanying error in posterior fossa development.

Anterior to the medulla is the premedullary cistern, which contains the bilateral vertebral arteries as they join to create the basilar artery. Working superiorly along the posterior part of the clivus is the prepontine cistern, which contains the basilar artery and the fifth and sixth cranial nerves. The former enters a CSF pocket called Meckel's cave, which contains the trigeminal ganglion and runs the branches of the trigeminal verve to their exiting foramina. The latter runs through the anterior pontine membrane just medial to Meckel's cave and through dural coverage toward the cavernous sinus [10]. Lateral to the brain stem lies the cerebellomedullary and cerebellopontine cisterns.

The cerebellopontine cistern is a notable cistern for intracranial surgery as it provides access to the middle cranial nerves and contains the cerebellopontine angle

(CPA), which is a common location for surgical pathology. Contained within the cerebellopontine cistern are cranial nerves seven and eight, the facial nerve, and vestibulocochlear nerve, respectively. These can be traced to their course through the internal auditory (acoustic) meatus.

Surrounding the midbrain are the perimesencephalic cisterns, which can be the site of non-aneurysmal, spontaneous, subarachnoid hemorrhage. Making up the perimesencaphlic cisterns anteriorly is the interpeduncular cistern, anterolaterally by the crural cisterns, posterolaterally by the ambient cisterns, and posteriorly by the quadrigeminal cistern.

Moving anteriorly from the interpeduncular cistern between the underside of the brain and the anterior skull base is the suprasellar or chiasmatic cistern which contains the circle of Willis, the optic chiasm, and the pituitary stalk, or infundibulum. The floor of the suprasellar cistern is the diaphragm sella, which is a dural continuation of the roof of the cavernous sinus that overlies the sella turcica with a small opening for the pituitary stalk. The dura then folds under itself and descends into the sella turcica to surround the pituitary gland. In radiographic evaluations of concern for intracranial hypertension, the suprasellar cistern can be seen to protrude through the diaphragm sella and consume the space in the sella turcica. This is a route to expand the fixed volume of the skull and displace CSF in abnormal spaces. On imaging this appears as the "empty sella sign" as the pituitary gland is pushed to the side and the hypodense CSF fills the cavity instead.

An important surgical component of the diaphragm sella is whether parasellar pathology has violated it and opened the sella to communications with the CSF-filled basal cisterns. If not, CSF leak is unusual during endoscopic, endonasal approaches to sella pathology. If the diaphragm sella is compromised either by pathology or during a surgical case, the risk of CSF leak postoperatively increases, and there is increased importance on the repair of the skull base defect created during surgery as well as perioperative, prophylactic measures to decrease CSF leak.

Moving superior from the suprasellar cistern is the cistern of the lamina terminalis. This lies just anterior to the third ventricle, and approach to the third ventricle can be obtained via the posterior border of this cistern, aptly named the lamina terminalis. This cistern is entered during approaches to anterior cerebral arteries, as the A1 and A2 segments of the anterior cerebral arteries and the anterior communicating artery are found within the cistern of the lamina terminalis.

Other cisterns exist in sulci between cerebral gyri and in the divisions between separate lobes. The most prominent is the Sylvian cistern which exists in the Sylvian fissure that separates the frontal lobe from the temporal lobe. This cistern contains the middle cerebral artery and is frequently opened during neurosurgical procedures to access portions of the middle cerebral artery, distal intracranial internal carotid artery, and lesions at the skull base.

CSF Resorption

Resorption of CSF from the subarachnoid space back into the circulating blood volume is primarily thought to occur via protrusions of the subarachnoid space, called arachnoid villi, through the dura mater into the main drainage spaces of the brain, named dural venous sinuses. Additional resorption is known to happen via the lymphatic system from CSF-filled spaces along the cranial and spinal nerve sheaths, including the cribriform plate [11]. There is also additional drainage in the adventitia and perivascular spaces of cerebral blood vessels [3]. Resorption is a dynamic process, partially dependent on the local pressure gradient, as the pressure in the subarachnoid space roughly equals the intracranial pressure – which is much higher than the venous or lymphatic pressures. The change in resorption based on pressure is also observed in alterations to local pressure dynamics caused during position adjustments. For example, there is increased CSF resorption in the lumbosacral nerve roots when standing or upright [12]. Additionally, in normal circumstances, cervical lymph is 10% CSF, but during times of elevated pressure, CSF can make up 80% of cervical lymph contents [13].

Venous Sinuses

Venous sinuses collect all of the venous blood in the brain and return it to the heart via the jugular system in the neck, as detailed in Fig. 3.5. They are called sinuses rather than veins because they are channels or spaces created between two layers of dura mater. They collect blood from draining cerebral veins, both cortical and deep. The flow of this blood goes from the superior sagittal sinus at the top of the head, midline, and superior to the falx cerebri—which is a dural fold that splits the two cerebral hemispheres. The superior sagittal sinus runs from anterior to posterior and joins deep drainage of the brain and posterior fossa drainage at the confluence of sinuses, or torcula. From the torcula split bilateral transverse sinuses, which run laterally and join the superior petrosal sinus drainage of the cavernous sinus and cerebellum to become the sigmoid sinus near the mastoid bone. The sigmoid sinus meets additional cavernous sinus and cerebellum drainage via the inferior petrosal sinus at the jugular bulb in the jugular foramen, which then transitions to the internal jugular vein. The cavernous sinus lies on either side of the pituitary fossa and is thus commonly encountered during endoscopic, endonasal approach to sellar pathology and can be a difficult area to control bleeding if there is tumor or iatrogenic invasion. It receives venous drainage from the eye.

The inferior sagittal sinus mirrors the superior sagittal sinus by running from anterior to posterior, but inferior to the falx cerebri along the corpus callosum. The vein of Galen is formed by the conjoining of two pairs of veins, the basal veins of Rosenthal and the internal cerebral veins. The basal vein of Rosenthal drains the mesial temporal lobe and runs along the medial surface of the temporal lobe and

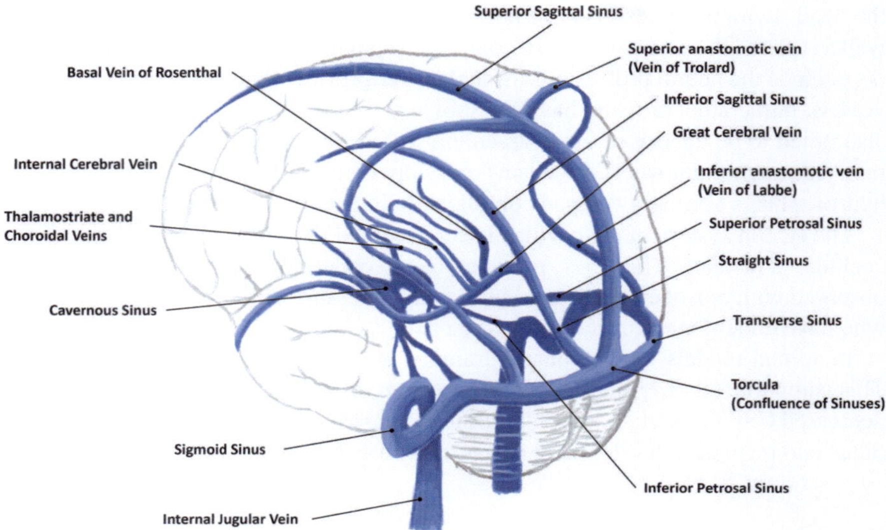

Fig. 3.5 Dural venous sinuses. (Image courtesy of Dr. Michelle Paff, University of California Irvine, Neurosurgery Department, 2021)

laterally around the midbrain in the ambient cistern. The internal cerebral vein drains the choroid plexus and thalamus via the choroidal vein and thalamostriate vein, respectively, which join at the foramen of Monro and run as the internal cerebral vein along the roof of the third ventricle until meeting with the basal vein of Rosenthal at the vein of Galen.

The deep drainage system ends in the straight sinus that runs midline near the falx cerebri and connects to the torcula. The straight sinus anteriorly receives cortical drainage from the inferior sagittal sinus and from the deep structures via the great cerebral vein or vein of Galen.

Arachnoid villi, also known as arachnoid granulations, are endothelium lined, finger-like protrusions of the arachnoid mater through the dura mater of the dural venous sinuses to allow the subarachnoid space to communicate with the draining blood volume. These have been shown to grow and shrink to alter the surface area for modifiable CSF resorption based on the pressure [3]. They are most commonly found in the superior sagittal sinus and transverse sinus, commonly next to the confluence of a cerebral vein into the sinus.

Lymphatics

The importance of lymphatic drainage in CSF resorption into the bloodstream is a more novel idea than the findings of arachnoid granulations in the dural venous sinuses, but many studies are connecting CSF to the draining lymphatic system of the head. Lymphatic vessels have been found in the dural covering of the brain, as well as around the nerve sheaths of cranial and spinal nerves [3, 11]. When researchers occlude the neural protrusions through the cribriform plate or the cervical lymph vessels, intracranial pressure has been shown to rise [14, 15]. Lymphatic drainage is also noted to be decreased in subarachnoid hemorrhage and ischemic strokes, currently through unknown mechanisms, possibly contributing to the development of hydrocephalus seen as a delayed complication in these conditions [16].

The lymph system of the cochlea is connected to the subarachnoid space via the cochlear aqueduct. This may provide the association of auditory disturbances observed with episodes of elevated intracranial pressure or those seen with patients who have undergone ventricular shunting [3].

In animal models, the lymphatic drainage of CSF is seen to decrease with age. This supports the hypothesis of age leading to decreased CSF turnover from decreased CSF production and resorption leading to increased toxic cerebral metabolites and increased development of neurocognitive disorders [11].

Perivascular Pathway

As CSF fills the perivascular spaces and interfaces with neuronal interstitial fluid, increased importance of the perivascular drainage has been noted. The interface between the interstitial fluid, CSF, and perivascular drainage is a convective process with bidirectional flow. This is increased during sleep, highlighting the importance of sleep in clearing toxic waste products of cerebral metabolism [17]. This drainage is associated with a protein membrane channel called aquaporin-4 (AQ-4). AQ-4 knockouts in mice studies are observed to have less CSF drainage via the perivascular system. The consequences are decreased resorption of dangerous cerebral metabolites, such as tau and beta amyloid proteins [18]. AQ-4 is also found to be decreased in chronic or repetitive traumatic brain injuries, connecting the increasing neurocognitive disorders found in this condition [16].

Pathology

Intracranial pathology is best understood in the context of a principle called the Monro-Kellie doctrine. This states the skull is a fixed, finite volume and the pressure within is made up of the volume of its constituents, namely, the brain, blood, and CSF. All methods to modulate intracranial pressure are geared toward modulating one of those three elements. Ultimately, if intracranial pressure was left untreated and continued to increase, those three components would look for routes outside the fixed space of the skull. This is what leads to cerebral herniation, and eventually all blood would be squeezed out of the intracranial space—leading to brain death.

Modulating intracranial pressure is an important consideration in skull base pathology, as elevated pressure can worsen skull base CSF leaks and disrupt skull base reconstructions. The reverse is true as skull base surgery and pathology can affect intracranial pressure with mass lesions taking up intracranial space or altering CSF flow, intracranial seeding of malignancy or sinus infections, procedural hemorrhage, and post-procedural infection, including meningitis and disruption of CSF absorption.

Normal values for intracranial pressure (ICP) in adults are typically 5–15 cm H_2O, while in infants <5 cm H_2O. There are normal physiologic processes that can temporarily increase ICP, such as any activity that increases cardiac output like exercise or any process that decreases venous return like Valsalva maneuvers. Also, the concept that the cranial vault is a fixed volume is not true in children, as the sutures separating the individual skull bones have not fused and can expand, allowing for increased volume. This is seen commonly in infants with hydrocephalus or increased CSF. The size of the head and the openings around the bones in children, such as the fontanelles, allow a window into evaluating intracranial pressure.

We will explore each intracranial constituent and how it is modulated in controlling intracranial pressure and also how skull base pathology can influence each of those elements. However, full depth discussion of the skull base pathology and some of the therapies to counter elevated ICP will be found in chapters later in this book. In general, approaches to managing intracranial pressure follow a tiered management approach targeting the etiology of the elevated pressure and moving from the least invasive to the most invasive. The obvious exception is in the cases of a mass lesion (intracranial hemorrhage, enlarged CSF spaces, or cerebral neoplasms) where invasive surgery is often required, urgently in the setting of elevated intracranial pressures.

Altering Brain

The most direct way to alter the volume of the brain is to physically remove certain components. This can become necessary during processes where increases in brain volume have raised the intracranial pressure and are putting the rest of the brain at risk. Cerebral edema during ischemic stroke or traumatic brain injury is the most common etiology. These lead to increased brain volume with the development of cytotoxic edema. This is a temporary process, and the affected brain will eventually shrink in size to smaller than the original size due to the apoptosis and necrotic cell death that occurs. During this temporary increase in edema and intracranial pressure, a procedure called a decompressive craniectomy can be performed to increase the volume of the previously fixed and finite cranial compartment. In addition to this, lobectomy can be performed if cerebral swelling is expected to exceed the additional volume created. During traumatic brain injury, the anterior non-dominant frontal lobe (usually the right side) is the safest target without long-term neurologic deficits. During ischemic stroke, portions of the affected brain can be removed if necessary [19].

Another approach to decrease brain volume in these two pathologic entities is to counter the cerebral swelling by increasing the osmolality of the blood to encourage interstitial fluid to re-enter the bloodstream. This impacts the affected tissue, but also the currently unaffected brain tissue, so there are limits of this approach before neurologic side effects occur. The two most common approaches to increase osmolality are to use mannitol or hypertonic saline injected intravenously. These will make the blood hypertonic in comparison to cerebral tissue and decrease brain volume through fluid migration from the brain to the bloodstream. An additional approach to counter cerebral swelling is the use of steroids for vasogenic edema caused by tumors. Decreasing brain volume will improve ICP through an additional benefit of improved CSF circulation and resorption by opening the cisterns and subarachnoid spaces.

Altering Blood

When considering how to alter the blood component in the intracranial space, we have to separate the blood contained in the cerebral vasculature from any blood that has violated the barriers in the brain and taken up valuable real estate. This adds volume to the fixed compartment and may require surgery to remove the foreign collection. Hemorrhage can occur in any of the intracranial compartments that have been created by the meninges of the brain. These compartments are detailed in Fig. 3.6.

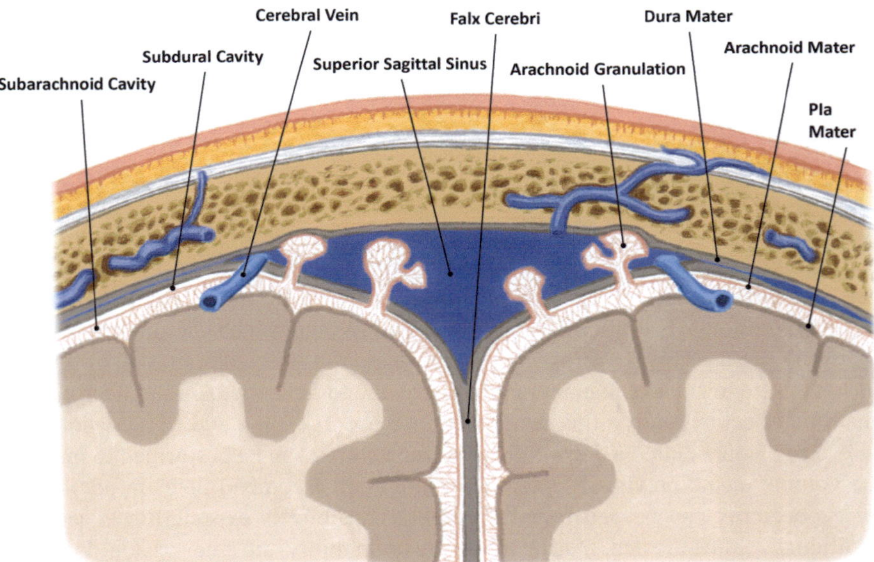

Fig. 3.6 Intracranial spaces. (Image courtesy of Dr. Michelle Paff, University of California Irvine, Neurosurgery Department, 2021)

- Epidural hemorrhage, between the dura and the skull, is most often caused by trauma and rupture of a dural vessel/sinus or bleeding from the bone. This is often a convex shape as the epidural space is separated in areas where the dura attaches to the inside of the skull.
- Subdural hemorrhage would be between the dural layer and the arachnoid layer and is also most frequently caused by trauma. It is a convex shape that forms along the outside of the brain and follows the contouring. Other causes include rupture of vascular malformation or even spontaneous hemorrhage from cerebral sag pulling the brain parenchyma away from the skull and stretching the veins that bridge from the parenchyma to the dural sinuses. This etiology can occur with age and brain shrinkage or even from over drainage of CSF from a lumbar puncture or lumbar drain.
- Subarachnoid hemorrhage is between the arachnoid layer and the pial layer – or the layer right on top of the parenchymal surface. This can occur from trauma, but is traditionally attributed to rupture of a cerebral aneurysm. This layer is where CSF production, circulation, and absorption occur and is in communication around the entire brain. Typically surgery isn't performed to drain the blood as it rarely forms a focal mass lesion, but blood in this space can cause a host of issues with CSF circulation as well as irritation of the cerebral vasculature.

Outside of surgical evacuation of blood that has formed a mass lesion in the brain, sometimes it becomes necessary to decrease the amount of blood in the cerebral vasculature in order to decrease intracranial pressure. The least invasive of these methods is positioning to maximize venous blood return from the brain. This includes elevating the head, ensuring no compression of the major neck veins by external devices (such as a cervical collar), and preventing increased abdominal or thoracic pressure that would decrease venous return. This is most relevant during surgery when positive pressure ventilation results in an increase in thoracic pressure and reduced venous return. In an effort to minimize this effect, use of high peep should be avoided. In addition, if the peak pressures are elevated, the tidal volume is usually reduced, and the respiratory rate increased. Obese patients also have significantly increased intrathoracic pressure in the supine position, so reverse Trendelenburg is used to minimize this effect.

Altering CSF

Managing CSF as an intracranial component relies on understanding the tenets discussed earlier in this chapter. Therapeutic aims to decrease the amount of CSF focus on decreasing production, improving circulation, or increasing resorption. The body has developed some means to develop an equilibrium between the CSF volume and the intracranial pressure, such as decreased production from the choroid plexus and increased resorption at the arachnoid villi when ICP is elevated. External intervention is required when these intrinsic processes cannot overcome the pathologic disturbances.

CSF production naturally decreases as we age, and consequently so does the resorption as outflow will equal inflow to keep a steady volume of CSF intracranially. The vessels "feeding" the choroid plexus are similar to the types of vessels that first get affected with the calcifications and atherosclerotic changes that come with age. This small vessel disease is often not visualized on vessel imaging and usually manifests in magnetic resonance imaging. Also, the lymphatic component of CSF resorption has also been shown to undergo age-related degeneration, resulting in decreased resorption [11]. If one comes first and causes the other, or they share a similar process, there is no certainty. But the result is decreased turnover, and one of the purposes of CSF reviewed earlier in this chapter is maintaining delicate homeostasis of the neuronal environment and eliminating waste from utilized products. The decreased turnover leads to increased concentrations of toxic metabolites and development of neuron loss as the subsequent neurocognitive disorders [3].

Not all disease processes altering CSF dynamics can be categorized into just affecting production, circulation, or resorption of CSF. Neither do they always result in elevated pressure. One example of this is normal pressure hydrocephalus, which develops later in life as a consequence of reduced production, reduced resorption, increased CSF volume, and decreased brain volume. Despite there being normal pressure when tested invasively, some prove to benefit from CSF diversion [20].

Production

Pathology that increases production of CSF involves tumors of the choroid plexus, including choroid plexus papilloma and choroid plexus carcinoma, which are both treated surgically. Due to their origin in the choroid plexus, which is an intraventricular substance, these tumors can also cause hydrocephalus via impaired circulation.

There aren't many treatments that are targeted at modulating CSF production, but the most common medical treatment is acetazolamide. Acetazolamide is a carbonic anhydrase inhibitor, which is an important protein in the production of CSF at the choroid plexus. This medication has been used commonly in the treatment of idiopathic, intracranial hypertension (IIH) to decrease CSF production and ICP in a chronic manner. Many patients do not tolerate the side effects of this medication.

Surgical approach to decrease CSF production involves cauterizing the choroid plexus. This is most commonly done in conjunction with a treatment titled endoscopic third ventriculostomy, which aims to treat obstructive hydrocephalus by improving circulation via a new route from the ventricular system to the cisternal system. This combined approach has been utilized to help children with hydrocephalus avoid shunts, particularly in developing countries where access to healthcare is less reliable and shunt failure is common and can have dire consequences [21]. This technique is yet to be fully investigated in adults.

Circulation

Any substance that can disrupt the path from CSF production to CSF resorption can cause elevated ICP and development of hydrocephalus. When there is impairment of CSF circulation, it is known as obstructive hydrocephalus, where a focal point of compression in the ventricular system is causing upstream dilation. Impairment of resorption, or communicating hydrocephalus, will be discussed next. Obstructive hydrocephalus can occur from congenital causes, such as aqueductal stenosis, or developed causes, such as mass effect from a para- or intraventricular tumor causing closure of a ventricle. At times, the etiology of hydrocephalus can cause either obstructive or communicating hydrocephalus and sometimes a combination of the two. One example is intraventricular hemorrhage. Intraventricular hemorrhage and subarachnoid hemorrhage are the most common causes of hydrocephalus. If the blood traps CSF circulation at the cerebral aqueduct, this is likely to cause a picture of obstructive hydrocephalus with upstream dilation of the ventricular system. This is a common etiology of hydrocephalus in the pediatric population. However, subarachnoid hemorrhage causing hydrocephalus in adults is most commonly from ruptured cerebral aneurysm. This blood is outside the ventricular system and most closely associated with CSF absorption sites. Thus it causes a communicating hydrocephalus, where the entire ventricular system is enlarged [22]. This is not uncommon, known to occur 20–30% of the time after aneurysm rupture [23].

Intraventricular tumors are known to cause obstruction of the ventricular system when large enough. These can be categorized by which parts of the ventricular system they affect. Choroid plexus tumors were mentioned previously and include choroid plexus papilloma (80% of primary choroid plexus tumors) and choroid plexus carcinoma, which typically occur in the first 5 years of life but only accounts for a small percentage of pediatric brain tumors (1–5%) [24, 25]. Other intraventricular tumors grow from the lining or walls of the ventricles. These include ependymoma, subependymoma, central neurocytoma, and subependymal giant cell astrocytoma. Lastly, the most common tumor found inside the ventricle does not come from ventricular components. This is the colloid cyst, which is almost always found at the foramen of Monro and is made up of primitive neuroepithelium.

Tumors can also grow from other cerebral tissues and obstruct the ventricular system when large enough. Third ventricular compression can occur from skull base lesions, including pituitary adenomas, craniopharyngiomas, and anterior skull base meningiomas. Pineal region tumors may also cause hydrocephalus but putting pressure on the tectum resulting in narrowing/obstruction of the cerebral aqueduct. Due to the constrictive size of the posterior fossa, masses in that region can cause obstructive hydrocephalus from fourth ventricle compression. In adults, the most common posterior fossa mass is metastasis, and the most common primary tumor in the posterior fossa is a hemangioblastoma. In children, posterior fossa masses are the most common site for brain tumors [26]. Medulloblastoma accounts for 30–40% of all posterior fossa tumors, followed by pilocytic astrocytoma accounting for 25–35% [27]. Other less common pediatric posterior fossa masses include ependymoma, atypical teratoid/rhabdoid tumor, brain stem glioma, and teratoma. Other etiologies that can cause compression of the ventricular system and obstructive hydrocephalus include traumatic brain injury with the associated swelling and cerebral edema, as well as ischemic and hemorrhagic stroke, particularly in the posterior fossa.

There is currently no medication designed to treat the mechanical problem of obstructive hydrocephalus, so the mainstays have been surgical and mechanical diversion or re-routing of CSF. An external ventricular drain (EVD) is a common measure to quickly alleviate hydrocephalus and is one of the first procedures learned by training neurosurgeons. This will be discussed in a later chapter in detail. But in brief, a catheter is placed through a small burr hole (or twist drill hole)craniotomy into the lateral ventricle. This diverts fluid to an external drainage bag and alleviates the buildup of hydrocephalus and intracranial pressure. At times, obstructive hydrocephalus is known to be permanent, such as in congenital causes or inoperable tumors, or the hydrocephalus fails to resolve after obstruction removal. This necessitates a new permanent alternative to circulation, which can come in the form of a ventricular shunt. This is a catheter that is placed in a similar fashion to an EVD, but the tubing is tunneled under the skin and CSF diverted to another body system to be reabsorbed. Most commonly the site is the peritoneal space, but the cardiac atrium, pleural space, urinary bladder, and even gall bladder have been used [28, 29].

As mentioned above, ventricular shunts can have frequent problems with clotting and infection, and attempts to surgically introduce new routes of circulation have been utilized. The most common is the endoscopic third ventriculostomy. This is where a hole is made in the floor of the third ventricle into the suprasellar cistern. This bypasses the normal route of CSF from the ventricular system to the cisternal system, which usually occurs at the foramen of Magendie or Luschka in the fourth ventricle. Another procedure that also attempts to connect the ventricles to the cisterns is fenestration of the lamina terminalis. As a reminder, the lamina terminalis is the anterior wall of the third ventricle, and fenestration of it would connect the third ventricle to the cistern of the lamina terminalis which freely communicates with other subarachnoid cisterns. This is a common maneuver in the surgical approach to clipping anterior circulation aneurysms and has the additional benefit in that surgery of providing increased brain relaxation and decreased harmful brain retraction. A randomized control trial is evaluating whether this can decrease development of hydrocephalus following aneurysmal subarachnoid hemorrhage [30] after meta-analyses have shown the maneuver to decrease shunt-dependent hydrocephalus from 15.3% to 11.4% [31].

Resorption

As mentioned earlier in this chapter, CSF is constantly made, and the system experiences turnover about four times daily. This is reliant on a robust and intact CSF resorption system, the details of which we have covered. As the final pathway in this system, there are many pathologies that can collect at resorption sites and cause disturbances. This can be seen in traumatic brain injury, when inflammatory mediators are released from injured brain into surrounding fluid, which then circulate around the brain impacting normal tissue and leading to a cascade that can cause hydrocephalus [16, 32]. A similar process can occur in both ischemic and hemorrhagic stroke [16], and we have already reviewed how subarachnoid hemorrhage often leads to hydrocephalus via decreased resorption in 20–30% of cases.

Skull base surgery can also be the etiology of hydrocephalus, as one study showed 8% of cranial base surgery patients developed shunt-dependent hydrocephalus due to postoperative hemorrhage or meningitis from postoperative CSF leak. Anything that can settle in, obstruct, or inflame the resorption sites can lead to hydrocephalus. Some tumors approached through skull base surgery must be completely removed en bloc, as CSF spread has been known to cause aseptic meningitis and postoperative hydrocephalus [33]. In addition, some of these processes such as meningitis may affect cerebral compliance which can lead to hydrocephalus without a significant increase in intracranial pressure.

Similar to obstructive hydrocephalus, the mainstay of treatment for elevated ICP and communicating hydrocephalus from impaired CSF resorption is surgical. Unlike obstructive hydrocephalus, these cases almost always require internal shunting, as creating new circulation routes doesn't address the primary problem of decreased resorption. Novel techniques to establish new connections from the subarachnoid space to the venous sinuses are being developed and trialed, but none are in mainstream use [34–36].

Conclusion

- Reviewed the details of cerebrospinal fluid physiology including the production, circulation, and resorption and when those processes malfunction
- Reviewed an introduction to intracranial pressure and how the three constituents that make up ICP are modulated
- Set the framework for understanding the intracranial spaces associated with skull base surgery and potential pitfalls
- Set up later chapters that will dive into diagnosis, imaging, and treatment of CSF leaks, as well as associated repairs of skull base defects

References

1. Rink C, Khanna S. Significance of brain tissue oxygenation and the arachidonic acid cascade in stroke. Antioxid Redox Signal. 2011;14(10):1889–903. https://doi.org/10.1089/ars.2010.3474.
2. Hofman FM, Chen TC. Chapter 3—Choroid plexus: structure and function, the choroid plexus and cerebrospinal fluid. Cambridge: Academic Press; 2016. p. 29–40, ISBN 9780128017401

3. Sakka L, Coll G, Chazal J. Anatomy and physiology of cerebrospinal fluid. Eur Ann Otorhinolaryngol Head Neck Dis. 2011;128(6):309–16. https://doi.org/10.1016/j.anorl.2011.03.002. Epub 2011 Nov 18

4. Tumani H, Huss A, Bachhuber F. The cerebrospinal fluid and barriers—anatomic and physiologic considerations. Handb Clin Neurol. 2017;146:21–32. https://doi.org/10.1016/B978-0-12-804279-3.00002-2.

5. Oldendorf WH, Hyman S, Braun L, Oldendorf SZ. Blood-brain barrier: penetration of morphine, codeine, heroin, and methadone after carotid injection. Science. 1972;178(4064):984–6. https://doi.org/10.1126/science.178.4064.984.

6. Nau R, Sörgel F, Prange HW. Lipophilicity at pH 7.4 and molecular size govern the entry of the free serum fraction of drugs into the cerebrospinal fluid in humans with uninflamed meninges. J Neurol Sci. 1994;122(1):61–5. https://doi.org/10.1016/0022-510x(94)90052-3.

7. Harary M, Dolmans RGF, Gormley WB. Intracranial pressure monitoring-review and avenues for development. Sensors (Basel). 2018;18(2):465. https://doi.org/10.3390/s18020465.

8. Xu Q, Yu SB, Zheng N, Yuan XY, Chi YY, Liu C, Wang XM, Lin XT, Sui HJ. Head movement, an important contributor to human cerebrospinal fluid circulation. Sci Rep. 2016;19(6):31787. https://doi.org/10.1038/srep31787.

9. Miller AD, Leslie RA. The area postrema and vomiting. Front Neuroendocrinol. 1994;15(4):301–20. https://doi.org/10.1006/frne.1994.1012.

10. Sabancı PA, Batay F, Civelek E, Al Mefty O, Husain M, Abdulrauf SI, Karasu A. Meckel's cave. World Neurosurg. 2011;76(3–4):335–41; discussion 266-7. https://doi.org/10.1016/j.wneu.2011.03.037.

11. Ahn JH, Cho H, Kim JH, Kim SH, Ham JS, Park I, Suh SH, Hong SP, Song JH, Hong YK, Jeong Y, Park SH, Koh GY. Meningeal lymphatic vessels at the skull base drain cerebrospinal fluid. Nature. 2019;572(7767):62–6. https://doi.org/10.1038/s41586-019-1419-5. Epub 2019 Jul 24

12. Brierly JB, Field EJ, Yoffey JM. Passage of indian ink particles from the cranial subarachnoid space. J Anat. 1949;83(Pt 1):77.

13. Silver I, Li B, Szalai J, Johnston M. Relationship between intracranial pressure and cervical lymphatic pressure and flow rates in sheep. Am J Phys. 1999;277(6):R1712–7. https://doi.org/10.1152/ajpregu.1999.277.6.R1712.

14. Mollanji R, Bozanovic-Sosic R, Zakharov A, Makarian L, Johnston MG. Blocking cerebrospinal fluid absorption through the cribriform plate increases resting intracranial pressure. Am J Physiol Regul Integr Comp Physiol. 2002;282(6):R1593–9. https://doi.org/10.1152/ajpregu.00695.2001.

15. Földi M, Csillik B, Zoltán OT. Lymphatic drainage of the brain. Experientia. 1968;24(12):1283–7. https://doi.org/10.1007/BF02146675.

16. Bothwell SW, Janigro D, Patabendige A. Cerebrospinal fluid dynamics and intracranial pressure elevation in neurological diseases. Fluids Barriers CNS. 2019;16(1):9. https://doi.org/10.1186/s12987-019-0129-6.

17. Xie L, Kang H, Xu Q, Chen MJ, Liao Y, Thiyagarajan M, O'Donnell J, Christensen DJ, Nicholson C, Iliff JJ, Takano T, Deane R, Nedergaard M. Sleep drives metabolite clearance from the adult brain. Science. 2013;342(6156):373–7. https://doi.org/10.1126/science.1241224.

18. Iliff JJ, Wang M, Liao Y, Plogg BA, Peng W, Gundersen GA, Benveniste H, Vates GE, Deane R, Goldman SA, Nagelhus EA, Nedergaard M. A paravascular pathway facilitates CSF flow through the brain parenchyma and the clearance of interstitial solutes, including amyloid β. Sci Transl Med. 2012;4(147):147ra111. https://doi.org/10.1126/scitranslmed.3003748.

19. Schwake M, Schipmann S, Müther M, Stögbauer L, Hanning U, Sporns PB, Ewelt C, Dziewas R, Minnerup J, Holling M, Stummer W. Second-look strokectomy of cerebral infarction areas in patients with severe herniation. J Neurosurg. 2019;132(1):1–9. https://doi.org/10.3171/2018.8.JNS18692.

20. Wu EM, El Ahmadieh TY, Kafka B, Caruso J, Aoun SG, Plitt AR, Neeley O, Olson DM, Ruchinskas RA, Cullum M, Batjer H, White JA. Ventriculoperitoneal shunt outcomes of

Normal pressure hydrocephalus: a case series of 116 patients. Cureus. 2019;11(3):e4170. https://doi.org/10.7759/cureus.4170.

21. Warf BC. Comparison of endoscopic third ventriculostomy alone and combined with choroid plexus cauterization in infants younger than 1 year of age: a prospective study in 550 African children. J Neurosurg. 2005;103(6 Suppl):475–81. https://doi.org/10.3171/ped.2005.103.6.0475.

22. Golanov EV, Bovshik EI, Wong KK, Pautler RG, Foster CH, Federley RG, Zhang JY, Mancuso J, Wong ST, Britz GW. Subarachnoid hemorrhage - induced block of cerebrospinal fluid flow: role of brain coagulation factor III (tissue factor). J Cereb Blood Flow Metab. 2018;38(5):793–808. https://doi.org/10.1177/0271678X17701157. Epub 2017 Mar 28

23. Germanwala AV, Huang J, Tamargo RJ. Hydrocephalus after aneurysmal subarachnoid hemorrhage. Neurosurg Clin N Am. 2010;21(2):263–70. https://doi.org/10.1016/j.nec.2009.10.013.

24. Custodio G, Taques GR, Figueiredo BC, Gugelmin ES, Oliveira Figueiredo MM, Watanabe F, Pontarolo R, Lalli E, Torres LF. Increased incidence of choroid plexus carcinoma due to the germline TP53 R337H mutation in southern Brazil. PLoS One. 2011;6(3):e18015. https://doi.org/10.1371/journal.pone.0018015.

25. Grygotis LA, Chew FS. Choroid plexus carcinoma of the lateral ventricle. AJR Am J Roentgenol. 1997;169(5):1400. https://doi.org/10.2214/ajr.169.5.9353468.

26. Kornienko VN. Diagnostic Neuroradiology. In: Igor Nikolaevich Pronin. New York: Springer. ISBN:3540756523.

27. Kerleroux B, Cottier JP, Janot K, Listrat A, Sirinelli D, Morel B. Posterior fossa tumors in children: radiological tips & tricks in the age of genomic tumor classification and advance MR technology. J Neuroradiol. 2020;47(1):46–53. https://doi.org/10.1016/j.neurad.2019.08.002. Epub 2019 Sep 18

28. West KW, Turner MK, Vane DW, Boaz J, Kalsbeck J, Grosfeld JL. Ventricular gallbladder shunts: an alternative procedure in hydrocephalus. J Pediatr Surg. 1987;22(7):609–12. https://doi.org/10.1016/s0022-3468(87)80110-0.

29. Morosanu CO, Filip GA, Nicolae L, Florian IS. From the heart to the bladder-particularities of ventricular shunt topography and the current status of cerebrospinal fluid diversion sites. Neurosurg Rev. 2020;43(3):847–60. https://doi.org/10.1007/s10143-018-1033-2. Epub 2018 Oct 18

30. Tao C, Fan C, Hu X, Ma J, Ma L, Li H, Liu Y, Sun H, He M, You C. The effect of fenestration of the lamina terminalis on the incidence of shunt-dependent hydrocephalus after aneurysmal subarachnoid hemorrhage (FISH): study protocol for a randomized controlled trial. Medicine (Baltimore). 2016;95(52):e5727. https://doi.org/10.1097/MD.0000000000005727.

31. Mao J, Zhu Q, Ma Y, Lan Q, Cheng Y, Liu G. Fenestration of lamina terminalis during anterior circulation aneurysm clipping on occurrence of shunt-dependent hydrocephalus after aneurysmal subarachnoid hemorrhage: meta-analysis. World Neurosurg. 2019;129:e1–5. https://doi.org/10.1016/j.wneu.2019.01.270. Epub 2019 Feb 16

32. Illes S. More than a drainage fluid: the role of CSF in signaling in the brain and other effects on brain tissue. Handb Clin Neurol. 2017;146:33–46. https://doi.org/10.1016/B978-0-12-804279-3.00003-4.

33. Kato K, Ujiie H, Higa T, Hayashi M, Kubo O, Okada Y, Hori T. Clinical presentation of intracranial epidermoids: a surgical series of 20 initial and four recurred cases. Asian. J Neurosurg. 2010;5(1):32–40.

34. Kralick F, Oh J, Medina T, Noh HM. Micro-fabricated shunt to mimic arachnoid granulations for the treatment of communicating hydrocephalus. Acta Neurochir Suppl. 2012;114:239–42. https://doi.org/10.1007/978-3-7091-0956-4_47.

35. Heilman CB, Basil GW, Beneduce BM, Malek AM. Anatomical characterization of the inferior petrosal sinus and adjacent cerebellopontine angle cistern for development of an endovascular transdural cerebrospinal fluid shunt. J Neurointerv Surg. 2019;11(6):598–602. https://doi.org/10.1136/neurintsurg-2018-014445. Epub 2019 Jan 9

36. Malek A, Heilman C. E-020 design of an endovascular transdural cerebrospinal fluid shunt implant to MIMIC arachnoid granulation function. J NeuroInterventional Surgery. 2018;10:A57.

Chapter 4
Diagnosis of CSF Leak

Charles C. L. Tong

Introduction

Cerebrospinal fluid (CSF) rhinorrhea is defined by the presence of CSF in the nasal cavity as a result of a bony defect and disruption of the dura in the anterior or middle cranial fossae. The etiology of the breakdown of the barriers separating the sub-arachnoid space and the extracranial space can be classified into traumatic, sponta-neous, or neoplastic. Historically, repairs of CSF leak in the anterior and middle cranial fossae were performed by neurosurgeons using open intracranial approaches, but subsequent development and widespread adoption of endoscopic approach have become the standard of care, with high success rates and decreased morbidity. This chapter explores the diagnostic work up and preoperative tests for CSF leaks.

History and Physical Exam

The etiology of anterior skull base CSF leak is often revealed through careful his-tory taking and physical examination with nasal endoscopy. The exact location of bony defect with dural disruption and the presence of a meningoencephalocele can be further characterized with imaging.

C. C. L. Tong (✉)
Department of Otolaryngology - Head and Neck Surgery, Lenox Hill Hospital/Northwell Health System, New York, NY, USA
e-mail: ctong1@northwell.edu

© The Author(s), under exclusive license to Springer Nature Switzerland AG 2023
E. C. Kuan et al. (eds.), *Skull Base Reconstruction*,
https://doi.org/10.1007/978-3-031-27937-9_4

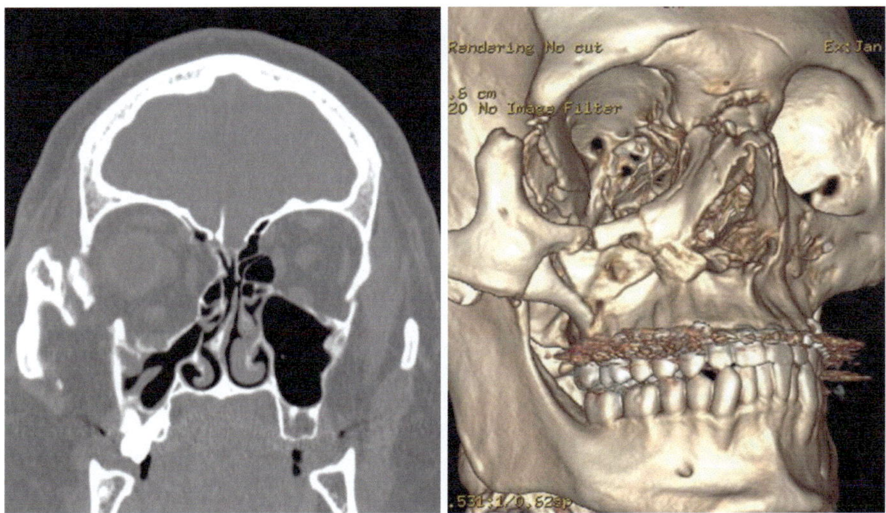

Fig. 4.1 Intoxicated young male ejected from the driver's seat without his seat belt fastened at twice the legal highway speed limit. Non-contrast computed tomography and three-dimensional reconstruction showing multiple midface fractures including a severely comminuted zygomatico-maxillary complex fracture, medial orbital wall fracture, frontal sinus fracture, and mandible fracture (not shown). Initial exam revealed a Glasgow score of 8, severe epistaxis, periorbital hemorrhage, and various musculoskeletal injuries. His nasal drainage collected on day 2 of admission was positive for beta-2 transferrin

Traumatic CSF Leak

Traumatic CSF leaks may result from blunt head trauma (accidental, Fig. 4.1) or penetrating trauma (most often iatrogenic). The incidence of a skull base fracture can be as high as 20% among patients with a skull fracture, most commonly in the anterior cranial fossa (ACF) [1]. The most common causes of ACF injury are motor vehicle accidents and mechanical falls, and risk factors include male gender (>70%) and young age (<35 years old) [2, 3]. In recent reports, post-traumatic CSF leaks have seen a reduction in rates in adults compared to the past, dropping from 10–30% to more recently 2.3%, possibly due to widespread use of safety belt and improved vehicle safety features [4, 5]. The most notable reason that the ACP is more vulnerable than the middle cranial fossa or posterior cranial fossa is the variable depth of the cribriform plate and the thin lateral lamellae which can be less than 1 mm thick. The depth of the cribriform plate is dictated by the length of the lateral lamellae of the ethmoid bone, as classified by Keros in 1962: Type I (1–3 mm depth), Type II (4–7 mm depth), and Type III (8–16 mm depth) [6]. Although functional endoscopic sinus surgery and neurosurgical procedures are most common surgeries leading to iatrogenic ACF CSF leaks, the actual incidence is quite low, estimated between 0.2 and 0.57% [7, 8]. Nevertheless, proper presurgical planning and patient counseling identify patients most at risk for iatrogenic CSF leaks.

Table 4.1 Symptoms and signs of ACF CSF leak

Traumatic (accidental or Iatrogenic)	Non-traumatic (spontaneous, neoplastic)
Epistaxis, rhinorrhea	*Rhinorrhea*
Meningitis	*Meningitis*
Ocular or periorbital hemorrhage	*Hyposmia or anosmia*
Other motor or sensory nerve deficits	

For patients with ACF fractures and CSF leaks, over 95% of them present early in their clinical course (within 48 h) with associated alarming symptoms (Table 4.1) [9–11]. Delayed presentations due to limited access to healthcare services or lack of initial symptoms usually present with meningitis or intermittent rhinorrhea, most often unilateral. The most common sites leading to CSF rhinorrhea after trauma are frontal sinus (31%), followed by sphenoid (11–31%) and ethmoid sinuses (15–19%) [12]. Temporal bone fractures can also present with rhinorrhea via the Eustachian tube.

Spontaneous CSF Leak

The cerebrospinal fluid is a clear fluid produced mainly by the choroid plexus. It consists of glucose (about 60–80% of serum concentration), electrolytes, proteins (including beta-2 transferrin), and a few cells. At baseline, this fluid is clear and colorless, without significant concentration of immune infiltrates. As the CSF is being produced by the plasma passing through the epithelial cells of the choroid plexus, it circulates from the lateral ventricles into the cisterns and the subarachnoid space prior to being resorbed into the venous system at the level of the arachnoid villi. Approximately 500 mL of CSF is produced daily at a rate of 18-24 mL per hour, with the total CSF volume being circulated at 90–150 mL in adults [13–15]. This equilibrium of production and resorption establishes the hydrostatic pressure, which ranges from 5 to 25 cmH_2O [16].

Historically, patients with spontaneous CSF leaks have been related to normal intracranial pressure, but they are increasingly found to have elevated ICP in lumbar punctures measured in recent studies [11, 17–19]. Elevated CSF pressure in the absence of a space-occupying lesion or dilated ventricles is most commonly found in idiopathic intracranial hypertension (IIH), also known as pseudotumor cerebri. Patients with IIH can present with symptoms of pressure-type headaches, pulsatile tinnitus, papilledema, visual disturbances, and clear rhinorrhea. They are most commonly seen in females of childbearing age and overweight [12, 20–23]. Radiographically, IIH patients can have partial or total empty sella syndrome with the diaphragma herniating into the sella and displacing the pituitary gland (Fig. 4.2). Of patients with sphenoid sinus fistula, over 90% had extensive pneumatization of the lateral recess, 60% with arachnoid pits (arachnoid granulations that penetrate the dura but do not communicate with the venous system), with a similar number with empty sella syndrome [24]. A smaller proportion of patients (30%) was also

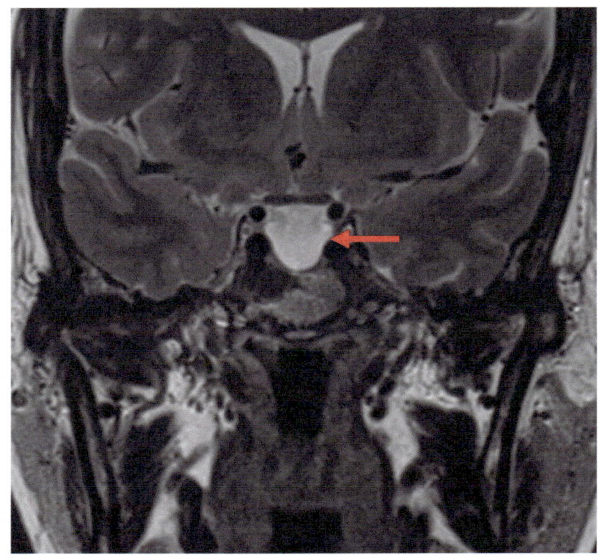

Fig. 4.2 MRI brain, T2-weighted image showing CSF replacing an enlarged and empty sella

found to have erosion of the dorsum sellae in a separate study, which all support the diagnosis of intracranial hypertension [25].

While the exact pathophysiology is not well understood, three main mechanisms have been described that could lead to increased ICP: increased venous sinus pressure, decreased CSF resorption, and increased CSF production. Fundamentally, the resorption rate of CSF depends on the pressure gradient between the CSF and the venous sinus system. A rise in venous sinus pressure stemming from venous sinus stenosis is commonly observed in patients with IIH, especially in the transverse sinus [26]. Reduction in ICP via CSF diversion has shown to relieve the venous stenosis, suggesting another process in causing IIH [27]. Other early studies have investigated the potential role for increased CSF production in IIH, but in cases where hypersecretion of CSF is known to occur such has choroid plexus papilloma, hydrocephalus and ventricular enlargement are observed which are rare in IIH [28]. In contrast, obesity is a common risk factor for developing IIH, with majority of patients with BMI over 30 [29–32]. Some theorized that excess weight leads to increased abdominal mass, thus raising intrathoracic pressure and venous pressure [33]. This theory is supported by clinical observations that weight loss improves this condition, and subsequent studies have confirmed objective reduction in ICP and papilledema in patients with significant weight loss [34, 35]. The mechanism by which weight loss improves IIH is not known, and by this theory alone, obese men should be equally affected. Inflammatory mediators have become the focus of recent investigations as cytokines produced by adipose tissue are found to be significantly higher in CSF of IIH patients compared to controls [36, 37]. Concentrations of CSF estrone were also found higher in patients with IIH than in controls, although contribution of hormonal factors remains observational [38, 39]. Regardless of the

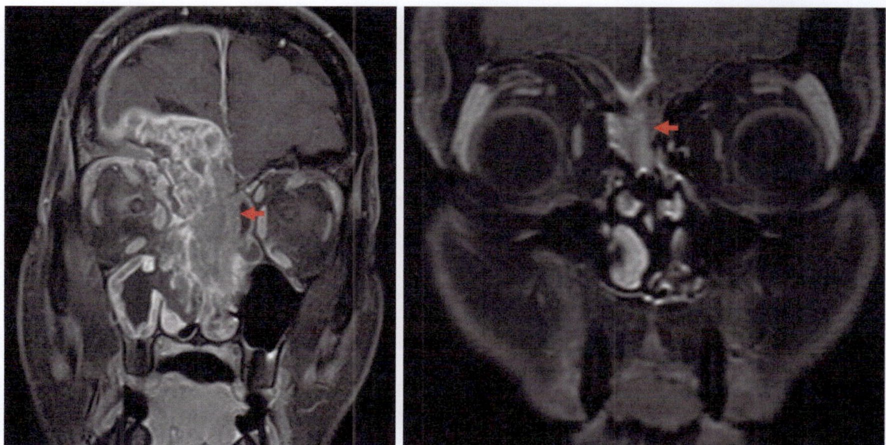

Fig. 4.3 MRI brain, T1-weighted images with contrast. Left image shows a patient with sinonasal Ewing sarcoma with extensive intracranial extension. Right image shows a patient with an olfactory groove meningioma

proposed mechanisms leading to increased ICP, it is generally accepted that the constant pulsatile pressure exerted on the skull base would ultimately lead to erosions and defects over sites of inherent weakness.

Neoplastic CSF Leak

CSF leak related to anterior skull base neoplasm can occur through direct erosion of the surrounding bone or, most commonly, during resection of the lesion. Tumor burden, location, and degree of intracranial extension often dictate the size of the dural defect and the difficulty in achieving a water-tight seal (Fig. 4.3). Please refer to Sect. 4 and 5 for reconstruction techniques.

Labs: Halo Sign, Beta-2 Transferrin, Beta-Trace Protein

Diagnosing CSF rhinorrhea has been, and remains, a diagnostic challenge. Advanced imaging, such as the high-resolution computed tomography (CT) and magnetic resonance imaging (MRI), has greatly enhanced the ability to localize the defect, but small fistulas may not be detectable (Fig. 4.4). Nevertheless, the presence of CSF in sinonasal drainage is sufficient to support the diagnosis. Historically, the "halo sign," "target sign," or "double ring sign" has been noted on absorbent surfaces (dressing, bedsheets, pillow covers) in patients with active serosanguinous rhinorrhea or otorrhea. Since the drainage contains plasma, a central blood stain is

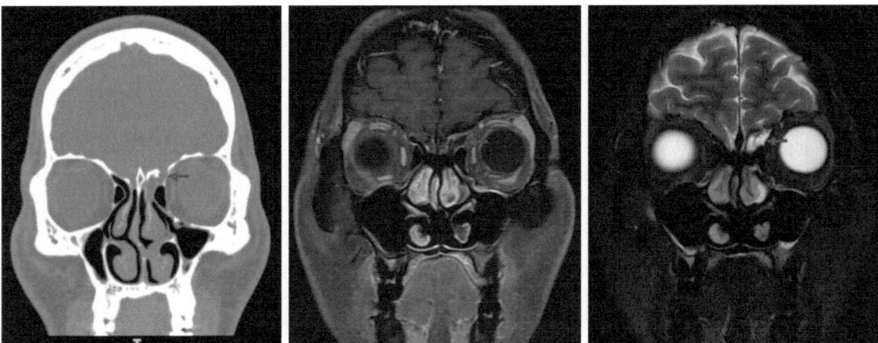

Fig. 4.4 Healthy young male presented to a rhinology practice for persistent perennial allergy symptoms and clear rhinorrhea. Initial consultation reveals a significant history of hospitalization 7 years ago in which he presented to a local emergency department with fever, headache, and altered mental status. He has poor recollection of the events but recall that he was diagnosed with meningitis and was admitted to the intensive care unit. No definitive etiology was determined. On nasal endoscopy, a smooth pulsating lesion was identified in the anterior ethmoid cavity. The red arrow denotes the bony dehiscence in the anterior skull base as identified on the CT scan and the meningoencephalocele on MRI

often observed and is surrounded by a clear or lightly stained ring around it. This finding often represents a basilar skull fracture, but it is not specific for CSF, and further testing is required for confirmation. If an aspirate of the nasal secretions can be collected, further analysis can be performed. As normal CSF glucose concentration is lower compared to serum glucose (50–80 mg/100 mL or 2/3 of serum glucose), the CSF/plasma glucose ratio has been used to confirm the presence of a leak, but it is subject to patient's glycemic status. Other chemical tests also have limited clinical utility due to low specificity and unreliability.

The single most commonly used assay today is the Beta-2-transferrin assay to detect the presence of CSF in sinonasal fluid. Also known as the tau protein, β-2 transferrin is a molecule found only in CSF, perilymph, and aqueous humor but not in nasal secretions [40]. It has a high sensitivity approaching 99% and specificity of 97%; thus it is currently the gold standard in detecting CSF rhinorrhea [41]. In patients able to cooperate with examination, nasal secretions can be collected in a plain sterile tube by leaning forward or flexing the patient's head. Location of the drainage can suggest the laterality of the defect, but paradoxical rhinorrhea can occur due to anatomical obstruction. Occasionally, samples could not be collected at the time of exam but in a delayed fashion. It should be noted that β-2 transferrin could remain detectable for 14 days stored in room temperature [42]. The performance of the assay, which is qualitative, requires several hours to days to process contingent on the assay system.

Beta-trace protein is another noninvasive marker that has been used for diagnosis of CSF rhinorrhea. Also known as prostaglandin D synthase, it is synthesized mainly in the epithelial cells of the choroid plexus and is found in CSF concentrations of 35-fold higher than in plasma [43, 44]. Thus, it is of great interest for the protein to be used as a marker for diagnosis of CSF leak. The main advantage of the beta-trace protein assay is that it is quantitative, which can be automated with a reported sensitivity of 91% in diagnosing CSF leak [45]. It is certainly less time-consuming and labor-intensive than the β-2 transferrin assay, with results available in as few as 15 min [46]. However, the beta-trace protein assay is not always suitable, as CSF beta-trace levels are significantly decreased in the setting of bacterial meningitis [47]. Serum beta-trace protein is also altered by the presence of renal disease, although not known to significantly affect the results.

Fluorescein

One of the most significant advancements in localizing CSF leaks has been the use of intrathecal fluorescein (Fig. 4.5). While β-trace protein and β-2 transferrin have a high sensitivity and specificity for diagnosis of CSF leakage, the test does not provide information regarding the site or laterality of the defect. For patients with an unclear site of defect, a thorough endoscopic exam following the administration of intrathecal fluorescein can aid in identifying potential multiple small defects and ensuring successful closure at the end of the case. In small or low flow leaks, a blight light filter may be necessary for detection. It should be noted that fluorescein is widely used for CSF leak repair, it is not approved by the US Food and Drug Administration for intrathecal injection, as complications range from mild to severe (malaise, headaches, dizziness, seizures, and cranial nerve deficit) [48, 49]. It is generally accepted to mix 0.1 mL of 10% fluorescein with 10 mL of the patient's

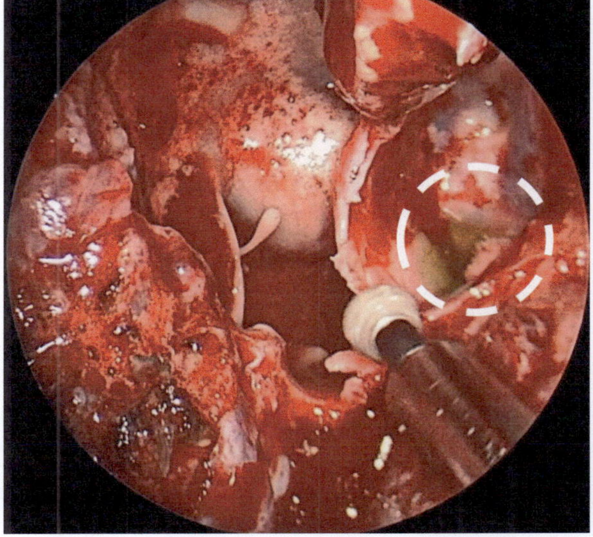

Fig. 4.5 Pterygopalatine fossa dissection for left lateral sphenoid recess encephalocele repair. White dotted circle indicates identification of intrathecal fluorescein

CSF and slowly injected over 10 min. Premedication with steroids and antihistamines should also be considered [48].

Complications: Meningitis and Pneumocephalus

The two most common complications of CSF rhinorrhea and ACF defects are meningitis and pneumocephalus. The incidence of meningitis and pneumocephalus is more widely reported following ACF, with known factors associated with increased risk of infection (GCS score <8, bony displacement over 1 cm, and prolonged CSF leak) [4, 50, 51]. While historically meningitis has been reported in as many as 50% of cases with CSF leak and mortality of up to 70% in the 1970s, the incidence of contemporary rates of meningitis and associated mortality has dropped below 10%, likely due to broad-spectrum antibiotics [52–54]. *Streptococcus pneumoniae* is the most common bacteria isolated, followed by *Haemophilus influenzae* [54]. CSF culture-directed antibiotics are often adequate to manage the acute meningitis followed by definitive closure of the defect. Pneumocephalus is almost only present in CSF rhinorrhea in the setting of a skull base fracture. This may present as a thin sliver of gas on the initial CT scan or with extensive subdural and intracranial air. While most injuries are managed conservatively, tension pneumocephalus can be observed with a characteristic "Mount Fuji sign" with the tips of the frontal lobes with a heaped-up appearance. The appearance of this sign often warrants immediate relief of the increased intracranial pressure.

References

1. Meco C, Oberascher G. Comprehensive algorithm for skull base dural lesion and cerebrospinal fluid fistula diagnosis. Laryngoscope. 2004;114:991–9.
2. Malham GM, Ackland HM, Jones R, et al. Occipital condyle fractures: incidence and clinical follow-up at a level 1 trauma Centre. Emerg Radiol. 2009;16:291–7.
3. Yalciner G, Kutluhan A, Bozdemir K, et al. Temporal bone fractures: evaluation of 77 patients and a management algorithm. Ulus Travma Acil Cerrahi Derg. 2012;18:424–8.
4. Brodie HA, Thompson TC. Management of complications from 820 temporal bone fractures. Am J Otol. 1997;18:188–97.
5. McCutcheon BA, Orosco RK, Chang DC, et al. Outcomes of isolated basilar skull fracture: readmission, meningitis, and cerebrospinal fluid leak. Otolaryngol Head Neck Surg. 2013;149:931–9.
6. Keros P. On the practical value of differences in the level of the lamina cribrosa of the ethmoid. Z Laryngol Rhinol Otol. 1962;41:809–13.
7. Stankiewicz JA, Lal D, Connor M, et al. Complications in endoscopic sinus surgery for chronic rhinosinusitis: a 25-year experience. Laryngoscope. 2011;121:2684–701.
8. Siedek V, Pilzweger E, Betz C, et al. Complications in endonasal sinus surgery: a 5-year retrospective study of 2,596 patients. Eur Arch Otorhinolaryngol. 2013;270:141–8.
9. Daele JJ, Goffart Y, Machiels S. Traumatic, iatrogenic, and spontaneous cerebrospinal fluid (CSF) leak: endoscopic repair. B-ENT. 2011;7(Suppl 17):47–60.

10. Loew F, Pertuiset B, Chaumier EE, et al. Traumatic, spontaneous and postoperative CSF rhinorrhea. Adv Tech Stand Neurosurg. 1984;11:169–207.
11. Schlosser RJ, Bolger WE. Nasal cerebrospinal fluid leaks: critical review and surgical considerations. Laryngoscope. 2004;114:255–65.
12. Banks CA, Palmer JN, Chiu AG, et al. Endoscopic closure of CSF rhinorrhea: 193 cases over 21 years. Otolaryngol Head Neck Surg. 2009;140:826–33.
13. Milhorat TH. The third circulation revisited. J Neurosurg. 1975;42:628–45.
14. McComb JG. Recent research into the nature of cerebrospinal fluid formation and absorption. J Neurosurg. 1983;59:369–83.
15. Davson H. Formation and drainage of the cerebrospinal fluid. Sci Basis Med Annu Rev. 1966:238–59.
16. Lee SC, Lueck CJ. Cerebrospinal fluid pressure in adults. J Neuroophthalmol. 2014;34:278–83.
17. Brainard L, Chen DA, Aziz KM, et al. Association of benign intracranial hypertension and spontaneous encephalocele with cerebrospinal fluid leak. Otol Neurotol. 2012;33:1621–4.
18. Schlosser RJ, Wilensky EM, Grady MS, et al. Elevated intracranial pressures in spontaneous cerebrospinal fluid leaks. Am J Rhinol. 2003;17:191–5.
19. Schlosser RJ, Wilensky EM, Grady MS, et al. Cerebrospinal fluid pressure monitoring after repair of cerebrospinal fluid leaks. Otolaryngol Head Neck Surg. 2004;130:443–8.
20. Alonso RC, de la Pena MJ, Caicoya AG, et al. Spontaneous skull base meningoencephaloceles and cerebrospinal fluid fistulas. Radiographics. 2013;33:553–70.
21. Butros SR, Goncalves LF, Thompson D, et al. Imaging features of idiopathic intracranial hypertension, including a new finding: widening of the foramen ovale. Acta Radiol. 2012;53:682–8.
22. Son HJ, Karkas A, Buchanan P, et al. Spontaneous cerebrospinal fluid effusion of the temporal bone: repair, audiological outcomes, and obesity. Laryngoscope. 2014;124:1204–8.
23. Quatre R, Attye A, Righini CA, et al. Spontaneous cerebrospinal fluid rhinorrhea: association with body weight and imaging data. J Neurol Surg B Skull Base. 2017;78:419–24.
24. Shetty PG, Shroff MM, Fatterpekar GM, et al. A retrospective analysis of spontaneous sphenoid sinus fistula: MR and CT findings. AJNR Am J Neuroradiol. 2000;21:337–42.
25. Giannetti AV, Guimaraes RE, Santiago AP, et al. A tomographic study of the skull base in primary spontaneous cerebrospinal fluid leaks. Neuroradiology. 2012;54:459–66.
26. Shiloah J, Covington JS, Schuman NJ. Reconstructive mucogingival surgery: the management of amalgam tattoo. Quintessence Int. 1988;19:489–92.
27. King JO, Mitchell PJ, Thomson KR, et al. Manometry combined with cervical puncture in idiopathic intracranial hypertension. Neurology. 2002;58:26–30.
28. Eisenberg HM, McComb JG, Lorenzo AV. Cerebrospinal fluid overproduction and hydrocephalus associated with choroid plexus papilloma. J Neurosurg. 1974;40:381–5.
29. Woodworth BA, Prince A, Chiu AG, et al. Spontaneous CSF leaks: a paradigm for definitive repair and management of intracranial hypertension. Otolaryngol Head Neck Surg. 2008;138:715–20.
30. Radhakrishnan K, Thacker AK, Bohlaga NH, et al. Epidemiology of idiopathic intracranial hypertension: a prospective and case-control study. J Neurol Sci. 1993;116:18–28.
31. Daniels AB, Liu GT, Volpe NJ, et al. Profiles of obesity, weight gain, and quality of life in idiopathic intracranial hypertension (pseudotumor cerebri). Am J Ophthalmol. 2007;143:635–41.
32. Seth R, Rajasekaran K 3rd, Luong A, et al. Spontaneous CSF leaks: factors predictive of additional interventions. Laryngoscope. 2010;120:2141–6.
33. Bloomfield GL, Ridings PC, Blocher CR, et al. A proposed relationship between increased intra-abdominal, intrathoracic, and intracranial pressure. Crit Care Med. 1997;25:496–503.
34. Sinclair AJ, Burdon MA, Nightingale PG, et al. Low energy diet and intracranial pressure in women with idiopathic intracranial hypertension: prospective cohort study. BMJ. 2010;341:c2701.
35. Kupersmith MJ, Gamell L, Turbin R, et al. Effects of weight loss on the course of idiopathic intracranial hypertension in women. Neurology. 1998;50:1094–8.

36. Dhungana S, Sharrack B, Woodroofe N. Cytokines and chemokines in idiopathic intracranial hypertension. Headache. 2009;49:282–5.
37. Ball AK, Sinclair AJ, Curnow SJ, et al. Elevated cerebrospinal fluid (CSF) leptin in idiopathic intracranial hypertension (IIH): evidence for hypothalamic leptin resistance? Clin Endocrinol. 2009;70:863–9.
38. Donaldson JO, Horak E. Cerebrospinal fluid oestrone in pseudotumour cerebri. J Neurol Neurosurg Psychiatry. 1982;45:734–6.
39. Markey KA, Uldall M, Botfield H, et al. Idiopathic intracranial hypertension, hormones, and 11beta-hydroxysteroid dehydrogenases. J Pain Res. 2016;9:223–32.
40. Skedros DG, Cass SP, Hirsch BE, et al. Beta-2 transferrin assay in clinical management of cerebral spinal fluid and perilymphatic fluid leaks. J Otolaryngol. 1993;22:341–4.
41. Warnecke A, Averbeck T, Wurster U, et al. Diagnostic relevance of beta2-transferrin for the detection of cerebrospinal fluid fistulas. Arch Otolaryngol Head Neck Surg. 2004;130:1178–84.
42. Zervos TM, Macki M, Cook B, et al. Beta-2 transferrin is detectable for 14 days whether refrigerated or stored at room temperature. Int Forum Allergy Rhinol. 2018;8:1052–5.
43. Meco C, Arrer E, Oberascher G. Efficacy of cerebrospinal fluid fistula repair: sensitive quality control using the beta-trace protein test. Am J Rhinol. 2007;21:729–36.
44. Melegos DN, Freedman MS, Diamandis EP. Prostaglandin D synthase concentration in cerebrospinal fluid and serum of patients with neurological disorders. Prostaglandins. 1997;54:463–74.
45. Bachmann G, Nekic M, Michel O. Clinical experience with beta-trace protein as a marker for cerebrospinal fluid. Ann Otol Rhinol Laryngol. 2000;109:1099–102.
46. Meco C, Oberascher G, Arrer E, et al. Beta-trace protein test: new guidelines for the reliable diagnosis of cerebrospinal fluid fistula. Otolaryngol Head Neck Surg. 2003;129:508–17.
47. Tumani H, Reiber H, Nau R, et al. Beta-trace protein concentration in cerebrospinal fluid is decreased in patients with bacterial meningitis. Neurosci Lett. 1998;242:5–8.
48. Placantonakis DG, Tabaee A, Anand VK, et al. Safety of low-dose intrathecal fluorescein in endoscopic cranial base surgery. Neurosurgery. 2007;61:161–5; discussion 165–6.
49. Moseley JI, Carton CA, Stern WE. Spectrum of complications in the use of intrathecal fluorescein. J Neurosurg. 1978;48:765–7.
50. Sakas DE, Beale DJ, Ameen AA, et al. Compound anterior cranial base fractures: classification using computerized tomography scanning as a basis for selection of patients for dural repair. J Neurosurg. 1998;88:471–7.
51. Yilmazlar S, Arslan E, Kocaeli H, et al. Cerebrospinal fluid leakage complicating skull base fractures: analysis of 81 cases. Neurosurg Rev. 2006;29:64–71.
52. Eljamel MS, Foy PM. Acute traumatic CSF fistulae: the risk of intracranial infection. Br J Neurosurg. 1990;4:381–5.
53. Eljamel MS, Foy PM. Post-traumatic CSF fistulae, the case for surgical repair. Br J Neurosurg. 1990;4:479–83.
54. MacGee EE, Cauthen JC, Brackett CE. Meningitis following acute traumatic cerebrospinal fluid fistula. J Neurosurg. 1970;33:312–6.

Chapter 5
Imaging for Detection of CSF Leaks

Marin Alisa McDonald

Introduction

A skull base cerebrospinal fluid (CSF) leak describes the egress of CSF from the intracranial subarachnoid space into the extracranial space via an osteodural defect, most commonly at the sinonasal or tympanomastoid cavities [1]. Leakage of CSF into either the nose or the ear, coined CSF rhinorrhea or otorrhea, was identified as pathologic entities over a century ago with a wide range of potential etiologies, including post-traumatic, surgical, neoplastic, and spontaneous causes. Subsequent decades have shown increasing recognition for the clinical importance of CSF leaks as sources of significant potential morbidity and mortality, with persistent CSF rhinorrhea carrying a 10 to 37% lifetime risk for meningitis [2–6], as well as increasing risk for seizures, cranial neuropathies, and headache [7].

Given the potential long-term consequences of missed diagnosis, the timely and accurate identification of a suspected CSF leak is of tremendous clinical import. β2-Transferrin protein testing remains the mainstay for confirmation of any suspected case of CSF rhinorrhea or otorrhea with reported sensitivity ranging from 87 to 100% and specificity of 71 to 94% [7–10]. Once confirmed, imaging plays a critical role in determining the site of a suspected or confirmed CSF leak, often using a combination of high-resolution computed tomography (HRCT) and magnetic resonance (MR) imaging, with or without the use of intrathecal contrast agents. Beyond the identification potential routes of CSF leak, radiological evaluation can also aid

M. A. McDonald (✉)
Division of Neuroradiology, Department of Radiology, University of California at San Diego, San Diego, CA, USA
e-mail: mamcdonald@health.ucsd.edu

E. C. Kuan et al. (eds.), *Skull Base Reconstruction*,
https://doi.org/10.1007/978-3-031-27937-9_5

in the diagnosis of any underlying causative etiology, such as spontaneous CSF leaks referable to idiopathic intracranial hypertension (IIH) or in the setting of skull base invasion from neoplastic or infectious etiologies [1, 7, 8, 11].

In the course of this chapter, we will review the imaging techniques used to diagnose and characterize the sites of CSF leak with an emphasis on noninvasive CT and MR imaging. We will highlight common imaging findings of confirmed CSF leaks and their causative factors, including traumatic, iatrogenic, and spontaneous leaks. We will then discuss potential mimics of CSF leak and common imaging pitfalls in this essential diagnosis.

Diagnostic Techniques

At our institution, initial imaging modalities in the evaluation of suspected or confirmed leaks are usually noninvasive, including high-resolution computed tomography (HRCT) and magnetic resonance cisternography (MRC). In complex or equivocal cases, more invasive techniques including computed tomography cisternography (CTC), contrast-enhanced magnetic resonance cisternography (CE-MRC), and radionuclide cisternography (RNC) are employed as problem-solving techniques (Table 5.1). Ultimately, the choice of imaging modality and diagnostic accuracy remains dependent on local experience, imaging expertise, and the technical capabilities at any individual institution.

Table 5.1 Proposed imaging algorithm for patients with confirmed CSF leak

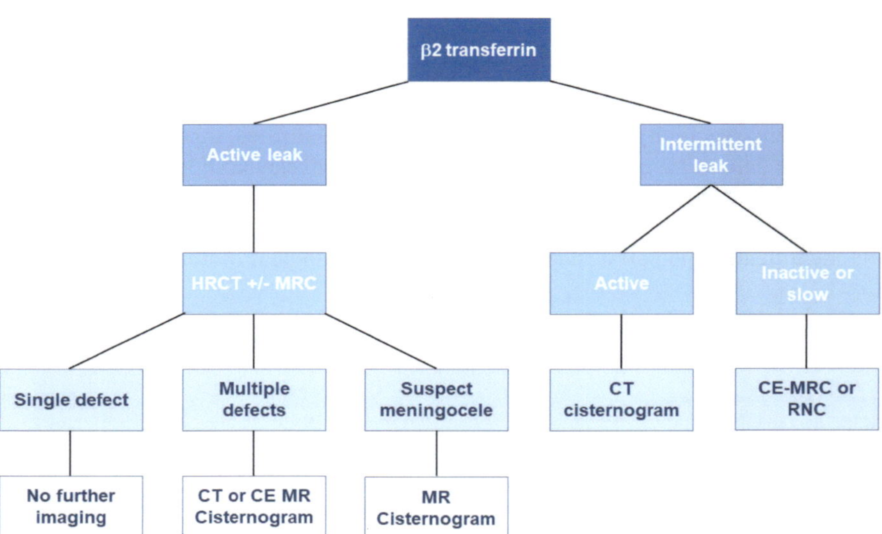

Computed Tomography

High-resolution CT (HRCT) of the paranasal sinuses and skull base is often the first-line imaging modality of choice in the setting of suspected CSF leak due to its relative clinical accessibility and short acquisition time. HRCT performed using submillimeter acquisition affords exquisite spatial resolution and superior delineation of osseous detail, making it ideal to identify potential regions of dehiscence of the anterior and posterolateral skull base [12–14]. In a recently meta-analysis, 12 published studies reported HRCT sensitivity over 80% in the identification of the site of a β2-transferrin-confirmed CSF leak [7]. Moreover, a recent investigation indicated that the size of the defect can be accurately predicted on HRCT to within 2 mm in 75% of cases [12] assuming minimum collimation and the ability to general multiplanar reformats. Adding to the potential utility of this technique, the identification of osseous dehiscence by HRCT is not dependent on the presence of an active leak at the time of imaging, making it ideal for the investigation of subtle abnormalities or slow-flowing leaks [11, 15]. Furthermore, dedicated HRCT of the paranasal sinuses and skull base affords the surgeon a detailed view of the remainder of the sinonasal cavity for surgical planning and intraoperative navigation during endoscopic repair [12, 14, 16].

HRCT performed for the identification of CSF leak should include minimum detector collimation, thin-section (0.5 mm or 0.625 mm) acquisition utilizing bone algorithms [1, 11, 17]. In general, axial images are considered superior for the evaluation of the vertically oriented structures of the skull base, including the posterior frontal and lateral sphenoid sinuses and in the evaluation of the mastoid air cells (Fig. 5.1). In distinction, coronal images offer advantage in the assessment of the

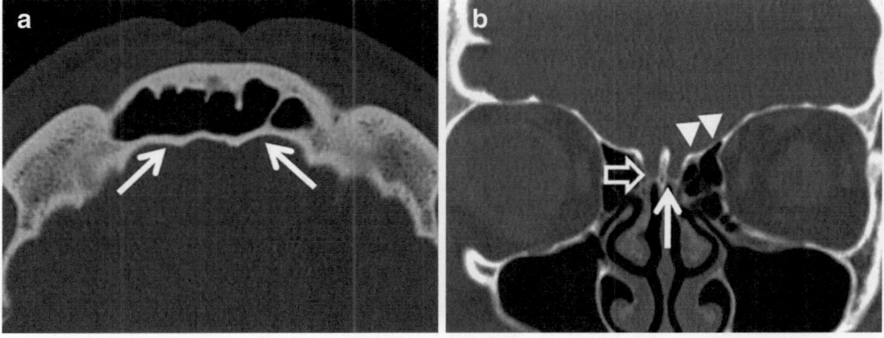

Fig. 5.1 High-resolution computed tomography (HRCT). Axial 0.625 mm direct acquisition (**a**) and reformatted coronal 1 mm (**b**) images of the anterior skull base obtained per HRCT protocol using bone algorithm reconstructions. In (**a**), axial views afford detailed evaluation of the vertically oriented components of the skull base, such as the posterior walls of the frontal sinus (arrows). Coronal reformats are ideally suited to assess the floor of the anterior cranial fossa, including common sites of CSF leak such as the olfactory fossa/cribriform plate (arrow), the lateral lamella (open arrow, shown near the attachment of the middle turbinate), and the fovea ethmoidalis (arrowheads)

longitudinally oriented cribriform plates, planum ethmoidale, planum sphenoidale, and temporal tegmen (Fig. 5.1). As such, historical acquisition parameters have included both axial and direct coronal planes for improved in-plane resolution, requiring prone positioning of the patient, significant neck extension within the gantry, and increased radiation dosage. Modern multi-detector CT now involves rapid, continuous volumetric acquisition with isotropic voxels, allowing for the creation of high-quality, high-resolution coronal and sagittal reformats from a single axial acquisition [1, 11]. Unless the location of a CSF leak is known, a thorough work up of CSF rhinorrhea requires HRCT imaging of the anterior, central, and posterolateral skull base as CSF leaking into the middle ear cavity can present as rhinorrhea via egress through the Eustachian tubes [18]. Therefore, the authors recommend a field-of-view inclusive of the sinonasal cavity, anterior and central skull base, and temporal bones for complete evaluation of suspected or confirmed CSF rhinorrhea.

Relative disadvantages of HRCT include the inability to assess for a concomitant dural defect in the setting of multiple regions of osseous thinning at the skull base. HRCT is also limited in the ability to discriminate between adjacent mucosal thickening and secretions from a suspected CSF collection in the paranasal sinuses [11, 16]. These limitations may contribute to the wide ranges of specificity of HRCT in the detection of a CSF leak reported in the literature, ranging from 57 to 100% [7, 19]. However, if only single osseous defect is identified on HRCT corresponding to the clinical symptoms, the patient can proceed to surgical repair without further imaging [12, 14].

Magnetic Resonance Cisternography

Magnetic resonance cisternography (MRC) is often performed as an adjunct or even a stand-alone imaging study in the setting of confirmed CSF leak due to superior soft tissue resolution and ability to increase the conspicuity of CSF based on the imaging technique utilized. Most MRC protocols exploit heavily T2-weighted (T2W) 3D-fast (turbo) spin echo (e.g., T2 SPACE, T2 CUBE) or steady-state-free precession (SSFP) sequences to highlight the intrinsic T2 prolongation of CSF relative to the adjacent neural and osseous elements, as well as facilitating the creation of multiplanar reformats from submillimeter acquisition [11, 20] (Fig. 5.2). In this manner, MRC can not only confirm but also identify the site of a CSF leak by visualizing a contiguous CSF column extending through a defect in the floor of the anterior cranial fossa, tegmen tympani, or tegmen mastoideum. Collectively, studies report a sensitivity of 56–94% for CSF leak detection, with a specificity of 57–100% [7].

A further advantage of MRC relative to HRCT is the ability to identify herniation of the meninges or neural elements (e.g., meningocele or meningoencephalocele) in association with an ongoing CSF leak [1, 11, 14]. Underlying meningoencephalocele should be considered in the setting of a skull base defect with downstream opacification of an adjacent sinus or mastoid air cell, particularly if the opacification

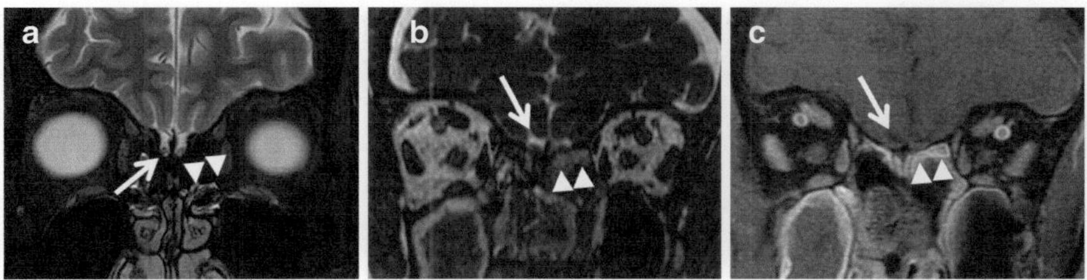

Fig. 5.2 Magnetic resonance cisternogram (MRC). Although various protocols exist, the mainstay of MRC is the use of a combination of multiplanar small field of view, thin section fast-spin-echo, and steady-state-free-precession (SSFP) imaging. In (**a**) coronal T2 fat-saturated images clearly depict the olfactory nerves in the olfactory groove (arrows), with easy differentiation from adjacent mucosal thickening of the ethmoid air cells (arrowheads). MRC performed to evaluate for recurrent leak after endoscopic nasal surgery (**b** and **c**) utilized both SSFP/FIESTA imaging (**b**) and thin section T1 fat-saturated post-contrast sequences (**c**) to clearly delineate the difference between native CSF signal (**b** and **c**, arrows) and adjacent mucosal thickening of the planum ethmoidale (**b** and **c**, arrowheads). No CSF leak was identified on the examination, and the patient continues to do well 2 years after surgery

is lobulated or anti-dependent. Although differentiation between fluid opacification and neural elements is often difficult by CT, the superior soft tissue resolution of MR easily distinguishes brain parenchyma from CSF, helping to aid surgical planning prior to repair (Fig. 5.2). The use of additional fast-spin echo and fast spoiled gradient-echo sequences, particularly with intravenous contrast and fat suppression, can further help identify potential complications related to CSF, such as retrograde meningitis and encephalitis.

One limitation of MRC is its dependence upon the presence of an active leak at the time of imaging to successfully identify the region of communication between the intracranial and extracranial compartments. Coupled with an inherently lower spatial resolution of the osseous skull base, many authors advocate use of both HRCT and MRC, with a combined reported accuracy of 92–100% in the current literature [21–23].

Contrast-Enhanced Cisternography

In contrast to the previously described imaging methodologies, contrast-enhanced CT and MR cisternography are invasive techniques, requiring the administration of intrathecal contrast, usually via lumbar puncture in the fluoroscopy suite. With improvements in both HRCT and MRC, intrathecal contrast-based imaging is utilized as a problem-solving tool at our institution, reserved for complex or equivocal cases after other imaging modalities have been employed.

CT cisternography (CTC) was previously the gold standard in the evaluation of potential CSF leaks, but now is predominantly used as a problem-solving technique, particularly to help pinpoint the site of an active leak in the setting of multiple

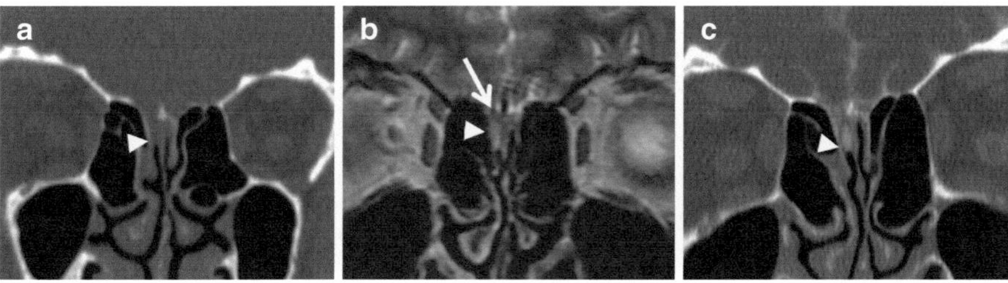

Fig. 5.3 Computed tomography cisternogram (CTC). 62-year-old patient presented with chronic but intermittent watery rhinorrhea, with β2 transferrin confirmed CSF leak at an outside institution. HRCT identified asymmetric opacification of the right superior meatus (**a**, arrowhead), although it was unclear if this was due to a low-lying right olfactory fossa or underlying osseous dehiscence. MRC revealed asymmetric opacification of the right superior meatus with otherwise appropriate localization of the right olfactory nerve (**b**, arrowhead). Of note, no clear CSF column could be identified on this study. In this setting, CTC was pursued as a problem-solving technique, demonstrating contrast accumulation through the right cribriform plate into the right nasal cavity (**c**, arrowhead) confirming CSF leak in this location

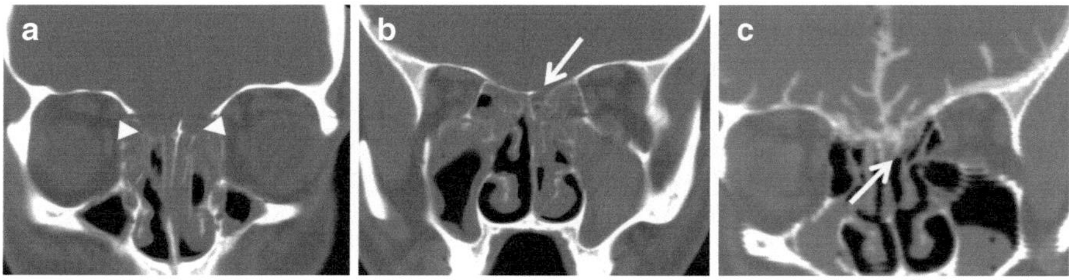

Fig. 5.4 CTC in the setting of complex skull base findings. In this patient with a history of prior facial trauma and β2 transferring positive rhinorrhea, multiple regions of thinning of the anterior skull base structures were noted, including involving the bilateral lateral lamella (**a**, arrowheads) and the left fovea ethmoidalis (**b**, arrow). Subsequent CTC performed with provocative maneuvering revealed contrast extravasation through the left fovea defect (**c**, arrow) as the site of the patient's ongoing CSF leak

osseous defects [14, 24] (Figs. 5.3 and 5.4). CTC protocol involves obtaining HRCT in both the prone and supine positions through the region of interest before and after low osmolality intrathecal contrast material is introduced. One advantage to CTC is the ability to perform provocative maneuvers at the time of imaging, such as sneezing or head hanging, to attempt to improve delineation of a leak. Evaluation of the obtained imaging requires comparison of the pre- and post-contrast scans, with a positive result considered if there is an increase in the attenuation of an opacified structure (sinus, nasal cavity, middle ear, etc.) adjacent to a skull base defect 50% or more above the baseline on the noncontrast examination [14]. The utility of a CTC is limited to patients in whom an active leak is present or elicited by provocative maneuvers. Additional pitfalls of this technique can include obscuration of small leaks by adjacent sclerotic changes of the paranasal sinuses or high-density, inspissated secretions, as well as the presence of blood. In combination, these factors may account for some degree of the disparity of reported sensitivities, ranging from 33% to 100% [7, 19, 22].

Intrathecal, contrast-enhanced techniques can also be combined with the MRC technique, utilizing thin-section, T1-weighted sequences obtained in multiple planes after the administration of gadolinium-based contrast. Similar to CTC, a positive study demonstrates contrast extravasation through an osseous and dural defect of the skull base and must be interpreted in conjunction with HRCT. Studies have shown enhanced sensitivity for detection of CSF leaks compared to both HRCT and standard MRC, with up to 100% sensitivity for high-flow leaks and 60% to 70% sensitivity for slow-flow leaks [20, 25, 26]. Some of this improved sensitivity may stem from the ability to perform delayed imaging up to 24 h after gadolinium administration, which can be particularly useful in slow-flowing or intermittent leaks [26]. As with all MR-based protocols, superior soft tissue resolution and increased conspicuity of CSF afford the ability to detect concomitant meningoceles as well as improved discrimination of leaking contrast from adjacent sclerotic or hypertrophied bony structures compared to CTC. Although several studies indicate good safety data using low-dose intrathecal gadolinium in other countries, intrathecal administration remains an off-label use of gadolinium by the US Food and Drug Administration (FDA), and long-term safety studies are still pending. As such, given the invasive nature of the study, the known neurotoxicity of gadolinium in high doses, and current off-label use, selective employment of this technique as a problem-solving tool only is recommended and only after thorough off-label use consent.

Nuclear Medicine Cisternography

Radionuclide cisternography (RNC) is a nuclear medicine diagnostic examination involving the intrathecal administration of technetium-99 or indium-111 radiotracer. Multiple pledglets are introduced to the nasal cavity followed by placing the patient in the Trendelenburg position to facilitate craniad tracer flow [1, 16]. Pledglet radioactivity is measured after 24 to 48 h to confirm the presence of a CSF leak, with a positive study heralded by a pledglet to serum plasma tracer ratio of 2:1 or 3:1 [1]. RNC is limited to the detection of active leaks and only offers minimal, if any, information about leak location given the inherent mixing of nasal secretions from side to side and the possibility of CSF rhinorrhea stemming from an underlying temporal bone process [1, 11, 14]. For these reasons, and due to its invasive nature, RNC is only selectively employed at our institution as a problem-solving measure for CSF leak confirmation.

Imaging Findings of CSF Leak

Imaging hallmarks of CSF leak on HRCT include an osseous defect in the skull base associated with an air-fluid level or opacification of the contiguous sinus, mastoid air cells, or middle ear cavity. The most common location for a skull base CSF leak is at the cribriform plate although several additional locations are also commonly implicated, including the anterior ethmoid, posterior ethmoid, sphenoid, and frontal sinuses [1] (Fig. 5.5). CSF leaks from the temporal bone tegmen are relatively less common but should be included in imaging protocol as CSF leakage into

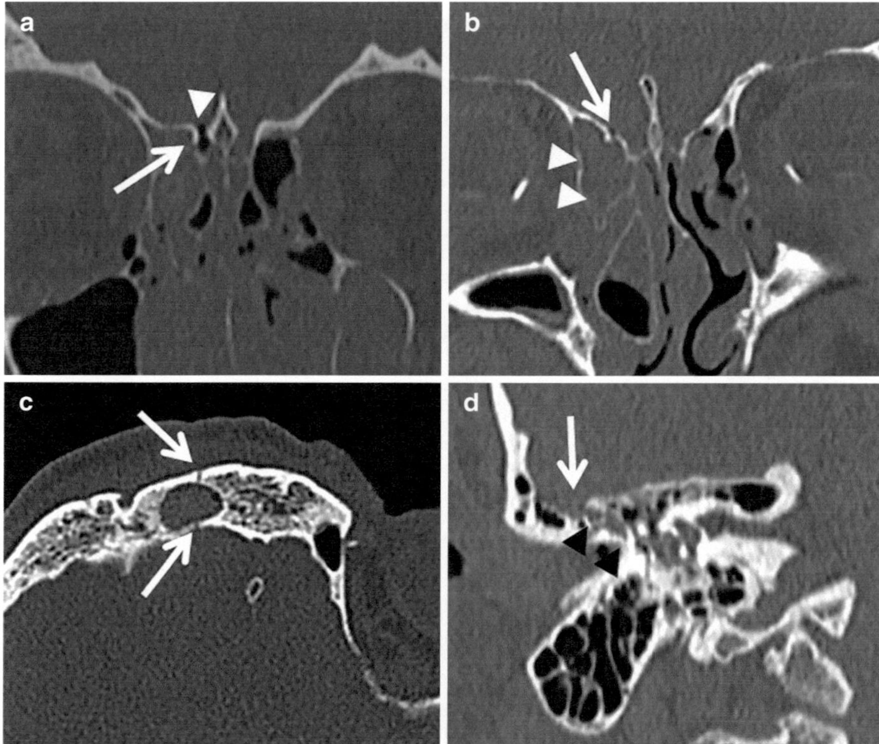

Fig. 5.5 Common sites of traumatic CSF leaks on HRCT. In (**a**), 1 mm bone algorithm coronal reformats clearly elucidate a focal region of pneumocephalus (arrowhead) adjacent to an otherwise subtle fracture of the right lateral lamella near the insertion of the middle turbinate. Focal pneumocephalus also heralds a subtle, minimally displaced fracture of the right fovea ethmoidalis (**b**, arrow) with associated CSF leak suspected based on downstream opacification of the adjacent superior ethmoid air cell (**b**, arrowheads). Bone algorithm axial 0.625 mm acquisition easily identifies a nondisplaced fracture extending through the anterior and posterior walls of the right frontal sinus (**c**, arrows) in the setting of facial trauma. In (**d**) coronal 1 mm bone algorithm reformats successfully resolve a mildly displaced fracture of the right tegmen mastoideum (arrow) with downstream opacification of the right-sided mastoid air cells, raising concern for post-traumatic CSF leak (arrowheads)

the middle ear can also manifest as rhinorrhea via egress through the Eustachian tubes [11, 14, 18] (Fig. 5.5). Anterior skull base defects are usually adjacent to the vertical insertion of the middle turbinate or at the lateral lamella, although normal thinning of these structures can make specific leak site detection difficult [1]. Identification is aided by comparing to the contralateral side, scrutinizing for subtle associated pneumocephalus adjacent to a fracture line, as well as identifying asymmetric mucosal thickening or soft tissue opacification beneath a suspected osseous defect as the first sign of an underlying meningoencephalocele (Figs. 5.6 and 5.7).

As adjunct imaging, or in the case of suspected meningoencephalocele, MRC may further help localize the leak by identifying a contiguous CSF column extending through a deficiency in the skull base and adjacent dura (Fig. 5.6), although this is contingent upon an active leak being present at the time of imaging. Further multiplanar T1- and T2-weighted imaging of the skull base is essential to detect the presence of an underlying meningocele/meningoencephalocele. Other indirect signs of CSF leak can also be revealed by MR, including variable degrees of encephalomalacia associated with an ongoing leak [11] (Fig. 5.6), associated dural enhancement (in the case of concurrent intravenous contrast administration), as well as the identification of potential intracranial complications, including meningitis/cerebritis (Fig. 5.8). Contrast-enhanced CT and MR cisternography evaluations are both based on identification of extravasated contrast via an osteodural defect in the skull base, often quantified in comparison to pre-contrast images, as previously described.

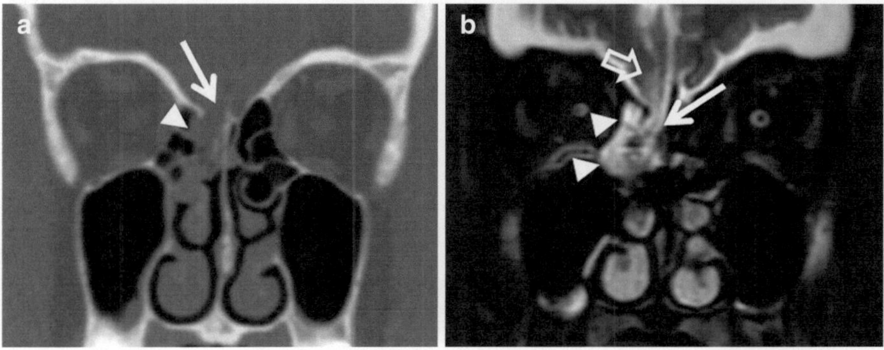

Fig. 5.6 Traumatic meningoencephalocele. 35-year-old male presents with new-onset seizures and watery nasal discharge for 1 year after assault. HRCT reveals focal dehiscence of the right cribriform plate (**a**, arrow) with polypoid opacification of the downstream ethmoid air cell (**a**, arrowhead). Concern for CSF leak and associated meningocele was raised and confirmed on MRC, with T2 fat-saturated sequences revealing herniation of the right gyrus rectus through the osteodural defect (**b**, arrow) and contiguous CSF column extending into the superior ethmoid air cells (**b**, arrowheads). Note associated gliosis of the right gyrus rectus, potentially contributing to the patient's ongoing seizure activity (**b**, open arrows)

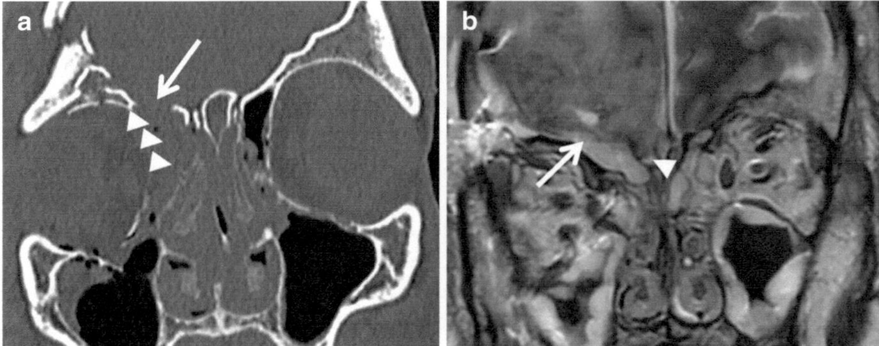

Fig. 5.7 Traumatic meningoencephalocele. In (**a**) 1 mm bone algorithm coronal reformats reveal comminuted fracture deformity of the superior, medial, and inferior right orbit extending through the floor of the frontal sinus and fovea ethmoidalis (**a**, arrow). Asymmetric opacification of the right superior meatus and anterior ethmoid air cells (**a**, arrowheads) raised concern for ongoing CSF leak and meningoencephalocele given proximity to the right frontal lobe. Subsequent MRC confirmed herniation of the adjacent anteroinferior frontal convexities into the frontal sinus defect (coronal T2 imaging in **b**, arrow) and into the olfactory fossa (**b**, arrowheads). Subsequent endoscopic and open repair of the skull base was performed with frankly gliotic brain noted herniating through the osteodural defect, which was successfully resected

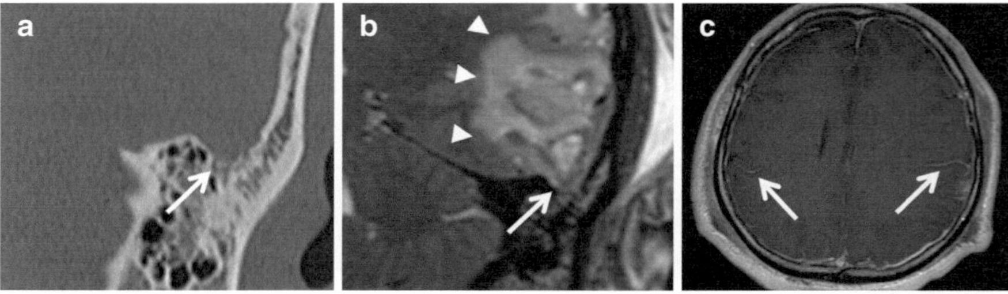

Fig. 5.8 Traumatic CSF leak with associated meningitis. 55-year-old male presenting as transfer from outside institution 1 month after left-sided head strike with persistent left-sided ear pain and constitutional symptoms. HRCT at our institution revealed a previously overlooked, subtle region of dehiscence of the left tegmen mastoideum (coronal reformats in **a**, arrow), prompting evaluation by MRC. In (**b**) T2 CUBE sequences were employed demonstrating a subtle meningoencephalocele through the queried defect (**b**, arrows). MRC also revealed asymmetric edema within the left inferolateral temporal lobe (**b**, arrowheads) with associated enhancement of the leptomeninges (axial T1 post-contrast in **c**, arrows) raising concern for superimposed meningitis due to ascending infection from the left middle ear cavity, later confirmed by lumbar puncture

With these general principles in mind, it is important to note that the imaging appearance of a CSF leak is dependent upon the underlying etiology, whether traumatic, iatrogenic, spontaneous, or secondary to underlying neoplastic, congenital, or infectious causes.

Traumatic CSF Leaks

The majority of skull base CSF leaks are associated with traumatic injuries, with 10% to 30% of skull base fractures complicated by concomitant CSF leak [14, 16, 27]. Tightly adherent dura along the inherently thin cribriform plates and planum ethmoidale/sphenoidale may explain the propensity for comminuted anterior cranial fossa fractures to result in CSF leak, although CSF from fractures of the posterior frontal sinus, lateral walls of the sphenoid sinus, or even the sella turcica have also been reported (Fig. 5.5). CSF leak frequency ranges from 11 to 45% of patients with underlying temporal bone fractures, more often in the setting of otic capsule violation [28]. Although displaced or comminuted fractures are rarely a clinical or diagnostic dilemma, subtle or nondisplaced fractures can be overlooked by routine CT; in this setting, the presence of intracranial pneumocephalus can be the first clue for a subtle osseous traumatic injury and should prompt careful interrogation of the adjacent skull base and/or repeat evaluation with HRCT (Fig. 5.5).

Iatrogenic CSF Leaks

CSF leak is a known complication of both neurosurgical and otolaryngologic procedures, with a reported overall incidence of 14% via endoscopic and endonasal approaches to the anterior and central skull base [29] (Fig. 5.9). As such, the timely reporting of variant anatomy of the anterior cranial fossa and central skull base is of critical importance on presurgical HRCT, including the Keros classification of the olfactory fossa and any associated asymmetry of the cribriform plate [30]. Variant sphenoid sinus pneumatization should also be reported, as well as any extension anteriorly into the clinoid process, laterally into the sphenoid wing, inferiorly into

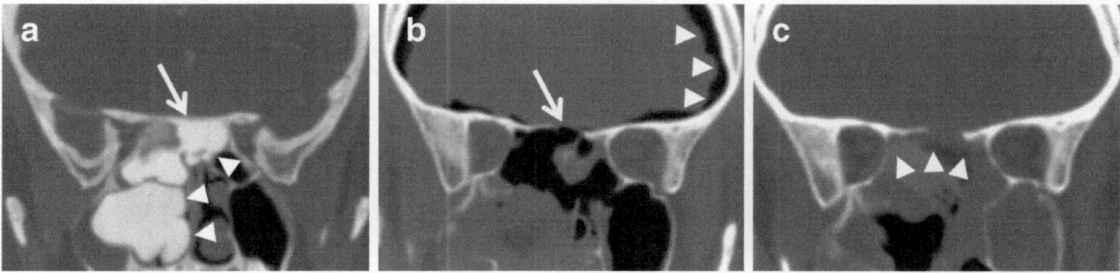

Fig. 5.9 Iatrogenic CSF leak. In (**a**) coronal reformatted images from CT angiography performed for surgical planning prior to resection of a transpatial sinonasal osteoma (**a**, arrowheads) demonstrating close approximation with and thinning of the planum sphenoidale (**a**, arrow). Although initially asymptomatic, the patient began to complain of watery rhinorrhea and worsening headaches on postoperative day 2. Subsequent HRCT demonstrated a focal osseous dehiscence of the left planum sphenoidale (**b**, arrow) with progressive pneumocephalus (**b**, arrowheads). Given concern for ongoing CSF leak, surgical exploration was performed revealing multiple dural tears and exposed brain in the region of osseous dehiscence, which was then repaired with an extensive nasoseptal flap (**c**, arrowheads)

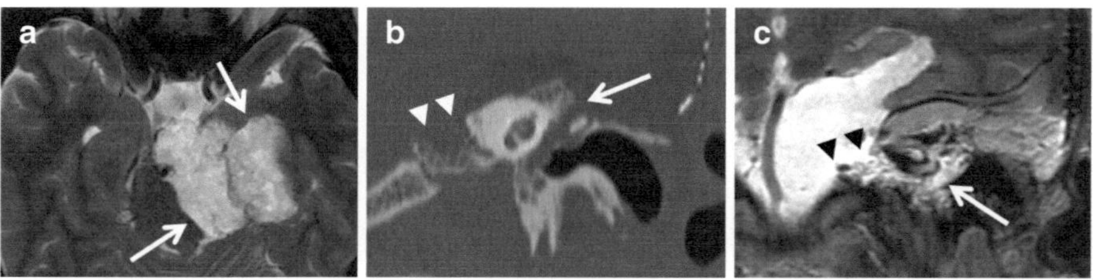

Fig. 5.10 Postsurgical CSF leak. 30-year-old female presented with copious clear rhinorrhea after left translabyrinthine approach epidermoid resection (show in **a**, axial T2 sequence, arrows). HRCT revealed several areas of potential osseous dehiscence involving the tegmen tympani (**b**, arrow), although fat-grafting material appeared to approximate the potential defect in this location. Instead, there was an additional 10 mm region of dehiscence of the left petrous ridge (**b** and **c**, arrowheads) with apparent contiguous CSF column extending from this defect through to the left middle ear cavity (T2-weighted coronal image in **c**, arrow), subsequently confirmed as the site of ongoing leak by surgical re-exploration

the pterygoid plate, or posteriorly into the clivus, as associated bony thinning can increase the risk of postoperative CSF leak [31]. Most iatrogenic leaks occur within the first 2 postoperative weeks and resolve spontaneously [14]; if repair is indicated, typically only preoperative HRCT is required as the location of the leak is assumed at the surgical site, although initial evaluation can be difficult in the immediate postoperative setting given adjacent post-surgical material and hemorrhage (Fig. 5.10).

Secondary CSF Leaks

In the absence of trauma or prior surgery, there are many additional potential causative etiologies of CSF leak at the skull base, including sinonasal or primary skull base malignancy (Fig. 5.11), prior radiation therapy/osteoradionecrosis, or congenital abnormalities, including encephaloceles, persistent craniopharyngeal canal, or primary empty sella syndrome.

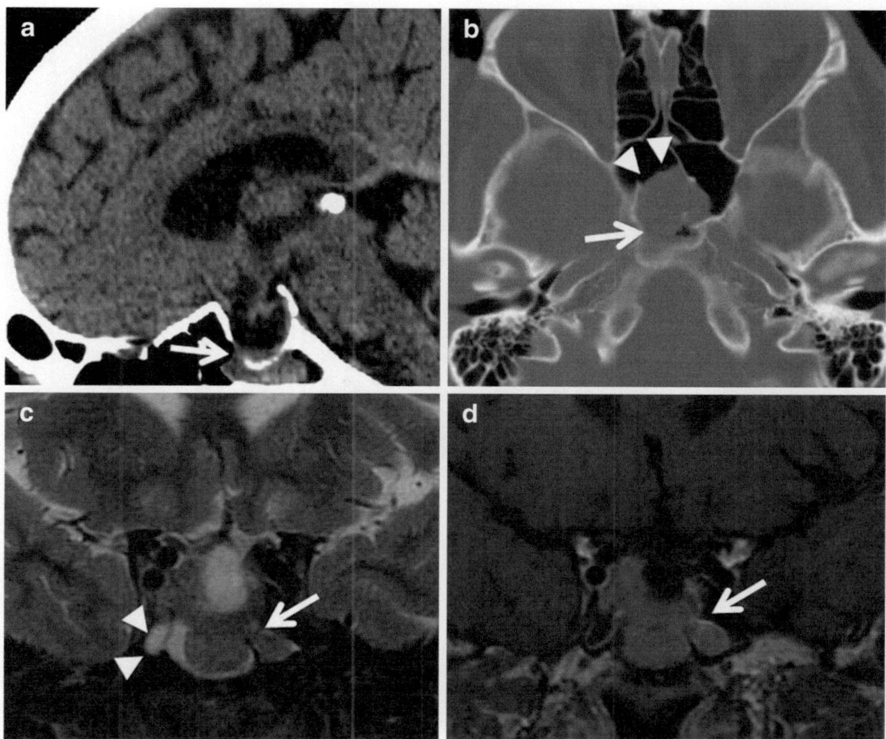

Fig. 5.11 CSF rhinorrhea related to neoplasia. 53-year-old female presenting with positional headaches and bilateral rhinorrhea. Screening head CT revealed a widened sella with a focal osseous defect of the anterior sella turcica and posterior wall of the sphenoid sinus (**a** and **b**, arrowheads). Internally, a polypoid, anti-dependent mass was noted without definite continuity with the brain parenchyma of the medial temporal lobes (**b**, arrowheads). Follow-up MRI demonstrated transpatial, T2 hypointense mass extending through the anteroinferior aspect of the sella turcica with low-level internal enhancement (coronal T2 fat-saturated in C and T1 post-contrast in **d**, arrows), compatible with underlying pituitary macroadenoma. Although no definite contiguous CSF column was identified through the osteodural defect of the central skull base, T2 hyperintense fluid in the adjacent sphenoid sinus (**c**, arrowheads) raised suspicion for subtle associated CSF leak as the cause of the patient's ongoing rhinorrhea

Spontaneous CSF Leaks

The last several decades have seen increased prevalence of idiopathic intracranial hypertension (IIH), a headache syndrome characterized by supranormal intracranial pressure without clear cause, classically seen in overweight women associated with visual disturbance, papilledema, and other potential neurologic stigmata [32]. Spontaneous CSF leaks are becoming a frequent presentation of IIH and one of the most common indications for imaging in the setting of CSF leak [33, 34]. In this cohort of patients, it is proposed that elevated intracranial pressures leads to increased magnitude of dural pulsations, weakening the

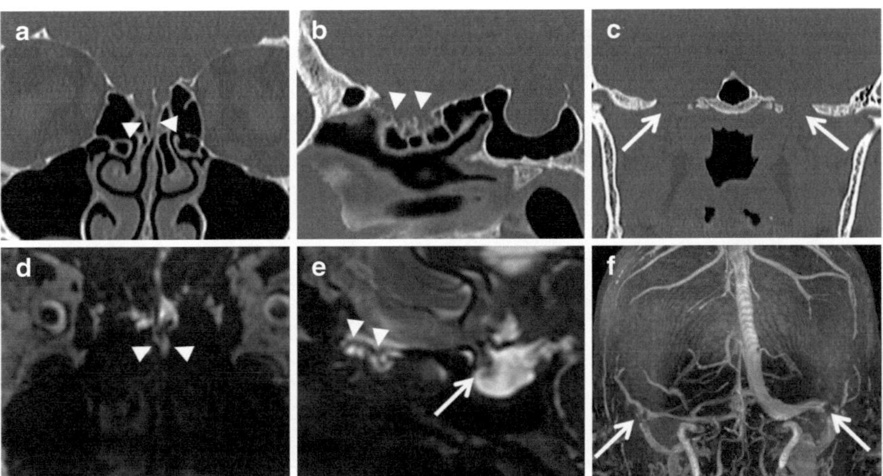

Fig. 5.12 Spontaneous CSF leak in the setting of idiopathic intracranial hypertension. 59-year-old female presenting with postural headaches and intermittent left-sided rhinorrhea. HRCT demonstrated thinning of both cribriform plates (**a**, arrowheads) with subtle downstream opacification of the left greater than right superior nasal cavity. Associated widening of the sella turcica (**b**, arrow) and foramen ovale (**c**, arrows) raised suspicion for elevated intracranial pressures. MRC (sagittal T2 CUBE sequences in **c** and **d**) confirmed active CSF leak on the left with contiguous CSF signal extending through the osteodural defect of the left cribriform plate (**c**, arrowheads). Associated meningoencephalocele with herniation of the olfactory bulb through the defect in the cribriform plate is best depicted on sagittal reformats (**d**, arrowheads). Additional stigmata of IIH were identified on the MRC, including widening of the sella turcica with flattening of the pituitary gland (**e**, arrow) and stenosis of the dural venous sinuses at the level of the transverse-sigmoid junctions (**f**, post-contrast MR venogram in **e**, arrows)

osseous skull base and resulting in multiple regions of thinning and dehiscence seen on HRCT [35, 36]. Loss of osseous integrity, coupled with elevated intracranial pressures, allows for the formation of multiple arachnoid pits/granulations and, eventually, dural tears with associated CSF leak. Although imaging findings are not in the diagnostic criteria for IIH, there are several MR imaging features that have been associated with IIH in the literature, including an expanded sella with a partially empty configuration, optic nerve sheath enlargement/tortuosity, flattening of the posterior globe, and/or papilledema [13, 37] (Figs. 5.12 and 5.13). Other works have described stenosis between the junction of the transverse and sigmoid sinuses as the most specific feature of IIH, although it remains unclear if this is a causative agent or secondary finding in this clinical diagnosis [38] (Fig. 5.12). Nevertheless, these imaging features in conjunction with clinical signs of papilledema and elevated opening pressure on lumbar puncture are strongly suggestive of the diagnosis of IIH. Given the propensity for multifocal regions of osseous thinning and the increased risk of meningocele/meningoencephalocele formation, patients with suspected or confirmed IIH often require multimodal imaging work up including both HRCT and MRC prior to any elective intervention.

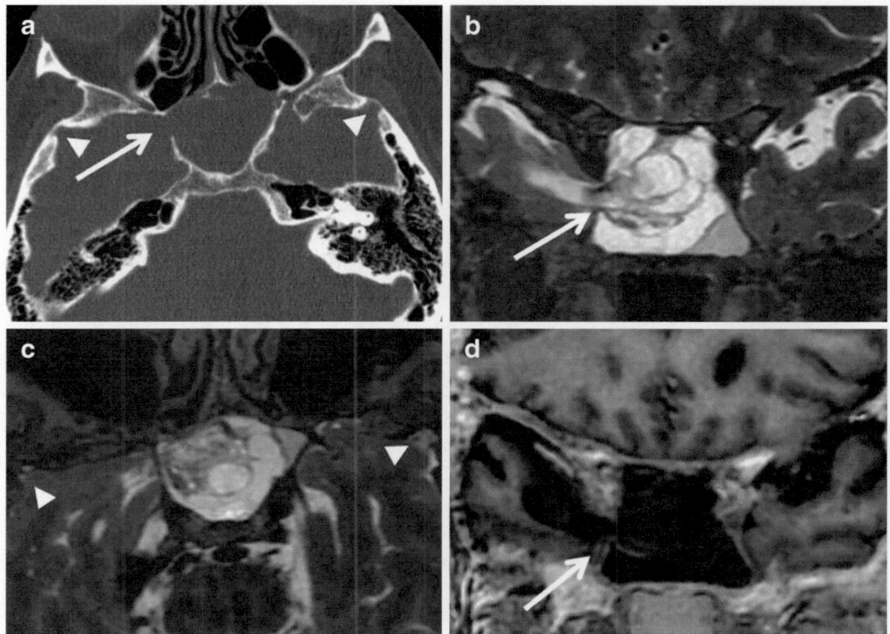

Fig. 5.13 Spontaneous CSF leak in the setting of idiopathic intracranial hypertension. 70-year-old female with 3-month history of intermittent vertigo, sinonasal congestion, and watery nasal discharge. An 8 mm defect was noted in the lateral wall of the right sphenoid sinus on HRCT (**a**, arrow) with polypoid opacification of the sinus lumen (**a**, open arrow) concerning for CSF leak and possible meningoencephalocele. Subsequent MRC demonstrated a large meningoencephalocele extending through the sphenoid sinus defect (**b** and **d**, arrows) with contiguous opacification of the sphenoid sinus with CSF as demonstrated by uniformly T2 hyperintense signal on heavily T2-weighted volumetric sequences (**b**). For this example, phase-sensitive-inversion-recovery (PSIR) sequences were also performed (**d**) which display native subarachnoid CSF signal as hypointense relative to the adjacent bony structures, which can be helpful in the discrimination between CSF and marrow signal. Also note additional focal regions of bony thinning of the inner margin of the middle cranial fossa (on HRCT in **a**, arrowheads), revealed as additional small meningoencephaloceles (**b**, arrowheads), in keeping with the diagnosis of IIH

Pitfalls and Mimics

There are numerous challenges in the imaging evaluation of patients with suspected or confirmed CSF rhinorrhea and otorrhea. Some of the more frequently encountered include:

- MRC, CTC, and contrast-enhanced MRC are dependent upon the presence of an active CSF leak at the time of imaging and, as such, may fail to detect intermittent or very-slow flow leaks at the time of imaging.
- Although HRCT can identify bony defects regardless of leak activity, thinning and irregularity of the skull base structures of the anterior and middle cranial

fossa are a relatively common finding in the population in the absence of clinical concern for CSF leak.
- Particularly in the setting of IIH or polytrauma, multiple osseous defects, and even multiple meningoceles, may be present in one patient, making the identification of the true site of active leakage difficult on HRCT. MR cisternogram can be helpful in this setting, but can result in the occasional false negative if the patient is not leaking at the time of imaging. In these cases, consideration of CTC or contrast-enhanced MRC is recommended, potentially with provocative maneuvers or delayed imaging, as problem-solving tools for better localization.
- Evaluation of contrast extravasation using CTC in the postoperative setting can be obscured by other high-density components, including hypertrophied osseous structures, inspissated secretions/blood products, and granulation tissue. Comparison between pre- and post-contrast images and careful windowing using soft tissue algorithms can be helpful to discriminate between artifact and true egress of contrast.

Although there is no real differential diagnosis for an underlying CSF leak, there are several imaging findings on HRCT that may mimic the opacification pattern of a CSF leak, yet belie a more insidious process. Ostiomeatal unit pattern sinonasal inflammatory disease, particularly if long standing, can result in various degrees of neo-osteogenesis and osseous thinning, although intact periosteum may be in place in the absence of symptoms referable to CSF rhinorrhea. Both CSF leaks and malignancy can present as unilateral opacification of the sinonasal cavity; in this case, frank osseous destruction of the intervening bony boundaries can tip the radiologist toward a diagnosis of underlying malignancy, which is easily confirmed by MRI (Fig. 5.14).

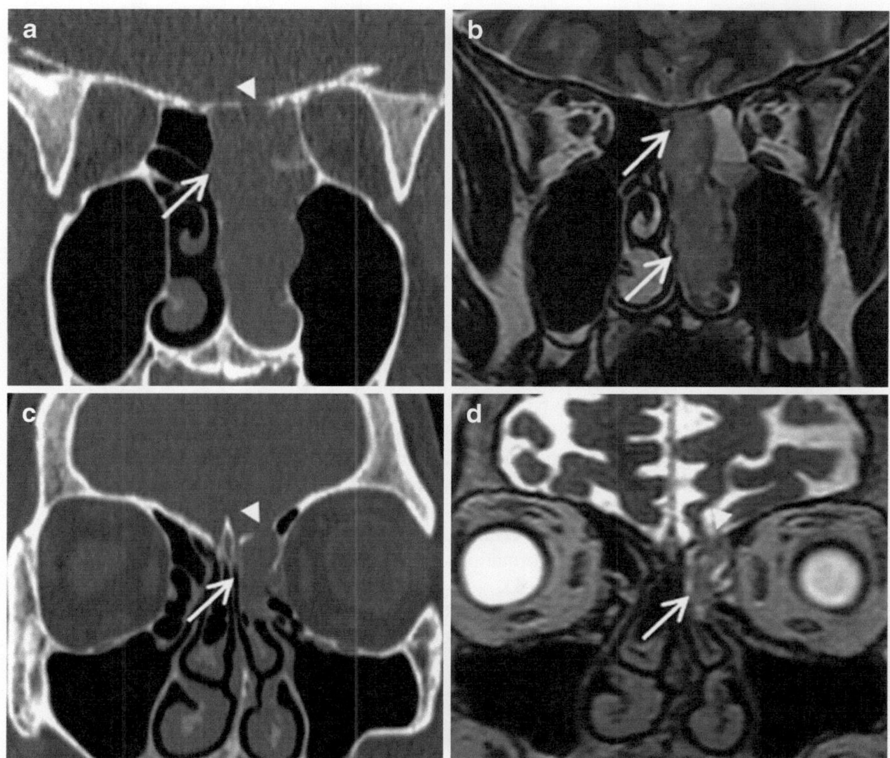

Fig. 5.14 Mimics of CSF leak. Coronal bone algorithm reformatted HRCT images (**a** and **c**) on two different patients, both of which demonstrate dehiscence of the floor of the anterior cranial fossa (**a** and **c**, arrowheads) with associated downstream opacification of the adjacent left ethmoid air cells (**a** and **c**, arrows). However, the follow-up MRI (coronal T2 weighted in **b**) in this patient with several months of long-standing left-sided nasal obstruction revealed a T2 hypointense mass extending from the superior meatus through the nasal cavity (**b**, arrows), now biopsy confirmed sinonasal neuroectodermal tumor (SNEC). In distinction, the patient in **c** presented with a history of remote trauma, chronic rhinorrhea, and recurrent meningitis, raising suspicion for an underlying CSF leak consequent to a previously undiagnosed fracture of the left lateral lamella. T2-CUBE sequences (coronal in **d**) were confirmatory, detailing a post-traumatic meningoencephalocele extending into the left anterior ethmoid air cells (**d**, arrow)

References

1. Lloyd KM, DelGaudio JM, Hudgins PA. Imaging of skull base cerebrospinal fluid leaks in adults. Radiology. 2008;248(3):725–36.
2. Daudia A, Biswas D, Jones NS. Risk of meningitis with cerebrospinal fluid rhinorrhea. Ann Otol Rhinol Laryngol. 2007;116(12):902–5.
3. Aarabi B, Leibrock LG. Neurosurgical approaches to cerebrospinal fluid rhinorrhea. Ear Nose Throat J. 1992;71(7):300–5.

4. Eftekhar B, Ghodsi M, Nejat F, Ketabchi E, Esmaeeli B. Prophylactic administration of ceftriaxone for the prevention of meningitis after traumatic pneumocephalus: results of a clinical trial. J Neurosurg. 2004;101(5):757–61.
5. Eljamel MS, Foy PM. Acute traumatic CSF fistulae: the risk of intracranial infection. Br J Neurosurg. 1990;4(5):381–5.
6. Friedman JA, Ebersold MJ, Quast LM. Post-traumatic cerebrospinal fluid leakage. World J Surg. 2001;25(8):1062–6.
7. Oakley GM, Alt JA, Schlosser RJ, Harvey RJ, Orlandi RR. Diagnosis of cerebrospinal fluid rhinorrhea: an evidence-based review with recommendations. Int Forum Allergy Rhinol. 2016;6(1):8–16.
8. Wang EW, Vandergrift WA, Schlosser RJ. Spontaneous CSF leaks. Otolaryngol Clin N Am. 2011;44(4):845–56. vii
9. Warnecke A, Averbeck T, Wurster U, Harmening M, Lenarz T, Stöver T. Diagnostic relevance of beta2-transferrin for the detection of cerebrospinal fluid fistulas. Arch Otolaryngol Head Neck Surg. 2004;130(10):1178–84.
10. Zapalac JS, Marple BF, Schwade ND. Skull base cerebrospinal fluid fistulas: a comprehensive diagnostic algorithm. Otolaryngol Head Neck Surg. 2002;126(6):669–76.
11. Hiremath SB, Gautam AA, Sasindran V, Therakathu J, Benjamin G. Cerebrospinal fluid rhinorrhea and otorrhea: a multimodality imaging approach. Diagn Interv Imaging. 2019;100(1):3–15.
12. La Fata V, McLean N, Wise SK, DelGaudio JM, Hudgins PA. CSF leaks: correlation of high-resolution CT and multiplanar reformations with intraoperative endoscopic findings. AJNR Am J Neuroradiol. 2008;29(3):536–41.
13. Alonso RC, de la Peña MJ, Caicoya AG, Rodriguez MR, Moreno EA, de Vega Fernandez VM. Spontaneous skull base meningoencephaloceles and cerebrospinal fluid fistulas. Radiographics. 2013;33(2):553–70.
14. Reddy M, Baugnon K. Imaging of cerebrospinal fluid rhinorrhea and otorrhea. Radiol Clin N Am. 2017;55(1):167–87.
15. Lloyd MN, Kimber PM, Burrows EH. Post-traumatic cerebrospinal fluid rhinorrhoea: modern high-definition computed tomography is all that is required for the effective demonstration of the site of leakage. Clin Radiol. 1994;49(2):100–3.
16. Prosser JD, Vender JR, Solares CA. Traumatic cerebrospinal fluid leaks. Otolaryngol Clin N Am. 2011;44(4):857–73. vii
17. Schuknecht B, Simmen D, Briner HR, Holzmann D. Nontraumatic skull base defects with spontaneous CSF rhinorrhea and arachnoid herniation: imaging findings and correlation with endoscopic sinus surgery in 27 patients. AJNR Am J Neuroradiol. 2008;29(3):542–9.
18. Saim L, McKenna MJ, Nadol JB. Tubal and tympanic openings of the peritubal cells: implications for cerebrospinal fluid otorhinorrhea. Am J Otol. 1996;17(2):335–9.
19. Stone JA, Castillo M, Neelon B, Mukherji SK. Evaluation of CSF leaks: high-resolution CT compared with contrast-enhanced CT and radionuclide cisternography. AJNR Am J Neuroradiol. 1999;20(4):706–12.
20. Algin O, Hakyemez B, Gokalp G, Ozcan T, Korfali E, Parlak M. The contribution of 3D-CISS and contrast-enhanced MR cisternography in detecting cerebrospinal fluid leak in patients with rhinorrhoea. Br J Radiol. 2010;83(987):225–32.
21. Shetty PG, Shroff MM, Sahani DV, Kirtane MV. Evaluation of high-resolution CT and MR cisternography in the diagnosis of cerebrospinal fluid fistula. AJNR Am J Neuroradiol. 1998;19(4):633–9.
22. Mostafa BE, Khafagi A. Combined HRCT and MRI in the detection of CSF rhinorrhea. Skull Base. 2004;14(3):157–62; discussion 62
23. Tuntiyatorn L, Laothammatas J. Evaluation of MR cisternography in diagnosis of cerebrospinal fluid fistula. J Med Assoc Thail. 2004;87(12):1471–6.
24. Vimala LR, Jasper A, Irodi A. Non-invasive and minimally invasive imaging evaluation of CSF Rhinorrhoea - a retrospective study with review of literature. Pol J Radiol. 2016;81:80–5.

25. Selcuk H, Albayram S, Ozer H, Ulus S, Sanus GZ, Kaynar MY, et al. Intrathecal gadolinium-enhanced MR cisternography in the evaluation of CSF leakage. AJNR Am J Neuroradiol. 2010;31(1):71–5.
26. DelGaudio JM, Baugnon KL, Wise SK, Patel ZM, Aiken AH, Hudgins PA. Magnetic resonance cisternogram with intrathecal gadolinium with delayed imaging for difficult to diagnose cerebrospinal fluid leaks of anterior skull base. Int Forum Allergy Rhinol. 2015;5(4):333–8.
27. Baugnon KL, Hudgins PA. Skull base fractures and their complications. Neuroimaging Clin N Am. 2014;24(3):439–65, vii-viii
28. Johnson F, Semaan MT, Megerian CA. Temporal bone fracture: evaluation and management in the modern era. Otolaryngol Clin N Am. 2008;41(3):597–618. x
29. Naunheim MR, Sedaghat AR, Lin DT, Bleier BS, Holbrook EH, Curry WT, et al. Immediate and delayed complications following endoscopic Skull Base surgery. J Neurol Surg B Skull Base. 2015;76(5):390–6.
30. García-Garrigós E, Arenas-Jiménez JJ, Monjas-Cánovas I, Abarca-Olivas J, Cortés-Vela JJ, De La Hoz-Rosa J, et al. Transsphenoidal approach in endoscopic endonasal surgery for Skull Base lesions: what radiologists and surgeons need to know. Radiographics. 2015;35(4):1170–85.
31. Hamid O, El Fiky L, Hassan O, Kotb A, El Fiky S. Anatomic variations of the sphenoid sinus and their impact on trans-sphenoid pituitary surgery. Skull Base. 2008;18(1):9–15.
32. Kilgore KP, Lee MS, Leavitt JA, Mokri B, Hodge DO, Frank RD, et al. Re-evaluating the incidence of idiopathic intracranial hypertension in an era of increasing obesity. Ophthalmology. 2017;124(5):697–700.
33. Pérez MA, Bialer OY, Bruce BB, Newman NJ, Biousse V. Primary spontaneous cerebrospinal fluid leaks and idiopathic intracranial hypertension. J Neuroophthalmol. 2013;33(4):330–7.
34. Tam EK, Gilbert AL. Spontaneous cerebrospinal fluid leak and idiopathic intracranial hypertension. Curr Opin Ophthalmol. 2019;30(6):467–71.
35. Stevens SM, Rizk HG, Golnik K, Andaluz N, Samy RN, Meyer TA, et al. Idiopathic intracranial hypertension: contemporary review and implications for the otolaryngologist. Laryngoscope. 2018;128(1):248–56.
36. O'Connell BP, Stevens SM, Xiao CC, Meyer TA, Schlosser RJ. Lateral Skull Base attenuation in patients with anterior cranial fossa spontaneous cerebrospinal fluid leaks. Otolaryngol Head Neck Surg. 2016;154(6):1138–44.
37. Bathla G, Moritani T. Imaging of cerebrospinal fluid leak. Semin Ultrasound CT MR. 2016;37(2):143–9.
38. Farb RI, Vanek I, Scott JN, Mikulis DJ, Willinsky RA, Tomlinson G, et al. Idiopathic intracranial hypertension: the prevalence and morphology of sinovenous stenosis. Neurology. 2003;60(9):1418–24.

Chapter 6
Conservative and Medical Therapy for Cerebrospinal Fluid Leaks

Jacob G. Eide and Michael A. Kohanski

Introduction

Cerebrospinal fluid (CSF) leaks and associated management are largely dependent on the volume, location, and etiology of the skull base defect. CSF leaks can broadly be separated into traumatic, spontaneous, and iatrogenic categories, which inform and guide the treatment pathways. Conservative medical treatment—focused on bed rest, treatment of comorbid intracranial hypertension, minimizing straining, and meningitis prophylaxis—and surgical repair of the skull base are the predominant treatment modalities. Conservative therapy relies on healing by secondary intention to close a skull base dehiscence and seal off the intracranial space, although permanent epithelialized tracts (fistulas) are unlikely to close with non-surgical therapy [1]. Of note, CSF diversion—either by lumbar drain, external ventricular device, or ventriculoperitoneal shunt—plays a prominent role for many physicians in the role of CSF leak therapy. CSF diversion will be discussed in detail in other chapters. In this chapter we highlight the indications for conservative medical management outside of CSF diversion and describe the current treatment paradigm.

J. G. Eide
Department of Otolaryngology - Head and Neck Surgery, Henry Ford Health, Detroit, MI, USA
e-mail: jeide1@hfhs.org

M. A. Kohanski (✉)
Department of Otorhinolaryngology-Head and Neck Surgery, Division of Rhinology, University of Pennsylvania, Perelman School of Medicine, Philadelphia, PA, USA
e-mail: michael.kohanski@pennmedicine.upenn.edu

E. C. Kuan et al. (eds.), *Skull Base Reconstruction*,
https://doi.org/10.1007/978-3-031-27937-9_6

Indications for Medical Management

Prior to decisions on treatment, the presence of a CSF leak must be confirmed, and the extent of the skull base defect delineated (please see preceding chapters for discussion on diagnosis and imaging modalities). The role of medical therapy for primary management of CSF leaks is controversial in the literature with some authors advocating for surgical repair of all leaks as soon as feasible [1]. There are, however, several scenarios where medical, nonoperative management has been utilized.

The most common indication for medical management is in cases of traumatic CSF leaks, where comorbid injuries to the central nervous system or resulting hemodynamic instability may delay operative repair while the patient is stabilized. The amount of time to delay operative management of a traumatic CSF leak is highly dependent on the patient's other injuries, overall prognosis, and goals of care. Some authors have proposed a short waiting period to see if small traumatic leaks will close spontaneously—with the ideal candidate having a small skull base defect, few comorbidities, and normal intracranial pressure [2]. An initial waiting period of 3–7 days has been suggested, noting that 3 days of conservative therapy has been effective in 39.5–68% of cases and improves to 85% after 7 days [3]. Conservative therapy must be balanced with increasing risk of meningitis with 5–11% risk of meningitis in the first week, which increases to 55–88% after 1 week [3, 4]. It should be noted that CSF leak from the middle cranial fossa is more likely to cease without surgical intervention (60%) than anterior cranial fossa fractures (26.4%), which may suggest that a shorter waiting period for the latter is appropriate [3].

The role for medical therapy, specifically acetazolamide, in spontaneous CSF rhinorrhea is even more controversial. Spontaneous CSF leak is thought to be associated with idiopathic intracranial hypertension leading to skull base erosion and often meningoencephaloceles [5]. Talik et al. completed a retrospective review of 16 patients with spontaneous CSF leaks treated with 250 mg acetazolamide twice daily instead of surgical repair and found that rhinorrhea abated in 31.3% of patients [6]. However, others noted that the resolution of rhinorrhea, while important for patient quality of life, does not decrease the risk of meningitis due to persistent skull base dehiscence and cessation of rhinorrhea would not promote healing of a fistulized CSF outflow tract [7]. The lifetime risk of meningitis in unclosed CSF leaks has been estimated to be as high as 19%, and accordingly the authors recommend surgical repair of all CSF leaks with medical therapy reserved as an adjunct to decrease intracranial pressure in the perioperative time period [7–9]. Indeed, in recent international recommendations for spontaneous CSF leak, the vast majority of experts recommended that patients should be operated on as soon as feasible, regardless of the defect size (88% agree or strongly agree), and that watchful waiting is supplementary and cannot replace surgical repair (94% agree or strongly agree) [1]. Taken together, there is likely insufficient evidence to support medical management as first-line therapy for spontaneous CSF leaks, given the small retrospective nature of the study by Tilak et al. [6] and the long-term risks of meningitis without operative repair of the CSF leak. However, in patients with significant comorbidities preventing operative repair or in cases where the patient refuses surgery, it may be an option to reduce CSF rhinorrhea and improve quality of life.

Iatrogenic leaks—either following endoscopic sinus or skull base surgery—are infrequently managed conservatively. Early intervention and return to the operating room (OR) is generally recommended for localization of the site of leak and repair, although there may be a limited role for CSF diversion. The role of CSF diversion will be discussed in other chapters. Figure 6.1 summarizes these findings and proposes an algorithm for operative vs medical therapy.

Active meningitis is also a relative indication for medical management. If the patient is actively infected, recommended treatment includes antibiotics, medical stabilization, and conservative measures for the CSF leak until the patient improves [10]. Similarly, active COVID-19 (SARS-CoV-2) infection may be an indication for a short course of medical management given data suggesting increased perioperative morbidity and mortality for patients who are actively infected [11–13]. While not previously reported on, there may be a role for medical therapy as a temporizing

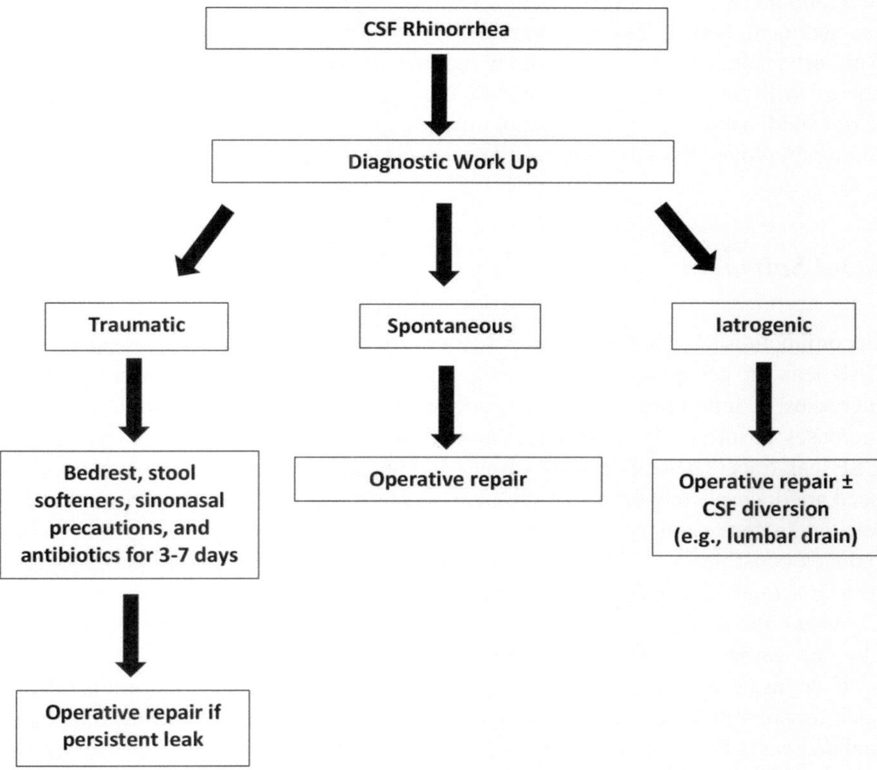

Fig. 6.1 Proposed treatment algorithm for CSF rhinorrhea medical vs surgical management

measure in resource-poor areas without access to dedicated skull base surgical care while plans for patient transfer are made. However, side effects of some of the therapeutics and associated need for close monitoring may make it challenging to initiate medical therapy for CSF leaks in resource-poor settings.

Medical Management Options

Bed Rest/Sinus Precautions

Bed rest is a common component of CSF leak management strategy to reduce straining and minimize intracranial pressure changes. Bed rest protocols vary widely with some keeping patients entirely in bed without bathroom privileges, while others allow for limited amounts of activity [14]. While bed rest is preferable for management of the CSF leak, the longer a patient is immobile, the higher the likelihood of deep vein thrombosis/pulmonary embolism, pneumonia, deconditioning, pressure ulcers, and patient dissatisfaction. There is no data to-date on the optimal amount of time for a patient to remain on bed rest as part of CSF leak medical management, although an initial period of 24–72 h is a relatively common practice. Similarly, sinus precautions, which include recommendations to the patient to sneeze with mouth open, avoid nose blowing, and minimize straining in order to avoid sudden changes in intracranial pressure and avoid pneumocephalus, are commonly employed but have not been extensively studied.

Stool Softeners

In conjunction with bed rest, stool softeners are often prescribed for patients with a CSF leak to decrease straining while having bowel movements and to reduce increases in intracranial pressure associated with straining. By avoiding sudden increases in intracranial pressure, the goal is to decrease CSF egress through the CSF leak tract. There are a wide variety of stool softeners, and the most commonly used are docusate and senna. Docusate works as a surfactant that lowers the surface tension in feces and promotes water and lipid absorption by the stool and thus reduces constipation [15]. Senna (also known as sennoside) is an anthraquinone derivative and stimulates luminal nerve endings causing colonic motility and reducing water absorption by the gut [16, 17]. Docusate and senna can be used individually or together given their complementary modes of action.

If docusate and senna are ineffective, other options include osmotic laxatives, such as polyethylene glycol, which forms hydrogen bonds with water molecules and decreases intestinal water reabsorption to soften stool [18]. More invasive methods of promoting bowel movements include suppositories such as bisacodyl, which also stimulates colonic neurons to promote motility and decrease salt/water excretion [19]. Finally, there are a variety of enema solutions which work mechanically to dilate the intestine and, depending on the type used, stimulate peristalsis and lubricate the stool. Table 6.1 outlines common laxatives, dosing, and side effects.

Table 6.1 Mechanism of action, side effects, and contraindications of commonly used therapies in medical management of CSF leak

Medication	Mechanism of action	Dosing	Side effects	Contraindication	Monitoring
Stool softener/laxatives					
Docusate	Surfactant stool softener	100 mg oral daily	Diarrhea, abdominal cramping	Intestinal obstruction, appendicitis, acute abdominal pain	None
Senna	Stimulant laxative	8.6–17.2 mg oral daily	Diarrhea	Intestinal obstruction, abdominal pain	None
Polyethylene glycol	Osmotic laxative	17 g oral daily	Diarrhea, rare reports of renal damage (primarily in topical/IV administration)	Intestinal obstruction, inflammatory bowel disease, electrolyte imbalance/renal impairment	Electrolyte monitoring if prolonged use or in cases of dehydration after use
Bisacodyl	Stimulant suppository	10 mg rectally PRN	Diarrhea, abdominal pain, headache	Has interactions with digoxin, antacids, and H2-receptor antagonists, bowel obstruction	Electrolyte monitoring if prolonged use
Antibiotics					
Ceftriaxone	Cell wall disruption via interaction with penicillin-binding proteins	1 mg IV every 24 h	Rare leukopenia, rash	Penicillin allergy	None
Metronidazole	Bacterial DNA strand breakage	500 mg IV or PO every 8 h	Headache, vaginitis, nausea, metallic taste, flushing/tachycardia when taken with alcohol	Pregnancy, active alcohol use, previous disulfiram use within 2 weeks	None

(continued)

Table 6.1 (continued)

Medication	Mechanism of action	Dosing	Side effects	Contraindication	Monitoring
Ampicillin-sulbactam	Cell wall disruption via interaction with penicillin-binding proteins with beta lactamase inhibitor	3000 mg IV every 6 h	Diarrhea, colitis, agranulocytosis, thrombocytopenia	Active *Clostridium difficile* GI infection due to concern for fulminant colitis and active mononucleosis due to rash, penicillin allergy	Consider renal, hepatic, and hematologic monitoring
Vancomycin	Cell wall disruption	15 mg/ kg IV every 24 h	Flushing, pruritus, erythematous rash, angiodema, phlepitis, rare Stevens-Johnson syndrome. Known to have nephrotoxic and ototoxic effects	Renal disease, hearing loss (relative), pregnancy, and advanced age	Daily vancomycin trough levels and adjustment of medication
Meropenem	Cell wall disruption via interaction with penicillin-binding proteins	1 mg IV every 8 h	Diarrhea, headache, rash, hypokalemia	Renal disease (relative)	Consider electrolyte monitoring
Levofloxacin	Inhibits bacterial DNA synthesis	250–750 mg oral daily	Photosensitivity, tendinitis, QT prolongation	Prolonged QT interval, pregnancy, pediatric patients (due to risk of cartilage damage), myasthenia gravis	Consider electrocardiogram to monitor QT interval, monitor for tendinitis
Amoxicillin-clavulanate	Cell wall disruption via interaction with penicillin-binding proteins with beta lactamase inhibitor	875–125 mg oral BID	Diarrhea, rash	Penicillin allergy, active mononucleosis due to rash	None

Antibiotics

The role of antibiotics in patients undergoing purely medical therapy is controversial. The International Consensus Statement on Spontaneous CSF leaks recommended against prescribing long-term antibiotics to patients without clinical signs of an infection as they have not been shown to reduce the incidence of meningitis [1]. However, following traumatic CSF leaks, there is mixed evidence on the use of antibiotics as part of medical management. One meta-analysis found a reduction in meningitis from 10% to 2.5% in patients treated with antibiotics [20], whereas a more recent meta-analysis of several randomized control trials investigating antibiotic prophylaxis for patients admitted for basilar skull fractures found no difference in rates of meningitis or need for surgical repair [21]. Based on the available evidence, antibiotic prophylaxis is recommended after traumatic CSF leak but not routinely administered for spontaneous CSF leaks. However, given the generalized increasing rates of antibiotic-resistant pathogens [22], further study is needed on the appropriate use of antibiotics.

While meningitis associated with CSF leak may be rare, given the risks of severe complications and poor outcomes associated with meningitis, antibiotics are commonly prescribed for CSF leaks and can be considered while the patient is undergoing medical therapy. A third-generation cephalosporin, such as ceftriaxone, delivered intravenously should be considered for inpatients given the excellent central nervous system penetration. The addition of metronidazole can also be considered if improved anaerobic coverage is desired [23].

For penicillin-allergic patients, fluoroquinolones (such as levofloxacin), vancomycin, or meropenem are alternatives that can provide prophylaxis against meningitis. The role for prolonged oral antibiotics is questionable; however amoxicillin-clavulanate and oral levofloxacin have been described for gram-positive and anaerobic coverage [24]. Please see Table 6.1 for details on dosing and mechanism of action for commonly used antibiotic regimens that provide CSF coverage [25–29].

Diuretic and Other Medical Options

Diuretics can reduce intracranial pressure through various pharmacologic mechanisms and are helpful adjuncts for management of CSF leaks, particularly CSF leaks associated with idiopathic intracranial hypertension (IIH). Diuretic use for CSF leak management is typically used as an adjunct to primary surgical repair and not as a primary modality of therapy. The most widely used diuretic therapy in spontaneous CSF leaks associated with IIH is acetazolamide—a carbonic anhydrase inhibitor that reduces the production of CSF and significantly decreases intracranial pressure [30]. As mentioned above, the evidence for using acetazolamide as a primary therapy for spontaneous CSF leak is based on one retrospective study by

Tilak et al. which reported a 31.3% resolution of CSF rhinorrhea, and the authors suggested a trial of 250 mg twice-daily acetazolamide prior to surgical repair of the skull base defect [6]. However, this regimen will not induce closure of an established CSF tract into the sinuses, and there remains a persistent risk for meningitis, which is the primary therapeutic indication for operative repair. Management of traumatic CSF leaks with acetazolamide has been examined in a randomized fashion. Acetazolamide treatment did not impact on the resolution of the CSF leak but did lead to increased rates of metabolic derangements including metabolic acidosis and hypokalemia and is therefore not routinely recommended in this cohort [31].

It should be noted that acetazolamide was previously used for glaucoma, heart failure, and epilepsy but treatment for CSF leak and intracranial hypertension is an off-label use. Currently, acetazolamide is not commonly used for any indication apart from IIH. The main side effects are metabolic derangements (especially hypokalemia, hyponatremia, and hyperchloremia), paresthesias of upper and lower extremities, and altered sense of taste with patients reporting bitter/metallic disturbances [32–34]. Ongoing monitoring of electrolyte levels, particularly sodium levels, are recommended while taking acetazolamide. The medication is also sulfonamide-based and contraindicated in patients with a known sulfa allergy. Acetazolamide is protein-bound and renally excreted, and adjustments for patients with creatinine clearance <50 mL/min are necessary [32].

Furosemide, a loop diuretic, has also been described in the treatment of intracranial hypertension, although the exact mechanism of CSF reduction is not well understood, and it is thought to be less potent at reducing intracranial pressures than acetazolamide [35]. Topiramate, an anticonvulsant medication, has also been investigated for intracranial hypertension. Animal models suggest that topiramate is more potent than acetazolamide, theorized to be due to its increased lipophilicity [35]. In open-label studies, topiramate was found to be comparable to acetazolamide for treating IIH with similar visual field outcomes but more prominent weight loss [36]. Table 6.2 summarizes common dosing of diuretics.

Table 6.2 Diuretic and other medical options for treating CSF rhinorrhea and comorbid intracranial hypertension

Medication name	Common dosing	Side effects	Recommended monitoring	FDA status
Acetazolamide	250 mg or 500 mg twice daily; must be renally dosed (if creatinine clearance <50 mL/min)	Paresthesias, electrolyte abnormalities, altered sense of taste	Electrolyte monitoring	Off label
Topiramate	50–100 mg orally twice daily	Weight loss, dizziness, paresthesias	Consider electrolyte monitoring	Off label
Furosemide	20–40 mg orally per day	Renal injury, electrolyte abnormalities, dizziness	Creatinine and electrolyte monitoring	Off label

Future Directions and Other Considerations

Medical management of CSF leaks has a limited role and is primarily constrained to traumatic CSF leak repairs. The current consensus statement on spontaneous CSF leak repairs advocates for skull base repair as soon as feasible for spontaneous leaks [1], and the potential role for primary medical therapy in these patients is controversial. Traumatic leaks have a reasonable chance of closure after medical therapy in the first week, with delayed operative closure for recalcitrant leaks. Many of the studies on nonoperative medical therapy for CSF leaks are limited in size and retrospective making broad recommendations difficult. Further research may provide new insights into the role of medical management for CSF leaks.

References

1. Georgalas C, Oostra A, Ahmed S, Castelnuovo P, Dallan I, van Furth W, et al. International consensus statement: spontaneous cerebrospinal fluid rhinorrhea. Int Forum Allergy Rhinol. 2021;11(4):794–803.
2. Bernal-Sprekelsen M, Bleda-Vázquez C, Carrau RL. Ascending meningitis secondary to traumatic cerebrospinal fluid leaks. Am J Rhinol. 2000;14(4):257–9.
3. Phang SY, Whitehouse K, Lee L, Khalil H, McArdle P, Whitfield PC. Management of CSF leak in base of skull fractures in adults. Br J Neurosurg. 2016;30(6):596–604.
4. Eljamel MS, Foy PM. Acute traumatic CSF fistulae: the risk of intracranial infection. Br J Neurosurg. 1990;4(5):381–5.
5. Woodworth BA, Palmer JN. Spontaneous cerebrospinal fluid leaks. Curr Opin Otolaryngol Head Neck Surg. 2009;17(1):59–65.
6. Tilak AM, Koehn H, Mattos J, Payne SC. Preoperative management of spontaneous cerebrospinal fluid rhinorrhea with acetazolamide. Int Forum Allergy Rhinol. 2019;9(3):265–9.
7. Geltzeiler M, Carrau R, Chandra R, Palmer J, Schlosser R, Smith T, et al. Management of spontaneous cerebrospinal fluid leaks. Int Forum Allergy Rhinol. 2019;9(3):330–1.
8. Daudia A, Biswas D, Jones NS. Risk of meningitis with cerebrospinal fluid rhinorrhea. Ann Otol Rhinol Laryngol. 2007;116(12):902–5.
9. Bernal-Sprekelsen M, Alobid I, Mullol J, Trobat F, Tomás-Barberán M. Closure of cerebrospinal fluid leaks prevents ascending bacterial meningitis. Rhinology. 2005;43(4):277–81.
10. Ter Horst L, Brouwer MC, van der Ende A, van de Beek D. Community-acquired bacterial meningitis in adults with cerebrospinal fluid leakage. Clin Infect Dis. 2020;70(11):2256–61.
11. Kayani B, Onochie E, Patil V, Begum F, Cuthbert R, Ferguson D, et al. The effects of COVID-19 on perioperative morbidity and mortality in patients with hip fractures. Bone Joint J. 2020;102-b(9):1136–45.
12. Knisely A, Zhou ZN, Wu J, Huang Y, Holcomb K, Melamed A, et al. Perioperative morbidity and mortality of patients with COVID-19 who undergo urgent and emergent surgical procedures. Ann Surg. 2021;273(1):34–40.
13. Jonker PKC, van der Plas WY, Steinkamp PJ, Poelstra R, Emous M, van der Meij W, et al. Perioperative SARS-CoV-2 infections increase mortality, pulmonary complications, and thromboembolic events: a Dutch, multicenter, matched-cohort clinical study. Surgery. 2021;169(2):264–74.
14. Schievink WI. Spontaneous spinal cerebrospinal fluid leaks and intracranial hypotension. JAMA. 2006;295(19):2286–96.

15. Hannoodee S, Annamaraju P. Docusate. StatPearls. Treasure Island (FL): StatPearls publishing. Copyright © 2021, StatPearls Publishing LLC; 2021.
16. Franz G. The senna drug and its chemistry. Pharmacology. 1993;47(Suppl 1):2–6.
17. Lemli J. Mechanism of action of sennosides. Bull Acad Natl Med. 1995;179(8):1605–11.
18. Dabaja A, Dabaja A, Abbas M. Polyethylene Glycol. StatPearls. Treasure Island (FL): StatPearls publishing. copyright © 2021, StatPearls Publishing LLC; 2021.
19. Lawrensia S, Raja A. Bisacodyl. StatPearls. Treasure Island (FL): StatPearls publishing. copyright © 2021, StatPearls Publishing LLC.; 2021.
20. Brodie HA. Prophylactic antibiotics for posttraumatic cerebrospinal fluid fistulae. A meta-analysis. Arch Otolaryngol Head Neck Surg. 1997;123(7):749–52.
21. Ratilal BO, Costa J, Pappamikail L, Sampaio C. Antibiotic prophylaxis for preventing meningitis in patients with basilar skull fractures. Cochrane Database Syst Rev. 2015;4:Cd004884.
22. Davies J, Davies D. Origins and evolution of antibiotic resistance. Microbiol Mol Biol Rev. 2010;74(3):417–33.
23. Weir CB, Le JK. Metronidazole. StatPearls. Treasure Island (FL): StatPearls publishing. copyright © 2021, StatPearls Publishing LLC.; 2021.
24. Hussein K, Bitterman R, Shofty B, Paul M, Neuberger A. Management of post-neurosurgical meningitis: narrative review. Clin Microbiol Infect. 2017;23(9):621–8.
25. Peechakara BV, Gupta M. Ampicillin/Sulbactam. StatPearls. Treasure Island (FL): StatPearls publishing. copyright © 2021, StatPearls Publishing LLC.; 2021.
26. Patel S, Preuss CV, Bernice F. Vancomycin. StatPearls. Treasure Island (FL): StatPearls publishing. copyright © 2021, StatPearls Publishing LLC.; 2021.
27. Margolin L. Impaired rehabilitation secondary to muscle weakness induced by meropenem. Clin Drug Investig. 2004;24(1):61–2.
28. Podder V, Sadiq NM. Levofloxacin. StatPearls. Treasure Island (FL): StatPearls publishing. copyright © 2021, StatPearls Publishing LLC; 2021.
29. Huttner A, Bielicki J, Clements MN, Frimodt-Møller N, Muller AE, Paccaud JP, et al. Oral amoxicillin and amoxicillin-clavulanic acid: properties, indications and usage. Clin Microbiol Infect. 2020;26(7):871–9.
30. Chaaban MR, Illing E, Riley KO, Woodworth BA. Acetazolamide for high intracranial pressure cerebrospinal fluid leaks. Int Forum Allergy Rhinol. 2013;3(9):718–21.
31. Gosal JS, Gurmey T, Kursa GK, Salunke P, Gupta SK. Is acetazolamide really useful in the management of traumatic cerebrospinal fluid rhinorrhea? Neurol India. 2015;63(2):197–201.
32. Van Berkel MA, Elefritz JL. Evaluating off-label uses of acetazolamide. Am J Health Syst Pharm. 2018;75(8):524–31.
33. Farzam K, Abdullah M. Acetazolamide. StatPearls. Treasure Island (FL): StatPearls Publishing. copyright © 2021, StatPearls Publishing LLC; 2021.
34. ten Hove MW, Friedman DI, Patel AD, Irrcher I, Wall M, McDermott MP. Safety and tolerability of acetazolamide in the idiopathic intracranial hypertension treatment trial. J Neuroophthalmol. 2016;36(1):13–9.
35. Scotton WJ, Botfield HF, Westgate CS, Mitchell JL, Yiangou A, Uldall MS, et al. Topiramate is more effective than acetazolamide at lowering intracranial pressure. Cephalalgia. 2019;39(2):209–18.
36. Celebisoy N, Gökçay F, Sirin H, Akyürekli O. Treatment of idiopathic intracranial hypertension: topiramate vs acetazolamide, an open-label study. Acta Neurol Scand. 2007;116(5):322–7.

Chapter 7
Cerebrospinal Fluid Diversion

Andrew K. Wong, Stephan Munich, and R. Webster Crowley

External Ventricular Drains

EVDs are catheters placed within the ventricles, allowings for CSF diversion into an external reservoir as well as continuous ICP monitoring. They can be placed in the operating room prior to the start of surgery, or they can be placed at the bedside when ICP needs to be emergently assessed, monitored, and controlled. The procedure is generally tolerated well utilizing conscious sedation and local anesthetic. A small incision is made in the skin followed by a small burr hole in the skull, typically at Kocher's point [1].Using surface anatomical landmarks, the catheter is guided to a predetermined depth, and placement within the ventricle is confirmed via brisk CSF flow, although this is occasionally not seen in cases of active CSF leaks which can result in low ventricular pressure. After placement of the catheter, it is connected to an external reservoir which allows for drainage and ICP pressure monitoring. The reservoir is placed at a height relative to the tragus, which approximates the foramen of Monro, to titrate drainage according to ICP.

In the management of skull base pathology and reconstruction, EVDs provide a means to control the flow of CSF and, as a result, ICP. This is particularly useful in the treatment of larger and deeper pathologies of the skull base in which the pathology prevents early access to the basal cisterns. These pathological processes may require significant manipulation and retraction of more superficial cortical structures which has shown to increase risk of surgery-related morbidity including venous congestion, contusions, postoperative seizures, and strokes [2–4]. CSF drainage allows for brain relaxation, minimizing the need for retraction. In cases of complex skull base pathology that either invades the skull base or requires violation of the skull base, an EVD may be placed also to facilitate subsequent repair of the

A. K. Wong · S. Munich · R. W. Crowley (✉)
Department of Neurosurgery, Rush University, Chicago, IL, USA
e-mail: stephan_munich@rush.edu; webster.crowley@rush.edu

© The Author(s), under exclusive license to Springer Nature
Switzerland AG 2023
E. C. Kuan et al. (eds.), *Skull Base Reconstruction*,
https://doi.org/10.1007/978-3-031-27937-9_7

skull base. By providing a low pressure CSF outlet, the EVD diverts CSF and subarachnoid pressure away from the repair site allowing it to heal.

EVD placement can generally be done safely and with low morbidity. However, as it necessitates passing the catheter through the cerebral cortex, there is a risk of intraparenchymal hemorrhage and infection. In a meta-analysis, the risk of overall hemorrhage has been reported to be 8.4%, with symptomatic hemorrhages at 0.7%, while the risk of infection has been reported to be 7.9% [5].

Lumbar Drains

LDs are placed in the enlarged subarachnoid space of the lumbar cistern that similarly allows for CSF diversion into an external reservoir. The procedure is generally tolerated well utilizing conscious sedation and local anesthetic. The patient is placed either in a lateral or sitting position with their back maximally flexed to allow for widening of the interlaminar space facilitating drain placement. Using surface landmarks or under fluoroscopic guidance, a trajectory to the L4/L5 interspace is used to obtain access to the lumbar cistern. The most commonly used surface landmark is the midline projection of the superior most aspect of the iliac crest which approximates the L4 spinous process. While the conus of the spinal cord typically terminates at L1, the dural sac ends in the sacral spine making this region safe for access during LD placement. The lumbar and sacral nerve roots which make up the cauda equina in the lumbar cistern are simply displaced rather than deformed during LD placement.

CSF diversion via a LD serves the same purpose as an EVD. Indications for LD placement in skull base surgery include the need for brain relaxation for surgical access, facilitating skull base repairs reducing CSF leak rates after various skull base approaches and in localizing CSF leaks. Approaches to deeper midline structures may require longer operative times and significant brain retraction. CSF diversion via a LD placed in the operating room prior to the start of surgery minimizes the need for such retraction reducing related morbidity.

Though the placement of a LD after various skull base procedures has shown to decrease overall CSF leak rates, proper patient selection to maximize benefit remains unclear. The use of vascularized nasoseptal flaps has dramatically improved the rates of CSF leak in the vast majority of uncomplicated endoscopic endonasal skull base surgeries such that the benefit of LD placement may be minimized to the point where it doesn't exceed the potential morbidity [6]. A recent randomized control trial demonstrated that patients with "high-flow" CSF leaks—as determined by dural defect and violation of ventricular or cisternal spaces—may benefit from LD placement [7]. CSF diversion away from a surgical repair site is believed to help with wound healing primarily through two mechanisms. By providing a low pressure egress, CSF is diverted away from the repair site allowing for adequate apposition of grafts and dura to allow for adequate sealing of the area. Furthermore, it has been suggested that CSF directly inhibits healing by potentially impairing cell migration and capillary formation [8, 9] .

In instances where the exact location of a CSF leak is unclear, intrathecal fluorescein instilled through the LD can be used to localize or confirm the area in question. This is particularly useful when the area of skull base defect is small or there are multiple areas of interest. Though the use of intrathecal fluorescein in this manner is off label, it has been shown to effectively localize areas of CSF leak with low morbidity. The sensitivity and specificity of intrathecal fluorescein have been reported to be as high as 93% and 100%, respectively [10].

LDs do not necessitate the direct brain contact that EVDs require. However, LDs are not an accurate means to measure and monitor ICP, and EVDs remain the gold standard. Significant variations of lumbar anatomy including scoliosis or severe lumbar stenosis are relative contraindications as they make cannulating the lumbar cistern challenging. Confirmed or suspected intracranial mass lesions are absolute contraindications for placement of LD due to potential for trans-tentorial downward herniation. Fundoscopic exam to evaluate for papilledema can be used as a means to screen for elevated ICP, though intracranial imaging to confirm potential mass lesions is typically obtained.

Complications from lumbar drain placement are relatively low with an overall rate of ~5% and include most commonly CSF leak at the insertion site (after removal), meningitis, and transient lower extremity numbness [11].

Shunts

Ventricular shunts are a form of permanent CSF diversion. They consist of a proximal catheter which accesses the ventricle and is connected to a shunt valve which sits on the calvarial surface and regulates the flow of CSF. The shunt valve is subsequently connected to a distal catheter which is placed in one of several spaces. The most common distal catheter placement site is the peritoneum. Atrial and pleural distal catheter sites can also be used and are often reserved for situations where there is significant compromise of the peritoneum, such as extensive prior abdominal surgeries that may incur scarring, or active peritoneal infection. Ventriculopleural shunts can be used for patients in which significant CSF shunting is required. The negative inspiratory pressure generated within the pleural space facilitates further CSF diversion.

Shunt valves regulate CSF flow through a shunt system by regulating the on-off function of the shunt depending on the pressure gradient across the valve. The pressure gradient threshold can be predetermined in fixed shunt valves or variable in programmable shunt valves. Anti-siphon devices within the shunt valves mitigate the effect of gravitational forces on the pressure gradient when the patient, and subsequently the shunt, changes from a recumbent to upright position [12].

Permanent CSF diversion is considered in CSF leaks when there is suspicion that the underlying etiology is elevated ICP, as seen in idiopathic intracranial hypertension (IIH) or pseudotumor cerebri. In such patients, the pathophysiology of the leak is not a mechanical defect that could be addressed via a simple repair of the skull base, but rather due to elevated ICP that requires resolution of the elevated pressure in order to adequately manage the leak. Clinical and radiographic correlates that suggest elevated ICP as the etiology are discussed in earlier chapters but include elevated BMI, obstructive sleep apnea, and an empty sella on MRI. There should be a high level of suspicion for underlying elevated ICP in patients with recurrent CSF leaks despite surgical repair. Confirmation can be achieved through a lumbar puncture and identification of elevated pressure, although this may be falsely depressed in cases of active CSF leak. While the cause of increased ICP remains unclear, a growing hypothesis is the presence of dural venous sinus stenosis which is discussed in the following section [13]. In placing the ventricular shunt and normalizing the pressure, the pulsatile stress within the subarachnoid space against weak areas of the skull base such as the tegmen tympani or lateral recess of the sphenoid is relieved, facilitating healing of the repair.

An alternative to ventricular shunts is a lumboperitoneal shunt in which the proximal catheter is placed in the lumbar cistern in a similar manner as a lumbar drain. Historically, this has been useful as patients with IIH typically have small, or slit, ventricles making successful cannulation with a catheter particularly challenging. However, with the advent of image guidance technology that has made ventricular access more reliable even in this subset of patients, lumboperitoneal shunts have fallen out of favor as they are more difficult to access and palpate. Given the nature of the area in which a lumboperitoneal shunt is placed, it is also more difficult to place an adjustable valve that can be accessed and reliably adjusted.

Ventriculoperitoneal shunts are relatively simple procedures but have known complications; particularly shunt infections, shunt malfunctions, and subdural hematomas from over-drainage. Of particular concern are shunt infections, as treatment typically involves removal of the entire shunt system, placement of a temporary EVD, and a course of antibiotics until the CSF is cleared of infection. The shunt system is then replaced, often through a different cranial location. This may require a prolonged intensive care unit stay for the duration of treatment. Shunt infection rates have been reported to be estimated at 8–15% [14]. Preventative measures include the use of antibiotic impregnated catheters, reducing operative time, and enhanced sterile techniques. Shunt malfunctions are relatively common, as it has been reported that 30–40% of shunts will need revision within the first year of insertion [15]. When done for assistance in skull base repair, malfunctioning shunts may not be clinically relevant if the malfunction occurs at a significant time interval from the shunt. However, for recently placed shunts, or in cases of underlying elevated intracranial pressure, shunt revision is often required, as failure to divert CSF generally results in recurrence of the leak. Subdural hematomas from overdrainage have been reported to be as high as 53% although symptomatic subdural hematomas were seen in 16% [14]. The etiology of subdural hematoma formation is straining and subsequent tearing of bridging veins when over-shunting leads to decompressed ventricles and thus contraction of the brain parenchyma. Programmable shunt valves have the advantage of adjusting the level of drainage to help titrate an appropriate amount of CSF diversion to prevent or treat subdural hematomas, and therefore are typically the authors' preferred valves in these cases.

Cerebral Venous Sinus Stenting

Dural venous sinus stenosis has been increasingly recognized as a potential etiology in the development of IIH and IIH-related spontaneous CSF leaks. While the exact mechanism may be unknown, it is believed that the reduction in venous outflow leads to venous hypertension proximal to the area of stenosis. As a result, the pressure needed to maintain CSF flow across the arachnoid villi from the subarachnoid space to the dural venous sinuses rises leading to an increase in ICP [16]. The increased pressure within the subarachnoid space along with the pulsatile nature of CSF flow leads to a gradual erosion of the skull base. In already diminutive areas of the skull base, such as the tegmen tympani or lateral recess of the sphenoid sinus, this can lead to defects within the skull base and subsequent CSF leaks with or without associated encephaloceles. Repair of the skull base without addressing the underlying elevated pressure risks recurrent CSF leak. Some have hypothesized that the development of a CSF leak is actually a compensating mechanism in which to offset and relieve the elevated ICP and that by repairing the defect without addressing the elevated pressure it closes off the system's ability to maintain normal pressure [17, 18].

CVSS, although not a form of CSF diversion, is aimed at improving CSF absorption through the arachnoid villi in order to achieve reduction in ICP. Workup and patient selection for CVSS is paramount in achieving good outcomes. Diagnosis of dural venous sinus stenosis can be made with a magnetic resonance venogram, although diagnostic cerebral angiogram remains the gold standard. Furthermore, determination of whether the stenosis is clinically significant should be made as it can be present and asymptomatic in a portion of the general population [19]. The trans-stenosis pressure gradient should be determined by obtaining femoral or upper extremity venous access and obtaining manometric pressure measurements at the pre-stenotic superior sagittal sinus as well as bilateral transverse sinuses, sigmoid sinuses, jugular bulb, and cervical internal jugular vein. Patients with a trans-stenosis pressure gradient of >8 mmHg may be candidates for CVSS placement.

Placement of the venous sinus stent is often completed under general anesthesia for patient comfort. The patient is typically started on aspirin 325 mg and clopidogrel 75 mg for 7 days prior to the procedure. Alternatively, if done in an acute setting, the patient can be bolused aspirin 325 mg and clopidogrel 600 mg immediately prior to the procedure. After obtaining access of the jugular vein through the femoral or antecubital vein, a stent is advanced over a guidewire to reach the area of sinus stenosis. The stent is then deployed to cover the entire area of stenosis. Resolution of the trans-stenosis pressure gradient is then confirmed. The patient then typically continues on dual antiplatelet therapy until eventually converting to aspirin 325 mg, alone.

CVSS has shown significant promise in the treatment of IIH with a technical success rate of 99.5% and a treatment failure rate (defined as need for conversion to a different treatment modality) of less than 3% [20]. While CVSS is a generally well-tolerated procedure and with low morbidity, it is not without known complications. A recent meta-analysis demonstrated an overall mortality rate of 0% and major complication rate, including intracranial hemorrhage, of 1.9% [21].

References

1. Morone PJ, Dewan MC, Zuckerman SL, Tubbs RS, Singer RJ. Craniometrics and ventricular access: a review of Kocher's, Kaufman's, Paine's, Menovksy's, Tubbs', Keen's, Frazier's, Dandy's, and Sanchez's points. Oper Neurosurg (Hagerstown). 2020;18(5):461–9.
2. Andrews RJ, Bringas JR. A review of brain retraction and recommendations for minimizing intraoperative brain injury. Neurosurgery. 1993;33(6):1052–63; discussion 63–4
3. Andrews RJ, Muto RP. Retraction brain ischaemia: cerebral blood flow, evoked potentials, hypotension and hyperventilation in a new animal model. Neurol Res. 1992;14(1):12–8.
4. Rosenørn J, Diemer NH. Reduction of regional cerebral blood flow during brain retraction pressure in the rat. J Neurosurg. 1982;56(6):826–9.
5. Dey M, Stadnik A, Riad F, Zhang L, McBee N, Kase C, et al. Bleeding and infection with external ventricular drainage: a systematic review in comparison with adjudicated adverse events in the ongoing clot lysis evaluating accelerated resolution of intraventricular hemorrhage phase III (CLEAR-III IHV) trial. Neurosurgery. 2015;76(3):291–300; discussion 1
6. Hadad G, Bassagasteguy L, Carrau RL, Mataza JC, Kassam A, Snyderman CH, et al. A novel reconstructive technique after endoscopic expanded endonasal approaches: vascular pedicle nasoseptal flap. Laryngoscope. 2006;116(10):1882–6.
7. Zwagerman NT, Wang EW, Shin SS, Chang YF, Fernandez-Miranda JC, Snyderman CH, et al. Does lumbar drainage reduce postoperative cerebrospinal fluid leak after endoscopic endonasal skull base surgery? A prospective, randomized controlled trial. J Neurosurg. 2018:1–7.
8. Goldschmidt E, Ielpi M, Loresi M, D'Adamo M, Giunta D, Carrizo A, et al. Assessing the role of selected growth factors and cytostatic agents in an in vitro model of human dura mater healing. Neurol Res. 2014;36(12):1040–6.
9. Babuccu O, Kalayci M, Peksoy I, Kargi E, Cagavi F, Numanoğlu G. Effect of cerebrospinal fluid leakage on wound healing in flap surgery: histological evaluation. Pediatr Neurosurg. 2004;40(3):101–6.
10. Raza SM, Banu MA, Donaldson A, Patel KS, Anand VK, Schwartz TH. Sensitivity and specificity of intrathecal fluorescein and white light excitation for detecting intraoperative cerebrospinal fluid leak in endoscopic skull base surgery: a prospective study. J Neurosurg. 2016;124(3):621–6.
11. El Ahmadieh TY, Wu EM, Kafka B, Caruso JP, Neeley OJ, Plitt A, et al. Lumbar drain trial outcomes of normal pressure hydrocephalus: a single-center experience of 254 patients. J Neurosurg. 2019;132(1):306–12.
12. Huang AP, Kuo LT, Lai DM, Yang SH, Kuo MF. Antisiphon device: a review of existing mechanisms and clinical applications to prevent overdrainage in shunted hydrocephalic patients. Biom J. 2022;45(1):95–108.
13. Farb RI, Vanek I, Scott JN, Mikulis DJ, Willinsky RA, Tomlinson G, et al. Idiopathic intracranial hypertension: the prevalence and morphology of sinovenous stenosis. Neurology. 2003;60(9):1418–24.
14. Paff M, Alexandru-Abrams D, Muhonen M, Loudon W. Ventriculoperitoneal shunt complications: a review. Interdiscip Neurosurg. 2018;13:66–70.

15. Crowley RW, Dumont AS, Asthagiri AR, Torner JC, Medel R, Jane JA Jr, et al. Intraoperative ultrasound guidance for the placement of permanent ventricular cerebrospinal fluid shunt catheters: a single-center historical cohort study. World Neurosurg. 2014;81(2):397–403.
16. Geisbüsch C, Herweh C, Gumbinger C, Ringleb PA, Möhlenbruch MA, Nagel S. Chronic intracranial hypertension after cerebral venous and sinus thrombosis - frequency and risk factors. Neurol Res Pract. 2021;3(1):28.
17. Ferrante E, Trimboli M, Petrecca G, Allegrini F. Cerebral venous thrombosis in spontaneous intracranial hypotension: a report of 8 cases and review of the literature. J Neurol Sci. 2021;425:117467.
18. Savoiardo M, Armenise S, Spagnolo P, De Simone T, Mandelli ML, Marcone A, et al. Dural sinus thrombosis in spontaneous intracranial hypotension: hypotheses on possible mechanisms. J Neurol. 2006;253(9):1197–202.
19. Durst CR, Ornan DA, Reardon MA, Mehndiratta P, Mukherjee S, Starke RM, et al. Prevalence of dural venous sinus stenosis and hypoplasia in a generalized population. J Neurointerv Surg. 2016;8(11):1173–7.
20. Leishangthem L, SirDeshpande P, Dua D, Satti SR. Dural venous sinus stenting for idiopathic intracranial hypertension: an updated review. J Neuroradiol. 2019;46(2):148–54.
21. Nicholson P, Brinjikji W, Radovanovic I, Hilditch CA, Tsang ACO, Krings T, et al. Venous sinus stenting for idiopathic intracranial hypertension: a systematic review and meta-analysis. J Neurointerv Surg. 2019;11(4):380–5.

Chapter 8
Anesthesia Considerations in Skull Base Reconstruction

Veronika Anufreichik and R. Ryan Field

Preoperative Evaluation

History of Present Illness

The anesthesiologist should know and understand the skull base reconstruction patient's original pathology, prior surgery performed, and current status of their neurological condition. This history will guide the appropriate medical optimization. A focused neurological exam, consisting of mental status, cranial nerve function, and a motor and sensory assessment, must also be performed. This information allows detection of any postoperative changes from baseline which can represent potentially significant complications. Risk for elevated ICP and seizures should be considered as this can change the anesthetic plan. Pertinent imaging must be reviewed with focus on signs of increased ICP and presence of lesions in close proximity to vital structures like vessels, sinuses, or cranial nerves.

Medical History

A full medical, surgical, family, and anesthetic history should be obtained with focus on prior intubations and anesthetic complications. Allergies, current medications, and social history should also be reviewed.

V. Anufreichik · R. R. Field (✉)
Department of Anesthesiology and Perioperative Care, University of California, Irivine, CA, USA
e-mail: fieldr@hs.uci.edu

E. C. Kuan et al. (eds.), *Skull Base Reconstruction*,
https://doi.org/10.1007/978-3-031-27937-9_8

Cardiovascular

It is important to assess patients for risk factors for perioperative cardiac events. In elective surgery, medical management should be optimized and further testing and work up performed if appropriate. With regard to time-sensitive surgery, the risks and benefits of delaying surgery to undergo indicated cardiac workup versus proceeding with surgery without further cardiac testing must be assessed by the surgeon, anesthesiologist, and cardiologist. Patients with acromegaly and Cushing's disease carry increased risk for hypertension, heart failure, and arrhythmias. In addition, these patients may develop right heart failure caused by pulmonary hypertension from chronic OSA.

Airway and Pulmonary

A careful airway assessment helps to predict the difficulty of ventilation and intubation. Special attention should be paid to cervical spine range of motion and any symptoms with range of motion. This information is not only useful for intubation but also for surgical position planning as certain neurosurgical approaches require significant neck flexion, rotation, or extension. Patients with acromegaly are at particularly increased risk for being difficult to ventilate and intubate. Chronic excess of growth hormone causes nasal and pharyngeal tissue hypertrophy, macroglossia, glossoptosis, and mandibular prognathism. Generalized airway swelling, an enlarged epiglottis, glottic narrowing, and recurrent laryngeal nerve dysfunction may also be present and could cause baseline hoarseness. Anesthesiologists should consider obtaining additional airway imaging in presence of dyspnea, orthopnea, stridor, or hoarseness. If above signs or symptoms of a potentially difficult airway are present, consider an awake intubation. Even when intubating asymptomatic acromegalics with a normal airway exam, it may be prudent to have emergency airway equipment available including oral and nasal airways, laryngeal mask airways (LMA), video laryngoscopes, fiber-optic bronchoscopes, and even a cricothyrotomy kit. Although Cushing's disease is not associated with a difficult airway, these patients may still be difficult to ventilate and intubate due to OSA and obesity.

Endocrine

Some of the patients presenting for skull base reconstruction may have previously undergone resection of a pituitary adenoma. It is important to understand the pathophysiology of these tumors as they can have major systemic effects via hormone secretion or mass effect. Patients should have serum and urine pituitary, thyroid, and adrenal hormone levels checked. Hypofunctioning hormones should be adequately replaced, and some functional adenomas may be medically treated while awaiting surgical resection. Additionally, in the presence of a pituitary adenoma, multiple endocrine neoplasia type 1 (MEN1) should be kept on the differential.

Functional (Hormone Secreting) Tumors

These pituitary adenomas primarily cause symptoms by the effects of the hormones they secrete. If they grow large enough, mass effect may also be seen.

Growth Hormone

Excess of this hormone in childhood causes gigantism (tall stature) and in adulthood causes acromegaly (increased growth of head and extremities) due to enlargement of the bone, connective tissue, and viscera. Besides potential difficult airway and cardiovascular complications, as mentioned earlier in this chapter, these patients may also have abnormal glucose tolerance, osteoarthritis, and increased sweating.

Adrenocorticotropic Hormone (ACTH)

Tumors secreting this hormone cause Cushing's disease by way of increased cortisol production by the adrenal cortex. In addition to the earlier mentioned cardiopulmonary complications of the condition, these patients can present with an increased intravascular volume, electrolyte abnormalities, and diabetes. Other manifestations of this disease include central obesity, proximal skeletal muscle weakness, fragile skin and veins, and abnormal wound healing. Therefore, the anesthesiologist must anticipate unpredictable effects of neuromuscular blockers, potentially difficult intravenous (IV) access, and increased infection risk.

Thyroid Secreting Hormone

These adenomas usually cause no symptoms but may occasionally cause hyperthyroidism or even thyrotoxicosis. Patients should be made euthyroid prior to surgery.

Prolactin

While this is the most common type of pituitary adenoma, its manifestations are the least likely to cause problems for the anesthesiologist. Symptoms can include galactorrhea, amenorrhea, infertility, and decreased libido.

Nonfunctional Tumors

Tumors that are not secreting hormones can still cause problems if they grow large enough to compress nearby structures like vessels and cranial nerves. Particularly large pituitary adenomas may even obstruct CSF drainage causing hydrocephalus and increasing ICP.

Hypopituitarism

This can be caused by tumor compression of the entire pituitary gland or its communication pathway with the hypothalamus. These patients lack all pituitary originating hormones and should be treated with pituitary replacement in the form of glucocorticoids, vasopressin, and thyroxine. Sensitivity to anesthesthetic drugs and need for extra vasopressor support are frequently seen in this population.

Visual Defects

Tumor compression of the optic chiasm most often causes bitemporal hemianopia. A careful preoperative visual field exam is imperative to be able to differentiate from other causes of potential perioperative visual disturbance.

Laboratory

In general, preoperative labs should only be obtained if an abnormal result is expected and if it will change management. A basic metabolic panel will be useful in patients on diuretics or with Cushing's disease as they may have significant electrolyte abnormalities. If a patient is anemic, has a bleeding disorder, or uses anticoagulants or large-volume blood loss is expected, baseline hemoglobin, coagulation studies, and platelet count would be valuable. A blood type and screen or cross-match should be obtained dependent on the likelihood of transfusion.

Anesthetic Management

Premedication

Administering sedating medications immediately preoperatively can benefit patients by reducing their anxiety and lowering potential sympathetic surge. However, many such medications can cause respiratory depression. This can be dangerous in patients with high ICP which would increase further from hypoventilation. Caution must also be used in acromegalics and any patients with OSA who have an increased risk of airway obstruction with such medications.

Induction

Standard IV anesthetic induction technique is appropriate without the presence of a difficult airway or increased ICP. In the setting of increased ICP, take extra caution to preserve normal systemic blood pressure and cerebral perfusion.

Airway Planning

Because most neurosurgical cases require general anesthesia with the head turned away from the anesthesiologist and secured in a particular position, an endotracheal tube is most often placed. Consider awake fiber-optic intubation with local anesthesia if anticipating difficult ventilation or intubation based on physical exam and history. The endotracheal tube should generally be secured in a direction away from the operative site. A wire-reinforced endotracheal tube may be used as it will be more resistant to kinking which can occur with certain degrees of neck rotation and flexion. If high peak pressures and/or an obstructive end-tidal carbon dioxide (CO_2) tracing is noted during a case, endotracheal tube obstruction must be ruled out. A suction catheter should pass freely through the endotracheal tube. If resistance is met, the surgeon should be notified that the endotracheal tube or neck must be repositioned.

Ventilation

Patients are usually ventilated with a controlled ventilator mode, and normocapnia is maintained. However, the end-tidal CO_2 goal can vary depending on the surgical approach. Maintaining normal tidal volumes of 6–8 ml/kg of ideal body weight, low airway pressures, and physiologic positive end expiratory pressure (PEEP) will promote normal brain venous drainage. Following are two examples of different ventilation goals to aid the surgeon.

Transsphenoidal Approach

This particular surgical approach usually requires mild permissive hypercapnia and intermittent Valsalva maneuvers. These techniques increase intracranial vascular volume and thus keep the sella sunken down and in good surgical view.

Retrosigmoid Approach

Surgeons may request hyperventilation to promote brain vasoconstriction which improves surgical visualization when operating in a small space.

Monitors

Standard American Society of Anesthesia monitors should be used in every anesthesia case, and this includes pulse oximetry, end-tidal CO_2 analysis, electrocardiogram, noninvasive blood pressure, and temperature monitoring. Additional monitors may be used depending on patient comorbidities and nature of surgery.

Arterial Blood Pressure

An anesthesiologist may elect to place this invasive catheter if rapid hemodynamic changes are expected such as brisk large-volume bleeding or the eliciting of the trigeminal cardiac reflex. It may also be warranted in a patient with a history of significant cardiac disease or a hemodynamically unstable patient from hypovolemia or septic shock. Furthermore, invasive blood pressure monitoring is useful if strict blood pressure control is necessary like when operating on an aneurysm. Of note, in acromegaly, the carpal ligament is often hypertrophied and may compress the ulnar artery. Allen's test, to confirm dual arterial blood supply of the hand, should absolutely be performed prior to radial artery cannulation in these patients.

Central Venous Pressure

This parameter may be useful to monitor based on patient comorbidities such as the presence of congestive heart failure. A specialized multiorifice central venous catheter may also be placed in patients at high risk for a VAE to be able to aspirate air if the embolism occurs.

Urine Output

This can provide information about renal function, volume status, and the presence of conditions such as diabetes insipidus (DI) or cerebral salt wasting syndrome (CSWS). Urine output should be monitored in longer surgeries and if large-volume resuscitation is anticipated.

Lumbar Drain

The provider may place this device to simultaneously monitor and manage ICP. Controlling ICP by removal or infusion of fluid could help to improve surgical visualization.

Vascular Access

Access should be established according to the expected need for large-volume resuscitation and prolonged administration of inotropes or vasopressors. Usually, one large bore IV line is adequate; however if significant bleeding is expected, it may be prudent to obtain additional access.

Positioning

Neurosurgical positioning can present many challenges to the anesthesiologist. Patients are often positioned 90–180 degrees away, significantly limiting access to the airway. Certain degrees of neck extension, flexion, and rotation can cause endotracheal tube kinking especially after the patient's body warmth softens it. Consider using the much more bend-resistant wire reinforced endotracheal tube in these situations. Because post intubation changes in head and neck position can advance or withdraw the endotracheal tube, its location should be confirmed after final positioning. All pressure points must be carefully padded and limbs positioned in a way to prevent peripheral nerve injury. Proper positioning should be periodically checked throughout the case as body parts can move with table position change. Special attention should also be paid to preventing patient movement, especially in the setting of microscopic dissection or operation near fragile vascular structures. To this end, the blood pressure cuff should ideally be placed away from the surgeon and the table adjusted only with the surgeon's notification. There are several unique positions used in skull base reconstruction surgery which present their own challenges.

Supine

This position is least likely to be associated with position-related injury. However, areas for concern include pressure injuries in heels, sacrum, and occiput.

Lateral

This approach can cause brachial plexus injury on the operative side secondary to contralateral head rotation, elevation of the ipsilateral shoulder, and ipsilateral arm downward traction. If the neck is excessively flexed, nerve over-stretching can cause cervical cord ischemia and even quadriplegia. Improper neck flexion can also impair venous drainage from the head and result in facial and glossal edema potentially precluding extubation for fear of airway obstruction. A gap of at least 1 inch should be maintained between the chin and suprasternal notch at all times to prevent these complications. Increased ventilation perfusion mismatch occurs in the lateral position, and this cause must be considered if oxygenation or ventilation problems arise.

Sitting

Sitting position causes the most hemodynamic changes secondary to reduced venous return to the heart from the limbs and torso. This may be circumvented by wrapping the lower extremities with elastic bandages to promote venous return, IV fluid administration to increase the vascular volume, and administration of vasopressors. Ideally this position is avoided in patients with reduced cardiac function and hypovolemia. Like lateral, the sitting position also increases risk of face and tongue swelling and cervical cord ischemia.

Prone

Because this position limits airway access the most, the endotracheal tube should be properly secured before positioning. Prone position also increases risk for blindness from direct orbital compression, retinal ischemia, or ischemic optic neuropathy. It should be checked that the eyes are free of pressure immediately after positioning and periodically throughout surgery. It is imperative that other pressure points are padded, including knees, iliac crests, genitals, breasts, and entire face. The abdomen must also remain without pressure to allow for respiration.

Anesthetic Choice

The ideal neurosurgery anesthetic is rapidly metabolized and eliminated to allow for a prompt postoperative neurological exam. To this end, anesthesia can be maintained with a low blood gas solubility inhalational anesthetic or IV agent like propofol supplemented with an opioid. Nitrous oxide is best avoided due to its property of rapid diffusion out of the blood into enclosed spaces and thus the potential risk of pneumocephalus. If Mayfield pins are used or microscopic surgery is performed, a completely still operating field is imperative. This can be achieved with adequate anesthesia or neuromuscular blockade. Neuromuscular blocker should be titrated to train-of-four testing in the setting of possible muscle weakness such as with Cushing's disease.

Blood Pressure and Fluid Management

Neurosurgical patient fluid management goals include maintaining euvolemia and adequate cerebral perfusion while avoiding cerebral edema. Hypoosmolar solutions should not be used because when administered in large volumes they reduce serum osmolality and cause fluid to shift to the intracerebral space. Fluids should be given to replace bleeding, insensible losses, and urine output.

Analgesia

Multimodal anesthesia should be instituted whenever possible. The surgeon should administer subcutaneous long-acting local anesthetic before making incision and re-administer it at the end of the surgery if enough time has elapsed for the effect to wear off. The total amount of local anesthetic administered by the surgeon and anesthesiologist should be communicated to avoid local anesthetic toxicity. Acetaminophen can be given preoperatively and re-dosed if not contraindicated based on comorbidities. If there is major concern for postoperative respiratory depression, an ultra-short-acting opioid like remifentanil can be administered intraoperatively. In most cases, it is appropriate to give a long-acting opioid before or shortly after emergence especially if only an ultra-short-acting opioid was used intraoperatively.

Antiemetic Plan

All patients should receive aggressive nausea and vomiting prophylaxis to avoid increasing ICP and potentially disrupting the reconstruction with retching. Of all the surgical approaches, lateral rectosigmoid craniotomies carry the greatest risk for postoperative emesis. Avoid anti-dopaminergic antiemetics like haloperidol, droperidol, metoclopramide, promethazine, and prochlorperazine in patients who may be taking dopamine agonist medications.

Unique Considerations

Transsphenoidal Approach

This surgical approach poses several unique challenges to the anesthesiologist.

Intranasal Pathway

Because the nasal cavity is highly vascularized, a topical intranasal vasoconstrictor like epinephrine or cocaine is frequently applied by the surgeon to reduce bleeding. Vascular absorption of this medication can cause rapid-onset intense systemic hypertension, arrhythmias, and possibly myocardial ischemia. The anesthesiologist must be vigilant during this time and treat the hemodynamic changes with short-acting medication if needed or wait it out if tolerated by the patient as the stimulus will only be present a short time. Despite local anesthetic application, this surgical approach can be extremely stimulating and may cause significant hypertension and increased ICP despite seemingly adequate anesthesia. The anesthesiologist can consider using an ultra-short-acting opioid or short-acting antihypertensive.

Sella Position

The anesthesiologist can perform several maneuvers to assist the surgeon in keeping the sella in good surgical view by slightly increasing ICP. Mild hypoventilation causes arterial vasodilation, while jugular compression and Valsalva maneuver increase intracranial venous pressure. Administration of intrathecal saline via a catheter would increase the CSF space pressure.

Bleeding

A throat pack may be placed by the surgeon for the duration of surgery to reduce the accumulation of gastric blood which can be significantly emetogenic. Careful vigilance must be taken to ensure removal of this item before emergence to prevent airway obstruction. Because the operative field is next to the carotid artery and cavernous sinus, rapid large-volume bleeding can occur suddenly. It is prudent to have adequate venous access and be prepared to transfuse blood if indicated.

Reduction of ICP

The goal of this is to improve surgical visualization for certain approaches and to reduce pressure-related ischemia. Simple measures include elevating the head of the bed to 30 degrees, maintaining normothermia, avoiding hyponatremia, and ensuring adequate sedation and pain control. Venous drainage can be optimized by upright head position, keeping neck veins free from compression and using low airway pressures and no or low PEEP. Hyperventilation may be used to promote neurovascular constriction, while diuretics and osmotherapy can be used to decrease intravascular volume. If present, hyponatremia can be aggressively treated with hypertonic saline. Furthermore, sedatives like propofol can be administered to quickly but temporarily reduce cerebral blood flow. Steroids are also used to help reduce swelling caused by vasogenic edema.

Neuroprotection

In the event of decreased oxygen supply to the brain such as during carotid artery occlusion, several steps are taken to increase brain oxygen delivery and reduce its demand. Crystalloid administration increases blood flow by decreasing blood viscosity as supported by Poiseuille's law. A hematocrit of approximately 30 is usually an appropriate target. Vasopressors should be administered to keep blood pressure 10–15% above baseline. Normoglycemia and hypothermia to 34 degrees Celsius should be maintained. Hypnotic agents can also be given to reduce brain metabolic activity.

Venous Air Embolism

This phenomenon occurs when air is entrained into the venous system and then travels to the right heart and potentially reduces or entirely blocks blood flow. The sitting and park bench positions particularly increase risk of VAE due to a lower venous pressure at the operative site because of its location above the heart. The anesthesiologist may be able to reduce this risk by several techniques that all increase venous pressure. Administering IV fluids and the use of PEEP will both increase central venous pressure. Of note, conversely, the release of PEEP poses an increased VAE risk due to the pressure changes. Moderate hypoventilation increases venous pressure by arterial vasodilation and increasing cerebral blood flow. However, this technique could worsen surgical exposure by increasing ICP and so may be controversial. If a VAE does occur, the anesthesiologist may notice a sudden decrease in end-tidal CO_2, hypoxia, and potentially cardiovascular collapse if the embolism is large enough. The first step of treatment involves immediate flooding of the surgical field with saline; thus it must always be readily available in surgeries carrying this risk. Other treatment includes administration of 100% FiO_2, jugular vein compression, lowering of the head, and placement of the patient in the left lateral position to displace the air from the right ventricular outflow tract. If cardiovascular collapse occurs, prompt initiation of advanced cardiovascular life support is imperative.

Emergence

Emergence from anesthesia and extubation is a critical time for the anesthesiologist with the potential for several complications. Ideally, this should occur timely, in order to perform an immediate postoperative neurologic assessment. However, emergence should also happen without coughing or bucking to prevent increasing ICP and potentially disrupting the reconstruction. Antihypertensive agents may need to be administered at this time to blunt the sympathetic reactivity. A deep extubation, which is performed with the patient adequately anesthetized, would prevent straining, although this may want to be avoided to ensure a normal neurologic exam prior to extubation. Also, caution must be taken with extubation if there is concern for cranial nerve damage which could impair airway reflexes or if there is presence of facial or tongue swelling. Transtracheal or IV lidocaine, small doses of opioids, or dexmedetomidine can help to facilitate a smooth yet awake extubation by blunting the patient's reaction to the presence of the endotracheal tube. Causes of a delayed emergence can include pharmacologic, metabolic, or intracranial pathology such as seizure, stroke, or bleeding and should be worked up immediately.

Extubation Criteria

Patients should only be extubated if extubation criteria are met. This reduces the chances of reintubation and of needing significant ventilatory or oxygen support. There should also be no major active surgical complications such as uncontrolled bleeding.

Neurologic

Ideally, patients should be at their baseline neurologic status and able to follow simple commands.

Airway and Pulmonary

Patients must keep their oxygen saturation and end-tidal CO_2 close to normal or baseline with minimal supplemental oxygen and ventilatory support. They should have a patent airway, strong cough, and intact airway reflexes and be swallowing their secretions. A leak should also be present around the endotracheal tube cuff at pressure below 20 cmH$_2$O with the cuff deflated. This must be checked in cases where surgical trauma may have caused airway tissue edema. Neuromuscular blockade should be reversed.

Cardiovascular

The heart rate and rhythm should be normal or baseline and not cause hemodynamic instability. Patients should not be on high or escalating doses of inotropes or vasopressors which could indicate tissue ischemia and impending decompensation in mental and respiratory status.

Normothermia

Patients need to have a normal core temperature.

Transsphenoidal Approach

Because this unique surgical approach involves the airway, it demands several extra precautions at time of extubation. Nasal packs are sometimes placed by the surgeon at the end of the case, and they may eliminate or limit breathing through the nose. Extubation should be performed when the patient is awake and able to maintain a patent airway. This is especially important because post extubation positive pressure ventilation with a face mask and the use of nasal airway devices must be avoided to prevent disrupting the surgical closure. If post extubation airway support is needed, an oropharyngeal airway or LMA can be used safely. An orogastric tube should also be used to empty the stomach of blood prior to extubation and the oropharynx suctioned well.

How to Handle Failed Extubation

When extubating patients at high risk for reintubation, consider placing an airway exchange catheter into the trachea prior to extubation. This provides a conduit to administer oxygen and a guide for an expedited reintubation.

Postoperative Care

The goals of postoperative care include close monitoring for complications, maintenance of cardiopulmonary stability, and prevention and treatment of pain and nausea. Continuing to prevent increases in ICP is imperative in the PACU where patients may become hypertensive secondary to pain, emesis, agitation, or delirium. The primary team should be made aware of any major changes in patient clinical status or any complications requiring prompt surgical re-exploration.

Monitoring

All patients should be frequently monitored for changes in mental status and neurologic exam. Cardiac rhythm and systemic blood pressure should be monitored as perioperative cardiovascular events can occur postoperatively. To prevent increasing ICP, keep the patient's head upright and administer antihypertensive medication if needed to maintain normotension. Avoid using vasodilators like nitroprusside, nitroglycerine, hydralazine, and calcium channel blockers to control the blood pressure as these agents actually increase cerebral blood flow. Oxygenation and ventilation must be continuously monitored and extra vigilance taken if the surgical approach involved the airway. Consider checking urine output and electrolytes if large-volume shifts are expected. Hemoglobin, platelets, and coagulation panel may be checked if there is concern for bleeding or coagulopathy.

Pain

Pain must be adequately controlled to prevent hypertension and tachycardia, which could put pressure on the reconstruction site and raise ICP. A multimodal pain regimen including non-opioids is best as long as there are no contraindications. Opioids must be carefully titrated to prevent respiratory depression, hypercapnia, and intracranial vasodilation. Consider administering an opioid reversal agent if an overdose is suspected.

Nausea

Aggressive antiemesis treatment must continue in the PACU as retching and vomiting will increase ICP and potentially disrupt the surgical repair. Certain antiemetics can cause sedation, especially when administered simultaneously with opioids.

Complications

Neurologic

Altered mental status, new neurologic deficit, or delayed emergence from anesthesia warrant immediate workup. Differential includes pharmacologic, metabolic, or intracranial causes. Consider prompt head imaging to look for bleeding or edema. If visual defects occur immediately postoperatively, they are usually caused by bleeding and hematoma development requiring emergent surgical exploration. If visual changes occur later, they are usually caused by edema which is treated with supportive care.

Pulmonary

Airway obstruction can occur from oversedation, hematoma formation, edema, or a retained surgical sponge. Administer reversal for any sedating agents if suspected. Inspect the airway for bleeding, secretions, or retained surgical equipment, and remove if possible. Attempt to relieve obstruction with head and neck position change, jaw thrust, or oral airways.

Bleeding

Superficial bleeding can occur at skin incisions or within the nasal mucosa. Bleeding in these locations usually will not cause hypovolemia or require transfusion. The more concerning intracranial bleeding can cause different symptoms depending on the location. A hematoma around the carotid artery can result in a stroke or increase ICP. An optic chiasm hematoma will immediately affect visual fields. Intracranial bleeding and hematomas require prompt imaging and may need emergent surgical evacuation.

CSF Leak

Postoperative rhinorrhea may be the first sign of this complication. The fluid should be tested for glucose, and concentration >30 mg/ml is consistent with CSF. Nasal mucus would not contain glucose. If left untreated, a CSF leak could cause tension pneumocephalus or meningitis. Treatment includes replacement of fat graft and possibly lumbar drain to decrease pressure on the repair.

Endocrine

Hypothalamic-pituitary axis malfunction can occur postoperatively and should be promptly diagnosed and treated. ACTH deficiency creates a cortisol deficit resulting in hypotension and potassium and sodium abnormalities. This is treated with hydrocortisone. Neurogenic DI, caused by decreased antidiuretic (ADH) hormone release, can occur in the first day after surgery and results in increased renal water loss. Electrolytes should be monitored and volume loss replaced with hypotonic fluid. Desmopressin is reserved for severe cases. Syndrome of inappropriate ADH release usually does not happen until 7 days postoperatively and is treated with fluid restriction.

Disposition

Intensive Care Unit (ICU)

Patients requiring frequent neurologic status monitoring or those with new neurologic deficits should be treated in a critical care unit. Hemodynamically unstable patients should also be admitted to the ICU for prompt resuscitation and titration of inotropes or vasopressors. Intubated patients or those with a tenuous airway also require close observation. Acromegalics and any patients at risk for OSA should be closely monitored in ICU for at least the first 24 h postoperatively.

Step Down Unit

This level of care is appropriate for patients who are currently stable but at moderate risk for deterioration in clinical status necessitating relatively frequent monitoring.

Patients not meeting the above criteria can recover safely in a regular postsurgical unit.

Recommended Reading

1. Amorocho MC, Fat I. Anesthetic techniques in endoscopic sinus and Skull Base surgery. Otolaryngol Clin N Am. 2016;49(3):531–47. https://www.sciencedirect.com/science/article/pii/S0030666516000335?via%3Dihub

2. Barash PG, Cullen BF, Stoelting RK, Cahalan MK, Stock MC, Ortega RA, et al. Anesthesia for neurosurgery. In: Clinical anesthesia. Philadelphia, PA: Wolters Kluwer; 2017. p. 1005–25.
3. Butterworth JF, Mackey DC, Wasnick JD. Anesthesia for neurosurgery. In: Morgan & Mikhail's clinical anesthesiology. New York, NY: McGraw-Hill Education; 2018. p. 593–611.
4. Ditzel Filho LFS, Prevedello DM, Patel MR, et al. Perioperative considerations: planning, intraoperative and postoperative management. Curr Otorhinolaryngol Rep. 2013;1:183–90. https://doi.org/10.1007/s40136-013-0030-9.
5. Dohi S. Perioperative challenges during pituitary surgery. In: Essentials of Neurosurgical Anesthesia & Critical Care. New York, NY: Springer; 2012. https://doi.org/10.1007/978-0-387-09562-2_25.
6. Horvat A, Kolak J, Gopcević A, Ilej M, Zivko G. Anesthetic management of patients undergoing pituitary surgery. Acta Clin Croat. 2011;50(2):209–16. https://core.ac.uk/download/pdf/14446753.pdf
7. Iida H. Anesthesia for pituitary surgery. In: Neuroanesthesia and cerebrospinal protection. Tokyo: Springer Japan; 2015. https://link.springer.com/chapter/10.1007/978-4-431-54490-6_38.
8. Jaffe RA, Schmiesing CA, Golianu B. Transsphenoidal resection of pituitary tumor. In: Anesthesiologist's manual of surgical procedures. Philadelphia, PA: Wolters Kluwer; 2020. p. 132–40.
9. Jellish WS, Murdoch J, Leonetti JP. Perioperative management of complex skull base surgery: the anesthesiologist's point of view. Neurosurg Focus. 2002;12(5):e5. https://thejns.org/focus/view/journals/neurosurg-focus/12/5/foc.2002.12.5.6.xml?body=pdf-16286
10. Nekhendzy V. Anesthesia for head and neck surgery. UpToDate https://www.uptodate.com/contents/anesthesia-for-head-and-neck-surgery
11. Paisansathan C, Ozcan M. Anesthesia for craniotomy. UpToDate. https://www.uptodate.com/contents/anesthesia-for-craniotomy
12. Schott M, Suhr D, Jantzen JPAH. Perioperative challenges during posterior fossa surgery. In: Essentials of neurosurgical anesthesia & critical care. New York, NY: Springer; 2012. https://doi.org/10.1007/978-0-387-09562-2_22.
13. Sekimoto K, Takazawa T. Anesthesia for posterior fossa tumor surgery. In: Neuroanesthesia and cerebrospinal protection. Tokyo: Springer Japan; 2015. https://doi.org/10.1007/978-4-431-54490-6_31.

Chapter 9
Allografts and Materials in Skull Base Reconstruction

C. Eric Bailey and Christopher H. Le

Introduction

While vascularized flaps have become standard for reconstruction of skull base defects with higher CSF flow or larger size [1], many materials have been used for repair of smaller or less complex defects, either as free grafts, as part of multilayer repairs, or as adjuncts for vascularized flaps. Materials may be divided into those derived from patient tissues (autologous) or from synthetic sources (non-autologous) [2]. Autologous materials include fat [3–8], free mucosal grafts [9–11], bone [12, 13], septal cartilage [5], and fascia lata [14, 15]. Alloderm [LifeCell, Branchburg, NJ, USA] [6, 11, 15], Gelfoam [Pfizer, New York, NY, USA] [3, 6], porcine small intestine submucosal grafts [16], polydioxanone [17–20], poly(D,L)lactide acid plate [21, 22], and collagen matrix [11] are non-autologous materials which have been used, occasionally in combination with sealants [23–28] or various packing materials for supporting reconstructions. While the relative lack of prospective comparisons, predominantly retrospective nature of available literature, and the use of materials in multiple combinations limit the ability to directly compare success rates for different materials, this chapter will review the autologous and non-autologous materials in widespread use for skull base reconstruction and the available data for their use.

Commercial products mentioned in this chapter are not intended to represent an endorsement of the product but are merely used to describe the specific formulation of materials used in the various studies reviewed.

C. E. Bailey · C. H. Le (✉)
Department of Otolaryngology, University of Arizona, Tucson, AZ, USA
e-mail: cebailey@hsc.wvu.edu; chle@oto.arizona.edu

© The Author(s), under exclusive license to Springer Nature Switzerland AG 2023
E. C. Kuan et al. (eds.), *Skull Base Reconstruction*,
https://doi.org/10.1007/978-3-031-27937-9_9

Autologous Grafts

Autologous graft materials are those which are derived from the patient's own tissues. Many autologous materials have been used for endonasal endoscopic repair of skull base defects, including fat [3–8], free mucosal grafts [9–11], bone [12, 13], septal cartilage [5], and fascia lata [14, 15].

Early techniques for repair of CSF fistula utilized autologous free grafts [29, 30], and autologous free grafts continue to be a viable option with good outcomes for small anterior skull base or sellar defects with low-flow CSF leaks [2, 31]. A recent meta-analysis and systematic review evaluated the effect of graft type on surgical outcomes and compared postoperative CSF leak rate, meningitis, and other major complications utilizing autologous vs. non-autologous grafts. In order to prevent confounding effects, studies utilizing both autologous and non-autologous grafts in combination or those using vascularized flaps were excluded. The authors identified 29 studies which met their inclusion criteria, including 1779 patients with repairs utilizing autologous grafts and 496 patients with repairs with non-autologous grafts. Among studies in which sufficient outcome data was available for adjusted systematic review, there were no significant differences in CSF leak rate between autologous and non-autologous materials. The rate of meningitis was lower for non-autologous materials. However, it is unclear whether this difference is related to graft type or to other factors such as lumbar drain placement [2]. The similar success rate between autologous and non-autologous grafts supports the findings of a previous systematic review [32], which also included studies that combined autologous and non-autologous grafts in multilayer repairs. High success rates have been reported whether the comparisons utilized allograft vs. xenograft or a combination of both [6, 14, 16, 33, 34].

While harvest of some autologous graft materials such as abdominal fat, fascia lata, split calvarial bone, or conchal cartilage requires a separate donor site with associated morbidity, other autologous materials such as free mucosal grafts, septal bone, and septal cartilage are readily available in the nasal cavity, precluding need for additional donor site, which negates one potential advantage of synthetic materials or xenografts (Table 9.1). Compared to synthetic materials or xenografts, autologous grafts have minimal cost aside from time required to harvest. Autologous grafts also have the potential for rapid rates of healing and integration into surrounding tissue. Experiments with free mucosal grafts demonstrated microscopic re-epithelialization by 12 days postoperatively, with adherence to the skull base surrounding the defect by the sixth postoperative day [35]. The biocompatibility of autografts can be beneficial in patients in whom long-term imaging follow-up is necessary, as decreased local inflammatory response may make interpretation of follow-up imaging more accurate [36].

Autologous grafts are not without disadvantages, however. Donor site morbidity must be considered in grafts which require a separate donor site [37], and while grafts harvested from the nasal cavity avoid a separate donor site, there can still be

Table 9.1 Sources of autologous free tissue grafts

Autologous free grafts from sinonasal cavity
Middle turbinate mucosa
Nasal floor mucosa
Inferior turbinate mucosa
Septal cartilage
Septal bone
Autologous free grafts from distant sites
Fascia lata
Conchal cartilage
Abdominal fat
Bone (mastoid, split calvarial)

significant crusting from the area of harvest. The amount of graft material may also be limited [36], particularly in the setting of revision surgery. The following sections will review individual autologous materials and the literature regarding their use in skull base reconstruction.

Fat

Fat grafts have a long history of use in skull base reconstruction. Fat is typically harvested from an abdominal donor site. The most common uses for fat autografts are to obliterate dead space in large resection cavities [37] in preparation for placement of other grafts [38] or in smaller areas such as the sella when there is a low-flow CSF leak [13]. Autologous dermal-fat graft composites have also been used and are reported to allow for easier manipulation of the fat graft [39]. Fat has also been used as a repair graft for small (<1 cm) low-flow intraoperative CSF leaks as an inlay graft or using a "bath plug" technique [1, 40, 41], whereby fat secured with suture was placed intracranially, with retraction on the suture to ensure snug fit prior to securing the fat with fibrin glue [42]. Interestingly, in one ex vivo porcine model, the "bath plug" technique performed favorably compared to standard fat graft or autologous mucosa overlay with Tisseel (Baxter Healthcare Corp, Deerfield, IL, USA) when tested for mean failure pressure. The "bath plug" technique was the only one of the three tested techniques that withstood adult physiologic supine cerebrospinal fluid (CSF) pressure [43].

An evidence-based review suggested that fat grafts are a good option for repair of many skull base defects with fistula closure rates from 82% to 100% [32], although it is noted that one of the cited studies found higher rates of meningitis and persistent CSF leak in patients who had fat and free mucosal graft closure for high-flow leaks compared to multilayer repair using fascia overlay and bone buttress

[44]. Similarly, a study published subsequent to this review reported a series of 551 endonasal endoscopic approaches for pituitary and parasellar tumors using abdominal fat to obliterate dead space prior to multilayer repairs. Moderate and high-flow CSF leaks were repaired in layered fashion, utilizing fat in the sella, suprasellar space, or clivus, respectively, before collagen matrix, bone or synthetic rigid buttress, and additional fat, collagen sponge, or nasoseptal flap. Postoperative leak rate for this repair type was 3.1% for moderate leaks and 4.8% for high-flow leaks [13]. Sanders-Taylor et al. described a series of 235 patients with sellar repair using fat to obliterate the sellar defect, prior to placement of septal bone or cartilage and biological glue with absorbable packing for reinforcement. Delayed CSF leak was reported to be 1.7%, with one patient requiring revision surgery [5]. A recent case series reported reconstruction of sellar defects in 380 patients with a combination of free abdominal fat graft with a synthetic plate or autologous cartilage or bone for reconstruction of the sellar floor. In this series, the indication for fat grafting was observed intraoperative CSF leak in 87% of cases; the remainder of cases used fat graft for closure of dead space, in the absence of observed CSF leak. The authors reported a 3.7% rate of persistent CSF leak requiring revision surgery. The rate of abdominal donor site complication was 1.1%. One weakness of this study is that categorization of CSF leak was not reported [8].

While most series report use of fat autografts for closure of dead space in preparation for multilayer repair, one case series reported the use of en bloc fat graft for repair of large anterior skull base defects following transcribriform endoscopic endonasal approach (EEA) for malignant skull base lesions. The repair of all defects ($n = 29$) was performed utilizing a single layer of autologous abdominal fat, supported in position by the surgeon until placement of fibrin glue. Subsequently, a bolster of silastic sheeting and non-absorbable nasal packs was placed. The mean defect size was reported to be 4.47 ± 2.9 cm^2. The authors report a 3.5% rate (one patient) of postoperative CSF leak which resolved with conservative management, as well as two cases (6.9%) of confirmed bacterial meningitis [7].

Advantages of using autologous fat are that it is readily available and has low cost. It does, however, have the disadvantage that a separate, non-regional harvest site is necessary, with potential for hematoma, seroma, or wound infection [39]. A separate issue is that fat also has a significant degree of atrophy with exposure to aerated sinus [3], which could potentially lead to graft failure. This is less of a concern when fat is used for closure of dead space or to bolster an overlay graft, but must be considered if fat is being used as a primary repair material.

Fascia Lata

Fascia lata has also seen widespread use as an autologous graft material for skull base reconstruction. The lack of an epithelial surface makes it suitable for inlay grafting [31] or onlay grafting [37]. The primary disadvantages of fascia lata are the need for a separate incision for harvest and the potential for postoperative complications, particularly in physically active patients [37]. Fascia lata has been suggested to be a suitable alternative to vascularized flaps for low-flow CSF leaks [1]. A fascia lata button technique has also been described for high-flow CSF leaks resulting from open cistern communication. This technique involves suturing two pieces of fascia lata together, which serve as a combined inlay/onlay graft. The inlay graft is approximately 30% larger than the defect, while the onlay graft is 5–10% larger than the defect. The authors subsequently placed either a nasoseptal flap or secured the onlay portion in place with biological glue. The authors report a CSF leak rate of 10% for open cistern high-flow CSF leaks using this technique, compared to 45% leak rate for the same patient population previously in their case series using fat obliteration, synthetic dural inlay, and onlay graft [45]. Fascia lata has also been used in combination with numerous other combinations of materials for multilayer repairs [14, 15, 44, 46]. The iliotibial tract, which is a continuation of the fascia lata, has also been described as an alternative source of fascia for repair. In one series of 62 patients who underwent endoscopic endonasal anterior skull base tumor resection that included dural resection, iliotibial tract fascia was used for an intradural layer, followed by another intracranial extradural fascia graft. Fat was used to fill any dead space between this extradural graft and a third extracranial onlay graft of fascia. Each layer was secured with fibrin glue. The authors report a 13% rate of postoperative CSF leak, with three cases that did not respond to conservative management and required revision of repair.

In summary, fascia lata provides a versatile autologous graft option that can be used as the sole repair material or in combination with other materials in multilayer repair or as an inlay graft in combination with vascularized repairs.

Bone

Bone grafts have been utilized for repair of skull base defects to provide rigid support in cases of large anterior skull base defects. Although indications for rigid reconstruction of skull base defects are not clearly defined, bone grafts are a nonsynthetic option for providing rigidity in skull base reconstruction. Bone graft options include both autologous sites such as lamella of middle turbinate [12, 47], vomer or septum [12, 48], mastoid bone [12], frontal bone [12], inferior turbinate bone [12], and non-autologous options such as cadaveric iliac crest [44]. A literature review identified five case series (including Germani et al. and Kong et al. described below) using bone grafts for CSF leak repair, with aggregate evidence of level C supporting use of bone as a graft material [32]. As with all autologous materials, a donor site is required; however, the bone can frequently be harvested locally from the sinonasal cavity precluding need for a separate incision. The numerous available donor sites in the nasal cavity as well as the availability of cadaveric iliac crest negate one of the advantages of synthetic rigid materials in that there is not additional donor site morbidity; however, there is still time required for graft harvest.

Bone grafts have been used in differing ways by many groups. Although not primarily evaluating the use of the bone as a grafting material, Germani et al. reported a series of 55 patients who had repair with a number of different materials. Twelve of these repairs utilized bone grafts of unspecified donor site. The success rate was 83%, with one of the persistent CSF leaks occurring in a patient with a small defect repaired with bone paste. Only one patient required revision surgery [33].

Several groups have suggested "gasket seal" type repairs using a rigid onlay graft approximately the size of the bony skull base defect "countersunk" into an inlay graft. Bone grafts have frequently been used in this reconstructive technique [38, 44, 46, 49]. Leng et al. described the "gasket seal" method in 2008 predominantly in a series of suprasellar and planum sphenoidale defects, and while bone grafts from vomer were used in their initial series, their description does not specify for which patients bone grafts were used as opposed to synthetic rigid materials [46]. Tabaee et al. reported a success rate of 87.5% using fat graft (if no ventricular communication), fascia lata inlay with bone graft onlay for repair of high-volume CSF leaks from suprasellar and anterior cranial fossa defects. Only one patient failed conservative management and required reoperation. The small sample size precluded comparison between repair types within the study. Kong et al. report using the gasket seal technique with cadaveric bone homografts for closure of sellar defects and extra-sellar defects with CSF leaks. Of 29 patients with intraoperative CSF leaks, 93.1% had successful closure of CSF fistula [44].

In a study which evaluated delayed postoperative CT imaging from 44 patients who underwent transsphenoidal sellar and parasellar surgery without bone graft placement, no appreciable bony regrowth over the skull base defect was identified on imaging (average of 12.4 months, range 6–24 months). By contrast, the authors report that among 13 patients who had anterior skull base reconstructions with free bone grafts, 84.6% had at least partial incorporation of the graft into the residual bony skull base on follow-up imaging [12], suggesting that if rigid reconstruction is necessary, free bone grafts may be an attractive option in patients not requiring postoperative radiation.

Different authors report varying indications for use of rigid materials in reconstruction. For repair of encephaloceles, non-traumatic CSF leaks, and meningoceles, Nyquist et al. [50] suggested use of a rigid reconstruction such as the bone with a vascularized flap if the defect size is greater than 1 cm. It is generally agreed that rigid reconstruction of bony skull base defects may be useful for patients with intracranial hypertension [51, 52]. However, concerns have been expressed regarding the use of bone grafts for reconstruction due to the risk of subsequent bony sequestra [53] or the possibility of osteoradionecrosis [54] in patients who may undergo radiation therapy. Others specifically avoid the use of rigid reconstruction with bone or alloplastic materials even in the setting of large defects after endoscopic endonasal tumor resection, due to concerns about infection or migration of the rigid graft [55]. To evaluate the necessity of rigid reconstruction of skull base defects, Eloy et al. evaluated changes in frontal lobe position after transcribriform resection of anterior skull base tumors. Defects were repaired with multilayer closure consisting of autologous fascia lata, acellular dermal allograft, and vascularized nasoseptal flap. Average defect size in their series was 9.3 cm^2. Displacement of the frontal lobe on postoperative imaging (mean follow-up 10.1 months) was compared to preoperative imaging. While there was significant variability in frontal lobe displacement between male and female patients, the mean postoperative frontal lobe displacement was 0.2 mm. The range of displacement of the inferior most portion of the frontal lobe from preoperative position was −3.9 to +2.9 mm, indicating either inferior displacement of the frontal lobes due to gravity or contraction of the graft leading to superior displacement. The authors were careful to mention the limitations of their study and suggest that the findings may not be generalizable to all areas of the anterior skull base or other reconstructive methods, but their findings do suggest that at least some locations of the anterior skull base may not require rigid support if multilayer repair is utilized [15].

Free Mucosa

Similar to bone and fat grafts, free mucosal grafts have a long history of use in skull base repair and closure of CSF fistula. While other reconstruction techniques such as pedicled flaps have gained prominence, free mucosal grafts are a viable option in selected patients. One recently published series reported outcomes of 158 consecutive patients who underwent endoscopic endonasal resection of pituitary adenomas. Nine patients in the series had reconstruction with nasoseptal flap due to opening into the suprasellar cistern during tumor removal. Twenty-seven patients early in the series had collagen matrix inlay with or without extradural onlay of oxidized cellulose. The remaining 122 patients had reconstruction with collagen matrix inlay graft with free mucosal onlay grafting. In the group with free mucosal onlay graft repair, the intraoperative leak rate was 39%, with a postoperative CSF leak rate of 0.82%. Postoperative CSF leak rates for the nasoseptal flap group and the group with collagen matrix inlay alone were 0% and 7.4%, respectively. The authors suggest that free mucosal grafts are an appropriate alternative to nasoseptal flaps for low-flow CSF leak repair in pituitary surgery [56]. Another recent case series reported results with 300 consecutive patients who underwent repair of sellar or parasellar defects. The repair algorithm utilized by the authors included use of free mucosal graft alone (if no intraoperative CSF leak), autologous fat (± rigid fixation with septal bone or resorbable plate) with free mucosal graft if low-flow CSF leak, or autologous fat with nasoseptal flap for high-flow CSF leaks. In the low-flow CSF leak group, which was repaired with free mucosal grafts, the authors report a postoperative CSF leak rate of 1.5%. Their findings in regard to high-flow CSF leaks were in agreement with previously published series, supporting the idea that pedicled flaps have a higher success rate for repair of high-flow CSF leaks [57, 58].

An evidence-based review of management of CSF leaks found 39 studies meeting their inclusion criteria, including one meta-analysis and two systematic reviews. While the overall level of evidence was judged to be low (grade C), there was not a notable difference found between free grafts and vascularized grafts [32]. There were several notable caveats, however. A systematic review by Soudry et al. evaluated repair of skull base defects following endoscopic endonasal skull base resection and identified 22 studies including 673 patients meeting inclusion criteria. The overall postoperative CSF leak rate was found to be 8.5%. Subgroup analysis was performed to evaluate the effect of location and degree of intraoperative CSF leak upon postoperative leak rates, and authors found that separately analyzing the subgroups proved difficult due to inter-relatedness of subsite and CSF leak rate for particular subsites such as tuberculum sella or clivus. The authors concluded that for low-flow CSF leaks (which in their analysis comprised exclusively sellar and parasellar defects), layered repair with free grafts (including mucosal free grafts) and/or synthetic materials resulted in high success rates. Consistent with the previously discussed studies, however, high-flow CSF leaks had better closure rates with vascularized grafts compared to free grafts (94% vs. 82%) [59]. A systematic review by Harvey et al. also supported the use of vascularized flaps for repair of high-flow CSF leaks, but further stratified repairs by the defect size. In 609 patients with large (>3 cm) dural defects from 38 studies, 54% of patients were repaired with free graft reconstruction, while 46% had repair with local or regional vascularized tissue flap. The persistent CSF leak rate for free grafts was reported to be 15.6%, while the leak rate for patients with vascularized repairs was 6.7%. This difference was statistically significant, suggesting that dural defects greater than 3 cm have lower leak rates following vascularized repair [57]. Nevertheless, the literature suggests that for small defects with no CSF leak or low-flow CSF leak, free mucosal grafts provide similar outcomes to vascularized repair.

Advantages of free mucosal grafts are that there is no tethering by the vascular pedicle and that free mucosal grafts are relatively easily harvested [60]. While readily available and frequently used, there are specific precautions relating to use of free mucosal grafts. If the mucosal side of the graft is not placed facing the nasal cavity, poor adherence and mucocele formation may be promoted [37]. This has led some to suggest marking the mucosal surface to prevent inadvertent placement of the mucosal surface facing away from the nasal cavity [52]. Graft size may also be limited by tissue availability. This is an important consideration in revision cases and can be problematic due to contracture of free mucosal grafts, which has been described to result in graft failure if the edge of the graft retracts prior to graft integration [36].

The nasal cavity offers multiple locations for harvest of free mucosal grafts, including the middle turbinate mucosa [9], inferior turbinate mucosa [10] or nasal floor mucosa [56]. Middle turbinate grafts are the most common free mucosal grafts [9], since the middle turbinate has frequently been removed to improve access for extended approaches [61, 62]. As middle turbinate preservation has been demonstrated to be feasible for many approaches [63], alternative sources for free mucosal grafts have been explored such as the nasal floor. An advantage of the nasal floor mucosa graft, include reported greater thickness of the graft compared to middle turbinate mucosa. Disadvantages of the nasal floor graft include transient numbness of the incisors due to injury to the nasopalatine nerve [56].

Tissue Glue

Migration of graft material after placement can lead to persistent CSF fistula. The narrow corridors in endoscopic skull base surgery limits ability to secure with skull base reconstruction material with sutures, and some graft materials are not durable enough for suturing. Accordingly, many surgeons use adjunct methods to stabilize grafts in appropriate position such as tissue sealants. Several types of tissue sealants are commercially available, which can generally be divided into fibrin-based, polyethylene glycol-based, and serum albumin-derived. Fibrin-based sealants include Beriplast (CSL Behring, King of Prussia, PA, USA), Tisseel/ Tissucol (human fibrin cryoprecipitate; Baxter Healthcare Corp, Deerfield, IL, USA), and Tachosil (human fibrin and thrombin-coated equine collagen sponge; Baxter Healthcare Corp, Deerfield, IL, USA). Bioglue (Cryolife, Kennesaw, GA, USA) is a serum albumin-derived sealant. PEG-derived sealants include Duraseal (Integra Life Sciences, Saint Priest, France) and Adherus (Stryker, Kalamazoo, MI USA).

There is data from in vitro and animal studies which suggests that sealants or glues may increase the stability of graft seal. One in vitro study utilizing fresh human cadaver dura tested four varieties of sealants or glues, with results showing that mean pressure at which leakage occurred was significantly increased for all four products, with differing pressures between the tested formulations [64]. In an in vivo porcine model, cribriform defects were created endoscopically and then repaired with free pericranial grafts with or without fibrin glue. The animals were euthanized 7 days postoperatively, and the burst pressure of the repair (hydraulic pressure at which leakage was visualized through the repair) was tested in blinded fashion. The pericranial repairs which included fibrin glue had statistically greater burst pressures and better adherence [65]. Another ex vivo porcine dura model tested the mean failure pressure of collagen matrix underlay grafts combined with polyethylene glycol (PEG) hydrogel sealant, collagen matrix underlay graft with fibrin glue, or fascia lata graft secured to dura with titanium clips. The collagen matrix underlay combined with PEG sealant was found to have significantly higher mean failure pressure than either collagen matrix with fibrin glue or fascia lata with titanium clips. No comparisons were made of the underlay graft mean failure pressure without sealant as a comparator, however [66].

Serum Albumin-Derived Sealants

Several studies have evaluated a bovine serum albumin and glutaraldehyde-based sealant. Some concerns were raised regarding release of glutaraldehyde from the sealant, with one study showing in vitro cytotoxicity in a human and mouse cell line as well as in vivo cytotoxicity in rabbit liver and lung tissue [67]. Another study found granulomatous inflammation at the site of adhesive use in ovine model of bronchial anastomosis and lung parenchymal repair, which was not present with hand-sutured anastomosis and repair [68]. However, an in vivo study in which the sealant was applied directly to rat cerebral cortex, intact pia, and arachnoid mater appeared to prevent inflammation of the brain parenchyma, suggesting that placement as a sealant over onlay grafting would be unlikely to provoke significant cortical inflammatory response [69]. Additional consideration should be given to avoid repetitive exposure to BSA-glutaraldehyde sealant per package insert, due to risk of possible sensitization and anaphylaxis [70].

Kumar et al. describe a prospective study of 32 patients who underwent transnasal transeptal transsphenoidal surgery with sellar reconstruction. Half of the patients had suprasellar extension. All repairs consisted of fat graft to obliterate the resection cavity and autologous bone graft to reconstruct the anterior sellar wall. The repair was then covered with bovine serum albumin-derived sealant and the nasal cavity packed with iodine-impregnated ribbon gauze. Intraoperative CSF leak was observed in nine patients, in whom lumbar CSF diversion was used postoperatively for 48 h. The authors reported no postoperative CSF leaks in this series [71].

Dusick et al. describe an industry-sponsored retrospective cohort study of 282 consecutive patients undergoing endonasal endoscopic sellar or parasellar surgeries, 124 of which had bovine serum albumin-derived sealant used to reinforce repair of intraoperative CSF leak. Repairs consisted of collagen sponge with sealant for reconstruction if no leak was present; titanium mesh sandwiched with collagen sponge inlay and onlay with sealant for low-flow leaks; abdominal fat graft with collagen sponge and intrasellar titanium mesh for moderate leaks; and abdominal fat graft with collagen sponge and intrasellar titanium mesh with 48 h of lumbar drain for large diaphragmatic or dural defects from extended transsphenoidal approaches. Although no control group was included in the study, the authors compare the results with their previously reported results which did not utilize sealant. In patients with low and moderate flow intraoperative CSF leaks, postoperative CSF leak rate was 0% in this series, which is comparable to rates reported in the literature [72]. For 31 patients in this study with high-flow CSF leaks, the rate of postoperative CSF leak was 6.5%, which is lower than the same authors' previously reported rate of 21% [73]. While this may be from beneficial effect of the sealant, it could also be explained by greater surgical experience and improved technique over time.

Fibrin-Derived Sealants

Fibrin-based sealants rely on the activity of thrombin to convert fibrinogen to fibrin. Fibrin-based sealants have been evaluated as replacement for fat or muscle grafts for closure of the sella and parasellar region after sublabial transsphenoidal approach [25, 74]. Seda et al. reported a series 64 patients with intraoperative CSF leak following sublabial transsphenoidal approach who underwent repair using only oxidized cellulose polymer and fibrin sealant. One patient (1.6%) had a postoperative CSF leak, with another patient developing meningitis but no identifiable CSF leak. All patients had lumbar CSF diversion for 5 days postoperatively [74]. As techniques shifted from microsurgical approaches to endoscopic endonasal approaches, interest in the use of sealants as adjuncts in endoscopic repair developed. One early rodent in vivo study evaluated the use of fibrin glue as a substitute for muscle patches or as an adjunct combined with muscle patch repair for experimentally produced cribriform CSF leaks. The authors reported that the control group (no repair) had an 89% rate of persistent CSF leak at 3 weeks. The group repaired with fibrin sealant alone had a 59% CSF leak rate, while the group with muscle patch repair had a 33% rate of CSF leak. The rats treated with muscle patch and fibrin sealant had a 22% rate of persistent CSF leak at 3 weeks [75].

More recent studies have focused on the use of fibrin sealants in multilayer skull base reconstruction. Cappabianca et al. used Tissucol fibrin sealant with or without collagen fleece (combined with a polyester-silicone dural substitute) for closure of sellar defects following endoscopic endonasal transsphenoidal surgery. They found that fibrin sealant with collagen fleece ($n = 13$) had lower rate of CSF leak (0% leak rate) compared to fibrin sealant ($n = 16$) alone (12.5% leak rate). The patients in each group had intraoperative CSF leak. The authors note that CSF diversion via lumbar drain was used when repair was not considered watertight, with extended approach to planum sphenoidale or clivus, or if "copious" CSF leak was noted intraoperatively. In the fibrin sealant group (leak rate of 12.5%), 6 of 16 patients had postoperative CSF diversion, compared to no patients in the collagen fleece + fibrin sealant group (leak rate of 0%) [26]. In another paper, the same group reports the use of fibrin-based sealant in place of autologous fat for filling dead space in the sella prior to multilayer repair in 40 patients with intraoperative CSF leaks. The authors mention that four patients who underwent transsphenoidal surgery had postoperative CSF leaks managed by applications of fibrin glue every 48 h until closure of the fistula, with 1–5 applications [27].

Additionally, Cavallo et al. report the use of repeated applications of fibrin-based sealant Tisseel in nine patients while awake in outpatient OR for CSF leak after extended transsphenoidal surgery as a nonoperative intervention. Four of the patients also required lumbar CSF diversion due to severity of the leak. All patients had undergone multilayer repair at the time of original procedure. The sealant was applied daily in patients with moderate or severe leaks, or every 2–3 days for "weeping" leaks. Sealant was applied between 1 and 5 times. Leaks were diagnosed between POD 3 and POD 33 [76]. A separate group report on a series of 18 consecutive patients with use of fibrin glue and polyglactin acid sheet for repair of CSF leak following endoscopic endonasal pituitary surgery. The authors compare their results to their previous 38 patients treated either with fibrin glue alone or with pedicled mucosal grafts and fibrin glue. In the six patients treated with fibrin glue alone, the postoperative CSF fistula rate was 33.3% (2 leaks), while for the 32 patients with mucosal graft and fibrin glue, the postoperative CSF fistula rate was 15.6%. Among the 18 patients with polyglactin acid sheet and fibrin glue, there were no reported postoperative CSF leaks with 7-month follow-up [77].

While fibrin-based sealants have been widely studied, there are potential concerns with their use. One of these is the potential for spread of infectious disease, as the majority of fibrin-based sealants are derived from pooled human donor plasma [31]. IgE-mediated hypersensitivity reactions and anaphylaxis have also been reported with the use of fibrin-based sealants in other types of surgery [78], reportedly in relation to the bovine protease inhibitor aprotinin [79], which is used to prevent degradation during storage. Aprotinin is used in cardiac surgery as well, and 1 study of 12,403 patients in which aprotinin was used found that even for those previously exposed to aprotinin ($n = 801$), the rate of reactions was 1.5%, with less than half of reactions being severe [80], suggesting that severe reactions would be unlikely with fibrin-based sealants.

PEG-Derived Sealants

Burkett et al. describe a series of 204 consecutive patients undergoing endonasal endoscopic pituitary surgery. The first 107 patients were repaired using fibrin sealant and Gelfoam for grades 0 (no noticeable leak) and 1 CSF leaks (small weeping CSF leak without visible defect). Grade 2 leaks (visible diaphragmatic defect with associated leak) were repaired with fibrin sealant, Gelfoam, abdominal fat graft, nasal packing, and 5 days of lumbar drain. For the second group comprising 97 patients, collagen matrix covered with PEG dural sealant was utilized for grades 0 and 1, while collagen matrix and PEG dural sealant with nasal packing was used for grade 2 CSF leaks. Therefore, in group 2, all repairs incorporated PEG hydrogel sealant. Among the patients whose repairs incorporated PEG dural sealant, overall postoperative CSF leak rate was 1%, representing one patient with grade 2 leak with persistent CSF leak. In group 1, which utilized fibrin sealant, the overall leak rate was 1.9% [24].

In another study of closure of sellar defects following transsphenoidal pituitary surgery, 74 patients with Grade I CSF leaks ("weeping" CSF leak or small arachnoid defect) were repaired with gelatin sponge packing with PEG hydrogel sealant overlay. Reported persistence of CSF leak was 2.7%, with 1.4% incidence of meningitis [81]. A larger study reported outcomes for 250 patients undergoing endoscopic endonasal pituitary surgery. Of these patients, 180 repairs included a PEG hydrogel (Duraseal) sealant and 70 repairs without PEG hydrogel. The leak rate reported between the groups with and without PEG hydrogel was not statistically different. However, in addition to the retrospective nature of the study, interpretation of the results is hampered by the variability in repair materials utilized, including autologous fat, gelatin sponge, gelatin/thrombin foam in addition to the PEG-hydrogel, or fibrin-based sealants, which represented 20 separate combinations of materials reported [82].

PEG hydrogel materials are known to swell with hydration. There have been case reports from neurosurgical literature reporting complications due to this effect when PEG hydrogel materials were used in confined areas [83, 84], leading to caution in the use of hydrogel materials in enclosed areas.

The need for a glue or sealant in all cases has been questions, however. A case-control study comparison was made between patients with high-flow CSF leaks repaired with nasoseptal flap with ($n = 42$) or without ($n = 32$) dural sealant. Dural sealants used included either a polyethylene hydrogel (Duraseal) or a fibrin sealant (Tisseel; or Evicel; Ethicon, Somerville, NJ, USA). The difference in postoperative CSF leak between the groups (0% without sealant and 2.4% with sealant) was not statistically significant. The authors note, however, that in this retrospective study, the proportion of suprasellar/planum sphenoidale defects (an area with potentially greater risk of high-flow CSF leaks) was greater in the group utilizing dural sealant (14 patients) than in the group without sealant (three patients). Still, this retrospective study suggests that sealant may not be necessary with vascularized repairs even for high-flow CSF leaks, although the authors caution that randomized prospective trials are necessary [23].

Homologues and Xenografts

While free grafts with various autologous materials such as mucosa and fascia lata have a long history of use in skull base reconstruction, homologues and xenografts are now frequently used in situations where autologous free grafts would have been used previously. Similar success rates have been reported with allografts or xenografts for repair of CSF leaks [2, 32].

Duragen, Alloderm, and Collagen Matrix

For endoscopic skull base surgery for resection of intracranial lesions requiring resection of dura, subsequent reconstruction of dura is critical. Collagen matrix is often used as an inlay graft in multilayer skull base reconstruction (Fig. 9.1), and a number of dural replacement products based on acellular collagen have been introduced. Duragen (Integra Life Sciences, Princeton, NJ, USA) composed of bovine Achilles tendon [36] has been used as an epidural or subdural inlay graft [39, 85]. Duramatrix (Stryker, Kalamazoo, MI, USA) and Duraform (Codman & Shurtleff, Raynham, USA) are other collagen matrices derived from bovine Achilles tendon.

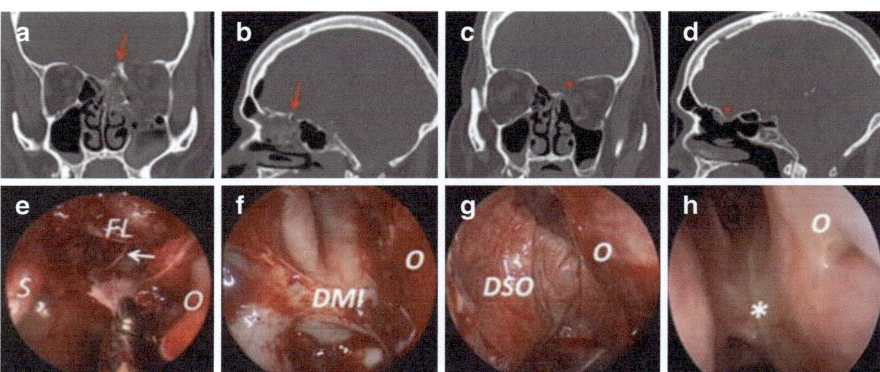

Fig. 9.1 Collagen matrix inlay graft and SIS onlay graft: 49-year-old male presenting with fractures of the left posterior frontal sinus and ethmoid skull base after ground-level fall. (**a**) Collagen dural matrix inlay graft, porcine small intestinal submucosa (SIS) onlay graft. (**b**) Patient suffered ground-level fall with resulting left posterior table frontal sinus and ethmoid fractures with displacement of bony fragment (arrow). (**c**, **d**) Postoperative scans with asterisk over site of EEA repair. (**e**) Endoscopic view of skull base fracture. (**f**) Endoscopic view of skull base fracture with collagen dural matrix inlay (DMI). (**g**) Endoscopic view demonstrating completed repair of skull base defect with porcine small intestinal submucosa as dural substitute onlay graft (DSO). (**h**) Postoperative repair with asterisk marking site of healed skull base reconstruction. *FL* frontal lobe, *S* septum, *O* orbit

TissuDura (Baxter, Vienna, Austria) is an impermeable collagen matrix composed of minced equine Achilles tendon.

A small series reported by Yoo et al. used either acellular dermis (Alloderm) or bovine Achilles tendon collagen (Duramatrix) for reconstruction of large (>2 cm in largest diameter) in a single layer underlay technique. The authors report that the Duramatrix group had a shorter period of postoperative crusting, less time to remucosalization, and fewer postoperative debridements necessary compared to the Alloderm group. Neither group had postoperative CSF leak, although the small sample size ($n = 2$ for Alloderm group and $n = 3$ for Duramatrix group) limits generalizability [86].

Oakley et al. reported a series of 120 patients with transdural surgery either for intracranial or paranasal sinus pathology. All patients were repaired using collagen matrix (Duragen) as an intracranial inlay graft in the subdural or arachnoid space. Additional layers were utilized depending on defect size (free mucosal graft for defects <1 cm, vascularized mucoperiosteal flap [nasoseptal flap for 69.2%], or combination for large defects). The authors report a 3.3% rate of postoperative CSF leak, 3.3% rate of meningitis, and 1.7% intracranial bleeding. The authors concluded that collagen matrix combined in a two-layer repair provided a viable skull base repair which, while having increased cost compared to autologous grafts, has advantages as no harvest time or donor site is necessary [85].

Cappabianca et al. [87] report a series of 72 patients undergoing endonasal endoscopic transsphenoidal pituitary surgery, of whom 15 underwent repair with equine

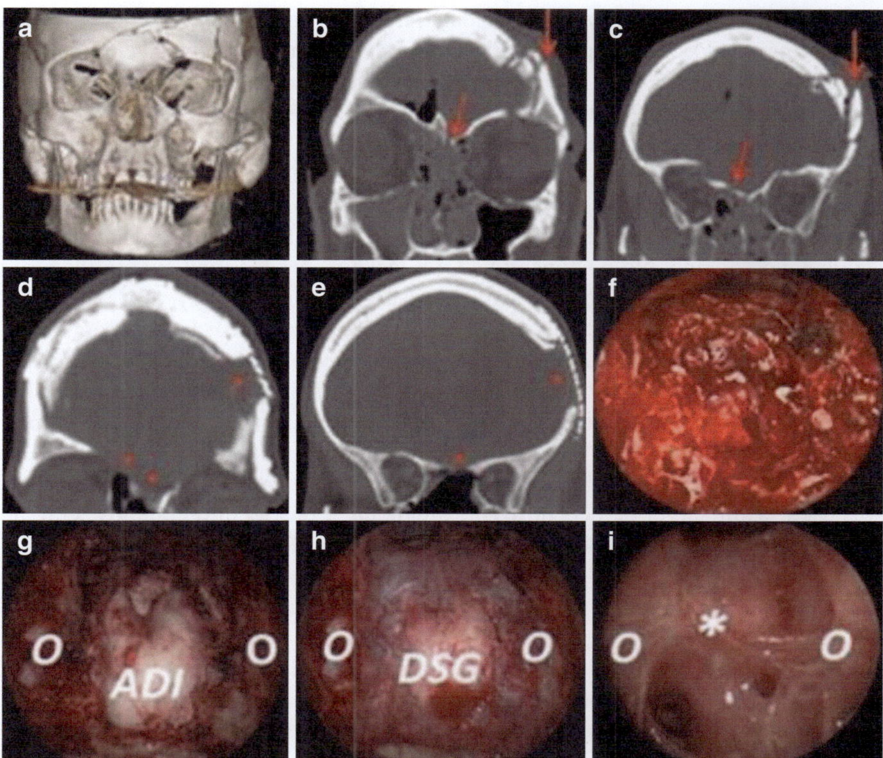

Fig. 9.2 Acellular dermal inlay graft and SIS onlay graft: 24-year-old male presented with highly comminuted fractures involving entirety of anterior skull base after gunshot wound to the head. Combined open and endoscopic approaches were used. (**a**) 3D reconstruction of maxillofacial CT. Patient presented with highly comminuted fractures involving the entirety of the anterior skull base following gunshot wound to head (**b**, **c**) Comminuted anterior skull base fractures. Arrows denote sites of dural injury and cerebrospinal fluid leak (arrow). (**d**, **e**) Postoperative scans with asterisk over site of repairs. (**f**) Endoscopic view of skull base fractures prior to repair. (**g**) Endoscopic view of skull base reconstruction after open and endoscopic approaches with a pedicled pericranial flap covered by acellular dermal inlay (ADI) centrally and orbits (O) laterally. (**h**) Endoscopic view of skull base reconstruction after placement of porcine SIS as dural substitute graft (DSG). (**i**) Endoscopic view of postoperative repair with asterisk marking the site of healed skull base reconstruction. *O* orbit

collagen matrix. Of these, nine were performed for CSF leak (six of which extended into the suprasellar cistern, in which case collagen matrix was placed intradurally) and six to reconstruct the diaphragma sellae without CSF leak. The postoperative CSF leak rate was 6.7% ($n = 1$). The authors felt the material was safe and biocompatible, but the small sample size limits conclusions.

Acellular dermis is another homograft which has been widely used for skull base reconstruction (Fig. 9.2), both following endoscopic skull base surgery and for repair of iatrogenic or spontaneous CSF leaks. Lorenz et al. describe a series of 24 patients who underwent transsphenoidal transseptal hypophysectomy via hybrid microscopic-endoscopic approach. Eleven (45.8%) of these patients had intraoperative CSF leaks. There were also eight patients diagnosed with CSF leaks following skull base surgery, sinus surgery, or trauma. The authors describe the use of acellular dermis as an intracranial extradural graft, bolstered by septal bone or cartilage placed intracranially. A second acellular dermal allograft was positioned intracranially over the bone/cartilage graft. A free mucosal graft was then placed as an overlay and secured with fibrin glue and micofibrillar collagen before placement of gelatin sponge and packing. No postoperative CSF leaks were identified among the eight patients with CSF leak following skull base surgery, sinus surgery, or trauma. Two of the hypophysectomy patients developed postoperative CSF leak. Overall CSF leak rate was 6.3%, with leak rate among hypophysectomy patients of 8.3% [34].

Germani et al. reported a retrospective series of 55 patients who underwent endonasal endoscopic pituitary surgery. A subset of 30 of these patients had repair utilizing acellular dermis (Alloderm), either alone ($n = 12$) or in combination with free mucosal graft, bone, or cartilage. For defects less than 2 cm, overlay technique was used, while larger defects utilized a single layer tucked intracranially with the edges placed against the bony defect. The remainder of patients had repairs utilizing primarily free mucosal grafts or bone and free mucosal grafts. Failure rate for the acellular dermis group was 3%, with a failure rate for the other group was 8% [33].

A larger study by the same senior author extended these results with a series of 429 patients with sellar floor repair after pituitary adenoma resection (endonasal endoscopic 43.3%; sublabial microsurgical 41.4%). This retrospective cohort study utilized a historic comparison group repaired with fat autograft. The intraoperative leak rate was 35.5%. Of patients with intraoperative CSF leaks, 95 (59%) had repair with acellular dermis (Alloderm), while the remainder were repaired with fat autograft. In cases with CSF leak, acellular dermis was used both as inlay and onlay grafts. Overall CSF leak was 3.9%. In the acellular dermis group, there were eight CSF leaks (8.4%). The fat autograft group had seven CSF leaks (15.2%) [6].

In a comparison of reconstructive materials, Prickett et al. report a series of 40 CSF leak repairs in 37 patients. Repair materials which varied between repairs included mucosal grafts ($n = 17$), acellular dermis ($n = 10$), and collagen matrix grafts (Duraform or Duragen; $n = 13$). Repair technique involved either a single layer of graft material under investigation supported by bone graft or multiple layers of the study graft material, at surgeon's discretion. Other materials for multilayer repair included fibrin glue and absorbable packing material, which were used for all repairs. The authors reported no differences in CSF fistula closure rate between the materials used. Other primary endpoints evaluated included weeks of graft crusting and time to mucosalization of graft. There was a significantly longer period of crusting and time to remucosalization in the acellular dermis group compared to collagen matrix grafts or mucosal grafts. There was no reported crusting at repair site by first postoperative visit for the mucosal graft group; however, donor site crusting (which due to lack of donor site was not present in the other groups) persisted for an average of 6.5 weeks [11].

As discussed earlier in the section on fibrin-based sealants, Cappabianca et al. have described the use of a polyester-silicone dural substitute used with Tissucol fibrin sealant with or without collagen fleece for closure of sellar defects with intra-operative CSF leak following endoscopic endonasal transsphenoidal surgery [26, 88]. The polyester-silicone dural substitute was used for all intraoperative CSF leaks. They found that polyester-silicone dural substitute and fibrin sealant with addition of collagen fleece ($n = 13$) resulted in a lower CSF leak rate (0% leak rate) compared to polyester-silicone and fibrin sealant ($n = 16$) alone (12.5% leak rate). The authors note that CSF diversion via lumbar drain was used when repair was not considered watertight, with extended approach to planum sphenoidale or clivus, or if "copious" CSF leak was noted intraoperatively. No patients in the collagen fleece + fibrin sealant group required lumbar drain [26].

Homologues and xenografts have enjoyed increasing use over time. A major reason cited for this is the avoidance of donor site morbidity [32]. Additional advantages are that no operative time is needed for graft harvest and preparation and that graft size is not limited by available tissue or previous surgical treatment. A further potential advantage is the multifunctional nature of several of the non-autologous materials. Human acellular dermis (Alloderm) has variously been used as an inlay graft [34, 89], to obliterate dead space in a manner analogous to fat for reconstruction of sellar defects [6], as an overlay graft [14, 90], or as a single layer graft for reconstruction of large anterior skull base defects [33]. Collagen matrix is most commonly utilized as a dural replacement or as an inlay graft but has been also used to obliterate dead space [53]. As noted previously, success rates are similar for allografts and xenografts [2, 32], and these non-autologous materials provide the ability to replace multiple types of tissue in skull base repair, which can be particularly advantageous when autologous graft tissue is limited or absent.

Gelfoam, Surgiflo, Floseal

Visualization is paramount for endoscopic sinus and skull base surgery, making hemostasis a critical component of successful surgery and leading to trials of topical hemostatic agents, and flowable packing materials have been used for hemostasis in skull base surgery. Gelatin/thrombin hemostatic agents such as Surgiflo (Johnson & Johnson, Somerville, NJ, USA) have been reported to be successful in controlling bleeding in endoscopic sinus surgery [91]. While the use of thrombin-gelatin matrix in endoscopic sinus surgery has been controversial due to conflicting reports of the effect on synechiae formation [92, 93], various formulations of thrombin-gelatin matrix have been used as a hemostatic agent during extended endoscopic surgery. One series of 65 consecutive patients included 29 patients who had the use of thrombin-gelatin matrix for hemostasis. The authors found that thrombin-gelatin matrix (Floseal, Baxter Healthcare Corp, Deerfield, IL, USA) was useful for controlling mucosal oozing and focal bleeding [94]. Another series of 39 patients underwent endonasal endoscopic approach to sellar and parasellar lesions, with the need for lateral exposure. Human-derived thrombin and bovine-derived gelatin matrix (Floseal) was applied directly to sites of venous bleeding in the cavernous sinus to achieve hemostasis. The authors report average blood loss of 110 mL for pituitary adenoma cases ($n = 33$) and 370 mL for expanded skull base cases ($n = 6$), although there was no control group to allow for comparison of blood loss [95]. Porcine gelatin matrix/human thrombin mix has also been used for hemostasis in superior intercavernous sinus and cavernous sinus venous bleeding [96].

Gelatin sponge has frequently been used for filling the sella following endonasal endoscopic sellar surgery when no CSF leak is detected [3, 24, 82], but has also been used in combination with fibrin sealant for repair of sellar defects and CSF leak. In one report of 120 cases of endoscopic endonasal pituitary surgery, there were 28 intraoperative CSF leaks. Gelatin sponge was placed as an underlay and secured with fibrin sealant. An additional layer of gelatin sponge, followed by additional fibrin glue and a third layer of gelatin sponge were used as overlay to complete the repair. The authors reported a 3.6% failure rate for the described repair [97].

Gelatin sponge has also been used in combination with fibrin sealant-coated collagen fleece and autologous bone graft for sellar reconstruction, with or without CSF leak. Of the 50 cases reviewed in one series which utilized this repair, ten had intraoperative CSF leaks. No patients had postoperative CSF leak [98].

Some formulations of gelatin agents have enough structural stability to use for support of grafts in place of more traditional nonabsorbable packing. While foley catheters have been used for supporting nasoseptal flaps and other pedicled grafts, purified porcine gelatin (Gelfoam) has been reported to be a potential alternative. In 1 series of 73 patients undergoing endoscopic endonasal transsphenoidal surgery, there were 36 intraoperative CSF leaks, including 30 high-flow CSF leaks. Rolled purified porcine gelatin was packed into the sphenoid cavity to hold the nasoseptal flap against the cranial base. There was one postoperative CSF leak in the series (1.4%), which is in line with rates reported in the literature for studies utilizing foley catheters [58, 99, 100]. The authors note that the gelatin material swells with moisture, which would accentuate the effect of packing. The absorbable nature of gelatin packing can also be advantageous to provide a dissolvable layer between the skull base repair and non-dissolvable packing placed as a bolster, to decrease the potential for dislodgement of the graft with removal of non-dissolvable packing.

Resorbable Plates

Several studies have reported on the use of absorbable plates for reconstruction of skull base defects. After being reported in the repair of craniosynostosis [101], poly (D,L) lactic acid (PDLLA) was trialed as an option for repair of sellar defects [21]. PDLLA is an absorbable polymer that retains strength for approximately 10 weeks and absorbs over approximately 72 weeks [101]. Potter et al. described a series of 28 patients in 2005 who underwent repair of sellar defects ($n = 20$), anterior skull base defects secondary to meningocele repair ($n = 7$), or frontal sinus defects ($n = 1$).

The authors report that for the majority of cases ($n = 25$), a layer of dural substitute was placed as an epidural inlay graft, after which the PDLLA plate was placed as a second extradural inlay graft. Additional overlay grafts were used, including cellulose sponge ($n = 21$), free mucosal or fat graft ($n = 6$), and nasoseptal flap ($n = 1$). The eight patients with intraoperative CSF leak had lumbar drains. The reported CSF leak rate was 3.7% ($n = 1$) with the one reported leak occurring in a patient who had revision open craniotomy 2 days post-op to remove residual tumor [21]. Seaman et al. [22] reported a retrospective series of 24 patients who also had repair using PDLLA plate for repair of extrasellar skull base defects. Two patients had nasoseptal flap as additional repair, and two patients had free mucosal grafts. The authors reported no CSF leaks with mean follow-up of 30 months.

Polydioxanone (PDS) is a second absorbable material that has been used to provide semi-rigid support for repair of sellar defects [18, 19] and anterior skull base defects [17, 20]. Mohd Slim et al. described the use of 0.15 mm thickness perforated PDS plate as an extradural underlay for reconstruction of the sella following transsphenoidal pituitary surgery. Following placement of the PDS plate, a nasoseptal flap was used as an overlay, with reinforcement with fibrin glue and non-absorbable packing. Among the 13 patients they report, eight had intraoperative CSF leaks and four had postoperative lumbar drains. No postoperative CSF leaks were reported through 3 months of follow-up [18]. Zeden et al. also reported the use of PDS plate for repair of sellar floor following endonasal endoscopic transsphenoidal surgery. In their series of 30 patients, they utilized PDS plate placed into the epidural space behind the edges of the bony defect. Gelatin foam, collagen matrix, oxidized cellulose, or an abdominal fat graft were used to fill the sella prior to placement of the PDS, which material choice dictated by presence and rate of CSF leak or herniation of the diaphragm into the sella. Ten of the patients (33%) had intraoperative CSF leak. Twenty-five of the patients had pituitary macroadenoma, with the remaining five patients having Rathke cysts. The postoperative CSF leak rate in this series was 3.3% ($n = 1$), which was associated with graft displacement in one patient with Rathke cyst.

Al-Asousi et al. report a series of seven patients who had repair of either posterior table frontal sinus CSF leaks or ethmoid roof CSF leaks from a variety of etiologies. Mean defect size was 16.4 × 11.4 mm. All repairs utilized a non-perforated PDS sheet as an inlay graft. Additional multilayer repair with onlay graft utilizing either porcine small intestine submucosal graft or free mucosal autograft were also used. The authors reported no postoperative CSF leaks [17]. Jolly et al. report a small series of three patients with large skull base defects (average size not reported) following resection of skull base lesions in which they utilized 0.5 mm thickness PDS plate deployed using what the authors describe as a "PDS wrap" technique. The rationale for this method was that herniation of the brain through large defects can make placement of intradural underlay grafts challenging. The authors initially placed an intradural underlay dural graft (Duragen) noting that the amount of graft able to be placed between the brain and native dura was limited by brain herniation through the large defects. Subsequent to this, the PDS plate was wrapped in a second dural graft and the edges sutured together. The PDS plate was then used to elevate the brain while placing the PDS extradurally beneath the bony ledge of the defect. The sutures were then cut, allowing the dural graft "wrap" to unfold while being held in place by the PDS plate. This second dural graft was positioned as an extradural underlay. A nasoseptal flap, layers of tissue glue, and nonabsorbable packing were used to complete the repair. The authors advocated this technique for repair of large defects, as they felt the PDS plate facilitated placement of the second dural underlay by anchoring the graft during placement, retracting the brain parenchyma, as well as providing a rigid support to limit brain herniation through the defect [20].

Polyglactin acid has been used both for repair of sellar defects [77] and parasellar defects [102]. A series of 18 consecutive patients with use of fibrin glue and polyglactin acid sheet for repair of CSF leak following endoscopic endonasal pituitary surgery are reported by Yano et al. The authors compare their results to their previous 38 patients treated either with fibrin glue alone or with pedicled mucosal grafts and fibrin glue. In the six patients treated with fibrin glue alone, the postoperative CSF fistula rate was 33.3% (2 leaks), while for the 32 patients with mucosal graft and fibrin glue, the postoperative CSF fistula rate was 15.6%. Among the 18 patients with polyglactin acid sheet and fibrin glue, there were no reported postoperative CSF leaks with 7-month follow-up [77]. The same authors describe their series of 74 endoscopic endonasal approaches consisting of 55 anterior extended approaches, 10 clival approaches, and 9 cavernous approaches. Multilayer repair of defects was performed using fat graft with polyglactin sheet underlay, covered by septal bone set within the edges of the bony defect. A mucosal flap was then placed and secured with fibrin glue and Foley balloon. Postoperative CSF leak rate was reported to be seven patients (9.5%) with median follow-up of at least 12.6 months. The authors attribute four of the postoperative CSF leaks to absence or inadequacy of nasoseptal flap [102].

Absorbable plates have been proposed as an option for providing rigid reconstruction of the skull base. While the necessity of rigid reconstruction has been debated, there may be advantages to the use of a synthetic material compared to autologous or homologous bone grafts, which have been the traditional option for rigid reconstruction. While autologous bone grafts are less expensive and may potentially be harvested from the nasal cavity, synthetic options such as PDLLA or PDS are available in a range of sizes and thicknesses. Synthetic rigid reconstruction options also may address the concerns about the potential for osteoradionecrosis in patients who will undergo postoperative radiation therapy [55], prolonged healing time, potential for formation of bony sequestra [46], and potentially increased risk of infection with the use of bone grafts [54]. PDS sheet has been used in nasal septal reconstruction [103], and in vivo animal models have suggested that PDS foil remains stable for at least 10 weeks and is absorbed by 25 weeks [104]. This suggests that PDS may be useful in providing rigid support in the initial postoperative period without the risk of osteoradionecrosis or bony sequestra formation. However, the nature of the data (retrospective case series) limits ability to answer this question.

Packing

Migration of the graft can lead to failure of skull base repair with CSF leak, regardless of repair type. Various strategies have been used to maintain graft position during the perioperative period. In addition to sealants and biologic glues as discussed above, nasal packing has been frequently employed, both for pedicled flaps [99, 100] and for free grafts [60]. Both absorbable and non-absorbable packing has been used. Absorbable packing types have included Nasopore [Stryker, Kalamazoo, MI USA] [55, 85, 86], Gelfoam [14, 33], and Merogel sponges [Minneapolis, MN, USA] [31]. These tend to be used to directly support the graft prior to placement of non-absorbable packing. Non-absorbable packing has included bismuth iodine paraffin-embedded gauze [85], foley catheter balloons [85, 90], and Merocel [Minneapolis, MN, USA] [14, 16, 33, 55, 86]. One early meta-analysis reported that 61% of groups routinely used nasal packing [105], but some large series of repair of smaller defects such as after pituitary surgery have avoided the use of nasal packing except in cases of epistaxis [106]. Evidence regarding the indications for use of nasal packing and outcomes is limited. A meta-analysis by Hegazy et al. evaluated 14 studies representing 204 surgeries. Of these cases, 61% utilized nasal packing, and no significant effect was found depending on packing type or use [105]. A later evidence-based review did not find sufficient data to make a recommendation regarding the use of nasal packing. The authors mention the lack of evidence for benefit and the possibility of toxic shock syndrome, patient discomfort, and the potential for graft dislodgement during packing removal as potential harms [32]. A later evidence-based review also identified limited evidence for the use of nasal packing in endoscopic skull base surgery but suggested nasal packing may be used as an adjunct based on surgeon preference [31]. There is data, however, from a series of 100 endoscopic transsphenoidal surgeries for pituitary lesions that use of nasal packing negatively affects patient-reported sinonasal quality of life at 3 months postoperatively [107]. While there is not much data supporting their use, the rational for nasal packing in reconstruction is to prevent graft migration while protecting the graft from airflow. Absorbable packing also provides a barrier between the graft and any non-absorbable packing that will be removed postoperatively to prevent traction on the repair with inadvertent dislodgement. Additionally, absorbable packing may help to distribute pressure more evenly over the skull base and graft [90].

Biodesign and Other Impermeable Grafts

Data from a canine model [108] and a subsequent clinical trials following Chiari decompression or tumor resection [109] suggested that porcine small intestinal submucosa (SIS) graft could be a suitable dural replacement graft (Fig. 9.3). Porcine small intestinal submucosa (SIS) graft has FDA approval for use as a dural

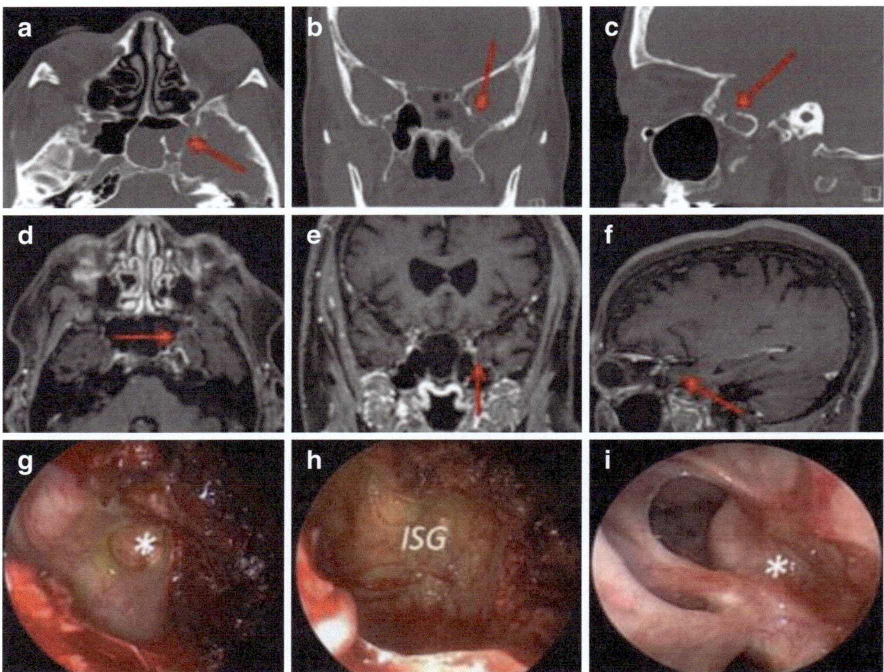

Fig. 9.3 SIS onlay graft: 62-year-old female with encephalocele and CSF leak following ground-level fall, repaired via EEA. (**a–c**) CT scan in axial, coronal, and sagittal planes with red arrow at location of encephalocele in left sphenoid sinus lateral recess, lateral to the foramen rotundum. Focal cortical thinning and fluid filling; the left sphenoid sinus is suggestive of CSF leak. (**d–f**) T1 post contrast MRI with arrows demonstrating location of left sphenoid sinus lateral recess encephalocele. (**g**) Exposure of 5 mm encephalocele (*) after transpterygoid approach. (**h**) Skull base reconstruction with porcine SIS graft (ISG) following reduction of encephalocele. (**i**) 6-month postoperative appearance with asterisk marking site of repair

substitute [16], but it is also frequently used as an onlay graft (see Figs. 9.1 and 9.2), similar to fascia lata.

An ovine transfrontal durotomy model utilized SIS and vascularized mucosal flaps during validation of their model of skull base reconstruction. Bilateral trans-frontal craniotomies and durotomies were performed in six sheep, with bilateral vascularized mucosal flaps for repair. SIS was used as subdural inlay graft on the left side. Although no differences in postoperative CSF leak rates were reported between the vascularized mucosal flap side and the side with SIS inlay in this open model of skull base repair (as there were no CSF leaks for either repair type), histologic analysis showed grossly thicker repair on the SIS side without increased inflammatory response or alterations in graft healing or integration [110].

Illing et al. reported the use of porcine small intestinal submucosal (SIS) graft in series of 155 patients undergoing 170 surgeries for repair of skull base defects following surgery for neoplasm, traumatic, congenital, or spontaneous causes. The repair technique utilized SIS grafts for placement as inlay graft (when defect size allowed) and an onlay graft, with 79% of patients also receiving an additional nasal septal flap onlay. The authors report a 94.7% first-repair success rate for repair of defects in various locations, with central sphenoid, posterior table of frontal sinus, cribriform plate, and ethmoid roof being the most common locations [16]. This success rate is similar to previously published rates with nasoseptal flap utilizing adjunctive autologous (fascia) onlay [99].

SIS graft has also been reported to have stable mechanical properties with repeated stress [111], suggesting it would be appropriate for situations such as skull base repair where recurrent stress (such as Valsalva maneuvers) would increase pressure [16].

Conclusions

This chapter has reviewed the commonly used allografts and materials in skull base repair. The majority of the available data is retrospective, and generalizations regarding material use are difficult as most materials are used in combination for multilayer repairs, making it difficult to make definitive statements about the properties and effectiveness of a single material. However, some broad conclusions are supported by the literature. As there were no significant differences in CSF leak rate between autologous and non-autologous materials [2], either may be used depending upon the specific clinical situation. The balance between cost of non-autologous materials versus potential for donor site morbidity and time for harvest of autologous materials are factors which may be decisive in specific clinical scenarios. Additionally, the availability, quality, or quantity of autologous tissue may be limited depending upon extent of disease in cases of malignancy, prior radiation, or previous sinonasal surgery. In these situations, the potential to substitute homologues or xenografts for one or more different layers of reconstruction can be useful (Table 9.2), particularly with the potential of some non-autologous materials to substitute for multiple types of tissue/layers in a multilayer reconstruction. Low-flow CSF leaks identified intraoperatively may be repaired with similar outcomes by use of vascularized flaps or multilayer repair with autologous free grafts or non-autologous materials [59]. Finally, independent of the graft material chosen for repair, the experience of the surgeon and surgical technique are critical factors in the success of the repair [2].

Table 9.2 Comparison of autologous and non-autologous graft materials

Autologous graft	Comparable non-autologous material
Bone/cartilage	Absorbable plate
Fascia lata	Acellular dermis
Free mucosa	SIS
Fat	Acellular dermis, collagen matrix, gelatin

Case Examples
Case 1: Collagen matrix inlay graft and SIS onlay graft
A 49-year-old male presented with fractures of the left posterior frontal sinus and ethmoid skull base after ground-level fall while intoxicated. Defect was measured to be 1.8 mm × 11.4 mm with a fragment of bone protruding into the frontal lobe near the olfactory groove (see Fig. 9.1). Endoscopic endonasal approach was used for repair with placement of engineered collagen matrix inlay and porcine SIS onlay graft. Patient had no recurrence of CSF leak.

Case 2: Acellular dermal matrix inlay graft with SIS inlay graft
A 24-year-old male who presented with highly comminuted fractures involving the entirety of the anterior skull base after gunshot wound to the head. His defect was measured to 3.5 cm × 5.4 cm with an additional large defect in the left temporal skull (see Fig. 9.2). Open craniotomy was performed for placement of pericranial flap, aided by endoscopic endonasal approach for placement of acellular dermal matrix inlay and porcine SIS onlay grafts. He had no recurrence of CSF leak.

Case 3: SIS onlay graft
A 62-year-old female who presented with CSF leak after ground-level fall. Although there was minimal displacement of skull base fracture, she was found to have an approximately 5 mm left lateral sphenoid encephalocele (Fig. 9.3). After reduction of the encephalocele, the defect was repaired via EEA with SIS onlay graft. She had no recurrence of CSF leak.

References

1. Patel MR, Stadler ME, Snyderman CH, Carrau RL, Kassam AB, Germanwala AV, et al. How to choose? Endoscopic skull base reconstructive options and limitations. Skull Base. 2010;20(6):397–404.
2. Abiri A, Abiri P, Goshtasbi K, Lehrich BM, Sahyouni R, Hsu FPK, et al. Endoscopic anterior skull base reconstruction: a meta-analysis and systematic review of graft type. World Neurosurg. 2020;139:460–70.
3. Sciarretta V, Mazzatenta D, Ciarpaglini R, Pasquini E, Farneti G, Frank G. Surgical repair of persisting CSF leaks following standard or extended endoscopic transsphenoidal surgery for pituitary tumor. Minim Invasive Neurosurg. 2010;53(2):55–9.
4. Kuan EC, Yoo F, Patel PB, Su BM, Bergsneider M, Wang MB. An algorithm for sellar reconstruction following the endoscopic endonasal approach: a review of 300 consecutive cases. J Neurol Surg B Skull Base. 2018;79(2):177–83.
5. Sanders-Taylor C, Anaizi A, Kosty J, Zimmer LA, Theodosopoulos PV. Sellar reconstruction and rates of delayed cerebrospinal fluid leak after endoscopic pituitary surgery. J Neurol Surg B Skull Base. 2015;76(4):281–5.
6. Gaynor BG, Benveniste RJ, Lieberman S, Casiano R, Morcos JJ. Acellular dermal allograft for sellar repair after transsphenoidal approach to pituitary adenomas. J Neurol Surg B Skull Base. 2013;74(3):155–9.
7. Fonmarty D, Bastier PL, Lechot A, Gimbert E, de Gabory L. Assessment of abdominal fat graft to repair anterior skull base after malignant sinonasal tumor extirpation. Otolaryngol Head Neck Surg. 2016;154(3):540–6.
8. Roca E, Penn DL, Safain MG, Burke WT, Castlen JP, Laws ER. Abdominal fat graft for sellar reconstruction: retrospective outcomes review and technical note. Oper Neurosurg. 2019;16(6):667–74.

9. Fishpool SJ, Amato-Watkins A, Hayhurst C. Free middle turbinate mucosal graft reconstruction after primary endoscopic endonasal pituitary surgery. Eur Arch Otorhinolaryngol. 2017;274(2):837–44.
10. El-Banhawy OA, Halaka AN, Altuwaijri MA, Ayad H, El-Sharnoby MM. Long-term outcome of endonasal endoscopic skull base reconstruction with nasal turbinate graft. Skull Base. 2008;18(5):297–308.
11. Prickett KK, Wise SK, Delgaudio JM. Choice of graft material and postoperative healing in endoscopic repair of cerebrospinal fluid leak. Arch Otolaryngol Head Neck Surg. 2011;137(5):457–61.
12. Ramakrishnan VR, Terella AM, Poonia S, Chiu AG, Palmer JN. Osseous repair in minimally invasive reconstruction of anterior skull base defects. J Craniofac Surg. 2017;28(1):36–9.
13. Conger A, Zhao F, Wang X, Eisenberg A, Griffiths C, Esposito F, et al. Evolution of the graded repair of CSF leaks and skull base defects in endonasal endoscopic tumor surgery: trends in repair failure and meningitis rates in 509 patients. J Neurosurg. 2018;130(3):861–75.
14. Eloy JA, Patel SK, Shukla PA, Smith ML, Choudhry OJ, Liu JK. Triple-layer reconstruction technique for large cribriform defects after endoscopic endonasal resection of anterior skull base tumors. Int Forum Allergy Rhinol. 2013;3(3):204–11.
15. Eloy JA, Shukla PA, Choudhry OJ, Singh R, Liu JK. Assessment of frontal lobe sagging after endoscopic endonasal transcribriform resection of anterior skull base tumors: is rigid structural reconstruction of the cranial base defect necessary? Laryngoscope. 2012;122(12):2652–7.
16. Illing E, Chaaban MR, Riley KO, Woodworth BA. Porcine small intestine submucosal graft for endoscopic skull base reconstruction. Int Forum Allergy Rhinol. 2013;3(11):928–32.
17. Al-Asousi F, Okpaleke C, Dadgostar A, Javer A. The use of polydioxanone plates for endoscopic skull base repair. Am J Rhinol Allergy. 2017;31(2):122–6.
18. Mohd Slim MA, Jasem H, Melia L, McGarry G. Polydioxanone sheet as a rigid framework in skull-base repair: our experience in thirteen patients. Clin Otolaryngol. 2019;44(5):856–60.
19. Zeden JP, Baldauf J, Schroeder HWS. Repair of the sellar floor using bioresorbable polydioxanone foils after endoscopic endonasal pituitary surgery. Neurosurg Focus. 2020;48(6):E16.
20. Jolly K, Okonkwo O, Tsermoulas G, Ahmed SK. A novel technique for endoscopic repair of large anterior skull base defects: the PDS wrap. Am J Rhinol Allergy. 2020;34(1):70–3.
21. Potter NJ, Graham SM, Chang EH, Greenlee JD. Bioabsorbable plate cranial base reconstruction. Laryngoscope. 2015;125(6):1313–5.
22. Seaman SC, Moline MJ, Graham SM, Greenlee JDW. Endoscopic extrasellar skull base reconstruction using bioabsorbable plates. Am J Otolaryngol. 2021;42(1):102750.
23. Eloy JA, Choudhry OJ, Friedel ME, Kuperan AB, Liu JK. Endoscopic nasoseptal flap repair of skull base defects: is addition of a dural sealant necessary? Otolaryngol Head Neck Surg. 2012;147(1):161–6.
24. Burkett CJ, Patel S, Tabor MH, Padhya T, Vale FL. Polyethylene glycol (PEG) hydrogel dural sealant and collagen dural graft matrix in transsphenoidal pituitary surgery for prevention of postoperative cerebrospinal fluid leaks. J Clin Neurosci. 2011;18(11):1513–7.
25. Van Velthoven V, Clarici G, Auer LM. Fibrin tissue adhesive sealant for the prevention of CSF leakage following transsphenoidal microsurgery. Acta Neurochir. 1991;109(1–2):26–9.
26. Cappabianca P, Cavallo LM, Valente V, Romano I, D'Enza AI, Esposito F, et al. Sellar repair with fibrin sealant and collagen fleece after endoscopic endonasal transsphenoidal surgery. Surg Neurol. 2004;62(3):227–33; discussion 33.
27. Cappabianca P, Esposito F, Magro F, Cavallo LM, Solari D, Stella L, et al. Natura abhorret a vacuo--use of fibrin glue as a filler and sealant in neurosurgical "dead spaces". Technical note. Acta Neurochir (Wien). 2010;152(5):897–904.
28. Esposito F, Angileri FF, Kruse P, Cavallo LM, Solari D, Esposito V, et al. Fibrin sealants in dura sealing: a systematic literature review. PLoS One. 2016;11(4):e0151533.
29. Papay FA, Maggiano H, Dominquez S, Hassenbusch SJ, Levine HL, Lavertu P. Rigid endoscopic repair of paranasal sinus cerebrospinal fluid fistulas. Laryngoscope. 1989;99(11):1195–201.
30. Wigand ME. Transnasal ethmoidectomy under endoscopical control. Rhinology. 1981;19(1):7–15.

31. Wang EW, Zanation AM, Gardner PA, Schwartz TH, Eloy JA, Adappa ND, et al. ICAR: endoscopic skull-base surgery. Int Forum Allergy Rhinol. 2019;9(S3):S145–365.
32. Oakley GM, Orlandi RR, Woodworth BA, Batra PS, Alt JA. Management of cerebrospinal fluid rhinorrhea: an evidence-based review with recommendations. Int Forum Allergy Rhinol. 2016;6(1):17–24.
33. Germani RM, Vivero R, Herzallah IR, Casiano RR. Endoscopic reconstruction of large anterior skull base defects using acellular dermal allograft. Am J Rhinol. 2007;21(5):615–8.
34. Lorenz RR, Dean RL, Hurley DB, Chuang J, Citardi MJ. Endoscopic reconstruction of anterior and middle cranial fossa defects using acellular dermal allograft. Laryngoscope. 2003;113(3):496–501.
35. Hosemann W, Goede U, Sauer M. Wound healing of mucosal autografts for frontal cerebrospinal fluid leaks--clinical and experimental investigations. Rhinology. 1999;37(3):108–12.
36. Prickett KK, Wise SK. Grafting materials in skull base reconstruction. Adv Otorhinolaryngol. 2013;74:24–32.
37. Sigler AC, D'Anza B, Lobo BC, Woodard TD, Recinos PF, Sindwani R. Endoscopic skull base reconstruction: an evolution of materials and methods. Otolaryngol Clin N Am. 2017;50(3):643–53.
38. Garcia-Navarro V, Anand VK, Schwartz TH. Gasket seal closure for extended endonasal endoscopic skull base surgery: efficacy in a large case series. World Neurosurg. 2013;80(5):563–8.
39. Klatt-Cromwell CN, Thorp BD, Del Signore AG, Ebert CS, Ewend MG, Zanation AM. Reconstruction of skull base defects. Otolaryngol Clin N Am. 2016;49(1):107–17.
40. Wormald PJ, McDonogh M. 'Bath-plug' technique for the endoscopic management of cerebrospinal fluid leaks. J Laryngol Otol. 1997;111(11):1042–6.
41. Wormald PJ, McDonogh M. The bath-plug closure of anterior skull base cerebrospinal fluid leaks. Am J Rhinol. 2003;17(5):299–305.
42. Bhavana K, Kumar R, Keshri A, Aggarwal S. Minimally invasive technique for repairing CSF leaks due to defects of posterior table of frontal sinus. J Neurol Surg B Skull Base. 2014;75(3):183–6.
43. Lin RP, Weitzel EK, Chen PG, McMains KC, Majors J, Bunegin L. Failure pressures of three rhinologic dural repairs in a porcine ex vivo model. Int Forum Allergy Rhinol. 2015;5(7):633–6.
44. Kong DS, Kim HY, Kim SH, Min JY, Nam DH, Park K, et al. Challenging reconstructive techniques for skull base defect following endoscopic endonasal approaches. Acta Neurochir. 2011;153(4):807–13.
45. Luginbuhl AJ, Campbell PG, Evans J, Rosen M. Endoscopic repair of high-flow cranial base defects using a bilayer button. Laryngoscope. 2010;120(5):876–80.
46. Leng LZ, Brown S, Anand VK, Schwartz TH. "Gasket-seal" watertight closure in minimal-access endoscopic cranial base surgery. Neurosurgery. 2008;62(5 Suppl 2):ONSE342-3; discussion ONSE3.
47. Saafan ME, Albirmawy OA, Tomoum MO. Sandwich grafting technique for endoscopic endonasal repair of cerebrospinal fluid rhinorrhoea. Eur Arch Otorhinolaryngol. 2014;271(5):1073–9.
48. Tabaee A, Anand VK, Brown SM, Lin JW, Schwartz TH. Algorithm for reconstruction after endoscopic pituitary and skull base surgery. Laryngoscope. 2007;117(7):1133–7.
49. Nyquist GG, Anand VK, Mehra S, Kacker A, Schwartz TH. Endoscopic endonasal repair of anterior skull base non-traumatic cerebrospinal fluid leaks, meningoceles, and encephaloceles. J Neurosurg. 2010;113(5):961–6.
50. Fraser JF, Nyquist GG, Moore N, Anand VK, Schwartz TH. Endoscopic endonasal minimal access approach to the clivus: case series and technical nuances. Neurosurgery. 2010;67(3 Suppl Operative):ons150–8; discussion ons8.
51. Woodworth BA, Prince A, Chiu AG, Cohen NA, Schlosser RJ, Bolger WE, et al. Spontaneous CSF leaks: a paradigm for definitive repair and management of intracranial hypertension. Otolaryngol Head Neck Surg. 2008;138(6):715–20.

52. Zuniga MG, Turner JH, Chandra RK. Updates in anterior skull base reconstruction. Curr Opin Otolaryngol Head Neck Surg. 2016;24(1):75–82.
53. Harvey RJ, Nogueira JF, Schlosser RJ, Patel SJ, Vellutini E, Stamm AC. Closure of large skull base defects after endoscopic transnasal craniotomy. Clinical article. J Neurosurg. 2009;111(2):371–9.
54. Clavenna MJ, Turner JH, Chandra RK. Pedicled flaps in endoscopic skull base reconstruction: review of current techniques. Curr Opin Otolaryngol Head Neck Surg. 2015;23(1):71–7.
55. Snyderman CH, Wang EW, Zenonos GA, Gardner PA. Reconstruction after endoscopic surgery for skull base malignancies. J Neuro-Oncol. 2020;150(3):463–8.
56. Scagnelli RJ, Patel V, Peris-Celda M, Kenning TJ, Pinheiro-Neto CD. Implementation of free mucosal graft technique for sellar reconstruction after pituitary surgery: outcomes of 158 consecutive patients. World Neurosurg. 2019;122:e506–e11.
57. Harvey RJ, Parmar P, Sacks R, Zanation AM. Endoscopic skull base reconstruction of large dural defects: a systematic review of published evidence. Laryngoscope. 2012;122(2):452–9.
58. Zanation AM, Carrau RL, Snyderman CH, Germanwala AV, Gardner PA, Prevedello DM, et al. Nasoseptal flap reconstruction of high flow intraoperative cerebral spinal fluid leaks during endoscopic skull base surgery. Am J Rhinol Allergy. 2009;23(5):518–21.
59. Soudry E, Turner JH, Nayak JV, Hwang PH. Endoscopic reconstruction of surgically created skull base defects: a systematic review. Otolaryngol Head Neck Surg. 2014;150(5):730–8.
60. Ting JY, Metson R. Free graft techniques in skull base reconstruction. Basel: Karger; 2013.
61. Kassam A, Snyderman CH, Mintz A, Gardner P, Carrau RL. Expanded endonasal approach: the rostrocaudal axis. Part I. Crista galli to the sella turcica. Neurosurg Focus. 2005;19(1):E3.
62. de Divitiis E, Cavallo LM, Cappabianca P, Esposito F. Extended endoscopic endonasal transsphenoidal approach for the removal of suprasellar tumors: Part 2. Neurosurgery. 2007;60(1):46–58; discussion 9.
63. Nyquist GG, Anand VK, Brown S, Singh A, Tabaee A, Schwartz TH. Middle turbinate preservation in endoscopic transsphenoidal surgery of the anterior skull base. Skull Base. 2010;20(5):343–7.
64. Chauvet D, Tran V, Mutlu G, George B, Allain JM. Study of dural suture watertightness: an in vitro comparison of different sealants. Acta Neurochir. 2011;153(12):2465–72.
65. de Almeida JR, Ghotme K, Leong I, Drake J, James AL, Witterick IJ. A new porcine skull base model: fibrin glue improves strength of cerebrospinal fluid leak repairs. Otolaryngol Head Neck Surg. 2009;141(2):184–9.
66. Chorath K, Krysinski M, Bunegin L, Majors J, Weitzel EK, McMains KC, et al. Failure pressures of dural repairs in a porcine ex vivo model: novel use of titanium clips versus tissue glue. Allergy Rhinol. 2019;10:2152656719879677.
67. Fürst W, Banerjee A. Release of glutaraldehyde from an albumin-glutaraldehyde tissue adhesive causes significant in vitro and in vivo toxicity. Ann Thorac Surg. 2005;79(5):1522–8; discussion 9.
68. Herget GW, Kassa M, Riede UN, Lu Y, Brethner L, Hasse J. Experimental use of an albumin-glutaraldehyde tissue adhesive for sealing pulmonary parenchyma and bronchial anastomoses. Eur J Cardiothorac Surg. 2001;19(1):4–9.
69. Stylli SS, Kumar A, Gonzales M, Kaye AH. The biocompatibility of BioGlue with the cerebral cortex: a pilot study. J Clin Neurosci. 2004;11(6):631–5.
70. CryoLife, Inc. BioGlue® Surgical Adhesive. Summary of safety and effectiveness. Package insert for Bioglue (fda.gov). 2001. www.accessdata.fda.gov/cdrh_docs/pdf/P010003B.DOC.
71. Kumar A, Maartens NF, Kaye AH. Reconstruction of the sellar floor using Bioglue following transsphenoidal procedures. J Clin Neurosci. 2003;10(1):92–5.
72. Dusick JR, Mattozo CA, Esposito F, Kelly DF. BioGlue for prevention of postoperative cerebrospinal fluid leaks in transsphenoidal surgery: a case series. Surg Neurol. 2006;66(4):371–6; discussion 6.
73. Dusick JR, Esposito F, Kelly DF, Cohan P, DeSalles A, Becker DP, et al. The extended direct endonasal transsphenoidal approach for nonadenomatous suprasellar tumors. J Neurosurg. 2005;102(5):832–41.

74. Seda L, Camara RB, Cukiert A, Burattini JA, Mariani PP. Sellar floor reconstruction after transsphenoidal surgery using fibrin glue without grafting or implants: technical note. Surg Neurol. 2006;66(1):46–9; discussion 9.

75. Nishihira S, McCaffrey TV. The use of fibrin glue for the repair of experimental CSF rhinorrhea. Laryngoscope. 1988;98(6 Pt 1):625–7.

76. Cavallo LM, Solari D, Somma T, Savic D, Cappabianca P. The awake endoscope-guided sealant technique with fibrin glue in the treatment of postoperative cerebrospinal fluid leak after extended transsphenoidal surgery: technical note. World Neurosurg. 2014;82(3–4):e479–85.

77. Yano S, Tsuiki H, Kudo M, Kai Y, Morioka M, Takeshima H, et al. Sellar repair with resorbable polyglactin acid sheet and fibrin glue in endoscopic endonasal transsphenoidal surgery. Surg Neurol. 2007;67(1):59–64.

78. Scheule AM, Beierlein W, Lorenz H, Ziemer G. Repeated anaphylactic reactions to aprotinin in fibrin sealant. Gastrointest Endosc. 1998;48(1):83–5.

79. Shirai T, Shimota H, Chida K, Sano S, Takeuchi Y, Yasueda H. Anaphylaxis to aprotinin in fibrin sealant. Intern Med. 2005;44(10):1088–9.

80. Dietrich W, Ebell A, Busley R, Boulesteix AL. Aprotinin and anaphylaxis: analysis of 12,403 exposures to aprotinin in cardiac surgery. Ann Thorac Surg. 2007;84(4):1144–50.

81. Wang YY, Kearney T, Gnanalingham KK. Low-grade CSF leaks in endoscopic transsphenoidal pituitary surgery: efficacy of a simple and fully synthetic repair with a hydrogel sealant. Acta Neurochir. 2011;153(4):815–22.

82. Pereira EAC, Grandidge CA, Nowak VA, Cudlip SA. Cerebrospinal fluid leaks after transsphenoidal surgery - effect of a polyethylene glycol hydrogel dural sealant. J Clin Neurosci. 2017;44:6–10.

83. Blackburn SL, Smyth MD. Hydrogel-induced cervicomedullary compression after posterior fossa decompression for Chiari malformation. Case report. J Neurosurg. 2007;106(4 Suppl):302–4.

84. Han HJ, Jeong JH, Kim JW, Seung WB. Postoperative thecal sac compression induced by hydrogel dural sealant after spinal schwannoma removal. Korean J Neurotrauma. 2020;16(1):99–104.

85. Oakley GM, Christensen JM, Winder M, Jonker BP, Davidson A, Steel T, et al. Collagen matrix as an inlay in endoscopic skull base reconstruction. J Laryngol Otol. 2018;132(3):214–23.

86. Yoo F, Wang MB, Bergsneider M, Suh JD. Single layer repair of large anterior skull base defects without vascularized mucosal flap. J Neurol Surg B Skull Base. 2017;78(2):139–44.

87. Cappabianca P, Esposito F, Cavallo LM, Messina A, Solari D, di Somma LG, et al. Use of equine collagen foil as dura mater substitute in endoscopic endonasal transsphenoidal surgery. Surg Neurol. 2006;65(2):144–8; discussion 9.

88. Cappabianca P, Cavallo LM, Mariniello G, de Divitiis O, Romero AD, de Divitiis E. Easy sellar reconstruction in endoscopic endonasal transsphenoidal surgery with polyester-silicone dural substitute and fibrin glue: technical note. Neurosurgery. 2001;49(2):473–5; discussion 5–6.

89. Citardi MJ, Cox AJ III, Bucholz RD. Acellular dermal allograft for sellar reconstruction after transsphenoidal hypophysectomy. Am J Rhinol. 2000;14(1):69–73.

90. Zanation AM, Thorp BD, Parmar P, Harvey RJ. Reconstructive options for endoscopic skull base surgery. Otolaryngol Clin N Am. 2011;44(5):1201–22.

91. Woodworth BA, Chandra RK, LeBenger JD, Ilie B, Schlosser RJ. A gelatin-thrombin matrix for hemostasis after endoscopic sinus surgery. Am J Otolaryngol. 2009;30(1):49–53.

92. Chandra RK, Conley DB, Haines GK III, Kern RC. Long-term effects of FloSeal packing after endoscopic sinus surgery. Am J Rhinol. 2005;19(3):240–3.

93. Jameson M, Gross CW, Kountakis SE. FloSeal use in endoscopic sinus surgery: effect on postoperative bleeding and synechiae formation. Am J Otolaryngol. 2006;27(2):86–90.

94. Cappabianca P, Esposito F, Esposito I, Cavallo LM, Leone CA. Use of a thrombin-gelatin haemostatic matrix in endoscopic endonasal extended approaches: technical note. Acta Neurochir. 2009;151(1):69–77; discussion.

95. Bedi AD, Toms SA, Dehdashti AR. Use of hemostatic matrix for hemostasis of the cavernous sinus during endoscopic endonasal pituitary and suprasellar tumor surgery. Skull Base. 2011;21(3):189–92.
96. Liu JK, Christiano LD, Patel SK, Tubbs RS, Eloy JA. Surgical nuances for removal of tuberculum sellae meningiomas with optic canal involvement using the endoscopic endonasal extended transsphenoidal transplanum transtuberculum approach. Neurosurg Focus. 2011;30(5):E2.
97. Hobbs CG, Darr A, Carlin WV. Management of intra-operative cerebrospinal fluid leak following endoscopic trans-sphenoidal pituitary surgery. J Laryngol Otol. 2011;125(3):311–3.
98. Freyschlag CF, Goerke SA, Obernauer J, Kerschbaumer J, Thomé C, Seiz M. A sandwich technique for prevention of cerebrospinal fluid rhinorrhea and reconstruction of the sellar floor after microsurgical transsphenoidal pituitary surgery. J Neurol Surg A Cent Eur Neurosurg. 2016;77(3):229–32.
99. Hadad G, Bassagasteguy L, Carrau RL, Mataza JC, Kassam A, Snyderman CH, et al. A novel reconstructive technique after endoscopic expanded endonasal approaches: vascular pedicle nasoseptal flap. Laryngoscope. 2006;116(10):1882–6.
100. Kassam AB, Thomas A, Carrau RL, Snyderman CH, Vescan A, Prevedello D, et al. Endoscopic reconstruction of the cranial base using a pedicled nasoseptal flap. Neurosurgery. 2008;63(1 Suppl 1):ONS44-52; discussion ONS-3.
101. Acosta HL, Stelnicki EJ, Rodriguez L, Slingbaum LA. Use of absorbable poly (d,l) lactic acid plates in cranial-vault remodeling: presentation of the first case and lessons learned about its use. Cleft Palate Craniofac J. 2005;42(4):333–9.
102. Yano S, Hide T, Shinojima N, Hasegawa Y, Kawano T, Kuratsu J. Endoscopic endonasal skull base approach for parasellar lesions: initial experiences, results, efficacy, and complications. Surg Neurol Int. 2014;5:51.
103. Menger DJ, Tabink IC, Trenité GJ. Nasal septal abscess in children: reconstruction with autologous cartilage grafts on polydioxanone plate. Arch Otolaryngol Head Neck Surg. 2008;134(8):842–7.
104. Boenisch M, Mink A. Clinical and histological results of septoplasty with a resorbable implant. Arch Otolaryngol Head Neck Surg. 2000;126(11):1373–7.
105. Hegazy HM, Carrau RL, Snyderman CH, Kassam A, Zweig J. Transnasal endoscopic repair of cerebrospinal fluid rhinorrhea: a meta-analysis. Laryngoscope. 2000;110(7):1166–72.
106. Cappabianca P, Cavallo LM, Solari D, Stagno V, Esposito F, de Angelis M. Endoscopic endonasal surgery for pituitary adenomas. World Neurosurg. 2014;82(6 Suppl):S3–11.
107. Little AS, Kelly D, Milligan J, Griffiths C, Prevedello DM, Carrau RL, et al. Predictors of sinonasal quality of life and nasal morbidity after fully endoscopic transsphenoidal surgery. J Neurosurg. 2015;122(6):1458–65.
108. Cobb MA, Badylak SF, Janas W, Simmons-Byrd A, Boop FA. Porcine small intestinal submucosa as a dural substitute. Surg Neurol. 1999;51(1):99–104.
109. Bejjani GK, Zabramski J. Safety and efficacy of the porcine small intestinal submucosa dural substitute: results of a prospective multicenter study and literature review. J Neurosurg. 2007;106(6):1028–33.
110. Mueller SK, Scangas G, Amiji MM, Bleier BS. Prospective transfrontal sheep model of skull-base reconstruction using vascularized mucosa. Int Forum Allergy Rhinol. 2018;8(5):614–9.
111. Pui CL, Tang ME, Annor AH, Ebersole GC, Frisella MM, Matthews BD, et al. Effect of repetitive loading on the mechanical properties of biological scaffold materials. J Am Coll Surg. 2012;215(2):216–28.

Part II
Anterior Skull Base Pathology

Chapter 10
Traumatic and Iatrogenic CSF Leaks

Frederick Yoo

Introduction

Trauma is the most common cause of anterior skull base cerebrospinal fluid (CSF) leaks, making up 80–90% of these cases [1]. Traumatic CSF leaks can be further categorized base upon etiology of the injury. Non-iatrogenic injuries result from blunt force or penetrating craniofacial trauma involving the anterior skull base, with the vast majority of these cases being due to blunt trauma [2]. Iatrogenic injuries typically occur as a result of surgical procedures, namely, sinonasal, orbital, and neurosurgical procedures, and can be intentional or unintentional. Categorization of these injuries is helpful as evaluation and management of these patients can differ based on etiology (Fig. 10.1).

As the injuries sustained from the trauma causing the anterior skull base CSF leak may involve intracranial contents, as well as injury to other bodily systems, a multidisciplinary approach including otolaryngology, neurosurgery, and trauma specialists in evaluating and managing these patients is paramount. Identification and treatment of anterior skull base CSF leaks is important due to the risk of ascending meningitis which can be between 7 and 37%, with likely increasing rates with longer duration of active CSF leak [3]. In addition, a retrospective study of a traumatic brain injury registry in Taiwan revealed that patients with CSF leak associated with traumatic brain injury had significantly increased risk of mortality within a 1-year follow-up period, with subgroup analysis showing the highest mortality rate among those with CSF rhinorrhea at 10.9% [4].

It is evident that traumatic anterior skull base leaks are a significant and complex problem, with much nuance in the diagnostic and therapeutic considerations based upon mechanism of injury and characteristics of resultant defect. In this chapter, the

F. Yoo (✉)
Department of Head and Neck Surgery, Kaiser Permenente Orange County, Irvine, CA, USA
e-mail: Frederick.x.yoo@kp.org

© The Author(s), under exclusive license to Springer Nature Switzerland AG 2023
E. C. Kuan et al. (eds.), *Skull Base Reconstruction*,
https://doi.org/10.1007/978-3-031-27937-9_10

"

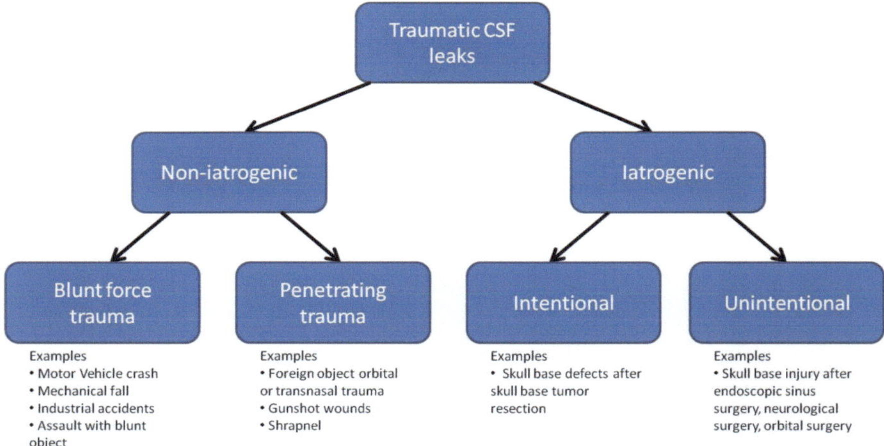

Fig. 10.1 Categorization of traumatic CSF leaks

pathophysiology, epidemiology, and diagnostic and therapeutic options for both non-iatrogenic (blunt and penetrating) and iatrogenic (unintentional) traumatic CSF leaks will be reviewed.

Non-iatrogenic Traumatic CSF Leaks

Pathophysiology, Epidemiology, and Diagnosis

As noted previously, non-iatrogenic traumatic CSF leaks can be divided into two groups based on mechanism of injury: blunt trauma and penetrating trauma. In the case of blunt trauma, CSF leaks may occur in approximately 2% of all closed head trauma and up to 30% of basilar skull fractures [5]. The thick frontal bone, air-filled sinuses, and partitions within the ethmoid skull base act as shock absorbers, requiring a significant amount of force required to cause a fracture in the skull base, thus contributing to the rarity of isolated skull base fractures without injury to the surrounding soft tissues and other bodily areas [6]. In one retrospective review of over 5000 head injury patients, skull base fracture was associated with moderate to severe head injuries 73.19% of the time [7]. The timing of presentation of CSF leaks can vary, with more than 50% presenting within 48 hours of injury, 70% within 1 week, and nearly all within 3 months [2]. There have been case reports of significantly delayed CSF leaks of up to 12 years following the traumatic event [8, 9]. Delays in leak presentation have been attributed to reduction in acute brain and soft tissue edema, devascularization of surrounding tissues, formulation of fistula tract, resorption of blood products/clots, and increases in intracranial pressure [1, 2]. Previous studies examining the location of anterior skull base leaks following non-iatrogenic trauma have found the most common sites to be the frontal sinus (30.8%), sphenoid sinus (11.4–30.8%), ethmoid roof (15.4–19.1%), cribriform plate (7.7%), frontoethmoid region (7.7%), and sphenoethmoid region (7.7%) [10, 11]. The presence of multiple skull base defects can occur commonly and was found to be present in 60% of accidental traumatic CSF leak cases in one series [9] (Figs. 10.2 and 10.3).

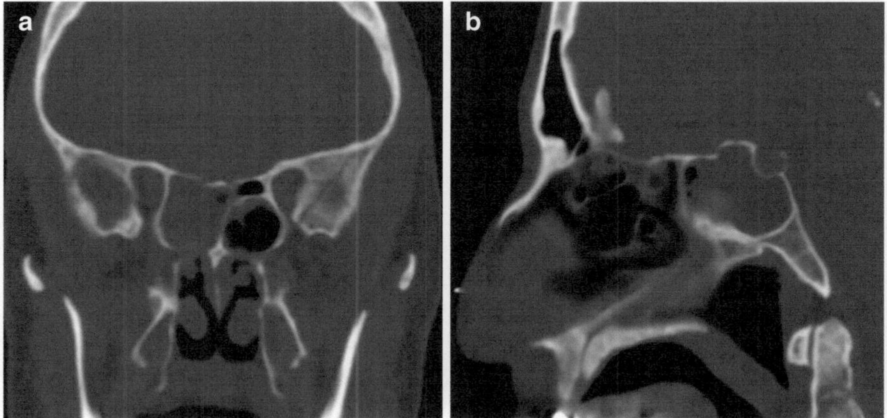

Fig. 10.2 Computed tomography (CT) imaging of a displaced planum sphenoidale fracture. CSF leak was noted 1 week after trauma and was repaired endoscopically. (**a**) Coronal plane CT image, (**b**) sagittal plane CT image (Image credit: Property of Edward Kuan, MD, used with permission)

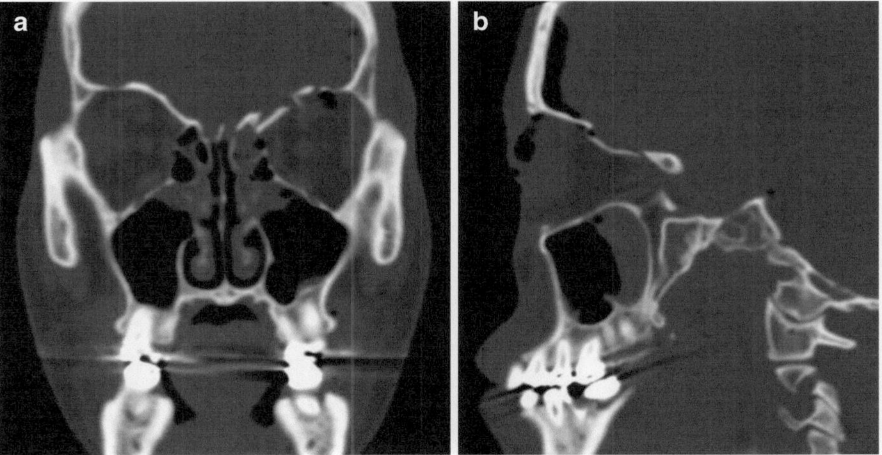

Fig. 10.3 Computed tomography (CT) imaging of orbital roof and ethmoid skull base displaced fracture with resultant CSF leak. Patient was managed with conservative management with resolution of CSF leak. (**a**) Coronal plane CT image, (**b**) sagittal plane CT image (Image credit: Property of Edward Kuan, MD, used with permission)

Penetrating trauma as the cause of anterior skull base injury and CSF leak is much rarer than blunt trauma. In one series of patients who had suffered traumatic skull base fractures over a 3-year period, only 3 out of 107 were due to penetrating injuries [12]. Due to the rarity of these injuries, no large case series or retrospective reviews of anterior skull base CSF leaks caused by penetrating trauma were identified in literature. Non-missile penetrating injuries of the anterior skull base via transnasal or transorbital injuries have been reported in numerous case reports [13–17]. In a literature review of 35 cases of transorbital and transnasal penetrating injuries, 47% of the cases were transnasal with 53% transorbital, and 66% of these cases were associated with CSF leak [15]. For missile injuries due to bullets or shrapnel, several case series presenting cases of anterior skull base injuries were identified [18–21]. One series reported 23 cases treated from military conflicts and peacekeeping operations, with the majority of 16 of them orbitocranial and three transethmoidal. CSF leak was noted in seven of these cases [18]. Another series of 116 penetrating craniocerebral injuries sustained in a wartime environment noted 13% of cases involving the anterior skull base, with a high mortality rate with only 49 survivors out of all cases [20]. Two other series presented cases of self-inflicted gunshot wounds involving the anterior skull base with resultant CSF leaks, 1 with 2 cases and the other with 11 cases reported [19, 21]. The paucity of literature for these types of injuries is likely secondary to the rarity of these cases and also the poor outcomes associated with these types of injuries. One common theme in the reports of penetrating traumatic CSF leaks is the risk of infection, with high rates of meningitis reported and reports of brain abscess formation in multiple patients [15, 18] (Fig. 10.4).

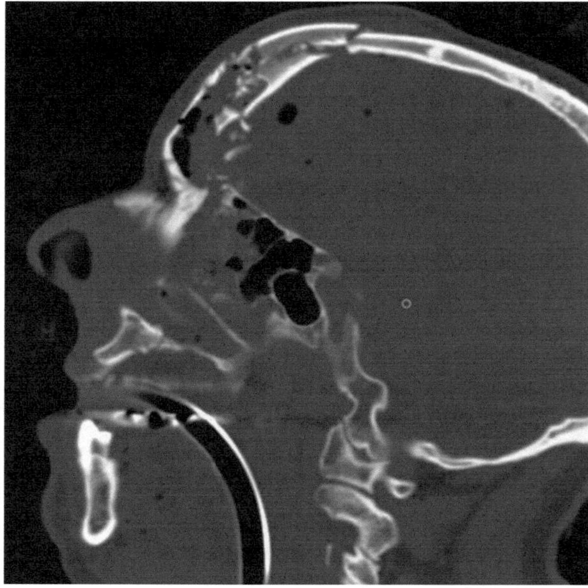

Fig. 10.4 Coronal CT image of self-inflicted gunshot wound to the anterior skull base with resultant delayed CSF leak repaired 2 months after injury (Image credit: Property of Edward Kuan, MD, used with permission)

Diagnostic workup of blunt and penetrating traumatic CSF leaks typically would start with imaging. As part of work up of traumatic brain injuries, computed tomography (CT) imaging of the head and skull base is typically employed as the American College of Surgeons recommends brain imaging in any patient with altered or depressed mental status, loss of consciousness, or significant post-traumatic amnesia [22]. With initial brain imaging, basilar skull base defects and fractures should be identified and can be further characterized with high-resolution CT scan of the anterior skull base (e.g., dedicated maxillofacial, sinus, orbit, or temporal bone cuts). Tri-planar, high-resolution CT scan with thin cuts (<1 mm), is rapid, requires no contrast, is inexpensive, has a high sensitivity (87%) for localizing CSF leak sites, and allows for evaluation of the skull base for any defects or other clues to a potential extracranial communication such as the presence of pneumocephalus [23]. As CSF leaks may not be clinically apparent at the time of presentation, vigilance with close monitoring for the development of clear, watery drainage from the nose or injury site is required. Collection of this fluid can then allow for beta-2 transferrin testing confirming presence of CSF. Beta-2 transferrin testing is highly sensitive (99%) and specific (97%) and is the gold standard for diagnosis of CSF leak [24]. Additional imaging modalities including CT cisternography, magnetic resonance imaging (MRI) with or without cisternography, and CT angiogram may be employed in certain situations to improve localization of the CSF fistula or to identify potential injuries to vascular structures in the skull base, especially with sphenoid sinus fractures.

Management of Non-iatrogenic Traumatic CSF Leaks

There are two pathways for management of non-iatrogenic traumatic CSF leaks, conservative/non-surgical and surgical. Anterior skull base CSF leaks associated with blunt or penetrating trauma are often associated with other significant injuries, including severe intracranial injuries. Thus, consultation with neurosurgical and trauma surgery colleagues and consideration of patient stability and overall prognosis should be taken prior to pursuing any surgical procedure. Should a neurosurgical intervention be required for addressing intracranial pathology, it is recommended that open repair of the skull base defect be performed simultaneously if possible [5, 25].

In other cases not requiring intracranial surgery, it is generally accepted in the literature that most non-iatrogenic traumatic CSF leaks are likely to spontaneously resolve without surgical management; thus, a more conservative initial approach utilizing bed rest, head of bed elevation, and reduction of spikes in intracranial pressure using anti-emetics and stool softeners is typically recommended. In addition, though CSF diversion with either lumbar drain or external ventriculostomy placement is invasive, it is typically grouped into the conservative/nonoperative management paradigm and may be an effective option [3]. A randomized-controlled trial by Albu et al. in patients with CSF rhinorrhea following close head trauma found that CSF diversion via lumbar drain reduced the CSF leak closure time to 4.83 ± 1.88 days compared to 7.03 ± 2.02 days in the conservative management (bed rest and head of bed elevation) group [26]. The duration of conservative management trial is somewhat controversial, with some advocating immediate surgical repair due to the risk of meningitis [27, 28]. As the risk of meningitis is generally considered to increase with duration of CSF leak, conservative management should not exceed a 7–10-day trial, with leaks that do not resolve within this time period proceeding to surgical management [5]. The use of prophylactic antibiotics after non-iatrogenic traumatic basilar skull fractures and CSF leaks is an option, but it must be noted that a recent review of studies on this topic found that the majority of studies did not find reduction in incidence of meningitis and recommended against the use of prophylactic antibiotics in basilar skull fracture and CSF leaks [3].

In the surgical management of non-iatrogenic anterior skull base CSF leaks, it should be noted that surgeon experience/expertise and hospital resources vary widely and should be a consideration when deciding to pursue surgical options and selecting an approach for repair. Though traditionally open transcranial approaches were the standard of care for addressing anterior skull base leaks, endoscopic approaches have been shown to be a safe and effective option in management of traumatic CSF leaks over the last two decades. Two systematic reviews, published in 2012 and 2016, have found the success rate of transnasal endoscopic approach to repair CSF rhinorrhea to be 90.1–90.6% effective, with low complication rates, and concluded that endoscopic repair should be considered the standard of care for most cases [29, 30]. Advances in endoscopic techniques for closure of CSF leaks with multilayer reconstruction utilizing a combination of homologous grafts (fat or fascia), allografts, xenografts, free mucosal grafts, and intranasal vascularized mucosal flaps have undoubtedly aided in the paradigm shift to endoscopic repair [31]. In cases of frontal sinus skull base defects, multiple studies have shown an endoscopic approach to be effective with high success rates (97.3–100%) [25, 32–34]. However, there are limitations in defects with extension far superiorly and laterally in the frontal sinus [34].

Open cranial approaches via craniotomy still play an important role in certain situations such as significant intracranial pathology necessitating neurosurgical intervention, comminuted or significantly displaced skull base fractures, large skull base defects, high-flow CSF leaks, open cranial trauma, superior and lateral frontal sinus defects, and previous failed endoscopic repair [5]. The advantages of open repair include wide visualization of the dural tear, option to treat any surrounding tissue injury, and use of a pericranial flap for coverage of the anterior skull base [1]. Large posterior table frontal sinus fractures can also be managed via osteoplastic flap or with cranialization through an open approach. Disadvantages include potential complications from frontal lobe retraction including anosmia, intracranial hemorrhage, edema, epilepsy, and long-term memory issues [35] (Fig. 10.5).

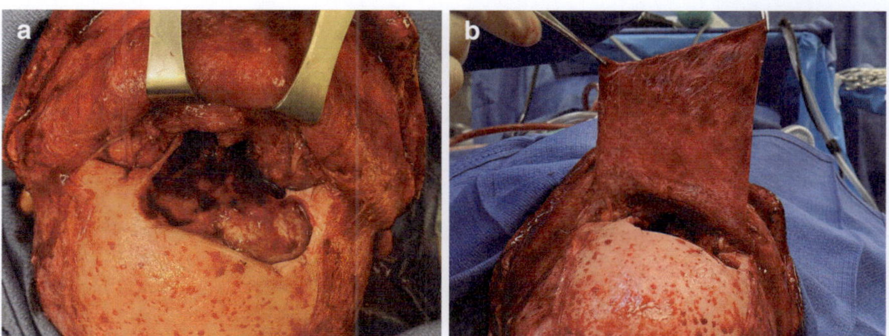

Fig. 10.5 (**a**) Osteoplastic flap approach for exposure of posterior table, (**b**) osteoplastic flap with pericranial flap harvested

Iatrogenic CSF Leaks

Pathophysiology, Epidemiology, and Diagnosis

Overall, unintentional iatrogenic CSF leaks are uncommon, and these complications make up only a small fraction of neurological, sinonasal, and orbital procedures. In terms of CSF leak as a complication of sinonasal surgery, a nationwide database retrospective review published in 2012 found the rate of CSF leak to be 0.17% following endoscopic sinus surgery [36]. Though rare, CSF leak can also be a complication of a "routine" surgery such as septoplasty, as several cases have been reported previously [37]. Additionally, reports of CSF leaks following balloon sinuplasty procedures have been reported [38, 39]. One study reviewing the Innovative OpenFDA Database for balloon sinuplasty complications noted that frontal sinus balloon procedures were most associated with CSF leaks [40]. More recently, with the increased utilization of nasal/nasopharyngeal swabs during the COVID-19 pandemic, there have been reports of CSF leaks as a complication of these procedures [41, 42]. For Graves' disease patients undergoing orbital decompression procedure, the rate of CSF leak was found to be 0.67% on the medial wall and 2.55% on the lateral wall [43]. In one retrospective study of 193 cases of CSF rhinorrhea, 50 of these cases were as a result of endoscopic sinus surgery, with the most common site of skull base defect in the ethmoid roof (62%), followed by cribriform (18%), frontal sinus (8%), and sphenoid sinus (4%) [10]. In this same series, only three CSF leaks were the result of neurosurgical procedures, with two of the defects located in the sphenoid sinus and one in the frontal sinus [10] (Fig. 10.6).

Ideally, identification of the CSF leak would occur at the time of injury, especially in the case of operative procedures; however, this is not always the case. Whether it is due to an excessively bloody surgical field obscuring view or lack of acute recognition by the operating surgeon, iatrogenic CSF leaks can often go unrecognized at the time of injury. Patients will typically report increased clear,

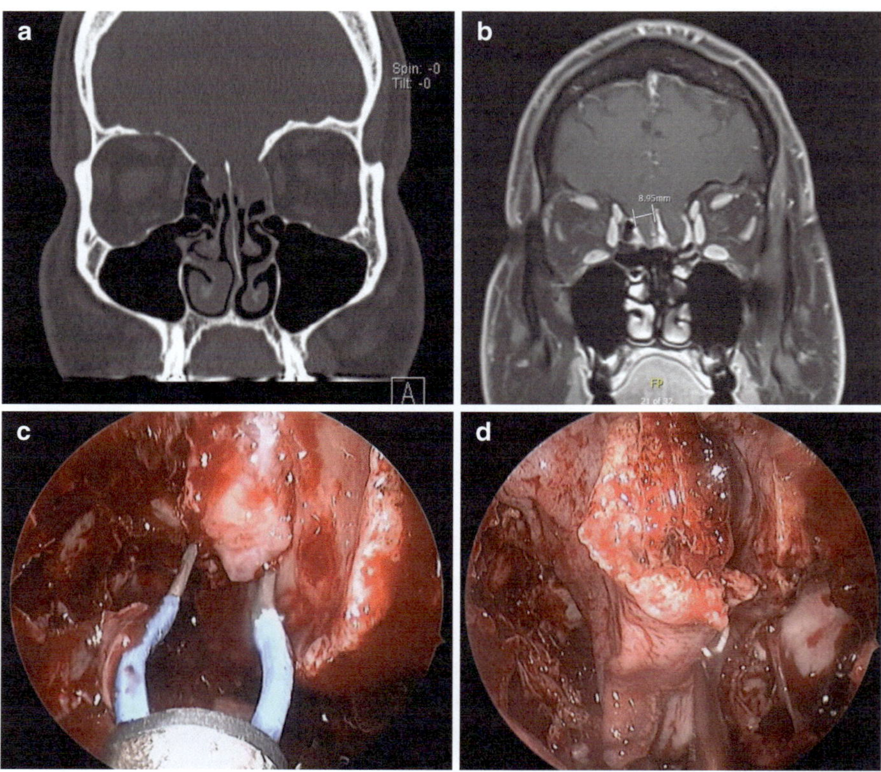

Fig. 10.6 Imaging with computed tomography (**a**) and magnetic resonance imaging (**b**) of a case of large bilateral ethmoid defects resulting in encephalocele formation and CSF leak. (**c**) Endoscopic photograph of right ethmoid encephalocele, (**d**) endoscopic photograph after placement of bilateral nasoseptal flaps for reconstruction (Image credit: Property of MUSC rhinology, used with permission)

watery nasal drainage, with possible salty or metallic tasting postnasal drainage in the early postoperative period. Surgeons must be vigilant to recognize these symptoms as potential signs of a CSF leak. Initial testing would involve collection of rhinorrhea fluid for beta-2 transferrin testing which is highly sensitive and specific and the gold standard for diagnosis of a CSF leak. Imaging with high-resolution CT scan of the sinuses and skull base will aid in localization of the skull base defect. Additional imaging may be employed to aid in localization as noted before, including CT cisternogram or MRI with or without cisternography. Though nuclear medicine cisternogram can localize the side of leak and has some utility in low and intermittent leaks, due to imprecise localization and high false-positive rate, it is generally not relied upon as a very useful imaging modality [35]. Additionally, intrathecal fluorescein can be utilized intraoperatively to aid in localization of the CSF leak site. However, it is used off label and has well-described neurological complications including seizures, headaches, and cranial nerve deficits, and full informed consent should be obtained prior to use [44]. Again, rapid diagnosis and treatment of the CSF fistula is important to minimize risk of meningitis which could have severe consequences.

Management of Iatrogenic CSF Leaks

Unlike in non-iatrogenic traumatic CSF leaks, iatrogenic CSF leaks are not likely to resolve with conservative management, and surgical repair is considered the first-line therapy [3]. As previously noted, in an ideal situation, the CSF leak would be identified at the time of injury and repaired at that time as well. However, surgeon experience/expertise and hospital resources vary widely; thus even with timely identification, immediate repair may not be possible. If a surgeon without adequate experience or expertise in addressing this complication encounters one, one option is to consult a colleague with expertise in this area intraoperatively. Another option would be to temporize the situation with nasal packing and arrange for transfer for a higher level of care. Other considerations to take into account in the decision to transfer the patient would be setting of the surgery (if at an outpatient surgery center), and hospital resources (accessibility to neurosurgical and intensive care resources which may be needed) as the patient should be monitored postoperatively.

Surgical repair of iatrogenic CSF leaks has been shown to be safe and effective via an endoscopic approach. Multiple studies have reported high success rates with a variety of reconstruction techniques, ranging from 86 to 100% in repair of traumatic CSF leaks, but most often these studies grouped iatrogenic and traumatic CSF leaks together [3]. One study which provided subgroup analysis found a 92% success rate with initial endoscopic repair for iatrogenic CSF leaks related to endoscopic sinus surgery [10]. Multilayer repair with a combination of homologous grafts (fat or fascia), allografts, xenografts, free mucosal grafts, and intranasal vascularized mucosal flaps is generally preferred, especially for larger defects, but smaller defects may be successfully reconstructed with a single-layer reconstruction using free mucosal grafts or vascularized flaps [31]. The patient should be monitored postoperatively in the inpatient setting for neurological assessment and potential persistent leak.

Summary

Traumatic anterior skull base CSF leaks, iatrogenic and non-iatrogenic, can be significant and complex problems which require timely identification and management. Persistent and untreated anterior skull base CSF leaks carry a high risk of ascending meningitis which increases over time with potentially serious consequences. The management of traumatic anterior skull base CSF leaks is dependent on the mechanism of injury and characteristics of the anterior skull base defect. For non-iatrogenic traumatic CSF leaks, conservative non-surgical management is an option as first-line treatment for most cases, with surgical treatment reserved for failures with non-surgical modalities and severe skull base injuries. For iatrogenic CSF leaks, surgical management is initially recommended.

References

1. Mathias T, Levy J, Fatakia A, McCoul ED. Contemporary approach to the diagnosis and management of cerebrospinal fluid rhinorrhea. Ochsner J. 2016;16(2):136–42.
2. Le C, Strong EB, Luu Q. Management of anterior skull base cerebrospinal fluid leaks. J Neurol Surg B Skull Base. 2016;77(5):404–11.
3. Wang EW, Zanation AM, Gardner PA, Schwartz TH, Eloy JA, Adappa ND, et al. ICAR: endoscopic skull-base surgery. Int Forum Allergy Rhinol. 2019;9(S3):S145–s365.
4. Liao KH, Wang JY, Lin HW, Lui TN, Chen KY, Yen DH, et al. Risk of death in patients with post-traumatic cerebrospinal fluid leakage--analysis of 1773 cases. J Chin Med Assoc. 2016;79(2):58–64.
5. Mourad M, Inman JC, Chan DM, Ducic Y. Contemporary trends in the Management of Posttraumatic Cerebrospinal Fluid Leaks. Craniomaxillofac Trauma Reconstr. 2018;11(1):71–7.
6. Donald PJ. Neurosurgery: Skull Base craniofacial trauma. J Neurol Surg B Skull Base. 2016;77(5):412–8.
7. Sivanandapanicker J, Nagar M, Kutty R, Sunilkumar BS, Peethambaran A, Rajmohan BP, et al. Analysis and clinical importance of Skull Base fractures in adult patients with traumatic brain injury. J Neurosci Rural Pract. 2018;9(3):370–5.
8. Guyer RA, Turner JH. Delayed presentation of traumatic cerebrospinal fluid rhinorrhea: case report and literature review. Allergy Rhinol (Providence). 2015;6(3):188–90.
9. Ibrahim AA, Okasha M, Elwany S. Endoscopic endonasal multilayer repair of traumatic CSF rhinorrhea. Eur Arch Otorhinolaryngol. 2016;273(4):921–6.
10. Banks CA, Palmer JN, Chiu AG, O'Malley BW Jr, Woodworth BA, Kennedy DW. Endoscopic closure of CSF rhinorrhea: 193 cases over 21 years. Otolaryngol Head Neck Surg. 2009;140(6):826–33.
11. Oh JW, Kim SH, Whang K. Traumatic cerebrospinal fluid leak: diagnosis and management. Korean J Neurotrauma. 2017;13(2):63–7.
12. Yellinek S, Cohen A, Merkin V, Shelef I, Benifla M. Clinical significance of skull base fracture in patients after traumatic brain injury. J Clin Neurosci. 2016;25:111–5.
13. Aydin S. Intracranial penetrating trauma caused by fishing sinker. World Neurosurg. 2019;129:237–40.
14. Bunevicius A, Bareikis K, Kalasauskas L, Tamasauskas A. Penetrating anterior Skull Base fracture inflicted by a Cow's horn. J Neurosci Rural Pract. 2016;7(Suppl 1):S106–s8.
15. Ghadersohi S, Ference EH, Detwiller K, Kern RC. Presentation, workup, and management of penetrating transorbital and transnasal injuries: a case report and systematic review. Am J Rhinol Allergy. 2017;31(2):29–34.
16. Hebecker R, Sola S, Lenz JH, Just T, Piek J. An unusual case of a penetrating skull-base injury caused by a wild deer's antler. Cen Eur Neurosurg. 2009;70(1):48–51.
17. Teng TS, Ishak NL, Subha ST, Bakar SA. Traumatic transnasal penetrating injury with cerebral spinal fluid leak. EXCLI J. 2019;18:223–8.
18. Bhatoe HS. Missile injuries of the anterior skull base. Skull Base. 2004;14(1):1–8; discussion

19. Kriet JD, Stanley RB Jr, Grady MS. Self-inflicted submental and transoral gunshot wounds that produce nonfatal brain injuries: management and prognosis. J Neurosurg. 2005;102(6):1029–32.
20. Levi L, Borovich B, Guilburd JN, Grushkiewicz I, Lemberger A, Linn S, et al. Wartime neurosurgical experience in Lebanon, 1982-85. I: penetrating craniocerebral injuries. Isr J Med Sci. 1990;26(10):548–54.
21. Reyes C, Solares CA. Endoscopic repair of frontal sinus cerebrospinal fluid leaks after firearm injuries: report of two cases. J Neurol Surg Rep. 2015;76(1):e8–e12.
22. Tominaga GTB, Aquino MR, Beckmann NM, Hanks SE, Spence SC, West OC, Burd RS, Falcone RJ Jr, Gaines BA, Jensen AR, Molik K, Cocanour CS, Cribari C, Fernandez FB, Jacobson L, Livingston DH, Mandell SP, Miller AN, Miller RS, Stassen NA. ACS TQIP best practices guidelines in imaging. Chicago: American College of Surgeons; 2018.
23. Zapalac JS, Marple BF, Schwade ND. Skull base cerebrospinal fluid fistulas: a comprehensive diagnostic algorithm. Otolaryngol Head Neck Surg. 2002;126(6):669–76.
24. Warnecke A, Averbeck T, Wurster U, Harmening M, Lenarz T, Stöver T. Diagnostic relevance of beta2-transferrin for the detection of cerebrospinal fluid fistulas. Arch Otolaryngol Head Neck Surg. 2004;130(10):1178–84.
25. Grayson JW, Jeyarajan H, Illing EA, Cho DY, Riley KO, Woodworth BA. Changing the surgical dogma in frontal sinus trauma: transnasal endoscopic repair. Int Forum Allergy Rhinol. 2017;7(5):441–9.
26. Albu S, Florian IS, Bolboaca SD. The benefit of early lumbar drain insertion in reducing the length of CSF leak in traumatic rhinorrhea. Clin Neurol Neurosurg. 2016;142:43–7.
27. Bernal-Sprekelsen M, Alobid I, Mullol J, Trobat F, Tomás-Barberán M. Closure of cerebrospinal fluid leaks prevents ascending bacterial meningitis. Rhinology. 2005;43(4):277–81.
28. Schoentgen C, Henaux PL, Godey B, Jegoux F. Management of post-traumatic cerebrospinal fluid (CSF) leak of anterior skull base: 10 years experience. Acta Otolaryngol. 2013;133(9):944–50.
29. Psaltis AJ, Schlosser RJ, Banks CA, Yawn J, Soler ZM. A systematic review of the endoscopic repair of cerebrospinal fluid leaks. Otolaryngol Head Neck Surg. 2012;147(2):196–203.
30. Sharma SD, Kumar G, Bal J, Eweiss A. Endoscopic repair of cerebrospinal fluid rhinorrhoea. Eur Ann Otorhinolaryngol Head Neck Dis. 2016;133(3):187–90.
31. Chin D, Harvey RJ. Endoscopic reconstruction of frontal, cribriform and ethmoid skull base defects. Adv Otorhinolaryngol. 2013;74:104–18.
32. Chaaban MR, Conger B, Riley KO, Woodworth BA. Transnasal endoscopic repair of posterior table fractures. Otolaryngol Head Neck Surg. 2012;147(6):1142–7.
33. Jones V, Virgin F, Riley K, Woodworth BA. Changing paradigms in frontal sinus cerebrospinal fluid leak repair. Int Forum Allergy Rhinol. 2012;2(3):227–32.
34. Woodworth BA, Schlosser RJ, Palmer JN. Endoscopic repair of frontal sinus cerebrospinal fluid leaks. J Laryngol Otol. 2005;119(9):709–13.
35. Illing EA, Woodworth BA. Management of Frontal Sinus Cerebrospinal Fluid Leaks and Encephaloceles. Otolaryngol Clin N Am. 2016;49(4):1035–50.
36. Ramakrishnan VR, Kingdom TT, Nayak JV, Hwang PH, Orlandi RR. Nationwide incidence of major complications in endoscopic sinus surgery. Int Forum Allergy Rhinol. 2012;2(1):34–9.
37. Venkatesan NN, Mattox DE, Del Gaudio JM. Cerebrospinal fluid leaks following septoplasty. Ear Nose Throat J. 2014;93(12):E43–6.
38. Sayal NR, Keider E, Korkigian S. Visualized ethmoid roof cerebrospinal fluid leak during frontal balloon sinuplasty. Ear Nose Throat J. 2018;97(8):E34–e8.
39. Tomazic PV, Stammberger H, Koele W, Gerstenberger C. Ethmoid roof CSF-leak following frontal sinus balloon sinuplasty. Rhinology. 2010;48(2):247–50.
40. Wright AE, Davis ED, Khan M, Chaaban MR. Exploring balloon sinuplasty adverse events with the innovative OpenFDA database. Am J Rhinol Allergy. 2020;34(5):626–31.

41. Paquin R, Ryan L, Vale FL, Rutkowski M, Byrd JK. CSF leak after COVID-19 nasopharyngeal swab: a case report. Laryngoscope. 2021;131(9):1927–9.
42. Rajah J, Lee J. CSF rhinorrhoea post COVID-19 swab: a case report and review of literature. J Clin Neurosci. 2021;86:6–9.
43. Sellari-Franceschini S, Dallan I, Bajraktari A, Fiacchini G, Nardi M, Rocchi R, et al. Surgical complications in orbital decompression for Graves' orbitopathy. Acta Otorhinolaryngol Ital. 2016;36(4):265–74.
44. Keerl R, Weber RK, Draf W, Wienke A, Schaefer SD. Use of sodium fluorescein solution for detection of cerebrospinal fluid fistulas: an analysis of 420 administrations and reported complications in Europe and the United States. Laryngoscope. 2004;114(2):266–72.

Chapter 11
Spontaneous CSF Leaks and Encephaloceles

Ashwini Tilak, Jessica W. Grayson, and Bradford A. Woodworth

Introduction

Spontaneous cerebrospinal fluid (sCSF) leaks occur in the absence of preceding trauma, skull base surgery, or congenital defect. They are commonly associated with a meningoencephalocele—a herniation of the meninges with or without brain tissue through the associated defect (referred to as either "encephaloceles" or "meningoencephaloceles" throughout the text). Historically, these were referred to as "idiopathic" CSF leaks. Today, it is widely accepted that sCSF leaks represent a variant of idiopathic intracranial hypertension (IIH) [1–6]. Patients with sCSF leaks share demographic characteristics with those with IIH, including predisposition for female gender, middle age, and obesity. They also share clinical characteristics including symptoms of pulsatile tinnitus, headache, visual disturbances, and balance issues. Radiographically, multiple studies have identified characteristics in sCSF leaks that are consistent with underlying IIH such as empty sella syndrome [1, 6–8]. A large majority of patients also suffer from elevated intracranial pressure, which are noted on opening pressure during lumbar

A. Tilak · J. W. Grayson
Department of Otolaryngology—Head and Neck Surgery, University of Alabama in Birmingham, Birmingham, AL, USA
e-mail: jgrayson@uabmc.edu

B. A. Woodworth (✉)
Department of Otolaryngology—Head and Neck Surgery, University of Alabama in Birmingham, Birmingham, AL, USA

Gregory Fleming James Cystic Fibrosis Research Center, Birmingham, AL, USA
e-mail: bwoodworth@uabmc.edu

E. C. Kuan et al. (eds.), *Skull Base Reconstruction*,
https://doi.org/10.1007/978-3-031-27937-9_11

163

puncture and following closure of the skull base defect. The success rate of sCSF leak repairs has improved in recent years when coupled with medical treatment for underlying IIH. This suggests that IIH drives skull base attenuation and formation of skull base defects resulting in CSF rhinorrhea [1, 4, 7, 9–11]. In this chapter, we describe the detailed approach to spontaneous CSF leak management, including preoperative imaging findings and other workup, intraoperative repair techniques to improve success rates, and postoperative treatment standards to mitigate chronically elevated ICP and thus decrease recurrence at the primary site and other skull base locations.

Preoperative Management

Patients should undergo both computed tomography (CT) and magnetic resonance imaging (MRI) in the evaluation and management of a sCSF leak. Preoperative imaging should include, at the least, an axial, thin-cut CT of the sinuses (≤1 mm slices) with coronal and sagittal reconstruction. CT delineates focal bone dehiscence and provides detailed images for intraoperative computer-assisted navigation. Fluid and soft tissue can look similar on CT imaging, and smaller meningoencephaloceles may be difficult to identify, particularly in the olfactory cleft. Inflammatory mucosal changes from pre-existing chronic rhinosinusitis also complicate the identification of encephaloceles. On MRI, meninges may be better seen herniating through the defect and confirm the presence of an encephalocele (Fig. 11.2) [7, 12, 13]. Neuroimaging findings consistent with intracranial hypertension are most readily identified with MRI scan as well [6, 12, 13].

Radiographic Features

Empty Sella

Eighty-five percent of patients with sCSF leaks will have concomitant presence of an empty sella on MRI [7, 9]. Dural herniation through the sellar diaphragm into the sella turcica leads to the radiographic appearance of an absent pituitary gland as the space fills with CSF and the pituitary gland is compressed against the floor (Fig. 11.1). Agid et al. [14] discovered empty sella to have a sensitivity of 26.7% and a specificity of 94.6% in IIH subjects. However, Bidot et al. [15] suggested that the appearance of empty sella in diagnostic imaging is also highly sensitive for IIH, with a pooled sensitivity of 80% and a pooled specificity of 83%.

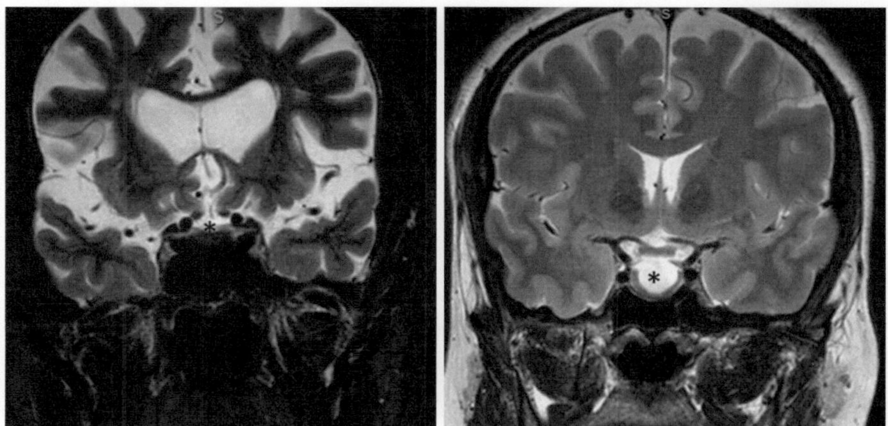

Fig. 11.1 Coronal T2-weighted MRI scan of a patient with normal pituitary gland and sella (left) and a patient with spontaneous CSF leak/IIH and an "empty sella," with pituitary gland compressed against the floor of the sella turcica with the remaining space filled with CSF (asterisk). (Image credit: Property of Bradford Woodworth, MD)

Orbital Findings

Dilation of the optic nerve sheath (ONS), optic nerve tortuosity, and protrusion and enhancement of the optic nerve head are commonly noted in patients with IIH [16, 17]. However, they are less often seen in the presence of an active CSF leak due to pressure valve release. Aaron et al. [18] identified that IIH patients with concurrent CSF leak did not present with papilledema and ICP was lower than a similar cohort of IIH patients. ICP measurements equalize across these groups after closure of the skull base defect. It is also thought that those with spontaneous CSF leaks are resistant to visual disturbances noted with elevated pressure. This may explain why the average age of diagnosis for IIH is in the 30s, while sCSF leaks occur on average in the 50s. Distension of the ONS on MRI is reflected as a ring of CSF surrounding the optic nerve and is considered one of the major indicators for IIH [19, 20]. Mallery et al. [21] reported a specificity of 83% and a sensitivity of 51%, while optic nerve head protrusion is highly specific for IIH with a specificity of 100% [14, 22]. Vertical tortuosity of the optic nerve is another commonly associated finding for elevated ICP with a specificity of 91.1% [14]. It is often associated with a "smear sign," where the mid-region of the optic nerve is obscured on T1-weighted images by orbital fat [23]. Finally, posterior globe flattening refers to a loss of curvature of the posterior sclera where the sclera merges with the outer layers of the optic nerve and is considered to be the most specific sign (97–100%) with a sensitivity of 43–57% [24]. ICP transmitted through the optic nerve to the posterior sclera leads to chorioretinal folds and acquired hyperopia [19]. While papilledema is best identified

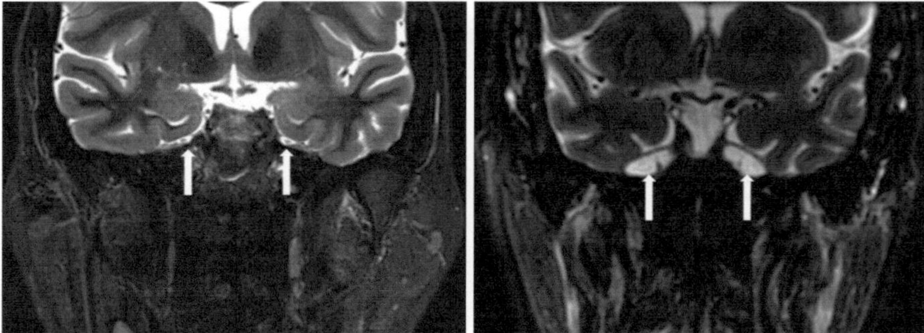

Fig. 11.2 T2-weight coronal MRI scans of a patient with normal Meckel's caves (left, arrows) and a patient with spontaneous CSF leak/IIH with dilated Meckel's caves (right, arrows). (Image credit: Property of Bradford Woodworth, MD)

clinically by fundoscopic examination, enhancement of the optic disc may also represent papilledema, although not specific, as it has been identified with other causes of optic disc edema [17].

Enlargement of Meckel's Cave

Meckel's cave enlargement may also be noted in patients with sCSF leaks [20, 25–27]. The elevated ICP is thought to compress the trigeminal ganglion in Meckel's cave leading to replacement with CSF, similar to CSF displacement in an empty sella. This is best identified on T2-weighted slices as an increase in intensity and dimensions of Meckel's cave (Fig. 11.2) [20]. This can also lead to the formation of petrous apex encephaloceles medial to Meckel's cave.

Transverse Venous Sinus Stenosis

Transverse venous sinus stenosis (TVSS) is best identified by magnetic resonance venography (MRV) [28]. It is identified in up to 90% of IIH patients, most commonly bilaterally. However, it is unclear whether TVSS causes IIH or vice versa. Patients suffering from IIH often experience pulsatile tinnitus due to turbulent blood flow. TVSS persists despite medical or surgical treatment of IIH [29]. However, endovascular shunting to manage transverse sinus stenosis has been successful in mitigating the visual symptoms of IIH and decreasing the need for medical therapy [30, 31].

Meningoceles and Meningoencephaloceles

Meningoencephaloceles are very common with spontaneous CSF leaks due to the underlying elevated ICP (Fig. 11.3) [15]. Current theory postulates that over time, the insult to the skull base caused by increased ICP leads to attenuation and eventually a defect with herniation [12].

Skull Base Attenuation and Arachnoid Pits

Skull base attenuation (thinning) on CT scan and multiple skull base defects are very common findings in spontaneous CSF leak patients (Fig. 11.4). Psaltis et al. identified significantly thinner skull base around the lateral lamella, ethmoid roof,

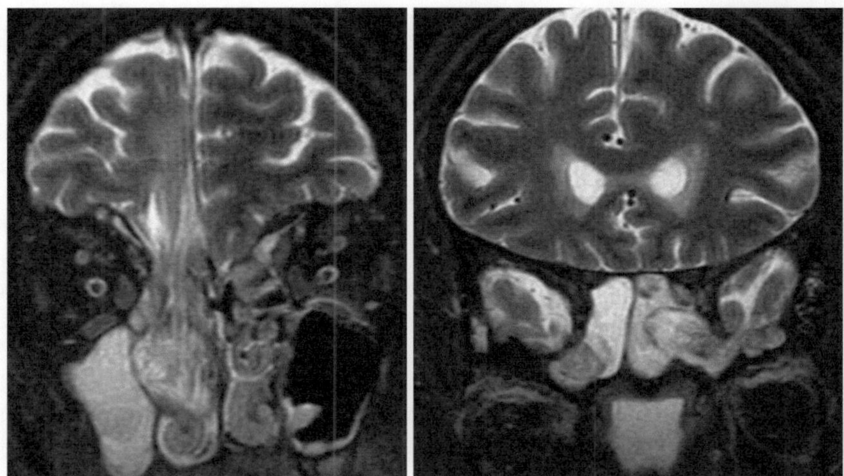

Fig. 11.3 T2-weighted MRI scans of a patient with a large frontoethmoidal encephalocele (left) and bilateral sphenoid lateral recess encephaloceles (right). (Image credit: Property of Bradford Woodworth, MD)

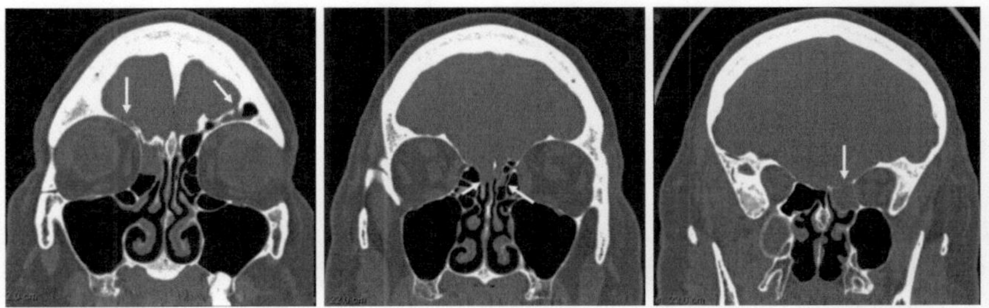

Fig. 11.4 Coronal CT scans of the sinuses of one patient with five separate skull base defects (arrows) in a patient with spontaneous CSF leaks and IIH. (Image credit: Property of Bradford Woodworth, MD)

and sella, all common sites of sCSF leaks in a case control study. Arachnoid pits are thought to represent arachnoid granulations which have penetrated the dura but failed to reach a venous sinus, leading to the appearance of lobulated or multilobulated bony "scalloped out" areas along the inner table of the skull base [6, 12]. In patients with IIH, the pulsatile increase in ICP leads to the formation of pits at the sites of arachnoid villi. These pits could lead to formation of bony defects through which the arachnoid/dura may herniate causing meningoencephalocele and CSF leak [32–34]. They appear isointense to CSF on MR imaging [12].

Sternberg's Canal Is Not Related to Spontaneous CSF Leaks

There is some controversy in the literature about the cause of spontaneous CSF leaks being linked to a persistent Sternberg's canal; however, current embryologic theory as well as radiographic evidence of leak location does not support this [6, 25, 35, 36]. In 1888, Maximilian Sternberg described the existence of a canal created during fusion of the alisphenoid, basisphenoid, and presphenoid ossification centers, which occurs near the lateral sphenoid sinus [6]. Sternberg examined dry skulls of 3–4-year-olds and saw that often the canal disappeared with age. Some adult skulls contained the defect, and thus he posited that failure of this fusion may lead to a persistent lateral craniopharyngeal canal. Since then, some authors erroneously posit that this canal is the cause of spontaneous lateral sphenoid CSF leaks [37–39]. However, given the evidence that sCSF leaks are related to intracranial hypertension, including demographic similarities as well as treatment failure when a leak is repaired and ICP is not addressed, this theory is not a plausible explanation for the etiology of these leaks. One paper quoting Sternberg's canal as a source of sCSF leak mentions a near 50% failure rate after repair, suggesting that the cause may have been IIH after all [37]. In addition, the canal is present medial to the superior orbital fissure, foramen rotundum, and V2; nearly all lateral sphenoid CSF leaks are located lateral to V2 [6]. In an imaging-based study, which examined 1000 sphenoid sinus CT scans and compared to a database of sCSF leaks, only one skull base defect traveling medial to V2 resembled the historical description of Sternberg's canal. All 25 pts. with lateral sphenoid CSF leaks had defects and arachnoid pits lateral to V2 [40]. Given the constellation of evidence, the authors argue that Sternberg's canal should be eliminated from the literature as a cause of spontaneous CSF leaks.

Surgical Management

The current standard of care of spontaneous CSF leaks includes endoscopic repair with treatment of underlying IIH, either surgically or medically [2–4, 7, 11, 41–45]. Historically, success rates for repair of spontaneous CSF leaks have been lower than those for iatrogenic or traumatic leaks; however this gap has closed as surgeons have started to manage ICP after repair, and currently endoscopic repair followed by ICP management is the recommended standard of treatment [5, 44, 46, 47].

A standard protocol is followed for treatment of spontaneous CSF leaks and encephaloceles at our institution. We approach these cases in combination with the neurosurgical team, which allows for multidisciplinary patient care in the setting of ICP management (lumbar drain, VP shunt placement) and management of potential, albeit rare, complications (intracranial hemorrhage) following resection of the encephalocele. Lumbar drains are placed intraoperatively, and opening pressure is measured [43]. As the patient already has a route of egress for CSF, the pressure does not represent the true extent of intracranial hypertension, but provides a good starting point measurement of relative pressure. Fluorescein is used intrathecally to identify occult leaks and confirm radiographic findings [48]. A mixture of 0.1 mL of 10% fluorescein diluted in 10 mL of sterile preservative free saline or the patient's own CSF is injected into the lumbar drain over 10 min. Consent is obtained from the patient prior to the case, as this is a non-FDA-approved use of fluorescein. The defect is then approached endoscopically with opening the sinuses on the side of the leak. Adjunct approaches such as the transpterygoid approach for sphenoid lateral recess leaks (Fig. 11.5) and periorbital suspension for supraorbital or far lateral

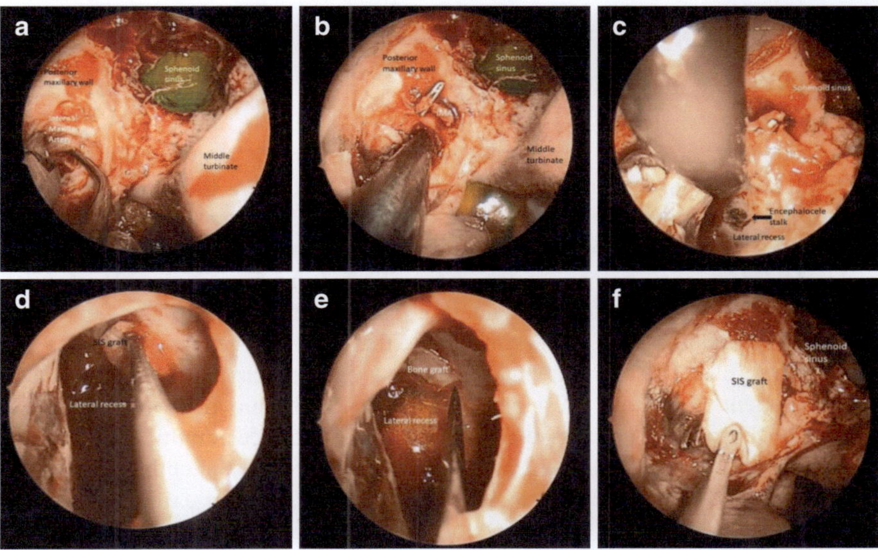

Fig. 11.5 Intraoperative endoscopic images for repair of lateral skull base encephalocele. (**a**) Right-sided FESS has been completed. Posterior wall of the maxillary sinus is removed, and the internal maxillary artery (IMA) is identified and clipped. Fluorescein is noted in the sphenoid sinus from the lateral recess CSF leak. (**b**) Once the IMA is clipped and divided, the pterygoid is removed to reveal the recess, inferior to V2. (**c**) The encephalocele is reduced with coblation until it is flush with the bony skull base. (**d**) After measurements are obtained, porcine small intestine submucosa (SIS) is placed into the epidural space. (**e**) A bone graft is next placed in the epidural space as the second layer. (**f**) A second layer of SIS is placed on top of the bone graft. (Image credit: Property of Bradford Woodworth, MD)

frontal sinus CSF leaks may be employed [11, 49–55]. If an encephalocele is present, it is fulgurated with radiofrequency coblation and bipolar until the base is level with the skull base [56]. A graft site is prepared by removing a cuff of normal mucosa surrounding the defect with a coblator. If there is a bony defect >2–3 mm, this is reconstructed using a bone graft harvested from the septum, turbinate, or posterior maxillary wall. Once the encephalocele is reduced, a porcine small intestine submucosal graft is placed in the epidural space, followed by a bone graft (if being used), followed by an overlay of porcine small intestine (Biodesign®, Cook Medical, Bloomington, In) or pedicled flap. The most often used pedicled flap is the nasoseptal flap; however, middle turbinate flaps can also be used [57–59]. We use a nasoseptal flap based on the posterior septal artery for cribriform, ethmoid, and planum sphenoidale leaks as there is evidence that this type of vascularized graft is superior when compared to free tissue grafts [60, 61]. In addition, bone grafts are not typically an option for cribriform leaks due to their size and location (leaks through olfactory filia), so we prefer vascularized tissue in this region for fast healing and support. Lateral sphenoid recess defects are repaired in three-layer fashion (porcine small intestine submucosa, bone, porcine small intestine submucosa) [6]. In order to maintain consistent pressure across the repair, iodoform bolsters are used to hold the repair in place [62]. We insert middle meatal spacers to provide support to the iodoform packing and prevent closure of the ethmoid cavity [63, 64].

Postoperative Management

Postoperatively, the patient is monitored in the neurologic ICU overnight. The lumbar drain is clamped at midnight on postoperative day 0. ICP is then measured 6–8 h later. If ICP is elevated at this time (typically >20 cm H_2O), acetazolamide 500 mg BID is started. The ICP is measured again 6–8 h after initiation to evaluate for post-acetazolamide response [65]. If the patient's pressure is significantly elevated (>30 cm H_2O) despite its use, VP shunting may be recommended as a permanent means of ICP control. It is important to note that these are general guidelines and not steadfast rules. Decisions are made regarding shunting based on team discussion and the patient's input and preference. Patients with chronic kidney disease, sulfa allergy, or those considered high risk (including recurrences, multiple defects, or extensive skull base attenuation on CT) are considered for shunting even if an appropriate response to acetazolamide is observed [43]. Adequate treatment of ICP post-repair is an extremely important component of management to prevent recurrence of CSF leak or further defects [47].

Approximately 2 weeks after surgery, postoperative packing is removed in the office under endoscopic guidance with topical anesthesia. If the patient was placed on long-term acetazolamide therapy, a basic metabolic panel is obtained to monitor for development of electrolyte abnormalities. Approximately 1 year after surgery, patients undergo a CT sinus without contrast to check incorporation of the bone graft and identify any new defects or attenuation that may develop.

Long-Term Medical Management

We recommend long-term use of acetazolamide unless patients undergo significant weight loss. In studies examining patients with IIH, decreased ICP was noted with even a modest 3–5% weight loss [66, 67]. Weight loss with a moderate diet and exercise program or bariatric surgery as indicated is an important way of treating IIH. Although there is limited data on topiramate, it may be used in place of acetazolamide to lower intracranial pressure, as it is also a carbonic anhydrase inhibitor [68, 69]. It also has the additional effect of decreasing appetite, which could help with weight loss.

Alternative Strategies: Dural Venous Stenting

Dural venous sinus stenting, a relatively new technique developed to treat IIH, has not been studied extensively in patients with sCSF leak. However, preliminary data for its use in patients with IIH without CSF leak demonstrates moderate symptom improvement in headache and visual acuity [30, 70–72]. Dural venous sinus stenting as a treatment for IIH is based on the theory that a stenosis between two sinuses increases CSF pressure. In dural venous sinus stenting (VSS), a patient is first started on dual antiplatelet therapy. Next, cerebral venography (via groin or other central venous access) is performed, and the pressure gradient across a sinus stenosis is measured; if the gradient is large (8 mm Hg most commonly used cutoff across several studies), a stent is inserted [72]. In several trials in the literature, a cohort of patients with medically refractory IIH (but no mention of leak) underwent VSS. While complication rates are low (~3%), complications have included intracranial hemorrhage and death in a small number of patients. The failure rate has been reported as 2.4% [71]. Published rates of improvement in clinical symptomatology are 40–69% [73]. One prospective trial, which involved measurement of ICP pre- and post stenting via lumbar puncture, actually saw a significant decrease in ICP after stenting, and a decreased dose of acetazolamide was required to control symptoms [30]. There is very little in the literature regarding VSS in patients with spontaneous CSF leak; however, one case report does mention a patient with IIH and a spontaneous CSF leak who underwent VSS without primary surgical repair of leak and clinically resolved their rhinorrhea; however, no skull base imaging was reported pre- or post stenting [70].

Conclusion

Spontaneous cerebrospinal fluid leaks, which occur in the absence of preceding trauma, skull base surgery, or congenital defect, are generally accepted to be sequelae of IIH. Adequate management of these skull base defects require identification on CT and MRI, adequate repair of the defect with uniform packing across the defect, and postoperative ICP management with weight loss, medical therapy, and possible VP shunting.

Disclosures Jessica W. Grayson has served on an advisory board for Glaxo-Smith-Kline. Bradford A. Woodworth serves as a consultant for Cook Medical, Smith and Nephew, and Medtronic.

References

1. Schlosser RJ, Woodworth BA, Wilensky EM, Grady MS, Bolger WE. Spontaneous cerebrospinal fluid leaks: a variant of benign intracranial hypertension. Ann Otol Rhinol Laryngol. 2006;115(7):495–500.
2. Chaaban MR, Illing E, Riley KO, Woodworth BA. Spontaneous cerebrospinal fluid leak repair: a five-year prospective evaluation. Laryngoscope. 2014;124(1):70–5.
3. Chaaban MR, Illing E, Riley KO, Woodworth BA. Acetazolamide for high intracranial pressure cerebrospinal fluid leaks. Int Forum Allergy Rhinol. 2013;3(9):718–21.
4. Teachey W, Grayson J, Cho D-Y, Riley K, Woodworth B. Intervention for elevated intracranial pressure improves success rate after repair of spontaneous cerebrospinal fluid leaks. Laryngoscope. 2017;127:2011–6.
5. Wang EW, Zanation AM, Gardner PA, et al. ICAR: endoscopic skull-base surgery. Int Forum Allergy Rhinol. 2019;9(S3):S145–365.
6. Woodworth BA, Palmer JN. Spontaneous cerebrospinal fluid leaks. Curr Opin Otolaryngol Head Neck Surg. 2009;17(1):59–65.
7. Woodworth BA, Prince A, Chiu AG, et al. Spontaneous CSF leaks: a paradigm for definitive repair and management of intracranial hypertension. Otolaryngol Head Neck Surg. 2008;138(6):715–20.
8. Vaphiades MS, Ranganath NK, Woodworth BA. Spontaneous cerebrospinal fluid otorrhea and rhinorrhea in idiopathic intracranial hypertension patients. J Neuroophthalmol. 2013;33(4):416.
9. Schlosser RJ, Bolger WE. Significance of empty Sella in cerebrospinal fluid leaks. Otolaryngol Head Neck Surg. 2003;128(1):32–8.
10. Wise SK, Schlosser RJ. Evaluation of spontaneous nasal cerebrospinal fluid leaks. Curr Opin Otolaryngol Head Neck Surg. 2007;15(1):28–34.
11. Illing EA, Woodworth BA. Management of Frontal Sinus Cerebrospinal Fluid Leaks and Encephaloceles. Otolaryngol Clin N Am. 2016;49(4):1035–50.
12. Settecase F, Harnsberger HR, Michel MA, Chapman P, Glastonbury CM. Spontaneous lateral sphenoid cephaloceles: anatomic factors contributing to pathogenesis and proposed classification. AJNR Am J Neuroradiol. 2014;35(4):784–9.
13. Alonso RC, de la Peña MJ, Caicoya AG, Rodriguez MR, Moreno EA, de Vega Fernandez VM. Spontaneous Skull Base meningoencephaloceles and cerebrospinal fluid fistulas. Radiographics. 2013;33(2):553–70.
14. Agid R, Farb RI, Willinsky RA, Mikulis DJ, Tomlinson G. Idiopathic intracranial hypertension: the validity of cross-sectional neuroimaging signs. Neuroradiology. 2006;48(8):521–7.
15. Bidot S, Saindane AM, Peragallo JH, Bruce BB, Newman NJ, Biousse V. Brain imaging in idiopathic intracranial hypertension. J Neuroophthalmol. 2015;35(4):400–11.
16. Bidot S, Levy JM, Saindane AM, et al. Spontaneous Skull Base cerebrospinal fluid leaks and their relationship to idiopathic intracranial hypertension. Am J Rhinol Allergy. 2021;35(1):36–43.

17. Hoffmann J, Huppertz HJ, Schmidt C, et al. Morphometric and volumetric MRI changes in idiopathic intracranial hypertension. Cephalalgia. 2013;33(13):1075–84.
18. Aaron G, Doyle J, Vaphiades MS, Riley KO, Woodworth BA. Increased intracranial pressure in spontaneous CSF leak patients is not associated with papilledema. Otolaryngol Head Neck Surg. 2014;151(6):1061–6.
19. Barkatullah AF, Leishangthem L, Moss HE. MRI findings as markers of idiopathic intracranial hypertension. Curr Opin Neurol. 2021;34(1):75–83.
20. Aaron GP, Illing E, Lambertsen Z, et al. Enlargement of Meckel's cave in patients with spontaneous cerebrospinal fluid leaks. Int Forum Allergy Rhinol. 2017;7(4):421–4.
21. Mallery RM, Rehmani OF, Woo JH, et al. Utility of magnetic resonance imaging features for improving the diagnosis of idiopathic intracranial hypertension without papilledema. J Neuroophthalmol. 2019;39(3):299–307.
22. Maralani PJ, Hassanlou M, Torres C, et al. Accuracy of brain imaging in the diagnosis of idiopathic intracranial hypertension. Clin Radiol. 2012;67(7):656–63.
23. Passi N, Degnan AJ, Levy LM. MR imaging of papilledema and visual pathways: effects of increased intracranial pressure and pathophysiologic mechanisms. AJNR Am J Neuroradiol. 2013;34(5):919–24.
24. Wong H, Sanghera K, Neufeld A, Maxner C, Shankar JJS. Clinico-radiological correlation of magnetic resonance imaging findings in patients with idiopathic intracranial hypertension. Neuroradiology. 2020;62(1):49–53.
25. Illing E, Schlosser RJ, Palmer JN, Curé J, Fox N, Woodworth BA. Spontaneous sphenoid lateral recess cerebrospinal fluid leaks arise from intracranial hypertension, not Sternberg's canal. Int Forum Allergy Rhinol. 2014;4(3):246–50.
26. Bialer OY, Rueda MP, Bruce BB, Newman NJ, Biousse V, Saindane AM. Meningoceles in idiopathic intracranial hypertension. AJR Am J Roentgenol. 2014;202(3):608–13.
27. Butros SR, Goncalves LF, Thompson D, Agarwal A, Lee HK. Imaging features of idiopathic intracranial hypertension, including a new finding: widening of the foramen ovale. Acta Radiol. 2012;53(6):682–8.
28. Rehder D. Idiopathic intracranial hypertension: review of clinical syndrome, imaging findings, and treatment. Curr Probl Diagn Radiol. 2020;49(3):205–14.
29. Chan W, Green AL, Mishra A, Maxner C, Shankar JJS. Transverse venous sinus stenosis in idiopathic intracranial hypertension: a prospective pilot study. Can J Ophthalmol. 2020;55(5):401–5.
30. Patsalides A, Oliveira C, Wilcox J, et al. Venous sinus stenting lowers the intracranial pressure in patients with idiopathic intracranial hypertension. J Neurointerv Surg. 2019;11(2):175–8.
31. Skyrman S, Fytagoridis A, Andresen M, Bartek J Jr. Idiopathic intracranial hypertension and transverse sinus stenoses. BMJ Case Rep. 2013;2013:bcr2013010082.
32. Silver RI, Moonis G, Schlosser RJ, Bolger WE, Loevner LA. Radiographic signs of elevated intracranial pressure in idiopathic cerebrospinal fluid leaks: a possible presentation of idiopathic intracranial hypertension. Am J Rhinol. 2007;21(3):257–61.
33. Almontasheri A, Al-Qahtani B, Aldajani N. Arachnoid pit and extensive sinus pnematization as the cause of spontaneous lateral intrasphenoidal encephalocele. J Clin Imaging Sci. 2012;2:1.
34. Shetty PG, Shroff MM, Fatterpekar GM, Sahani DV, Kirtane MV. A retrospective analysis of spontaneous sphenoid sinus fistula: MR and CT findings. AJNR Am J Neuroradiol. 2000;21(2):337–42.
35. Adepoju A, Carlstrom LP, Graffeo CS, et al. Sternberg's canal and defect: is the lateral Craniopharyngeal Canal a source of spontaneous cerebrospinal fluid leak? Anatomic and radiological analysis in pediatric and adult populations. Oper Neurosurg (Hagerstown). 2021;20(4):426–32.
36. Woodworth BA, Neal JG, Schlosser RJ. Sphenoid sinus cerebrospinal fluid leaks. Oper Tech Otolaryngol Head Neck Surg. 2006;17(1):37–42.
37. Tomazic PV, Stammberger H. Spontaneous CSF-leaks and meningoencephaloceles in sphenoid sinus by persisting Sternberg's canal. Rhinology. 2009;47(4):369–74.

38. Castelnuovo P, Dallan I, Pistochini A, Battaglia P, Locatelli D, Bignami M. Endonasal endoscopic repair of Sternberg's canal cerebrospinal fluid leaks. Laryngoscope. 2007;117(2):345–9.
39. Schick B, Brors D, Prescher A. Sternberg's canal--cause of congenital sphenoidal meningocele. Eur Arch Otorhinolaryngol. 2000;257(8):430–2.
40. Barañano CF, Curé J, Palmer JN, Woodworth BA. Sternberg's canal: fact or fiction? Am J Rhinol Allergy. 2009;23(2):167–71.
41. Alexander NS, Chaaban MR, Riley KO, Woodworth BA. Treatment strategies for lateral sphenoid sinus recess cerebrospinal fluid leaks. Arch Otolaryngol Head Neck Surg. 2012;138(5):471–8.
42. Allensworth JJ, Rowan NR, Storck KA, Woodworth BA, Schlosser RJ. Endoscopic repair of spontaneous skull base defects decreases the incidence rate of intracranial complications. Int Forum Allergy Rhinol. 2019;9(10):1089–96.
43. McCormick JP, Tilak A, Lampkin HB, et al. An expedited intracranial pressure monitoring protocol following spontaneous CSF leak repair. Laryngoscope. 2021;131(2):E408–12.
44. Oakley GM, Orlandi RR, Woodworth BA, Batra PS, Alt JA. Management of cerebrospinal fluid rhinorrhea: an evidence-based review with recommendations. Int Forum Allergy Rhinol. 2016;6(1):17–24.
45. Banks C, Grayson J, Cho DY, Woodworth BA. Frontal sinus fractures and cerebrospinal fluid leaks: a change in surgical paradigm. Curr Opin Otolaryngol Head Neck Surg. 2020;28(1):52–60.
46. Georgalas C, Oostra A, Ahmed S, et al. International consensus statement: spontaneous cerebrospinal fluid rhinorrhea. Int Forum Allergy Rhinol. 2020;11:794–803.
47. Teachey W, Grayson J, Cho DY, Riley KO, Woodworth BA. Intervention for elevated intracranial pressure improves success rate after repair of spontaneous cerebrospinal fluid leaks. Laryngoscope. 2017;127(9):2011–6.
48. Shahangian A, Soler ZM, Baker A, et al. Successful repair of intraoperative cerebrospinal fluid leaks improves outcomes in endoscopic skull base surgery. Int Forum Allergy Rhinol. 2017;7(1):80–6.
49. Bolger WE. Endoscopic Transpterygoid approach to the lateral sphenoid recess: surgical approach and clinical experience. Otolaryngol Head Neck Surg. 2005;133(1):20–6.
50. Tilak A, Purvis J, Peña-Garcia A, et al. Above and beyond: periorbital suspension for endoscopic access to difficult frontal sinus pathology. Laryngoscope. 2022;132(3):538–44.
51. Grayson JW, Jeyarajan H, Illing EA, Cho DY, Riley KO, Woodworth BA. Changing the surgical dogma in frontal sinus trauma: transnasal endoscopic repair. Int Forum Allergy Rhinol. 2017;7(5):441–9.
52. Conger BT Jr, Illing E, Bush B, Woodworth BA. Management of lateral frontal sinus pathology in the endoscopic era. Otolaryngol Head Neck Surg. 2014;151(1):159–63.
53. Chaaban MR, Conger B, Riley KO, Woodworth BA. Transnasal endoscopic repair of posterior table fractures. Otolaryngol Head Neck Surg. 2012;147(6):1142–7.
54. Jones V, Virgin F, Riley K, Woodworth BA. Changing paradigms in frontal sinus cerebrospinal fluid leak repair. Int Forum Allergy Rhinol. 2012;2(3):227–32.
55. Purkey MT, Woodworth BA, Hahn S, Palmer JN, Chiu AG. Endoscopic repair of supraorbital ethmoid cerebrospinal fluid leaks. ORL J Otorhinolaryngol Relat Spec. 2009;71(2):93–8.
56. Smith N, Riley KO, Woodworth BA. Endoscopic Coblator™-assisted management of encephaloceles. Laryngoscope. 2010;120(12):2535–9.
57. Conger BT Jr, Riley K, Woodworth BA. The Draf III mucosal grafting technique: a prospective study. Otolaryngol Head Neck Surg. 2012;146(4):664–8.
58. Virgin F, Barañano CF, Riley K, Woodworth BA. Frontal sinus skull base defect repair using the pedicled nasoseptal flap. Otolaryngol Head Neck Surg. 2011;145(2):338–40.
59. Virgin FW, Bleier BS, Woodworth BA. Evolving materials and techniques for endoscopic sinus surgery. Otolaryngol Clin N Am. 2010;43(3):653–72, xi
60. Harvey RJ, Parmar P, Sacks R, Zanation AM. Endoscopic skull base reconstruction of large dural defects: a systematic review of published evidence. Laryngoscope. 2012;122(2):452–9.

61. Kim-Orden N, Shen J, Or M, Hur K, Zada G, Wrobel B. Endoscopic endonasal repair of spontaneous cerebrospinal fluid leaks using multilayer composite graft and vascularized pedicled Nasoseptal flap technique. Allergy Rhinol (Providence). 2019;10:2152656719888622.
62. Chaaban MR, Woodworth BA. Complications of skull base reconstruction. Adv Otorhinolaryngol. 2013;74:148–62.
63. Banks CA, Palmer JN, Chiu AG, O'Malley BW Jr, Woodworth BA, Kennedy DW. Endoscopic closure of CSF rhinorrhea: 193 cases over 21 years. Otolaryngol Head Neck Surg. 2009;140(6):826–33.
64. Woodworth BA, Schlosser RJ, Palmer JN. Endoscopic repair of frontal sinus cerebrospinal fluid leaks. J Laryngol Otol. 2005;119(9):709–13.
65. Tilak AM, Koehn H, Mattos J, Payne SC. Preoperative management of spontaneous cerebrospinal fluid rhinorrhea with acetazolamide. Int Forum Allergy Rhinol. 2019;9(3):265–9.
66. Thurtell MJ, Wall M. Idiopathic intracranial hypertension (pseudotumor cerebri): recognition, treatment, and ongoing management. Curr Treat Options Neurol. 2013;15(1):1–12.
67. Rudnick E, Sismanis A. Pulsatile tinnitus and spontaneous cerebrospinal fluid rhinorrhea: indicators of benign intracranial hypertension syndrome. Otol Neurotol. 2005;26(2):166–8.
68. Çelebisoy N, Gökçay F, Şirin H, Akyürekli Ö. Treatment of idiopathic intracranial hypertension: topiramate vs acetazolamide, an open-label study. Acta Neurol Scand. 2007;116(5):322–7.
69. Meibodi R, Ali MA, Mohammad S, Mehrdad M, Abolfazl A. The effect of topiramate as an adjunct therapy to acetazolamide in Idiopathic intracranial hypertension patients. Bali Med J. 2018;7(1):4.
70. San Millán D, Hallak B, Wanke I, et al. Dural venous sinus stenting as a stand-alone treatment for spontaneous skull base CSF leak secondary to venous pseudotumor cerebri syndrome. Neuroradiology. 2019;61(9):1103–6.
71. Leishangthem L, SirDeshpande P, Dua D, Satti SR. Dural venous sinus stenting for idiopathic intracranial hypertension: an updated review. J Neuroradiol. 2019;46(2):148–54.
72. Kabanovski A, Kisilevsky E, Yang Y, Margolin E. Dural venous sinus stenting in the treatment of idiopathic intracranial hypertension: a systematic review and critique of literature. Surv Ophthalmol. 2022;67(1):271–87.
73. Satti SR, Leishangthem L, Spiotta A, Chaudry MI. Dural venous sinus stenting for medically and surgically refractory idiopathic intracranial hypertension. Interv Neuroradiol. 2017;23(2):186–93.

Chapter 12
Congenital Encephaloceles

Liam Gallagher, Amrita Ray, and David A. Gudis

Introduction

An encephalocele is a sac-like, soft tissue mass that occurs when intracranial contents herniate through a defect or structurally weakened area of the skull base. Encephaloceles may be identified as a congenital mass in infancy or present later in adult life secondary to trauma, surgery, tumors, or idiopathic skull base defects. In pediatric populations, the great majority of encephaloceles are congenital; however, they may also result secondarily from trauma, tumors, surgery, or craniofacial clefts [1]. Although encephaloceles may course through temporal, occipital, and even parietal bone defects, this chapter will emphasize congenital anterior/frontal encephaloceles.

The presentation and clinical significance of encephaloceles can vary widely depending on the location, size, and herniated contents of the defect. For example, posterior encephaloceles have a higher incidence of neurologic complications and lower survival rates. Large encephaloceles, particularly those with over 50% of brain tissue herniation, may cause intrauterine demise of the fetus [2]. At birth, encephaloceles may present with critical airway obstruction and/or obvious facial deformities. Occult encephaloceles often present later with symptoms related to nasal obstruction, respiratory distress, or recurrent meningitis. Alternatively, smaller defects may produce only subtle cosmetic deformities.

L. Gallagher · D. A. Gudis (✉)
Department of Otolaryngology, Columbia University Irving Medical Center, New York-Presbyterian Hospital, New York, NY, USA
e-mail: dag62@cumc.columbia.edu

A. Ray
Henry Ford Hospital, Detroit, MI, USA
e-mail: aray9@hfhs.org

E. C. Kuan et al. (eds.), *Skull Base Reconstruction*,
https://doi.org/10.1007/978-3-031-27937-9_12

Epidemiology

Encephaloceles are generally rare, but measurements of their incidence and type appear to vary by geography.

Overall, posterior congenital encephaloceles appear to be more common than anterior ones, with 70–90% of congenital encephaloceles involving the occipital region [3–5]. Worldwide prevalence of neutral tube defects is estimated to be 18 per 10,000 live births [6], with encephaloceles comprising approximately 10–20% of all neural tube defects. While occipital encephaloceles predominate among populations of European descent, anterior encephaloceles tend to be more common in Southeast Asia, Africa, and Russia, occurring in 1 in 3500–6000 live births [7, 8].

The incidence appears to be slightly lower in developed countries. In the USA, for example, congenital encephaloceles occur in an estimated 1 in 10,000 live births. Other estimates have ranged as widely as 1 in 2000 to 1 in 12,500 live births [9–11].

Neural tube defects appear to have a sex predominance in females, and this appears to hold true regarding encephaloceles as well [12]. Occipital encephaloceles [13] appear to occur in females in higher rates; alternatively, the sex predisposition for anterior encephaloceles is more nuanced, with some sources favoring a male predisposition, while others show similar incidence [14].

Etiology and Pathophysiology

While some cases of encephaloceles can be attributed to tumors, trauma, or iatrogenic injury, the majority of cases are isolated defects with a sporadic pattern of incidence, and the pathogenesis is not well understood. Posterior/occipital encephaloceles are considered to be a variant of neural tube defects [15]. The most accepted theory regarding anterior encephaloceles proposes that they result from an incomplete anterior fusion of neural folds and/or incomplete separation of neuroectoderm and surface ectoderm after fusion, preventing somatic mesoderm from interposing to develop into skull bone and meninges [16–21] (Fig. 12.1).

The early fetal brain is surrounded by layers of mesoderm and ectoderm, together referred to as the neurocranium. The mesodermal layer gives rise to the developing nasal and frontal bones. The fonticulus frontalis is a temporary space that develops between the nasal and frontal bones [23]. Contact between the dura and ectoderm results in a meningeal projection into the prenasal space. In normal development, this projection is obliterated, ultimately becoming the foramen cecum. An error in the involution of this projection is the common initial pathogenesis of gliomas, dermoids, and some encephaloceles [24]. In the case of encephaloceles, the lack of separation produces a mesodermal defect; since rostral neuropore closure is a focal process, rather than a smoothly progressive one, the defect may arise in various

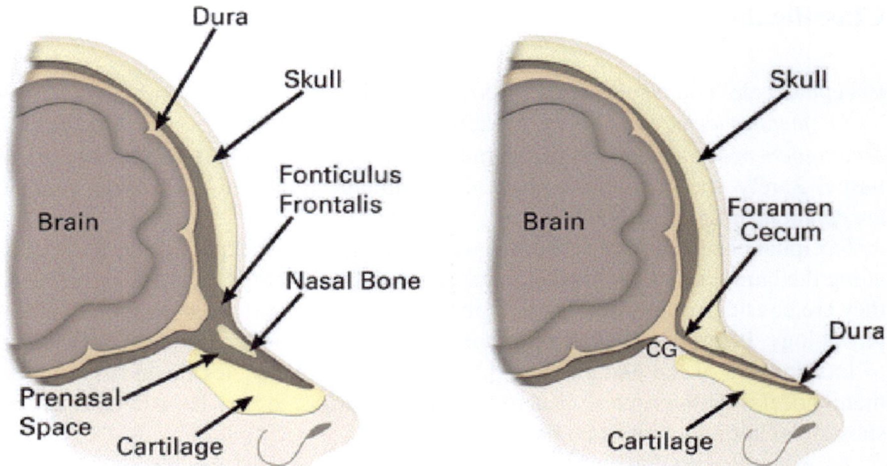

Fig. 12.1 Errors in the development of the nasal and frontal bone and rostral neuropore closure represent a common pathogenesis for anterior encephaloceles, gliomas, and dermoids. (Figure reprinted from [22])

locations. The anatomy of this bony defect ultimately defines the type and presentation of encephalocele.

Additional theories suggest abnormal gene signaling from the neural tube [25], malfunctions in the molecular sonic hedgehog pathway, as well as a sequalae of amniotic band syndrome [26–30]. Both anterior and posterior encephaloceles likely have multifactorial origins, including possible environmental, genetic, nutritional, and disease associations [23], although clear links have yet to be identified [27, 28]. Risk factors suggestive for congenital encephaloceles include those that may predispose for neural tube defects, which occur if the cranial neuropore is not fully closed by day 26 of gestation [25, 27, 31]. These risks include TORCH infections, family history of neural tube defects including anencephaly and spina bifida, insufficient prenatal folic acid intake, maternal rubella, and maternal diabetes [32].

Congenital encephaloceles have been associated with over 30 different diseases and syndromes including frontonasal dysplasia, Ehlers-Danlos syndrome, Meckel's syndrome, and amniotic band syndrome, among others; however, no identifiable specific genetic or familial inheritance pattern has been identified outside of a few isolated cases of autosomal dominant occipital encephaloceles [33]. Thus, the generally sporadic pattern of incidence and lack of strongly associated risk factors support the idea that these defects predominantly arise from mistakes in fetal skull development.

Classification

Encephaloceles can be classified by both their contents and location.

A *meningocele* describes a herniation that contains only meninges. *Meningoencephalocele* refers to a herniation that contains both meninges and brain tissue. Rarely, the herniation may be in communication with a ventricle, termed *encephalomeningocystocele*.

Occipital encephaloceles encompass up to 75% of all encephaloceles and occur along the lambdoid suture and foramen magnum [4, 15] (Fig. 12.2). As mentioned, they are considered a form of neural tube defects and arise through a similar pathophysiology. Parietal encephaloceles are rare and most commonly occur as a result of local atresia of the parietal bone [34]. These encephaloceles range from minor meningoceles, with primarily cutaneous manifestations, to very large defects which substantial herniation of brain tissue [35].

Anterior encephaloceles occur as a maldevelopment of the foramen cecum, which is a primitive tract between the anterior cranial fossa and nasal space [17, 24]. Anterior encephaloceles can be further classified by the location of protrusion from the skull base: these designations are *sincipital* and *basal* [36]. Sincipital encephaloceles are extranasal masses that occur near the forehead, glabella, or orbit, at the junction of the ethmoid and frontal bones near the root of the nose; these can be further classified into nasofrontal, naso-ethmoidal, and naso-orbital types. Basal encephaloceles occur as intranasal protrusions through the cribriform plate, ethmoid, or sphenoid sinuses and tend to be occult masses. These can be further subdivided into trans-ethmoidal, spheno-ethmoidal, spheno-orbital, spheno-maxillary, and transsphenoidal types [36]. Table 12.1 summarizes this classification system.

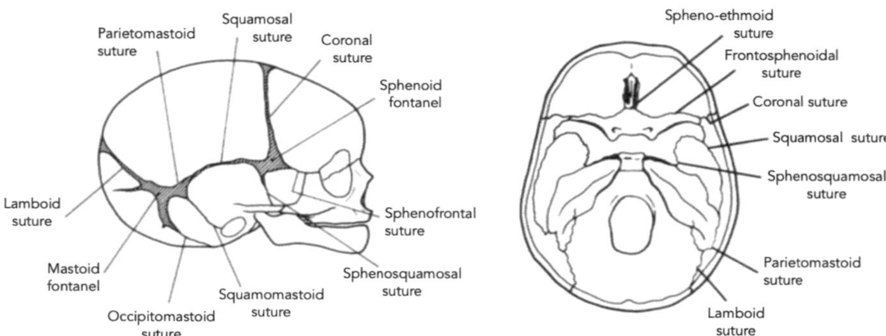

Fig. 12.2 Suture lines in the pediatric skull

Table 12.1 Classification of anterior encephaloceles. This table summarizes the classification of the two categories of anterior encephaloceles—sincipital and basal—by the course of the herniation and the clinical presentation

	Type	Course	Presentation
Sincipital	Nasofrontal	Through foramen cecum to come out between nasal and frontal bones	Glabellar mass
	Naso-ethmoidal	Through foramen cecum into prenasal space, between nasal bones and cartilages	Dorsal nasal mass
	Naso-orbital	At medial orbital wall, defect between defect in maxilla frontal process and ethmoid-lacrimal bone junction	Proptosis, visual issues
Basal	Trans-ethmoidal	Through cribriform into superior meatus, medial to middle turbinate	Nasal mass, nasopharyngeal mass
	Spheno-ethmoidal	Between posterior ethmoid and sphenoid, into nasopharynx	Nasal mass, nasopharyngeal mass
	Spheno-orbital	Through superior orbital fissure	Exophthalmos, diplopia
	Spheno-maxillary	Orbital fissures to pterygopalatine fossa	Facial mass, facial asymmetry
	Transsphenoidal	Sphenoid planum or sphenoclival defect into nasopharynx through craniopharyngeal canal [24]	Nasal mass, nasopharyngeal mass

Clinical Presentation

The clinical presentation of encephaloceles is widely variable and predominantly a function of three factors: the size of the defect, the location of the defect, and the herniated contents.

Large defects or significant parenchymal herniation may result in intrauterine demise. At birth, a large congenital nasal or nasopharyngeal mass of any origin, including encephaloceles, may cause respiratory distress and emergent airway obstruction [37]. Smaller encephaloceles may go undetected or cause vague, non-specific symptoms such as nasal obstruction or post-obstructive sinusitis. Cerebrospinal fluid (CSF) rhinorrhea may be mistaken for a runny nose [38]. A leaking hernia sac may also facilitate a route for commensal bacteria to enter the intracranial space [38–40]. Thus, one should consider an unidentified intranasal encephalocele particularly in cases of recurrent bacterial meningitis.

Many encephaloceles are visibly obvious at birth, particularly sincipital encephaloceles, which can present with a glabellar or dorsal nasal mass. Even small sincipital encephaloceles are likely to be visible because of their location. These facial masses often enlarge with crying, Valsalva, or the Furstenberg test, which involves compressing the jugular veins to increase subarachnoid pressure [23]. The exception among sincipital encephaloceles is a naso-orbital encephalocele, which may present more subtly with proptosis and vision disorders.

Basal encephaloceles tend to herniate into the nasal cavity, and therefore the presentation can be variable. The presentation of nasopharyngeal encephaloceles, such as trans-ethmoidal and spheno-ethmoidal, depends largely on the size and degree of obstruction. Proptosis and diplopia are common symptoms in spheno-orbital encephaloceles. Spheno-maxillary encephaloceles are exceedingly rare, but may present with a facial mass, swelling, or trismus in the region of the pterygopalatine fossa [41]. Also quite rare, transsphenoidal encephaloceles may involve pituitary or optic tissues resulting in hormonal or visual disturbance [42, 43]. Facial clues to the possible presence of an occult nasopharyngeal encephalocele include hypertelorism, cleft palate, and median cleft face syndrome [44].

Although the majority of encephaloceles are isolated defects, approximately one third of patients may have additional congenital structural malformations or complications, including Dandy-Walker or Chiari malformations, microcephaly, cleft lip, craniosynostosis, hydrocephalus [45], complex congenital heart disease, amniotic rupture sequence, or other systemic abnormalities [46].

Differential Diagnosis and Workup

Identification of a skull base encephalocele is based on symptoms, physical exam including nasal endoscopy, and imaging of the brain and skull base.

Differential Diagnosis

The clinician should consider the possibility of other sinonasal mass lesions, including nasal gliomas, dermoid cysts, and nasal polyps, which all can present as a nasal mass similar to encephaloceles, and thus a brief discussion on these masses is warranted [24].

Nasal gliomas and dermoids occur via the same pathophysiological aberration as anterior encephaloceles [17]. It should be noted that the term "glioma" is a bit of a misnomer, as nasal gliomas are not the same entity as intracranial gliomas; nasal gliomas are a developmental abnormality, rather than an intracranial glioma, which is a malignant neoplasm. The term "glioma" in this chapter will refer to the former, benign pathology.

Like encephaloceles, gliomas also develop secondary to an abnormal protrusion of intracranial tissue. However, unlike encephaloceles, the majority of the initial skull base defect eventually closes, resulting in ectopic, sequestered neurologic tissue [47]. Thus, gliomas contain nonfunctional, hamartomatous heterotopic glial tissue. While a small percentage of gliomas connect with dura, through either the foramen cecum or fonticulus, there is a lack of a continuous, patent connection to the intrathecal space or central nervous system [24], and thus the mass is not subject

Table 12.2 Differential diagnosis of external nasal and intranasal masses. This table presents the differential diagnoses for external nasal and intranasal masses with important clinical features

	Cause	Findings
External nasal mass	Sincipital encephaloceles	Transilluminate; Furstenberg (+)
	Gliomas	Transilluminate; Furstenberg (−)
	Dermoid	Non-compressible, non-pulsatile, often sinus tract or pit; Furstenberg (−)
	Hemangioma	T1 enhancement; Furstenberg (+)
Intranasal mass	Basal encephaloceles	Shiny smooth mass, midline or paramedian; Furstenberg (+)
	Nasal polyposis	Rare in infants, usually from middle meatus, Furstenberg (−)
	Lacrimal cyst	Bulges when pressure is applied to the lacrimal system
	Hemangioma	T1 enhancement; Furstenberg (−)

to intracranial pressure fluctuations. Therefore, gliomas are generally noncompressible masses that do not increase in size with crying or the Furstenberg test.

Gliomas may present as either an intranasal (30%), extranasal (60%), or both intra-/extranasal combined mass (10%) [48]. Extranasal gliomas are often at the glabella, but are not necessarily midline and may result in dystopia canthorum or hypertelorism. Intranasal gliomas may mimic nasal polyps and present high in the nasal cavity, often in association with the middle turbinate. Combined gliomas may have a dumbbell shape with a band separating the intra- and extranasal components. Gliomas may be unilateral and do not necessarily occur in the midline or attach to the skin or sinuses.

Nasal dermoids are the most common congenital midline lesion of the nose. These cystic lesions occur anywhere along the nasal dorsum or anterior cranial fossa secondary to failed regression of the neuroectodermal tract. They are comprised of ectoderm and mesodermal tissue [49] and may contain hair follicles, sebaceous glands, or eccrine glands within. Nasal dermoids may have an intracranial connection at the foramen cecum, frontalis, crista galli, or cribriform, and thus recurrent infections may track intracranially leading to brain abscesses or meningitis.

Additional masses that should be considered on the differential are included in Table 12.2.

Workup

Large encephaloceles may be identified on prenatal ultrasound imaging. Any concern for a congenital nasal or skull base lesion warrants a comprehensive physical exam including nasal endoscopy in addition to dedicated high-resolution imaging. Biopsy should not be performed before imaging is obtained and reviewed.

Diagnosis of extranasal encephaloceles is relatively straightforward based on physical exam and imaging. Internal encephaloceles are not as obvious or easily diagnosed in the absence of symptoms. Imaging routinely consists of computed tomography (CT) and/or magnetic resonance imaging (MRI). A high-resolution, non-contrasted CT scan allows for a detailed examination of the skull base and identification of any bony defects, as well as allows for surgical planning with the use of stereotactic navigation. MRI examines the soft tissue components of the mass to determine the nature of the herniated contents in addition to the presence or absence of an intracranial and/or intrathecal connection. Additionally, MRI may also demonstrate the presence of hydrocephalous, infection, or any other intracranial pathology that may be secondarily associated with a congenital encephalocele.

Angiography may demonstrate the presence of major arteries, such as an anterior cerebral artery, that may course through the encephalocele. While there are no published guidelines to describe the precise indications for angiography in this clinical context, it should be considered for any large encephalocele that contains a significant amount of parenchymal tissue. Generally, a CT angiography or MR angiography is sufficient to delineate the major skull base vasculature.

Combined CT and MR imaging modalities allow the clinician to elucidate the type of nasal mass, as well as identify the size, location, extent of bony destruction, and involvement of adjacent structures.

Additional Workup

Additional abnormalities or findings identified with imaging may warrant further workup to evaluate for an underlying chromosomal defect, syndrome, or inherited condition. Consultation with colleagues in genetics, neurology, cardiology, and nephrology, to name a few, may be needed to help optimize care for the patient. Craniopharyngeal canal defects may involve sellar structures and should prompt consideration of an endocrinologic evaluation.

Treatment

Diagnostic biopsy is generally not required and may lead to a CSF leak or provide a nidus for ascending infection and meningitis.

Surgical resection and skull base reconstruction is the primary treatment for congenital encephaloceles. The optimal timing of surgery varies based on the size, location, associated complications, and other potential comorbidities or craniofacial anomalies. Indications for urgent surgery include airway compromise, bacterial meningitis, CSF leak, and declining neurologic function. Expeditious treatment is always the goal, as the presence of an encephalocele represents an ongoing risk of meningitis.

Fundamental surgical goals include reduction of the encephalocele into the skull base and repair of the bony defect with a water-tight seal. Definitive surgical repair is often performed by a multidisciplinary team comprised of neurosurgical and oto-laryngology colleagues.

Extranasal masses may be excised with standard surgical excisions, although an intracranial component may necessitate neurosurgical involvement with an endo-scopic or open approach. For intranasal masses, depending on the location, surgical approaches may involve an open craniotomy approach versus a minimally invasive endoscopic endonasal approach. As endoscopic technology and techniques have developed in recent years, the endoscopic approach has become the preferred treat-ment route when possible, given the excellent visualization afforded with reduced morbidity. Our following surgical discussion will focus on the endonasal endo-scopic approach for internal nasal encephaloceles.

For an endoscopic, endonasal approach, stereotactic image guidance with either CT or MRI is routinely obtained for both preoperative evaluation and stereotactic surgical navigation.

Various endoscopic approaches for the skull base can be utilized depending on the location of the lesion and skull base defect. These may include a direct parasep-tal approach for lesions on the ethmoid or cribriform, a transsphenoidal approach, or a transpterygoid approach for lateral recess lesions. A transpalatal approaches is also a viable option, particularly in cases where the cleft palate provides a surgical window for access. However, in patients without an existing cleft palate, this approach is less popular, as palatal osteotomies and hard palate removal are not only technically challenging, but may also result in delayed healing and the need for enteral feeds.

During the approach, the surgeon should keep in mind a plan for reconstruction and save or harvest any tissue needed at that time. If there is a potential need for a vascularized tissue flap, most commonly a nasoseptal flap, this flap can either be harvested at the onset of the case or persevered during the dissection for future use.

Once the approach is complete and the lesion is in view, treatment steps first involve the reduction of the intranasal mass so that the bony skull base defect can be identified and visualized. Reduction of the intranasal mass can be done with a vari-ety of instruments including bipolar cautery and coblation. Given the open connec-tion with the intracranial space, powered instrumentation is generally avoided at the skull base.

Once the skull base defect is identified, the optimal repair is dictated by the size, location, and degree of CSF leak. Small defects with low-flow CSF leaks may require only a free mucosal graft, minimal patching with fat, free or vascularized mucosa, tensor fascia lata, and/or tissue glue. Larger or higher-flow defects may require more extensive, multilayer repairs, including any combination of fat, tensor fascia lata, vascularized pedicled mucosal flaps, or synthetic dural matrix.

Additional treatments may be necessary based on the individual's specific symp-toms and associated conditions. For example, craniofacial abnormalities or hydro-cephalous may require adjuvant interventions such as surgery, shunt placement, or other interventions. Symptomatic and supportive treatment may be needed for lifelong physical or cognitive deficits and may include medical, social, remedial education, and/or vocational services. Genetic counseling for families may also be warranted, depending on situation.

Prognosis

Important prognostic factors include the location of the defect, type, and amount of herniated contents, presence of hydrocephalus, low birth weight, preterm delivery, and presence of multiple defects.

The type of tissue in the herniated contents plays a significant role in ultimate prognosis, with patients with meningoceles faring considerably better than those with encephaloceles. A study of 24 patients with surgically treated encephaloceles found that presence of neural tissue in the hernia sac was the strongest predictor of mortality and functional outcome [50]. The prognosis of fetuses with meningoencephaloceles is poor and is often complicated by the presence of other CNS defects. Intrauterine demise usually occurs when over 50% of the cranial (i.e., neural) contents have been herniated [2]. Comparatively, patients with very large meningoceles tend to have excellent outcomes [42]; thus, although the size of the hernia sac is a statistically significant variable, it is an unreliable predictor of prognosis.

The prognosis for anterior encephaloceles is considerably better than for posterior encephaloceles, with 1 study of 83 cases reporting a mortality of 10% for anterior defects and 24% for posterior defects [3]. However, estimates of perinatal mortality may be affected by elective termination in the case of severe prenatally diagnosed defects. Case series of liveborn patients with anterior encephaloceles are limited and have reported mortality rates with a wide range of 0–20% [5]. For example, all 12 patients in one study from the Children's Hospital of Denver survived [46], while in an older report from Indiana University, one of five patients with anterior encephaloceles died [51]. A recent systematic review of 110 patients with anterior cranial fossa encephalocele noted a mortality rate of 4.8% [14]. The improved survival of anterior lesions reflects the fact that posterior encephaloceles tend to be larger and contain more neural contents than anterior encephaloceles.

The prognostic factors important for survival appear to be similarly influential in patients' functional outcomes as well. Children with congenital encephaloceles appear to have a greater risk of neurologic developmental delays. One small study of 12 patients with anterior encephaloceles reported normal development in 42% and severe disability in 25% of cases [46]. Patients with several defects have a worse prognosis compared to those with isolated encephaloceles.

The severity, size, and associated complications dictate the surgical management, timing, and likelihood of a successful intervention. Additionally, earlier surgical correction of encephaloceles often allows for the craniofacial bones to resume normal development and ultimately yields a better cosmetic outcome. Operative complications include intraoperative CSF leaks, which have been noted to occur in 18.5% of patients, versus postoperative leaks, which are noted in 6% of cases. Rates of meningitis and hydrocephalous were both low, ~3.7% [14]. Thus, the low incidence of complications favors surgical intervention for anterior encephalocele repair.

Although there is limited data regarding the risk of encephalocele recurrence, a recent systemic review over 110 patients identified a recurrence rate of 5.2% [14]. For comparison, the rate of recurrence of nasal gliomas has been estimated at 4–10% [52].

Conclusion

Congenital encephaloceles are rare malformations characterized by herniation of intracranial contents through defects in the bony skull base. These lesions can be categorized by their location and contents. Larger lesions may cause airway obstruction, and recurrent meningitis should prompt concern for a skull base defect. Endoscopic skull base surgery is the preferred method of repair, when possible, and allows for minimal morbidity and aesthetic disfiguration. Various techniques exist in approaching the lesion in an endoscopic fashion, and repair is tailored to the size, location, and leak status of the lesion. Endoscopic skull base reconstruction provides excellent visualization for surgery, repair, nominal cosmetic morbidity, and minimal impact on facial skeleton growth.

References

1. David DJ, Proudman TW. Cephaloceles: classification, pathology, and management. World J Surg. 1989;13(4):349–57.
2. Budorick NE, Pretorius DH, McGahan JP, Grafe MR, James HE, Slivka J. Cephalocele detection in utero: sonographic and clinical features. Ultrasound Obstet Gynecol. 1995;5(2):77–85.
3. Siffel C, Wong LYC, Olney RS, Correa A. Survival of infants diagnosed with encephalocele in Atlanta, 1979-98. Paediatr Perinat Epidemiol. 2003;17(1):40–8.
4. Arora P, Mody S, Kalra VK, Altaany D, Bajaj M. Occipital meningoencephalocele in a preterm neonate. BMJ Case Rep. 2012;2012:bcr2012006293.
5. Macfarlane R, Rutka JT, Armstrong D, Phillips J, Posnick J, Forte V, et al. Encephaloceles of the anterior cranial fossa. Pediatr Neurosurg. 1995;149:e828.
6. Blencowe H, Kancherla V, Moorthie S, Darlison MW, Modell B. Estimates of global and regional prevalence of neural tube defects for 2015: a systematic analysis. Ann N Y Acad Sci. 2018;1414(1):31–46.
7. Gump WC. Endoscopic endonasal repair of congenital defects of the anterior skull base: developmental considerations and surgical outcomes. J Neurol Surg B Skull Base. 2015;76:291.
8. Mahapatra AK, Agrawal D. Anterior encephaloceles: a series of 103 cases over 32 years. J Clin Neurosci. 2006;13(5):536–9.
9. Khoury MJ, Erickson JD, Cordero JF, McCarthy BJ. Congenital malformations and intrauterine growth retardation: a population study. Pediatrics. 1988;82(1):83–90.
10. Forrester M, Merz R. Epidemiology of neural tube defects, Hawaii, 1986–97. Hawaii Med J. 2000;59(8):323–7.

11. Feuchtbaum LB, Currier RJ, Riggle S, Roberson M, Lorey FW, Cunningham GC. Neural tube defect prevalence in California (1990–94): eliciting patterns by type of defect and maternal race/ethnicity. Genet Test. 1999;3(3):265–72.
12. Berry AD, Patterson JW. Meningoceles, meningomyeloceles, and encephaloceles: a neuro-dermatopathologic study of 132 cases. J Cutan Pathol. 1991;18(3):164–77.
13. Rehman L, Farooq G, Bukhari I. Neurosurgical interventions for occipital encephalocele. Asian J Neurosurg. 2018;13(2):233–7.
14. Lee JA, Byun YJ, Nguyen SA, Schlosser RJ, Gudis DA. Endonasal endoscopic surgery for pediatric anterior cranial fossa encephaloceles: a systematic review. Int J Pediatr Otorhinolaryngol. 2020;132:109919.
15. Lorber J, Schofield JK. The prognosis of occipital encephalocele. Z Kinderchir. 1979;28(4):347–51.
16. Hoving EW. Separation of neural and surface ectoderm in relation to the pathogenesis of encephaloceles. Z Kinderchir. 1990;45(Suppl):1–40.
17. Hoving EW. Nasal encephaloceles. Childs Nerv Syst. 2000;16(10–11):702–6.
18. Hoving EW, Vermeij-Keers C. Frontoethmoidal encephaloceles, a study of their pathogenesis. Pediatr Neurosurg. 1997;27(5):246–56.
19. Martínez-Lage JF, Poza M, Sola J, Soler CL, Montalvo CG, Domingo R, et al. The child with a cephalocele: etiology, neuroimaging, and outcome. Childs Nerv Syst. 1996;12(9):540–50.
20. Padget DH. Neuroschisis and human embryonic maldevelopment: new evidence on anencephaly, spina bifida and diverse mammalian defects. J Neuropathol Exp Neurol. 1970;29(2):192–216.
21. Gluckman TJ, George TM, McLone DG. Postneurulation rapid brain growth represents a critical time for encephalocele formation: a chick model. Pediatr Neurosurg. 1996;25(3):130–6.
22. Ginat DT, Robson CD. CT and MRI of congenital nasal lesions in syndromic conditions. Pediatr Radiol. 2015;45(7):1056–65.
23. Tirumandas M, Sharma A, Gbenimacho I, Shoja MM, Tubbs RS, Oakes WJ, et al. Nasal encephaloceles: a review of etiology, pathophysiology, clinical presentations, diagnosis, treatment, and complications. Childs Nerv Syst. 2013;29(5):739–44.
24. Rahbar R, Resto VA, Robson CD, Perez-Atayde AR, Goumnerova LC, McGill TJ, et al. Nasal glioma and encephalocele: diagnosis and management. Laryngoscope. 2003;113(12):2069–77.
25. Deora H, Srinivas D, Shukla D, Devi BI, Mishra A, Beniwal M, et al. Multiple-site neural tube defects: embryogenesis with complete review of existing literature. Neurosurg Focus. 2019;47(4):E18.
26. Lemire RJ. Neural tube defects. J Child Neurol. 1988;3(1):2–46.
27. Yengo-Kahn AM, Plackis AC, Bonfield CM, Reddy SK. Correction of a vertex encephalocele related to amniotic band syndrome. BMJ Case Rep. 2020;13(3):e234735.
28. Chen H, Gonzalez E. Amniotic band sequence and its neurocutaneous manifestations. Am J Med Genet. 1987;28(3):661–73.
29. Mishima K, Sugahara T, Mori Y, Sakuda M. Three cases of oblique facial cleft. J Craniomaxillofac Surg. 1996;24(6):372–7.
30. Da Silva A. Amniotic band syndrome associated with exencephaly: a case report and literature review. J Pediatr Neurosci. 2019;14(2):94–6.
31. Marin-Padilla M. Morphogenesis of experimental encephalocele (cranioschisis occulta). J Neurol Sci. 1980;46(1):83–99.
32. Yucetas SC, Uçler N. A retrospective analysis of neonatal encephalocele predisposing factors and outcomes. Pediatr Neurosurg. 2017;52(2):73–6.
33. Bassuk AG, McLone D, Bowman R, Kessler JA. Autosomal dominant occipital cephalocele. Neurology. 2004;62(10):1880–90.
34. Yokota A, Kajiwara H, Kohchi M, Fuwa I, Wada H. Parietal cephalocele: clinical importance of its atretic form and associated malformations. J Neurosurg. 1988;69(4):545–51.
35. Nayak A, Sharma S, Vadher RK, Dixit S, Batra RS. Congenital interparietal encephalocele: a case report. J Clin Diagn Res. 2015;9(4):9–10.

36. Suwanwela C, Suwanwela N. A morphological classification of sincipital encephalomeningoceles. J Neurosurg. 1972;36(2):201–11.
37. Yokota A, Matsukado Y, Fuwa I, Moroki K, Nagahiro S. Anterior basal encephalocele of the neonatal and infantile period. Neurosurgery. 1986;19(3):468–78.
38. Schick B, Draf W, Kahle G, Weber R, Wallenfang T. Occult malformations of the skull base. Arch Otolaryngol Head Neck Surg. 1997;123(1):77–80.
39. Schick B, Prescher A, Hofmann E, Steigerwald C, Draf W. Two occult skull base malformations causing recurrent meningitis in a child: a case report. Eur Arch Otorhinolaryngol. 2003;260(9):518–21.
40. Chen T, Chen H, Hu B, Hu H, Guo X, Guo L, et al. Characteristics of pediatric recurrent bacterial meningitis in Beijing Children's Hospital, 2006–2019. J Pediatr Infect Dis Soc. 2021;10:635.
41. Müller H, Slootweg PJ, Troost J. An encephalocele of the sphenomaxillary type. Case report. J Maxillofac Surg. 1981;9(C):180–4.
42. Pollack IF. Management of encephaloceles and craniofacial problems in the neonatal period. Neurosurg Clin N Am. 1998;9(1):121–39. https://doi.org/10.1016/S1042-3680(18)30285-7.
43. Tsutsumi K, Asano T, Shigeno T, Matsui T, Ito S, Kaizu H. Transcranial approach for transsphenoidal encephalocele: report of two cases. Surg Neurol. 1999;51(3):252–7.
44. Abdel-Aziz M, El-Bosraty H, Qotb M, El-Hamamsy M, El-Sonbaty M, Abdel-Badie H, et al. Nasal encephalocele: endoscopic excision with anesthetic consideration. Int J Pediatr Otorhinolaryngol. 2010;74(8):869–73. https://doi.org/10.1016/j.ijporl.2010.04.015.
45. Mahapatra AK. Anterior encephalocele – AIIMS experience a series of 133 patients. J Pediatr Neurosci. 2011;6(3):27–30.
46. Brown MS, Sheridan-Pereira M. Outlook for the child with a cephalocele. Pediatrics. 1992;90(6):914–9.
47. Younus M, Coode PE. Nasal glioma and encephalocele: two separate entities. Report of two cases. J Neurosurg. 1986;64(3):516–9.
48. Bradley P, Singh S. Nasal glioma. J Laryngol Otol. 1985;99(3):247–52.
49. Purnell CA, Skladman R, Alden TD, Corcoran JF, Rastatter JC. Nasal dermoid cysts with intracranial extension: avoiding coronal incision through midline exposure and nasal bone osteotomy. J Neurosurg Pediatr. 2020;25(3):298–304.
50. Date I, Yagyu Y, Asari S, Ohmoto T. Long-term outcome in surgically treated encephalocele. Surg Neurol. 1993;40(6):471–5.
51. Mealey J, Dzenitis A, Hockey A, et al. Neurol Surg. 1970;32:209–18.
52. Puppala B, Mangurten HH, McFadden J, Lygizos N, Taxy J, Pellettiere E. Nasal glioma: presenting as neonatal respiratory distress definition of the tumor mass by MRI. Clin Pediatr (Phila). 1990;29(1):49–52.

Chapter 13
Anterior Skull Base Surgical Approaches

Joseph S. Schwartz and Alex Tham

Introduction

Traditionally, skull base surgery involved open surgery either from above via a transcranial approach or from below via a transfacial approach. Often, both transcranial and transfacial approaches were required to adequately address skull base lesions. In this era of minimally invasive surgery, the endoscopic endonasal approach (EEA) has now superseded traditional open approaches.

Endonasal surgery of the skull base began with pituitary surgery. As skull base surgeons became more familiar and adept with this technique, extended skull base approaches were developed which provided exposures from the olfactory groove to C-2 and to the infratemporal region and jugular fossa laterally. Naturally, the sphenoid sinus is often the starting point for access to most of the skull base. The significance of the sphenoid sinus is also grounded in its proximity to critical anatomical structures, such as the optic nerves and internal carotid arteries (ICAs).

Extended approaches from the sphenoid sinus to adjacent areas of the anterior skull base can proceed in all directions. With the sphenoid as the epicenter, the approaches to the skull base can be divided along the sagittal and coronal planes (Table 13.1; Fig. 13.1). Within the scope of this chapter, only approaches to the anterior skull base will be discussed.

J. S. Schwartz (✉) · A. Tham
Department of Otolaryngology - Head and Neck Surgery, Jewish General Hospital, McGill University, Montreal, QC, Canada
e-mail: joseph.schwartz@mcgill.ca

E. C. Kuan et al. (eds.), *Skull Base Reconstruction*,
https://doi.org/10.1007/978-3-031-27937-9_13

Table 13.1 Classification of endoscopic endonasal approaches to the skull base

Sagittal plane
• Transfrontal
• Transcribriform
• Transsphenoidal
– Transplanum
– Transtuberculum (supersellar)
– Transsellar
• Transclival
– Superior: dorsum sellae
– Middle: mid-clivus
– Inferior: foramen magnum
• Transodontoid
Coronal plane
• Anterior (anterior cranial fossa)
– Medial supraorbital
– Transorbital
• Middle (middle cranial fossa)
– Medial transcavernous
– Transpterygoid
Medial petrous apex
Contralateral transmaxillary
– Suprapetrous
Meckel's cave
Lateral transcavernous
– Posterior (posterior cranial fossa)
Intrapetrous ("far medial")
Transjugular tubercle
Transcondylar
Parapharyngeal space/infratemporal skull base

Fig. 13.1 Endoscopic endonasal surgical approaches. (1) Transfrontal; (2) transcribriform; (3) transplanum; (4) transsellar; (5) transclival; (6) transodontoid

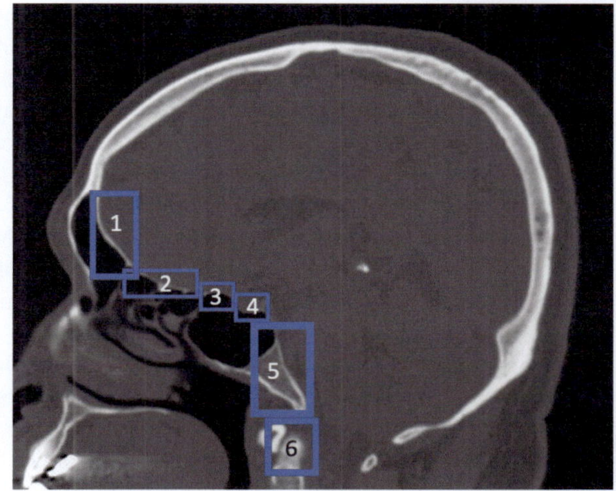

Sagittal Plane

Transfrontal

The transfrontal approach provides access to the ventral most anatomical subunit of the anterior skull base in the sagittal plane. The common indications for this approach include conditions involving the frontal sinuses such as mucocele, fibro-osseous tumor, and posterior frontal table fracture resulting in a cerebrospinal fluid (CSF) leak. This approach is also the preceding step in a transcribriform approach.

In this approach, an antero-superior septal window followed by a frontal sinus drillout (also known as a modified endoscopic Lothrop or Draf III) procedure is performed. The frontal neo-ostium serves to maximize the surgical corridor to optimize management of various frontal sinus conditions. During dissection, care should be taken to avoid injury to the olfactory fibers and cribriform plate which would otherwise negatively influence olfaction and may result in a CSF leak respectively.

The frontal sinus drill-out procedure was first described by Lothrop in 1914 [1] and modified by Draf in 1991 [2]. There are two approaches, the "inside-out" and the "outside-in." The inside-out approach is the traditional and first described technique for performing a frontal sinus drillout. Following a maxillary antrostomy and total sphenoethmoidectomy, the frontal recess is cleared of all bony partitions and cells creating a Draf IIa frontal sinusotomy. A 2 × 2 cm antero-superior septal window is then fashioned delimited posteriorly by the anterior face of the middle turbinate. Inferiorly, the window is made about 0.5 cm below the axilla of the middle turbinate so that instruments can pass trans-septally underneath the axilla of the contralateral middle turbinate. The roof of the nose forms the superior margin, and the anterior margin is about a centimeter from the frontal process of the maxilla.

The septal mucosa on both sides of the septal window can be harvested as free mucosal grafts which may be used to line the denuded bone of the frontal neo-ostium.

A high-speed drill is then used to remove the frontal process of the maxilla above the axilla. The zero-degree endoscope is used for the majority of the dissection, and both the scope and the burr are inserted via one nostril across the septal window so as to work on the contralateral frontal process. Starting from the frontal ostium, the burr is directed anteriorly toward the frontal process of the maxilla in a lateral and superior direction (inside-out). This is continued until the periosteum of the overlying skin is exposed, and this marks the lateral extent of the dissection. Drilling is now directed superiorly until the floor of the frontal sinus is reached and the frontal sinus is visualized. The dissection is repeated for the contralateral side until the contralateral frontal sinus is entered as well. It should be noted that dissection should not be directed medially prior to entering the frontal sinus to avoid injuring the olfactory filaments.

Dissection is now directed medially from both sides of the frontal sinuses, alternating from side to side, until the frontal intersinus septum is visualized. The two frontal sinuses are then connected by taking down the intersinus septum. Lastly, the frontal neo-ostium is further enlarged to achieve the largest possible anteroposterior and lateral dimensions. The frontal "T," which is comprised of the perpendicular plate of the ethmoid (long limb) and the posterior margin of the frontal sinus floor resection (short limbs), is lowered as much as possible without exposing the dura of the olfactory filaments. The mucosa of the olfactory cleft is first elevated and the position of the first olfactory filament identified prior to lowering of the frontal "T" region.

The 30-degree scope is now utilized to view the intersinus septum and frontal beak. The intersinus septum is completely removed up to the roof of the frontal sinus, and the frontal beak is drilled down until there is a smooth transition between the frontal sinus and nasal cavity. This completes the Draf III "inside-out" approach.

In the "outside-in" approach, the initial dissection of the frontal recesses is avoided. As opposed to the "inside-out" approach, the limits of the drill-out cavity are established at the outset of the procedure, and the dissection then proceeds toward the frontal recesses (outside-in). The zero-degree endoscope and high-speed drill is utilized for the majority of the dissection.

For this approach, the initial step involves the creation of a mucosal flap overlying the frontal beak, the frontal sinus floor, and the antero-superior septal window. Laterally the incision begins slightly anterior but at the level of the middle turbinate axilla. The incision is then carried superiorly onto the nasal roof and then brought down onto the anterior margin of the septal window. The septal incision is staggered by 0.5 cm relative to the lateral incision to prevent synechia formation. The septal incision is then brought down to the level of the upper one third and lower two thirds of the middle turbinate. The septal incision is then continued posteriorly to the anterior face of the middle turbinate. The flap is then raised posteriorly into the olfactory cleft. A small emissary nerve is often seen initially and is distinguished from the first olfactory filament by its lateral origin. The first olfactory filament originates medially and is often more difficult to dissect given the sleeve of periosteum that surrounds it as it enters the olfactory fossa.

An antero-superior septal window is then created, with the same boundaries mentioned earlier, to facilitate binostril access. Starting from the demucosalized frontal process of maxilla, dissection is continued laterally until the periosteum of the overlying skin is reached, and the procedure is repeated on the contralateral side. With the posterior (first olfactory filament) and lateral (periosteum of the frontal process of the maxilla) limits of the drill-out cavity now defined, bone removal between these landmarks can proceed rapidly without risk of iatrogenic skull base injury. The frontal sinus floor will appear in the midline, and transgression of the sinus mucosa should be avoided prior to complete bone removal to limit the exposure of bleeding mucosa. Once the remaining bone is removed and frontal sinus floor is entered, the frontal sinuses can then be connected with the frontal recesses using Kerrison rongeurs. An angled endoscope can now be used to inspect the frontal beak for any bony overhang, which should then be drilled down. Next, the interfrontal sinus septum is removed completely, and the final frontal neo-ostium is now achieved.

Transcribriform

The transcribriform approach, also known as a transnasal endoscopic anterior craniofacial resection (ACFR), is utilized for conditions such as esthesioneuroblastomas and olfactory groove meningiomas as well as midline sinonasal tumors and encephaloceles. The surgical access provided by this approach is not sufficient for tumors which extend far lateral over the orbital roof or involve the lateral part of the frontal sinuses.

In this approach, the intranasal portion of the tumor is debulked to identify the attachment to the cribriform plate. A complete full-house functional endoscopic sinus surgery (FESS) (maxillary antrostomy, total sphenoethmoidectomy, and Draf IIa frontal sinusotomy) is then performed bilaterally followed by a transfrontal approach to define the anterior limit of the dissection. The superior nasal septum is then removed along the sagittal plane, from the sphenoid rostrum posteriorly to the crista galli anteriorly. Following this, the sphenoid rostrum and the intersphenoidal septum are resected. The anterior and posterior ethmoidal arteries are then identified, cauterized, and transected.

The fovea ethmoidalis, at the periphery of the tumor, is then drilled along the sagittal plane bilaterally. These osteotomies are joined in the coronal plane with both an anterior and posterior osteotomy, providing the following resection margins: posterior table of the frontal sinus anteriorly, planum sphenoidale posteriorly, and the lamina papyracea laterally. Care should be taken to not violate the underlying dura while performing the osteotomies. The dura is then incised followed by mobilizing the crista galli. Following this, the falx cerebri is then identified and freed. Finally, the olfactory tracts are divided to deliver the tumor together with the anterior skull base en bloc. In certain cases, with small ipsilateral tumors, an ipsilateral resection of the anterior skull base can be performed, with preservation of olfaction on the contralateral side.

Transsphenoidal

For the transsphenoidal approach consisting of the transplanum, transtuberculum, and transsellar routes, the approach can be divided into the nasal phase and the sellar/tuberculum/planar phase. The nasal phase is similar for all these approaches.

For the nasal phase, the dissection first begins with out-fracturing of both inferior turbinates. Partial or complete middle turbinectomy, as required, is then performed, typically on the right side for a right-handed surgeon as this is the primary surgical corridor. The inferior half of the right superior turbinate is then resected followed by a posterior ethmoidectomy. The right sphenoid os is then identified, cannulated, and enlarged to the skull base superiorly and the medial orbital wall laterally. Next, the left superior turbinate is identified, and the inferior half of it is resected to allow for cannulation and enlargement of the natural sphenoid os which can be performed via a transnasal route so as to preserve the left middle turbinate. A posterior ethmoidectomy is also performed on the left side.

A posterosuperior septal window is then performed, to allow for a binostril approach to the sella. The posterior half of the bony nasal septum (vomer, clival keel) is then resected in a submucosal plane while avoiding injury to the posterior septal artery which courses along the inferior edge of the natural sphenoid os and provides vascular supply to the nasoseptal flap, the workhorse flap in endoscopic skull base reconstruction. The intersinus sphenoid septum is then resected to form a common sphenoid cavity. The mucosa of the sphenoid sinus is removed, completing the nasal phase of the dissection.

If a CSF leak is likely, a right-sided nasoseptal flap (NSF) may be harvested at the outset with the inferior incision coursing along the choanal arch and extending anteriorly at the junction of the nasal septum and nasal floor. Superiorly, care is taken to ensure the incision spares the superior centimeter of the nasal septum to avoid any potential olfactory injury. The inferior and superior incisions are then joined anteriorly at the mucocutaneous junction of the nasal septum. The NSF is then raised in a subperichondrial/subperiosteal plane, mobilized and tucked into the nasopharynx for use during the reconstructive phase of the procedure.

Should additional flap width be required, the nasal floor and lateral nasal wall region can be incorporated by altering the course of the inferior incision. Once the inferior incision completes the posterior edge of the nasal septum, it is then continued laterally along the coronal plane just anterior to the hard-soft palate junction. The incision is then carried into the inferior meatus and onto the lateral nasal wall just beneath the insertion of the inferior turbinate. The incision is then carried anteriorly taking care to not violate Hasner's valve. At the anterior head of the inferior turbinate, the incision is then carried medially in a coronal plane, just posterior to the maxillary alveolar process, and joined with the anterior incision at the mucocutaneous junction of the nasal septum.

If a CSF leak is less likely, the posterior septal artery and pedicle of the NSF can be inferiorly mobilized and thereby preserved in the event it is needed following tumor resection or revision surgery in the future. This maneuver has been coined the term "rescue flap" and essentially involves fashioning the posterior portion of both superior and inferior incisions without raising the anterior most portion of the NSF until it is certain it will be needed. The inferior incision terminates just anterior to the posterior border of the nasal septum, and the superior incision delineates the inferior and anterior borders of the posterosuperior septal window. Both inferior and superior incisions are performed to maximize pedicle mobilization and bony exposure of the sphenoid rostrum while minimizing the risk of flap tearing. In the event a NSF is deemed necessary, the incisions can be extended anteriorly and a traditional NSF with an intact vascular supply can be harvested.

Transplanum/Tuberculum (Suprasellar)

The transplanum approach is often performed in combination with the transcribriform and transsellar approaches for tumors involving the cribriform plate or suprasellar tumors (craniopharyngiomas, giant pituitary macroadenomas, meningioma, epidermoid, and gliomas) (Fig. 13.2).

In this approach, the anatomical landmarks of the optic nerves, medial opticocarotid recesses, and the chiasmatic groove are first identified. The bone overlying the tuberculum is drilled down using a diamond burr. This should be done with copious irrigation to avoid thermal injury to the optic nerves, particularly over the chiasmatic groove. The anterior limit of the resection is the posterior ethmoid sinuses and cribriform plates, up to the extent of the tumor. The posterior limit is the tuberculum sellae or chiasmatic groove overlying the superior intercavernous/circular sinus.

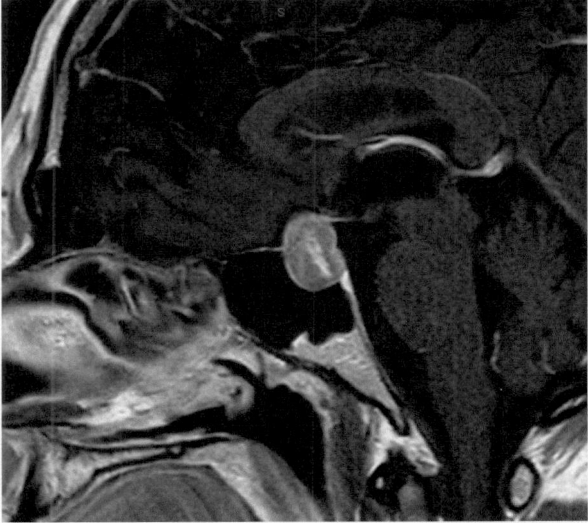

Fig. 13.2 Sella, suprasellar pituitary macroadenoma. Enhancing T1-weighted sella, suprasellar mass

With the underlying dura now exposed, two horizontal incisions are made in the dura, one above and the other below the superior intercavernous sinus. To widen the suprasellar space, the superior intercavernous sinus is exposed, coagulated, and transected. This provides adequate exposure of the pituitary stalk and optic chiasm. This concludes the planar/tuberculum phase of the dissection.

Transsellar

The transsellar approach is indicated for cases of pituitary micro- or macroadenoma situated within the sellar region. Extended approaches such as the transplanum or tuberculum (suprasellar) approaches are required if tumors extend superiorly above the sella. For tumors which extend inferiorly below the sella, a transclival approach can be utilized.

In the transsellar approach, after completion of the nasal phase of dissection, the following anatomical landmarks are identified: bilateral optic nerves, optico-carotid recesses, and ICAs.

In the midline, the sella, planum, tuberculum, and clivus (Fig. 13.3) are identified. The sphenoid cavity is then further exposed by removing the accessory septations within it, either using a diamond burr or through-cutting forceps. Next, the floor of the sphenoid is then lowered with a cutting burr to obtain adequate access to the sella. The anterior face and floor of the sella are then thinned out with a diamond burr until the bone is eggshell thin. The remaining thin bone is then removed with a Kerrison rongeur. An adequate exposure of the sella will allow us to identify the four blues, namely, the superior and inferior intercavernous sinuses and the cavernous sinuses on either side.

Fig. 13.3 Endoscopic view of the planum, tuberculum, sella, and clivus

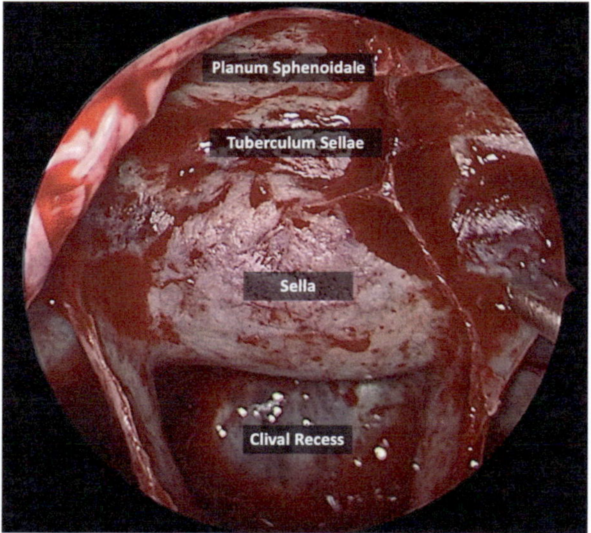

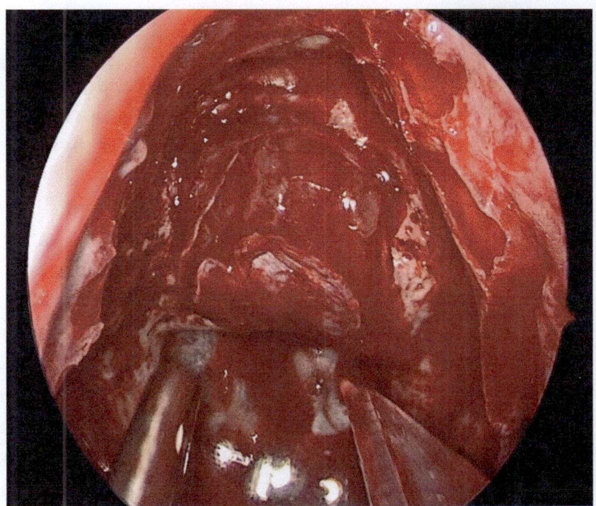

Fig. 13.4 U-shaped dural flap

With the sella exposed, the dura can be seen, comprised of two layers, the meningeal layer and the endosteal layer. The meningeal layer envelopes the brain and forms the diaphragm sellae, while the endosteal layer forms the periosteum of the sphenoid bone. The dura is then incised to expose the capsule of the pituitary gland. The incision can be cruciate in shape or U-shaped to create a flap (Fig. 13.4). This concludes the sella phase of the dissection.

Transclival

The clivus extends from the dorsum sellae to the foramen magnum, and it is divided into three parts:

- Upper clivus—extends from the dorsum sella to the floor of the sella
- Middle clivus—extends from the floor of the sella to the floor of the sphenoid sinus
- Lower clivus—extends from the floor of the sphenoid sinus to the foramen magnum

Depending on the portion of clivus involved, the transclival approaches can be divided into superior, middle, and inferior approaches. For all three transclival approaches, the nasal phase of the dissection is the same except for the NSF. Instead of tucking the NSF into the nasopharynx as for other skull base approaches, a wide maxillary antrostomy is performed on the side of the harvested NSF so that the flap can be stored in the maxillary sinus for use during the reconstructive phase of the procedure. This will ensure that the flap does not obstruct the surgical corridor during the course of the transclival approach.

Superior Clival Approach

The superior clival approach provides direct access to the brainstem and vertebro-basilar arterial system and is indicated for tumors situated in these regions, such as meningiomas, chordomas, craniopharyngiomas, chondromas, and chondrosarcomas.

In this approach, the floor of the sphenoid is drilled down to the level of the clivus, and the bone over the sella and tuberculum is drilled until eggshell thin and removed. This will reveal the underlying dura where the endosteal layer of the sella dura is incised along the floor of the sella and a U-shaped flap is elevated. The pituitary gland can be mobilized and transposed to access the upper clivus and posterior clinoids. Preservation of pituitary function can still be achieved despite the transposition [3, 4]. It is worth mentioning that the intradural transposition of the pituitary gland is no longer performed as it is associated with a high incidence of gland dysfunction. Interdural transcavernous exposure of the posterior clinoid process, with the gland still enveloped by the meningeal layer of dura, is now performed instead.

As popularized by the Pittsburgh group, the en bloc transposition technique [4], where the gland is completely transposed from the fossa, is achieved by resecting the lateral ligaments which anchor the gland to the cavernous sinus. It should be noted that the primary blood supply to the pituitary gland is the superior hypophyseal artery, and this should be preserved during the transposition. The inferior hypophyseal artery and ligaments are resected, and the same procedure is repeated on the contralateral side.

The dorsum sella located between the posterior clinoid processes is now exposed. The dorsum sella is then drilled down until the dura is exposed. The underlying dura is then excised, taking care to not injure the underlying basilar artery. Next, the posterior clinoid processes on both sides are drilled and removed, taking care not to injure the oculomotor nerves and the ICAs which are in close proximity.

Middle Clival Approach

In this approach, the middle third of the clivus is removed. First, the floor of the sphenoid is drilled down to the level of the clivus. At this level, the paraclival ICA lies laterally, and this will serve as the lateral extent of the dissection. Utilizing the anatomical landmarks of the Vidian canal [5] as well as following the floor of the sella laterally can facilitate the identification of the paraclival ICA.

Once the overlying mucosa of the clivus is removed, the middle third of the clivus (clival recess), between the sella superiorly and sphenoid floor inferiorly, is drilled down. Brisk bleeding may occur as the basilar venous plexus is encountered. This can be controlled with hemostatic agents such as Surgicel or Floseal. Care should also be taken to avoid injuring cranial nerve VI as it lies at the level of the paraclival carotids in Dorello's canal. For additional exposure, the pharyngeal fascia

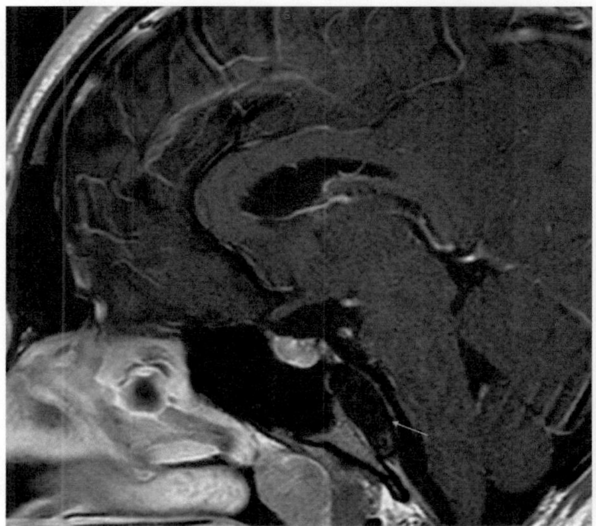

Fig. 13.5 Clival chordoma. T1-hypointense extra-axial cystic clival chordoma (green arrow)

and clival bone inferior to the sphenoid sinus can be removed as well. This might be required for certain clival chordomas (Fig. 13.5) which span both the middle and lower clivus.

Lower Clival Approach

In this approach, the vomer is drilled down to the level of the hard palate. The mucosa overlying the lower clivus is removed, preferably with a Coblator as bleeding can be brisk. With the mucosa removed, the underlying longus capitis and longus colli muscles are exposed. The buccopharyngeal fascia is then incised, and the longus capitis and longus colli muscles are dissected to expose the basisphenoid and basiocciput. The bone is then drilled away, taking care not to injure the petrous ICA laterally. The inferior limit of the dissection is formed by the arch of the atlas.

Transodontoid

The transodontoid approach may be utilized for conditions involving the craniovertebral junction, such as clival chordomas, meningiomas of the foramen magnum, or conditions affecting the upper cervical spine such as pannus formation, fracture of the odontoid process, and tumors of the upper cervical spine [6–8].

In this approach, dissection is commenced similar to the lower clival approach. However, the inferior limit of exposure in this approach is the body of C2. Having removed the clival bone to the inferior margin at the foramen magnum, the anterior ring of the C1 vertebra is visualized and drilled down. Care should be taken not to expose the condyle joint laterally as this is associated with an increased risk of infection. To avoid this, it is recommended that the bony opening is further enlarged laterally using the Kerrison rongeur, instead of drilling.

The odontoid process is now exposed, and it is removed from a superior to inferior direction, starting from the tip. This is to avoid detaching the neck of the odontoid inadvertently, leaving behind a free-floating tip still attached to the apical and transverse ligaments.

Coronal Plane

Medial Supraorbital

The medial supraorbital approach, also known as supramedial orbitotomy, is indicated for anterior skull base tumors which extend laterally over the orbital roof. Common tumors in this region include sinonasal tumors with lateral dural extension, fibro-osseous tumors, and meningiomas.

In this approach, an ipsilateral full-house FESS is first performed. Following that, the lamina papyracea is fractured and removed up to the skull base, exposing the underlying periorbita. Next, the anterior and posterior ethmoidal arteries are identified, cauterized, and transected. The periorbita is then freed from the orbital roof. Should there be a need for access to the lateral aspect of the orbital roof, this can be achieved by resecting the superior nasal septum so that a binostril approach can be utilized to improve the angle of reach.

Transorbital

The indications for the transorbital route to address orbital pathology have expanded over the years [9]. Common lesions which can be addressed via this approach include mucocele, meningioma, optic nerve glioma, and hemangioma. This approach may be extraconal or intraconal. Lesions which are sited lateral to the neuronal axis, however, are an absolute contraindication to this approach.

In this approach, similar to the medial supraorbital approach, an ipsilateral full-house FESS is first performed. Following that, the lamina papyracea is removed, exposing the underlying periorbita which is then incised with a sickle knife. To avoid transecting the medial rectus muscle, the incision should be made parallel to the direction of the muscle. If intraconal dissection is required, this is performed between the medial and inferior recti. To further facilitate intraconal dissection, external retraction of these muscles can be done via an external transconjunctival approach.

Pertinent anatomical structures run within the intraconal space, and knowledge of their location will keep us from injuring it inadvertently. The nerve supply to the muscle runs on the deep surface of the muscles, and the optic nerve is located superolaterally, while the retinal artery is inferior to the optic nerve.

Transpterygoid

The transpterygoid approach is the shared first step in accessing the surgical modules in the middle coronal plane. When performed alone, it provides access to the lateral recess of the sphenoid sinus. Common conditions involving the lateral recess include meningoceles, cerebrospinal fluid leaks, meningiomas, and schwannomas arising from the Vidian nerve, V2, and V3.

When performed to access the modules in the middle coronal plane, the transpterygoid approach serves to localize the petrous ICA and provides access to the anterior skull base both superior and inferior to the petrous ICA. In this approach, a wide maxillary antrostomy is performed, followed by a complete sphenoid-ethmoidectomy. The antrostomy can be converted to an endoscopic medial maxillectomy should access to the inferior aspect of the posterior maxillary wall be needed. This involves resection of the middle third of the inferior turbinate in addition to the adjacent medial maxillary wall until the nasal floor. The antrostomy can be extended further anteriorly via an endoscopic Denker's procedure or prelacrimal recess approach in order to augment visualization and surgical access to the anterolateral wall of the maxillary sinus, lateral compartment of the pterygopalatine fossa and the infratemporal fossa. The latter involves creating a bony window at the level of the pyriform aperture while preserving the distal portion of the nasolacrimal duct (NLD). The window can then be closed at the conclusion of the procedure by reapproximating the mucosa overlying the inferior turbinate with the anterolateral nasal wall. The former involves sacrificing the NLD as well as the remainder of the lateral nasal wall.

Next, the sphenopalatine arteries are identified at the sphenopalatine foramen, cauterized, and transected. The posterior maxillary wall is then taken down which exposes the underlying fascia of the pterygopalatine fossa. The boundaries of resection are the perpendicular plate of palatine bone medially, junction of the lateral and posterior wall laterally, and the orbital process of the palatine bone superiorly. When incising the fascia, care should be taken to not injure the underlying branches of the internal maxillary artery (IMA). Vascular structures (the IMA and its branches) are traditionally located inferomedially, whereas neural structures (V2, sphenopalatine ganglion) are located posterosuperiorly. The IMA is often buried in the fat of the pterygopalatine fossa. Pulsations may be seen which can help to identify the IMA. Should the vessel not be immediately identified, the pterygopalatine fossa can be defatted using a suction coagulator or bipolar cautery on a low setting. The IMA is then teased out with a blunt instrument, ligated with surgical clips, and divided at the midpoint of the posterior maxillary wall.

The contents of the pterygopalatine fossa are then dissected and displaced laterally to expose the base of the pterygoid bone. Relevant anatomical structures in this dissection include the Vidian (pterygoid) canal as well as the infraorbital nerve. The Vidian canal and the foramen rotundum are located inferolateral and superolateral to the lateral recess of the sphenoid sinus respectively. The foramen rotundum can be identified by tracing the infraorbital nerve proximally from along the orbital floor to the foramen rotundum. The intervening bone between the Vidian canal and foramen rotundum is then removed to expose the lateral recess.

Considerations in Pediatric Patients

While the principles of adult endoscopic skull base surgery are still applicable to pediatric patients, there are certain distinctive features of pediatric patients which should be recognized and addressed as these would affect the outcomes of the surgery.

Size and Tight Working Spaces

Naturally, the smaller anatomical dimensions in children will limit the working space. Firstly, the pyriform aperture is smaller. This can limit instrumentation which will necessitate the use of a smaller, 2.7 mm rigid scope. Banu et al. [10] found that the pyriform aperture increases in size with age from 6.7 mm in the 2–4 years age group to 8.3 mm in the 14–16 years age group. By downsizing the rigid scope, Tatreau et al. [11] found that the pyriform aperture may only limit surgical access in patients younger than 2 years of age. Care should be taken not to damage the bony pyriform aperture as it has been found to aid in the development of the upper midface in the first 10 years of life [11].

Next, the dimensions of the nasal cavity will also be smaller in pediatric patients, and the turbinates within the already reduced dimensions of the nasal cavity may further restrict access. This can be overcome by out fracturing the inferior turbinates as well as performing either partial or complete middle turbinectomies. Once surgical access has been enlarged, the pediatric 2.7 mm rigid scope can then be upsized to an adult 4 mm rigid scope which offers improved lighting and optics.

Pneumatization of Paranasal Sinuses

Sphenoid Sinus

The pneumatization of the paranasal sinuses should also be taken into consideration in the surgical approach. The sphenoid sinus, which serves as the epicenter of skull base surgery, may be pneumatized to various degrees depending on the age of the child. Pneumatization of the sphenoid sinus begins at the age of 1, and then rapid growth occurs between the age of 3 months and 5 years [12]. An adult-sized sphenoid sinus is reached by approximately 12 years of age [13, 14]. Limited pneumatization of the sphenoid sinus greatly increases the difficulty of establishing a working corridor, in view of the lack of landmarks such as the ICA and the optico-carotid recesses as well as the presence of cancellous bone which bleeds considerably when drilled. Nonetheless, these challenges can be overcome gradually with experience and with the assistance of an intraoperative image guidance system [15].

In addition, one should be mindful of the reduced distance between the nares and the sella in pediatric patients. This distance has been shown to increase by 15 mm from age 2 to the age 16 [10]. The intercarotid distance is another important anatomical consideration as it limits the size of the surgical window. The intercarotid distance has been shown to be significantly smaller in patients younger than 6 years of age as compared to adults (10.2 mm vs. 12.6 mm), but this difference becomes insignificant after 9 years of age [11]. A minimal intercarotid distance of 10 mm is generally required for performing transsphenoidal approaches safely.

Ethmoid Sinus

The ethmoid sinus is present from birth and is fully developed by age 1–3 years [12]. Care should be taken when performing ethmoidectomy. Interestingly, the majority of pediatric patients have a Keros Type I configuration of the olfactory fossa, making it less likely for the anterior skull base to be injured unintentionally.

Maxillary Sinus

The maxillary sinus is also present from birth, and it expands most rapidly transversely and vertically between 1 year and 8 years of age and between 1 year and 5 years of age, respectively [12].

Frontal Sinus

The frontal sinus is absent at birth and is the last paranasal sinus to develop. It is only visible from 6 years of age and reaches adult configuration by 16 years of age [13].

Craniocervical Junction

The distance between the nares and the odontoid process, in the pediatric age group, can vary by up to 19 mm as they mature [10]. Youssef et al. [16] have found that in about two thirds of pediatric patients, the inferior limit of the endoscopic transnasal approach is the upper one third of the odontoid process, while the remaining third may reach the inferior third. It is prudent to assess the level of the nasopalatal line preoperatively in a transodontoid approach. Should the transnasal route be inadequate, the transoral approach with retraction of the soft palate may be required to facilitate surgical access.

Reconstruction of the Skull Base and Postoperative Care

The size and reach of the NSF is occasionally a concern, particularly for defects which are very anterior and extensive or involve coverage of posterior fossa skull base defects [17, 18]. Firstly, the growth of the cranial vault precedes that of the facial growth, which then limits the reach of the flap, especially for children under 10 years of age. Secondly, it can be challenging to harvest the NSF due to the reduced size of the nasal cavity. However, this can be facilitated by resecting the middle turbinate which will increase the working space.

Postoperative debridement is a critical step in optimizing the postoperative course of patients undergoing endoscopic skull base procedures. Postoperative synechia, surgical site infection, sinus outflow obstruction, iatrogenic chronic sinusitis, and NSF failure resulting in CSF leak are all examples of postoperative complications that can be recognized and potentially avoided with serial postoperative endoscopic debridements in an office setting under local anesthesia. In-office postoperative debridements are generally well tolerated by adult patients, but this may be unattainable in pediatric patients. A pediatric patient's tolerance of postoperative debridement can often be predicted based on their tolerance of the preoperative nasal endoscopy and their age. A postoperative debridement and "second look" procedure under general anesthesia should be planned for patients less than 6 years of age and for those unable to tolerate preoperative nasal endoscopy. Depending on the child's age and level of maturity, in-office debridement can occasionally be performed in much the same way as adult patients.

Discussion

The various anterior skull base approaches have been presented. Each of these approaches is guided by the various anatomical bony, vascular, and neural landmarks. The sphenoid sinus forms the epicenter of these approaches, both in the sagittal and coronal planes, and naturally is the starting point of these approaches.

Depending on the size and site of the anterior skull base tumor, a combination of these surgical approaches may be required.

The ICA remains the most important structure in all of these approaches as it is the main limiting factor determining the extent of access in these approaches. Pediatric patients have their attendant distinctive anatomical differences to adults, which makes the surgical approaches more challenging. However, the general principles still apply, and these challenges can be overcome by firstly recognizing these challenges in our preoperative preparation and utilizing image guidance to aid us during the dissection.

Conclusion

The anterior skull base consists of multiple distinct anatomical regions. The surgical approaches to the anterior skull base can be classified into the various anatomical modules, oriented in the sagittal and coronal planes. With the sphenoid sinus as the epicenter, it forms the starting point for these surgical approaches. A combination of these surgical approaches may be needed, depending on the size and site of the tumor.

References

1. Lothrop HA. XIV. Frontal sinus suppuration: the establishment of permanent nasal drainage; the closure of external fistulae; epidermization of sinus. Ann Surg. 1914;59(6):937–57.
2. Draf W. Endonasal microendoscopic frontal sinus surgery, the Fulda concept. Oper Tech Otolaryngol Head Neck Surg. 1991;2(4):225–34.
3. Fernandez-Miranda JC, Gardner PA, Rastelli MM Jr, Peris-Celda M, Koutourousiou M, Peace D, et al. Endoscopic endonasal transcavernous posterior clinoidectomy with interdural pituitary transposition. J Neurosurg. 2014;121(1):91–9.
4. Kassam AB, Prevedello DM, Thomas A, Gardner P, Mintz A, Snyderman C, et al. Endoscopic endonasal pituitary transposition for a transdorsum sellae approach to the interpeduncular cistern. Neurosurgery. 2008;62(3 Suppl 1):57–72; discussion 4.
5. Vescan AD, Snyderman CH, Carrau RL, Mintz A, Gardner P, Branstetter BT, et al. Vidian canal: analysis and relationship to the internal carotid artery. Laryngoscope. 2007;117(8):1338–42.
6. Kshettry VR, Thorp BD, Shriver MF, Zanation AM, Woodard TD, Sindwani R, et al. Endoscopic approaches to the craniovertebral junction. Otolaryngol Clin N Am. 2016;49(1):213–26.
7. Kassam AB, Snyderman C, Gardner P, Carrau R, Spiro R. The expanded endonasal approach: a fully endoscopic transnasal approach and resection of the odontoid process: technical case report. Neurosurgery. 2005;57(1 Suppl):E213.
8. Liu JK, Patel J, Goldstein IM, Eloy JA. Endoscopic endonasal transclival transodontoid approach for ventral decompression of the craniovertebral junction: operative technique and nuances. Neurosurg Focus. 2015;38(4):E17.
9. Murchison AP, Rosen MR, Evans JJ, Bilyk JR. Endoscopic approach to the orbital apex and periorbital skull base. Laryngoscope. 2011;121(3):463–7.

10. Banu MA, Guerrero-Maldonado A, McCrea HJ, Garcia-Navarro V, Souweidane MM, Anand VK, et al. Impact of skull base development on endonasal endoscopic surgical corridors. J Neurosurg Pediatr. 2014;13(2):155–69.
11. Tatreau JR, Patel MR, Shah RN, McKinney KA, Wheless SA, Senior BA, et al. Anatomical considerations for endoscopic endonasal skull base surgery in pediatric patients. Laryngoscope. 2010;120(9):1730–7.
12. Shah RK, Dhingra JK, Carter BL, Rebeiz EE. Paranasal sinus development: a radiographic study. Laryngoscope. 2003;113(2):205–9.
13. Wolf G, Anderhuber W, Kuhn F. Development of the paranasal sinuses in children: implications for paranasal sinus surgery. Ann Otol Rhinol Laryngol. 1993;102(9):705–11.
14. Vidic B. The postnatal development of the sphenoidal sinus and its spread into the dorsum sellae and posterior clinoid processes. Am J Roentgenol Rad Ther Nucl Med. 1968;104(1):177–83.
15. Kuan EC, Kaufman AC, Lerner D, Kohanski MA, Tong CCL, Tajudeen BA, et al. Lack of sphenoid pneumatization does not affect endoscopic endonasal pediatric skull base surgery outcomes. Laryngoscope. 2019;129(4):832–6.
16. Youssef CA, Smotherman CR, Kraemer DF, Aldana PR. Predicting the limits of the endoscopic endonasal approach in children: a radiological anatomical study. J Neurosurg Pediatr. 2016;17(4):510–5.
17. Hadad G, Bassagasteguy L, Carrau RL, Mataza JC, Kassam A, Snyderman CH, et al. A novel reconstructive technique after endoscopic expanded endonasal approaches: vascular pedicle nasoseptal flap. Laryngoscope. 2006;116(10):1882–6.
18. Shah RN, Surowitz JB, Patel MR, Huang BY, Snyderman CH, Carrau RL, et al. Endoscopic pedicled nasoseptal flap reconstruction for pediatric skull base defects. Laryngoscope. 2009;119(6):1067–75.

Part III
Lateral Skull Base Pathology

Chapter 14
Traumatic and Iatrogenic CSF Leaks

Tina C. Huang

Cerebrospinal fluid leaks of the temporal bone are fairly uncommon and can be secondary to trauma, iatrogenic injury, and spontaneous leaks.

Temporal Fracture

Skull fractures comprise a small percentage of all head injuries and temporal bone fractures an even smaller percentage of those. Cannon et al. reported that 9% of all admitted head injuries had skull fractures with temporal bone fractures comprising 22% of those [1]. Another report found that for admitted head trauma, temporal bone fractures comprised 4.7% of all skull fractures and 35.9% of all skull base fractures [2]. A review from 2008 reported that 4–30% of admitted head injuries had skull base fractures with 18–40% of those with temporal bone fractures [3].

The classification scheme for temporal bone fractures has also changed over time. Previously, fractures were classified as either longitudinal, occurring parallel to the long axis of the temporal bone, or transverse, perpendicular to the long axis of the temporal bone. This resulted in the vast majority, 80–90% of fractures, being classified as longitudinal with 10–20% classified as transverse. However, many of the fractures did not follow either of those classifications and were then classified as mixed or oblique. Dahiya et al. reviewed their series of all admitted trauma with 69% having a closed head injury, 10.9% with a basilar skull fracture, and 4.3% with a temporal bone fracture. They proposed a new classification with fractures being classified as either otic capsule-sparing or otic capsule-violating as they found no

T. C. Huang (✉)

Department of Otolaryngology-Head and Neck Surgery, University of Minnesota, Minneapolis, MN, USA

e-mail: huang08@umn.edu

E. C. Kuan et al. (eds.), *Skull Base Reconstruction*, https://doi.org/10.1007/978-3-031-27937-9_14

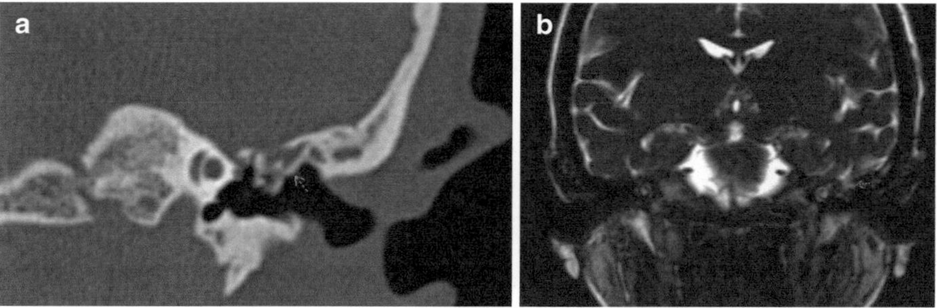

Fig. 14.1 (a) CSF leak from blunt trauma 10 years prior without meningitis (CT). (b) CSF leak from blunt trauma 10 years prior without meningitis (MRI)

true transverse fractures and only 38% were longitudinal with the rest having a mixed picture. The otic capsule-violating fractures had a much higher risk of facial nerve injury, sensorineural hearing loss, and CSF leak with a four times higher risk of CSF leak than otic capsule-sparing fractures [4]. Otic capsule-violating fractures were also the most predictive of significant injury [3].

The rate of CSF leak due to a temporal bone fracture ranged from 8.5 to 25% and presented as CSF otorrhea [5–7]. Alvi et al. reported that the most common cause of CSF otorrhea was injury which accounted for up to 3.6% of all hospitalized head injury, 6% of which were basilar skull fractures and 25% of which were temporal bone fractures. Ninety percent of the leaks stopped with conservative measures (bed rest, elevated head of bed, activity restrictions) [8]. Brodie et al. also found that 95% of the leaks stopped within 1 week with conservative measures. However, those that persisted longer than 7 days incurred a higher risk of meningitis [7] (Fig. 14.1a, b). For the leaks that did not stop with conservative measures, 7% stopped with lumbar drain placement, and an additional 10% did require surgical repair [9]. For those patients that required surgical repair, the approach was either middle fossa, transmastoid, or a combined approach. The success rate improved with support of a primary closure using either alloplastic or autologous grafts and may be even more successful with multilayered graft usage [9, 10]. For patients with persistent CSF leaks due to otic capsule-violating fractures, translabyrinthine repair or subtotal petrosectomy with mastoid obliteration was performed [11, 12].

Penetrating Trauma

A recent systematic review found that penetrating trauma comprised only 3% of temporal bone fractures and that they consist primarily of gunshot wounds (GSW). Gunshot wounds can be classified into those caused by low-velocity projectiles (<1000 m/s) and high-velocity projectiles (>1000 m/s) [13]. There is a high rate of cranial nerve injury, CSF leak, and vestibular and sensorineural hearing loss associated with such trauma. Facial nerve injury occurs in up to 50% of the injuries [14].

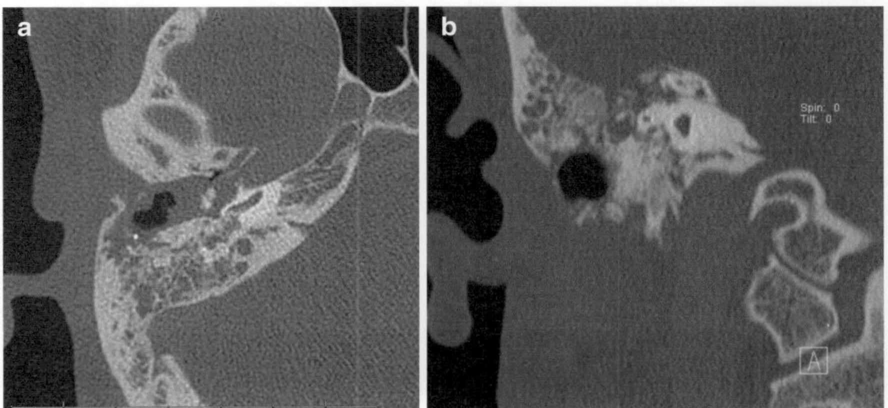

Fig. 14.2 (**a**) GSW with tegmen defect (CT axial). (**b**) GSW with tegmen defect (CT coronal)

CSF leak as a complication ranged from 8 to 12% [13]. With the increased availability of guns in the United States beginning in the 1970s, the incidence of low-velocity gunshot wounds began to increase. In a series of patients from 1989 to 1993, 25% of all missile injuries to the head and neck had temporal bone injury with 20% mortality. While CSF leak is not specifically mentioned, almost half of the injures were associated with intracranial injuries [15]. A literature review from a similar time period found 12 cases of GSW with facial nerve injury being the most common injury with a rate of 75% and 1 case of CSF otorrhea although dural repair was performed in 4 patients. Vascular injuries and hearing loss were also common [16]. A slightly earlier series from 1975 to 1984 found 22 cases with a 9% CSF leak rate [17]. The prevalence of gun violence had even begun to be noticed in the 1970s as a study from 1967 to 1978 identified 35 survivors of penetrating missile injuries, all of which were GSW [18]. Treatment of the injuries consisted of surgical intervention in all series ranging from middle ear exploration/tympanoplasty to mastoid obliteration (Fig. 14.2a, b).

Iatrogenic Injury

The incidence of CSF leak after iatrogenic injuries is higher than that for traumatic injuries. While the majority of the literature focuses on postoperative leaks after skull base surgeries, leaks and fistulas can occur after mastoid surgery as well (Fig. 14.3a, b). Wooten et al. had only a 1% rate of CSF leak after otologic surgery which rose to 33% if the patient had one prior surgery and 66% after multiple surgeries, and Feenstra et al. found that 74% of the patients requiring surgical treatment of temporal bone CSF leaks were due to iatrogenic causes but did not specify whether this included lateral skull base approaches whereas only 11% were secondary to trauma [19, 20]. Fifty-eight percent of patients required repair via a mastoid

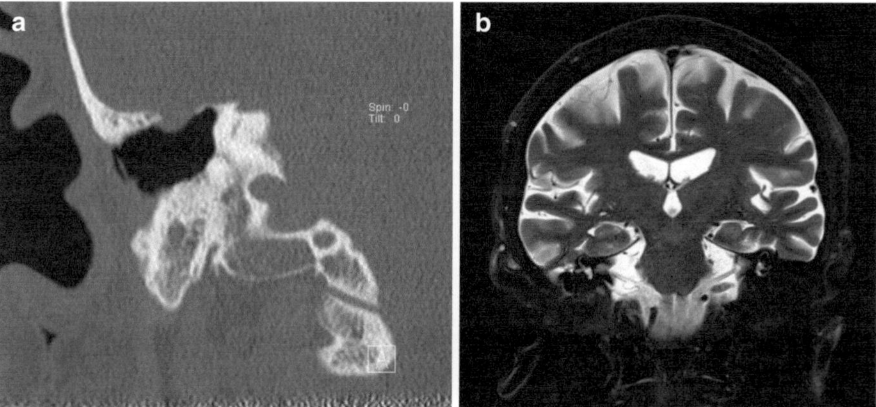

Fig. 14.3 (**a**) Iatrogenic CSF leak after canal wall down mastoidectomy (CT). (**b**) Iatrogenic CSF leak after canal wall down mastoidectomy (MRI)

approach only, 42% required a combined middle fossa and transmastoid approach, and 17% had a recurrent leak after repair [19]. A similarly high percentage of iatrogenic injury (67%) was the cause of patients requiring a combined middle fossa and transmastoid repair of CSF leak [21]. Interestingly, another study found that only 6.8% of the leaks requiring surgical repair were iatrogenic, whereas 21.4% were due to trauma [22].

CSF leak rates after vestibular schwannoma surgery range from 3 to 17% [23–38]. The middle fossa approach appears to have the lowest risk with rates ranging from 0 to 3% [25, 26]. Retrosigmoid approach rates ranged from 5.6 to 17% [27–30, 32, 36], and translabyrinthine rates were similar or slightly higher [23, 24, 33]. The leaks were primarily CSF rhinorrhea with the retrosigmoid approach versus an incision/flap leak in a higher percentage with the translabyrinthine approach [32, 38]. Several studies have found that increasing body mass index is associated with increasing rates of CSF leak [23, 34].

The majority of leaks were resolved with lumbar drain placement (LD) with 100% of the middle fossa leaks controlled with LD [25, 28, 32, 35, 38]. Leaks originating at the incision or under the flap were all controlled with either oversewing plus replacement of the dressing or LD [32]. For leaks requiring surgical intervention, there was found to be no difference in success rate with graft material or with single-layer versus multi-layer closure [22, 28]. However, bone wax alone as an intervention had a 38% rate of failure [31].

Several authors found that their leak rates decreased over time which was attributed to a change in technique with closure such as removing residual air cells, waxing residual air cells, packing with abdominal fat, and using a Palva flap and a change in surgical approach [24, 27, 38]. There was only one group who had an increased rate over time which was attributed to increased removal of the lateral bone over the internal auditory canal with exposure of pericanalicular air cells [31].

In summary, CSF leaks of the temporal bone and lateral skull base, whether caused by traumatic or iatrogenic injury, can often resolve with conservative measures. However, a minority will require surgical repair, often with combined approaches or obliteration. The leaks typically present within the first week of injury, but those which present later are at increased risk for the development of meningitis and other complications.

References

1. Cannon CR, Jahrsdoerfer RA. Temporal bone fractures. Review of 90 cases. Arch Otolaryngol. 1983;109(5):285–8. In: Ovid MEDLINE(R).
2. Schubl SD, Klein TR, Robitsek RJ, Trepeta S, Fretwell K, Seidman D, Gottlieb M. Temporal bone fracture: evaluation in the era of modern computed tomography. Injury. 2016;47(9):1893–7. In: Ovid MEDLINE(R).
3. Johnson F, Semaan MT, Megerian CA. Temporal bone fracture: evaluation and management in the modern era. Otolaryngol Clin North Am. 2008;41(3):597–618, x. In: Ovid MEDLINE(R).
4. Dahiya R, Keller JD, Litofsky NS, Bankey PE, Bonassar LJ, Megerian CA. Temporal bone fractures: otic capsule sparing versus otic capsule violating clinical and radiographic considerations. J Trauma. 1999;47(6):1079–83. In: Ovid MEDLINE(R).
5. Yalciner G, Kutluhan A, Bozdemir K, Cetin H, Tarlak B, Bilgen AS. Temporal bone fractures: evaluation of 77 patients and a management algorithm. Ulus Travma Acil Cerrahi Derg. 2012;18(5):424–8. In: Ovid MEDLINE(R).
6. Lancaster JL, Alderson DJ, Curley JW. Otological complications following basal skull fractures. J R Coll Surg Edinb. 1999;44(2):87–90. In: Ovid MEDLINE(R).
7. Brodie HA, Thompson TC. Management of complications from 820 temporal bone fractures. Am J Otol. 1997;18(2):188–97. In: Ovid MEDLINE(R).
8. Alvi A, Bereliani A IV. Trauma to the temporal bone: diagnosis and management of complications. J Craniomaxillofac Trauma. 1996;2(3):36–48. In: Ovid MEDLINE(R).
9. Savva A, Taylor MJ, Beatty CW. Management of cerebrospinal fluid leaks involving the temporal bone: report on 92 patients. Laryngoscope. 2003;113(1):50–6. In: Ovid MEDLINE(R).
10. Hoang S, Ortiz Torres MJ, Rivera AL, Litofsky NS. Middle cranial fossa approach to repair tegmen defects with autologous or alloplastic graft. World Neurosurg. 2018;118:e10–7. In: Ovid MEDLINE(R).
11. Arnaboldi L, De Micheli G, Dorizzi A, Marella V, Monolo L, Tarfani A. Surgical treatment of cerebrospinal fluid otorrhea. Translabyrinthine approach in posterior petrous bone fractures. J Neurosurg Sci. 1983;27(3):167–70. In: Ovid MEDLINE(R).
12. Magliulo G, Ciniglio Appiani M, Iannella G, Artico M. Petrous bone fractures violating otic capsule. Otol Neurotol. 2012;33(9):1558–61. In: Ovid MEDLINE(R).
13. Kennedy KL, Cash E, Petrey J, Lin JW. Temporal bone fractures caused by ballistic projectiles: a systematic review. Otolaryngol Head Neck Surg. 2021;164(6):1160–5. In: Ovid MEDLINE(R).
14. Kilty S, Murphy PG. Penetrating temporal bone trauma. J Trauma. 2009;66(3):E39–41. In: Ovid MEDLINE(R).
15. Stack BC Jr, Farrior JB. Missile injuries to the temporal bone. South Med J. 1995;88(1):72–8. In: Ovid MEDLINE(R).
16. Haberkamp TJ, McFadden E, Khafagy Y, Harvey SA. Gunshot injuries of the temporal bone. Laryngoscope. 1995;105(10):1053–7. In: Ovid MEDLINE(R).
17. Duncan NO III, Coker NJ, Jenkins HA, Canalis RF. Gunshot injuries of the temporal bone. Otolaryngol Head Neck Surg. 1986;94(1):47–55. In: Ovid MEDLINE(R).

18. Hagan WE, Tabb HG, Cox RH, Travis LW. Gunshot injury to the temporal bone: an analysis of thirty-five cases. Laryngoscope. 1979;89(8):1258–72. In: Ovid MEDLINE(R).
19. Wootten CT, Kaylie DM, Warren FM, Jackson CG. Management of brain herniation and cerebrospinal fluid leak in revision chronic ear surgery. Laryngoscope. 2005;115(7):1256–61. In: Ovid MEDLINE(R).
20. Feenstra L, Sanna M, Zini C, Gamoletti R, Delogu P. Surgical treatment of brain herniation into the middle ear and mastoid. Am J Otol. 1985;6(4):311–5. In: Ovid MEDLINE(R).
21. Jeevan DS, Ormond DR, Kim AH, Meiteles LZ, Stidham KR, Linstrom C, Murali R. Cerebrospinal fluid leaks and encephaloceles of temporal bone origin: nuances to diagnosis and management. World Neurosurg. 2015;83(4):560–6. In: Ovid MEDLINE(R).
22. Stenzel M, Preuss S, Orloff L, Jecker P, Mann W. Cerebrospinal fluid leaks of temporal bone origin: etiology and management. ORL J Otorhinolaryngol Relat Spec. 2005;67(1):51–5. In: Ovid MEDLINE(R).
23. Copeland WR, Mallory GW, Neff BA, Driscoll CL, Link MJ. Are there modifiable risk factors to prevent a cerebrospinal fluid leak following vestibular schwannoma surgery? J Neurosurg. 2015;122(2):312–6. In: Ovid MEDLINE(R).
24. Fishman AJ, Marrinan MS, Golfinos JG, Cohen NL, Roland JT Jr. Prevention and management of cerebrospinal fluid leak following vestibular schwannoma surgery. Laryngoscope. 2004;114(3):501–5. In: Ovid MEDLINE(R).
25. Lipschitz N, Kohlberg GD, Tawfik KO, Walters ZA, Breen JT, Zuccarello M, Andaluz N, Dinapoli VA, Pensak ML, Samy RN. Cerebrospinal fluid leak rate after vestibular schwannoma surgery via middle cranial fossa approach. J Neurol Surg B Skull Base. 2019;80(4):437–40. In: Ovid MEDLINE(R) PubMed-not-MEDLINE.
26. Leonetti JP, Anderson D, Marzo S, Moynihan G. Prevention and management of cerebrospinal fluid fistula after transtemporal skull base surgery. Skull Base. 2001;11(2):87–92. In: Ovid MEDLINE(R) PubMed-not-MEDLINE.
27. Falcioni M, Romano G, Aggarwal N, Sanna M. Cerebrospinal fluid leak after retrosigmoid excision of vestibular schwannomas. Otol Neurotol. 2008;29(3):384–6. In: Ovid MEDLINE(R).
28. Arlt F, Trantakis C, Krupp W, Renner C, Winkler D, Strauss G, Meixensberger J. Cerebrospinal fluid leak after microsurgical surgery in vestibular schwannomas via retrosigmoidal craniotomy. Neurol Res. 2011;33(9):947–52. In: Ovid MEDLINE(R).
29. Li D, Wang H, Fan Z, Fan Z. Complications in retrosigmoid cranial nerve surgery. Acta Otolaryngol (Stockh). 2010;130(2):247–52. In: Ovid MEDLINE(R).
30. Bani A, Gilsbach JM. Incidence of cerebrospinal fluid leak after microsurgical removal of vestibular schwannomas. Acta Neurochir (Wien). 2002;144(10):979–82; discussion 982. In: Ovid MEDLINE(R).
31. Nutik SL, Korol HW. Cerebrospinal fluid leak after acoustic neuroma surgery. Surg Neurol. 1995;43(6):553–6; discussion 556–7. In: Ovid MEDLINE(R).
32. Hoffman RA. Cerebrospinal fluid leak following acoustic neuroma removal. Laryngoscope. 1994;104(1 Pt 1):40–58. In: Ovid MEDLINE(R).
33. Celikkanat SM, Saleh E, Khashaba A, Taibah A, Russo A, Mazzoni A, Sanna M. Cerebrospinal fluid leak after translabyrinthine acoustic neuroma surgery. Otolaryngol Head Neck Surg. 1995;112(6):654–8. In: Ovid MEDLINE(R).
34. Mantravadi AV, Leonetti JP, Burgette R, Pontikis G, Marzo SJ, Anderson D. Body mass index predicts risk for complications from transtemporal cerebellopontine angle surgery. Otolaryngol Head Neck Surg. 2013;148(3):460–5. In: Ovid MEDLINE(R).
35. Magliulo G, Sepe C, Varacalli S, Fusconi M. Cerebrospinal fluid leak management following cerebellopontine angle surgery. J Otolaryngol. 1998;27(5):258–62. In: Ovid MEDLINE(R).
36. Millen SJ, Meyer G. Surgical management of CSF otorhinorrhea following retrosigmoid removal of cerebellopontine angle tumors. Am J Otol. 1993;14(6):585–9. In: Ovid MEDLINE(R).

37. Fishman AJ, Hoffman RA, Roland JT Jr, Lebowitz RA, Cohen NL. Cerebrospinal fluid drainage in the management of CSF leak following acoustic neuroma surgery. Laryngoscope. 1996;106(8):1002–4. In: Ovid MEDLINE(R).
38. Brennan JW, Rowed DW, Nedzelski JM, Chen JM. Cerebrospinal fluid leak after acoustic neuroma surgery: influence of tumor size and surgical approach on incidence and response to treatment. J Neurosurg. 2001;94(2):217–23. In: Ovid MEDLINE(R).

Chapter 15
Spontaneous CSF Leaks and Encephaloceles

Joe Walter Kutz Jr.

Introduction

Spontaneous cerebrospinal fluid (sCSF) leaks and encephaloceles of the temporal bone are uncommon causes of hearing loss, middle ear effusion, tympanostomy tube otorrhea, meningitis, and, rarely, seizures. The risks factors for sCSF leaks include obesity, idiopathic intracranial hypertension, and obstructive sleep apnea [1–3]. With the increasing incidence of obesity in the United States, sCSF leaks are becoming more common [2]. Because other conditions such as eustachian tube dysfunction and chronic otitis media more commonly cause these symptoms, diagnosis is often delayed by months and sometimes years. Delayed diagnosis should be avoided since a sCSF leak places the patient at risk for meningitis, although the incidence of meningitis has not been determined. This chapter will review the presentation, risk factors, radiographic findings, and management of sCSF leaks and encephaloceles of the temporal bone.

Presenting Signs and Symptoms

Patients with sCSF leaks most commonly present with a chronic middle ear effusion. Initial treatment by their primary care physician or otolaryngologist is directed towards eustachian tube dysfunction and may include oral steroids, nasal steroid

J. W. Kutz Jr. (✉)
Department of Otolaryngology, University of Texas Southwestern Medical Center,
Dallas, TX, USA
e-mail: walter.kutz@utsouthwestern.edu

© The Author(s), under exclusive license to Springer Nature
Switzerland AG 2023
E. C. Kuan et al. (eds.), *Skull Base Reconstruction*,
https://doi.org/10.1007/978-3-031-27937-9_15

sprays, and antihistamines. The diagnosis is often suspected once medical management fails, a tympanostomy tube is placed, and the patient develops copious, clear otorrhea. The patient with a sCSF leak and a tympanostomy tube or perforation will describe soaking cotton balls and noticing spotting on their pillow when sleeping. The fluid can be collected and sent for beta-2 transferrin; however, the history of copious clear otorrhea and supporting imaging can usually make a definitive diagnosis of a sCSF leak without laboratory confirmation.

There are subtle differences between a middle ear effusion related to eustachian tube dysfunction and CSF in the middle ear space. Chronic serous otitis media usually appears amber in color compared to the clear appearance of CSF. Serous otitis media is often associated with a retracted tympanic membrane, which is uncommon with a CSF effusion. If CSF is suspected, a 1 cc syringe and 25-gauge needle can be used to aspirate the middle ear fluid and sent for beta-2 transferrin. A positive beta-2 transferrin is diagnostic for CSF.

In our study of patients presenting with sCSF leaks, 12.5% presented with a history of meningitis [4]. The incidence of meningitis in the setting of a sCSF leak or encephalocele is unknown; however, this is often the primary reason to repair the defect causing the leak. Once a diagnosis of a sCSF leak is made, the patient should be informed about the signs and symptoms of meningitis. The patient should be vaccinated against streptococcus pneumoniae, which includes both the pneumococcal conjugate vaccine (PCV13) and the pneumococcal polysaccharide vaccine (PPSV23). The patient should be counseled to avoid nose blowing and to sneeze with their mouth open to prevent possible pneumocephalus.

Temporal bone encephaloceles are a rare cause of seizures. We have repaired three encephaloceles that presented with seizures (unpublished data) without an active CFS leak, and none of the patients continued to have seizures after repair of the encephalocele.

A thorough history should inquire about the possibility of multiple simultaneous leaks. In patients with extremely elevated CSF pressure, simultaneous leaks may occur from different anatomical areas such as the temporal bone and the anterior skull base or bilateral temporal bone. Schwartz et al. reported a 3.8% incidence of simultaneous leaks from different anatomical sites. These patients were more likely to be morbidly obese (mean BMI 46.2 kg/m^2 vs. 31.5 kg/m^2), African American, and female [5].

Risk Factors for sCSF Leaks

It is important to elicit risk factors and treat conditions that increase the risk of developing a sCSF leak or encephalocele. Conditions that cause chronically elevated intracranial pressure include obesity, obstructive sleep apnea, and idiopathic intracranial hypertension. If these conditions are not recognized and treated after repair, recurrent leaks are common.

Role of Obesity

Most, but not all, patients who present with sCSF leaks are obese, as defined by a body mass index (BMI) of $\geq$30 kg/m^2. In a series of 50 patients with sCSF leaks, 70% were obese with a mean BMI of 35.0 kg/m^2, and 32% had a BMI $\geq$40 kg/m^2 [4].

It is thought obesity causes increased intracranial pressure by the following mechanism. Obesity causes increased abdominal pressure that leads to increased lung intrapleural pressure. This in turn decreases cardiac filling, decreases venous return, and increases intracranial venous pressure [3].

Weight loss has been shown to decrease intracranial pressure, so referral for weight loss or bariatric surgery should be considered in patients that are morbidly obese [6].

Idiopathic Intracranial Hypertension

Idiopathic intracranial hypertension is a risk factor for the development of sCSF leaks and encephaloceles [7, 8] Obesity and obstructive sleep apnea are risks factors for elevated CSF pressure [9]. Signs and symptoms of IIH include headaches, blurry vision, nausea, neck stiffness, and dizziness [10]. Untreated, IIH can lead to permanent vision loss [10]. Papilledema is common in the setting of IIH; however, papilledema does not occur in the setting of an active leak [11]. Lumbar puncture is used to make a definitive diagnosis. An opening pressure greater than 25 mm/H$_2$O is diagnostic of IIH [12].

Obstructive Sleep Apnea

Obstructive sleep apnea (OSA) has been associated with a higher incidence of sCSF leaks. Nelson et al. found the rate of OSA in patients with sCSF leaks to be 14.8% nationally and 37.1% at their institution [2]. A systematic review investigating the association between OSA and sCSF leaks by Bakhsheshian et al. concluded an overall prevalence of OSA of 16.7% in patients with cSCF leaks. They estimate the odds of having OSA in a patient with a sCSF leak to be 4.73 times higher than controls [1].

Obstructive sleep apnea causes apneic episodes that result in hypoxia and hypercapnia, which leads to cerebral vasodilation and transient increased in intracranial pressure [9]. This cycle of increased intracranial pressure may lead to a sCSF leak.

One may argue obesity has a higher risk of both sCSF leaks and OSA, so an independent association of OSA and sCSF leaks may be present since both conditions are more commonly seen in obese patients. However, Nelson et al.

demonstrated that obese patients with sCSF were 13.7 times likely to have a sCSF leak than a similar control group of obese patients with a cochlear implant [13].

Congenital Defects

Congenital defects occur when there is an abnormal communication between the arachnoid space and the air-containing space of the temporal bone. The most common defects encountered include a persistent Hyrtle's fissure and defects in the stapes footplate. Often the inner ear will be abnormal with an open cochlear aperature and incomplete partition of the cochlea. Careful review of the CT may show soft tissue around the footplate that represents soft tissue protruding through the footplate [14].

Workup

Most often a CSF leak of the temporal bone presents with a unilateral effusion or copious otorrhea after placement of a tympanostomy tube. A history of copious otorrhea is often enough to diagnose a sCSF leak; however, in the case of a unilateral effusion or intermittent otorrhea, laboratory testing and imaging may be necessary.

Laboratory Findings

If a CSF leak is suspected, fluid can be sent for beta-2 transferrin, which has 97% sensitivity and 99% specificity for CSF [15]. A tympanocentesis can be performed to collect fluid through an intact tympanic membrane or collected if otorrhea is occurring through a tympanostomy tube or perforations. Occasionally, not enough fluid is present to collect and send for laboratory analysis, but if the history, exam findings, and radiographic findings are convincing, beta-2 transferrin confirmation of a CSF leak may not be necessary.

CT

High-resolution, fine-cut CT of the temporal bone and skull base is the best initial radiographic study to identify the location of a CSF leak (Fig. 15.1a–c). The most common locations are along the tegmen tympani and tegmen mastoideum, which

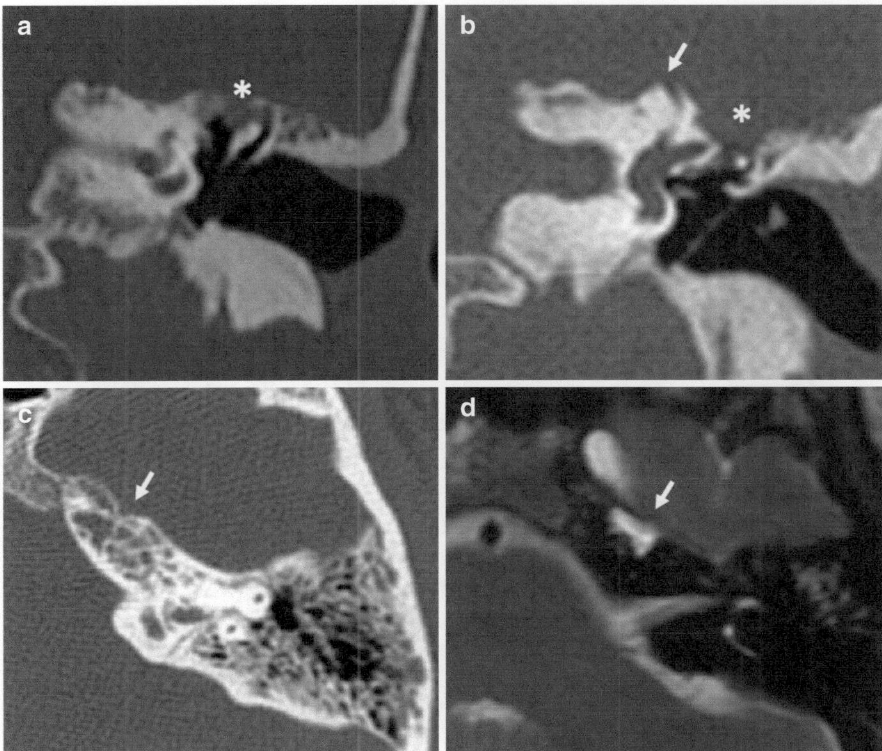

Fig. 15.1 (**a**) Coronal CT showing an encephalocele (*) contacting the ossicles. (**b**) Coronal CT with arrow pointing to superior semicircular canal dehiscence in the setting of an encephalocele (*). (**c, d**) Axial CT showing a less frequent defect of the petrous apex. T2-weighted MRI showing a meningocele of the petrous apex

are best visualized using a coronal CT scan. Less common locations for a leak include the posterior fossa plate and the petrous apex. Wick et al. reported that 5.6% of sCSF leaks originating from the temporal bone were from the posterior fossa [16]. Axial CT should be viewed to evaluate for leaks in these less common locations. At our institution, we reported multiple defects in 52.7% of patients with sCSF leaks. Because multiple leak sites are common, reviewing both coronal and axial scans is necessary for all cases [4]. CT also allows accurate evaluation of the superior semicircular canal, which was found to be dehiscent in 12.5% of patients with sCSF leaks in our series [4].

MRI

If CT shows the location of the defect(s), a MRI may not be necessary. MRI is most useful to confirm the presence of an encephalocele. A heavily weighted, fine-cut T2 image in the coronal plane will often show an encephalocele that will be hypointense against the hyperintense background of the CSF fluid (Fig. 15.1d). MRI cisternogram imaging may be useful for cases when a CSF leak is suspected on history and CT imaging, but more information is needed. MRI is also useful in the evaluation of findings associated with IIH including an empty sella, flattening of the posterior optic globe, tortuous optic nerves, and stenosis of the transverse sinuses [17].

Long-Term Follow-Up and Management

The underlying cause of the cerebrospinal fluid leak should be determined. A lumbar puncture 4–6 weeks after surgery with measurement of opening cerebrospinal fluid pressure and a sleep study testing for obstructive sleep apnea should be obtained. If a lumbar puncture is obtained before repair of the CSF leak or too soon after repair of the leak, the opening pressure may be falsely low. If the lumbar puncture opening pressure is greater than 25 mm/H_2O, treatment for idiopathic intracranial hypertension should be considered. Opening pressure between 20 and 25 mm/H_2O is borderline elevated, and referral to neurology or neuro-ophthalmology should be considered. Idiopathic intracranial hypertension is typically treated with acetazolamide, topirimate, or a ventriculoperitoneal shunt in cases that do not respond to medical management.

If the sleep study shows obstructive sleep apnea, treatment should be initiated.

Meningitis Risk

The incidence of meningitis before and after repair of the cerebrospinal fluid leak has not been established but would be expected to be higher before surgical repair. The Centers for Disease Control and Prevention recommends both the pneumococcal conjugate vaccine (PCV13) and the pneumococcal polysaccharide vaccine (PPSV23) for patients with cerebrospinal fluid leaks. (Available from: https://www.cdc.gov/vaccines/vpd/pneumo/hcp/recommendations.html.)

In certain situations, a patient may decline surgical repair for personal or health reasons and must be informed about the risk of meningitis. Rao and Redleaf reported on nine patients with spontaneous cerebrospinal fluid leaks or encephaloceles who did not undergo surgical repair or had persistnet leakage after repair with a follow-up time between 6 and 132 months, and none of these patients developed meningitis during the observationn time. In addition, they reported on ten patients with encephalcoeles and an infected mastoid who did not undergo repair, and none developed meningitis [18, 19].

Although the incidence of meningitis has not been established, patients with skull base defects do present with meningitis, so meningitis precautions should be discussed with the patient during the initial visit and during subsequent visits.

Conclusions

sCSF leaks and encephaloceles are an uncommon but important cause of chronic otorrhea or a middle ear effusion. If the fluid tests positive for beta-2 transferrin, the diagnosis is confirmed. A high-resolution CT of the temporal bone can identify most defects causing the sCSF leak. Multiple defects are present in greater than half of cases, and less common locations such as the petrous apex and posterior fossa should be carefully viewed (Fig. 15.2). After repair, idiopathic intracranial hypertension and obstructive sleep apnea should be investigated since these are the two most common underlying causes of elevated cerebrospinal fluid pressure (Fig. 15.3). Vaccination for bacterial meningitis is recommended by the CDC and may provide protection from subsequent meningitis.

Fig. 15.2 Preoperative and postoperative considerations

Mechanisms for increased intracranial pressure

Obesity	**Sleep apnea**
↑ abdominal pressure	Hypoxia and hypercapnia
▼	▼
↑ intrapleural lung pressure	Cerebral vasodilation
▼	▼
↓ cardiac filling, venous return	↑ intracranial pressure
▼	
↑ intracranial pressure	

Preoperative and postoperative considerations for patients with a spontaneous CSF leak

Preoperative	**Postoperative**
Testing	Lumbar puncture with measurement of opening pressure
Audiogram	If opening pressure elevated or suspicion for IIH, refer to neurology or neuro-ophthalmology
Collect fluid for beta-2 transferrin if possible	Recommend sleep study
High resolution CT of the temporal bones and skull base	Confirm administration of pneumococcal conjugate vaccine (PCV13) and the pneumococcal polysaccharide vaccine (PPSV23)
Consider MRI to evaluate for encephalocele or findings of IIH	Discuss meningitis precautions
Counseling	
Avoid nose blowing and sneeze with mouth open to prevent possible pneumocephalus	
Recommend pneumococcal conjugate vaccine (PCV13) and the pneumococcal polysaccharide vaccine (PPSV23)	
Discuss meningitis precautions	

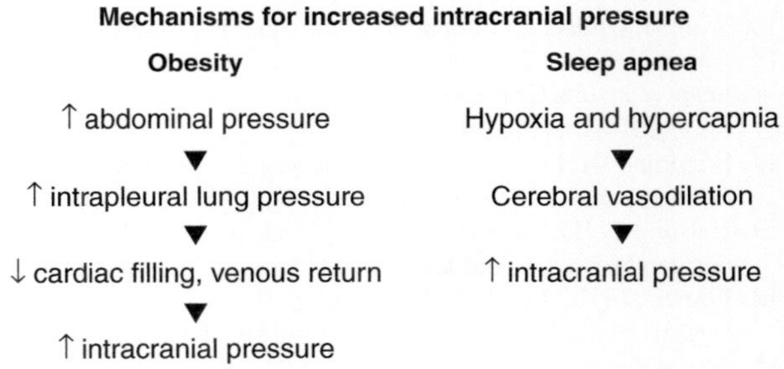

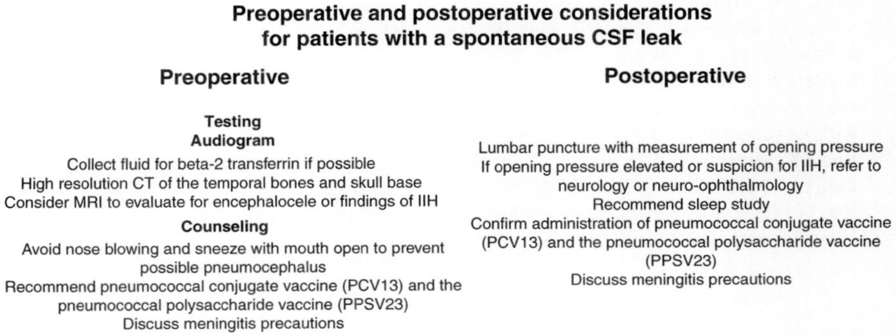

Fig. 15.3 Proposed mechanisms of action for the development of increased intracranial pressure in the settings of obesity and obstructive sleep apnea [12, 13]

References

1. Bakhsheshian J, Hwang MS, Friedman M. Association between obstructive sleep apnea and spontaneous cerebrospinal fluid leaks: a systematic review and meta-analysis. JAMA Otolaryngol Head Neck Surg. 2015;141(8):733–8.
2. Nelson RF, Gantz BJ, Hansen MR. The rising incidence of spontaneous cerebrospinal fluid leaks in the United States and the association with obesity and obstructive sleep apnea. Otol Neurotol. 2015;36(3):476–80.
3. Sugerman HJ, DeMaria EJ, Felton WL III, Nakatsuka M, Sismanis A. Increased intra-abdominal pressure and cardiac filling pressures in obesity-associated pseudotumor cerebri. Neurology. 1997;49(2):507–11.
4. Kutz JW Jr, Johnson AK, Wick CC. Surgical management of spontaneous cerebrospinal fistulas and encephaloceles of the temporal bone. Laryngoscope. 2018;128(9):2170–7.
5. Schwartz N, Brown KD, Sasaki-Adams D, Morgan SA, Zanation AM, Thorp BD, et al. Multifocal skull base defects with associated spontaneous cerebrospinal fluid leaks. Otol Neurotol. 2021;42(5):e624–8.
6. Kupersmith MJ, Gamell L, Turbin R, Peck V, Spiegel P, Wall M. Effects of weight loss on the course of idiopathic intracranial hypertension in women. Neurology. 1998;50(4):1094–8.
7. Bidot S, Levy JM, Saindane AM, Narayana KM, Dattilo M, DelGaudio JM, et al. Spontaneous skull base cerebrospinal fluid leaks and their relationship to idiopathic intracranial hypertension. Am J Rhinol Allergy. 2021;35(1):36–43.
8. Perez MA, Bialer OY, Bruce BB, Newman NJ, Biousse V. Primary spontaneous cerebrospinal fluid leaks and idiopathic intracranial hypertension. J Neuroophthalmol. 2013;33(4):330–7.
9. Jennum P, Borgesen SE. Intracranial pressure and obstructive sleep apnea. Chest. 1989;95(2):279–83.
10. Wall M. Update on idiopathic intracranial hypertension. Neurol Clin. 2017;35(1):45–57.
11. Aaron G, Doyle J, Vaphiades MS, Riley KO, Woodworth BA. Increased intracranial pressure in spontaneous CSF leak patients is not associated with papilledema. Otolaryngol Head Neck Surg. 2014;151(6):1061–6.
12. Friedman DI, Liu GT, Digre KB. Revised diagnostic criteria for the pseudotumor cerebri syndrome in adults and children. Neurology. 2013;81(13):1159–65.
13. Nelson RF, Hansen KR, Gantz BJ, Hansen MR. Calvarium thinning in patients with spontaneous cerebrospinal fluid leak. Otol Neurotol. 2015;36(3):481–5.
14. Ehmer DR Jr, Booth T, Kutz JW Jr, Roland PS. Radiographic diagnosis of trans-stapedial cerebrospinal fluid fistula. Otolaryngol Head Neck Surg. 2010;142(5):694–8.
15. Warnecke A, Averbeck T, Wurster U, Harmening M, Lenarz T, Stover T. Diagnostic relevance of beta2-transferrin for the detection of cerebrospinal fluid fistulas. Arch Otolaryngol Head Neck Surg. 2004;130(10):1178–84.
16. Wick CC, Killeen DE, Clark M, Kutz JW, Isaacson B. Posterior fossa spontaneous cerebrospinal fluid leaks. Otol Neurotol. 2017;38(1):66–72.
17. Mallery RM, Rehmani OF, Woo JH, Chen YJ, Reddi S, Salzman KL, et al. Utility of magnetic resonance imaging features for improving the diagnosis of idiopathic intracranial hypertension without papilledema. J Neuroophthalmol. 2019;39(3):299–307.
18. Rao AK, Merenda DM, Wetmore SJ. Diagnosis and management of spontaneous cerebrospinal fluid otorrhea. Otol Neurotol. 2005;26(6):1171–5.
19. Rao N, Redleaf M. Spontaneous middle cranial fossa cerebrospinal fluid otorrhea in adults. Laryngoscope. 2016;126(2):464–8.

Chapter 16
Lateral Skull Base Surgical Approaches

Rance J. T. Fujiwara, Mehdi Abouzari, Hamid R. Djalilian, and Kevin A. Peng

Middle Cranial Fossa Approach

Encephaloceles and CSF leaks, whether posttraumatic, infectious, iatrogenic, or spontaneous, most commonly occur through the floor of the middle cranial fossa and may involve the tegmen tympani, tegmen mastoideum, petrous apex, or any combination thereof [1–3]. As such, the middle cranial fossa (MCF) approach remains the primary surgical approach to access these defects from above for CSF leak repairs of the lateral skull base. It is sometimes combined with a transmastoid approach with or without elevation of a tympanomeatal flap and middle ear dissection to gain inferior access.

R. J. T. Fujiwara
David Geffen School of Medicine at UCLA, Los Angeles, CA, USA

M. Abouzari
University of California Irvine Medical Center, Orange, CA, USA
e-mail: mabouzar@hs.uci.edu

H. R. Djalilian
Otolaryngology-Head and Neck Surgery, University of California, Irvine, Irvine, CA, USA
e-mail: hdjalili@hs.uci.edu

K. A. Peng (⌧)
House Institute, Los Angeles, CA, USA
e-mail: kpeng@houseclinic.com

© The Author(s), under exclusive license to Springer Nature Switzerland AG 2023
E. C. Kuan et al. (eds.), *Skull Base Reconstruction*,
https://doi.org/10.1007/978-3-031-27937-9_16

Incision and Flap Elevation

One common incision used for access to the squamous portion of the temporal bone is in the shape of a reverse question mark. The incision starts just anterior to the tragus and is carried superiorly, passing 3–4 cm posterior to the external auditory meatus, superiorly for 5–6 cm, and finally anteriorly to the temporal hairline. The skin and soft tissue are incised sharply to the level of the temporoparietal fascia. At this point, a large temporalis fascia graft may be harvested in the usual fashion for reconstruction of the skull base defect. A cuff of fascia should be preserved along the rim of the muscle flap for closure at the conclusion of the case. An inferiorly based temporalis muscle flap is then elevated off the calvarium using monopolar cautery and periosteal elevators, exposing the squamous portion of the temporal bone. The inferior extent of dissection is the zygomatic root, which should be readily palpable through the inferior aspect of the incision. If it cannot be palpated, additional relaxing incisions are made until exposure is adequate.

During the incision and flap elevation, care should be taken near the proximal aspect of the temporalis muscle at the zygoma, where the frontal branch of the facial nerve is located within the temporoparietal fascia and can be injured if one is not in the appropriate plane or if monopolar cautery is used inappropriately. To minimize the risk of facial nerve injury, intraoperative facial nerve monitoring is employed in all cases.

Craniotomy

Having exposed the squamous temporal bone, a craniotomy measuring approximately 5 × 5 cm is performed with cutting followed by diamond burrs. If desired, the craniotome may also be used. The dura can be visualized through transparent bone once it is thinned enough, at which point a diamond burr is used to complete the craniotomy. The craniotomy window should be centered at the root of the zygoma, with roughly two thirds of the window anterior to the external auditory canal and its lower edge roughly at the level of the floor of the middle cranial fossa. Once this is complete, the bone flap can be carefully separated from the underlying dura, with great attention to avoid lacerating the dura.

The dura is then elevated off the floor of the middle cranial fossa in lateral to medial and posterior to anterior direction (to prevent injury to the greater superficial petrosal nerve) under the microscope until the area of dehiscence is visualized. Often, an encephalocele may protrude through dehiscent tegmen. This is thought to be secondary to trauma, idiopathic intracranial hypertension, or dural and bone weakness in areas of aberrant arachnoid granulations [4–7]. Careful dissection in the tegmen tympani is required to avoid iatrogenic injury to the ossicular chain if the encephalocele is abutting or impinging upon the ossicles [4, 8]. The base of the encephalocele herniation can be visualized from the extradural approach with retraction of the temporal lobe, and the encephalocele can often be reduced back into the middle cranial fossa [9]. If reduction is impossible, transection at the stalk of the encephalocele can be performed. If no encephalocele is present, the area of meningeal defect leading to leak must be positively identified.

As the dura is elevated from the floor of the middle cranial fossa, there are several key anatomic landmarks of note. Posteriorly, the arcuate eminence is often the first landmark identified and is a relative bony landmark for the superior semicircular canal, which may sometimes be dehiscent in suspected cases of idiopathic intracranial hypertension with concurrent encephalocele [10, 11]. It is important to note that the arcuate eminence may not lie directly over the superior semicircular canal, and it consequently cannot be regarded as a foolproof landmark. Anteriorly, the greater superficial petrosal nerve is identified. The bisection of the angle formed by the arcuate eminence and greater superficial petrosal nerve may be used to approximate the location of the internal auditory canal [12]. Drilling of the internal auditory canal, such as that done for a middle fossa resection of a vestibular schwannoma, is rarely necessary. If necessary, dissection may be carried as medially as the ridge of the petrous apex medially, with attention paid to avoid laceration of the superior petrosal sinus. During elevation, bony vascular channels are obliterated with bone wax, and dural attachments may be addressed with bipolar electrocautery and sharp transection.

Repair of Skull Base Defect

Depending on the size of the dehiscence or CSF leak, the previously harvested fascia graft with or without a bone or cartilage graft may be used for reconstruction in a multilayer fashion. Both intradural and extradural approaches have been described, and each may be used alone or in conjunction with the other. Options for meningeal repair include previously harvested temporalis fascia, synthetic dural substitute, and other autologous tissue (such as fascia lata). In an intradural repair, a dural incision is made, the repair material is placed intradurally to cover the area of meningeal dehiscence and/or encephalocele, and the dura is reapproximated. For an extradural repair, the repair material is placed in onlay fashion between the bony middle fossa floor and the native dura, taking care to cover areas of dehiscence. Fibrin sealant is often utilized.

If desired, a bone graft may be used. The bone graft is usually a split calvarial graft from the previously harvested bone flap and can be placed over the bony defect on the floor of the middle cranial fossa floor in the extradural space. This may be necessary in cases of large dehiscence with concern for continued soft tissue prolapse. Rarely, an inferiorly based temporalis muscle flap may be utilized, traversing the craniotomy via the inferior border. Cartilage is rarely utilized for lateral skull base CSF leak repairs, and even bone grafts and temporalis rotational flaps are rarely necessary.

Translabyrinthine Approach

The translabyrinthine approach to the lateral skull base is most often used to access tumors of the cerebellopontine angle in patients with non-serviceable hearing. It was popularized in the 1960s following several publications by William F. House illustrating successful outcomes in vestibular schwannoma resections via this approach [13, 14]. The approach gives ample access to the cerebellopontine angle and internal auditory canal, as well as improved exposure of areas of the middle and posterior cranial fossa. Cerebrospinal fluid leaks originating from the posterior cranial fossa are very rare, with the largest case series documenting five cases in a 10 year period [15, 16]. In these cases, a translabyrinthine approach may be considered.

Simple Mastoidectomy and Facial Nerve Identification

A simple mastoidectomy is first performed [17]. Briefly, the mastoid cortex is first removed in a systematic fashion using a cutting burr. Surface landmarks include the temporal line superiorly (which delineates the superior extent of the dissection and approximates the tegmen tympani and floor of the middle cranial fossa) and the spine of Henle representing the posterior aspect of the bony ear canal. The tegmen tympani is skeletonized with careful attention to any defects or encephaloceles which may be encountered. The posterior ear canal is then thinned appropriately, and finally the sigmoid sinus is located by continuing the mastoid dissection posteriorly. For the purposes of the translabyrinthine approach, skeletonization of the sigmoid sinus, tegmen, and sinodural angle is necessary for a wide exposure of the labyrinth and ultimately the internal auditory canal. Koerner's septum, a thin bony plate at the petrosquamous suture line, is encountered as the dissection is continued. The mastoid antrum will be encountered deep to Koerner's septum and the horizontal semicircular canal and incus visualized. Additional drilling anterior to the horizontal semicircular canal will allow for identification of the second genu and the vertical segment of the facial nerve.

Postauricular Labyrinthectomy

The three semicircular canals are then fenestrated in a systematic manner, beginning with the horizontal canal and followed by the posterior and superior canals. One must pay close attention to the close proximity of the second genu of the facial nerve to the anterior aspect of the horizontal canal while opening the labyrinth. The medial wall of the horizontal and superior canals also abuts the labyrinthine segment of the facial nerve. The vestibule can then be widely opened. Remnant bone overlying the posterior and middle fossa dura can be removed with diamond burr drills and rongeur instruments. In vestibular schwannoma surgeries, the internal auditory canal is then exposed by identification of its superior landmark (approximated by the ampulla of the superior canal) and inferior landmark (retrofacial air cells superior to the jugular bulb).

Repair of Skull Base Defect

When a translabyrinthine approach is performed for CSF leak repair, the mastoidectomy and labyrinthectomy cavity is typically obliterated in order to close the dural defect and CSF leak. Abdominal fat is the grafting material of choice. The middle ear is first obliterated with muscle or fat, and the Eustachian tube is packed with a combination of muscle, bone wax, woven oxidized regenerated cellulose, and fat. The incus can be separated from the stapes and malleus, and the long process can be used to hold the packing material in the Eustachian tube. The abdominal fat graft is placed into the mastoidectomy and labyrinthectomy cavity, and a craniotomy plate is placed over the abdominal fat graft to ensure consistent pressure to maximize chances of sealing the leak.

Transmastoid Approach

The choice of approach of CSF leak depends on the location and multitude of defects. The initial approach to the repair of small (<1 cm) or a few tegmen mastoideum defects or posterior fossa defects is the transmastoid approach [18]. For larger (>1 cm) defects or multiple (>3) tegmen mastoideum defects, the transmastoid approach [19, 20], MCF approach [1, 21], and the combined approach [22, 23] have been advocated by different authors throughout the literature.

Postauricular Cortical Mastoidectomy

A classic postauricular incision is made. The cortical mastoidectomy is then performed, and the tegmen defect(s) is exposed. In cases with associated meningocele or meningoencephalocele, the stalk of the herniated tissue is cauterized with bipolar cautery on a low setting (10–15 W) and amputated at its base which can be subsequently sent for pathologic analysis to confirm diagnosis. In mastoidectomy, the goal is to expose the dural defect without creating a considerable opening of the mastoid antrum. Bone wax is used to obliterate all the facial recess, retrofacial air cells, and mastoid tip cells to prevent communication between the mastoid and the middle ear. The sole use of bone wax is not adequate for long-term control of CSF leakage. A large temporalis fascia can be used to cover all the air cells and the mastoid antrum to separate the middle ear from the mastoid. The goal of this step is to prevent communication of the CSF leak (in case of surgical failure) with the middle ear. Fibrin glue is then used to cover the fascia to adhere it better and prevent motion.

Repair of Tegmen Defect

Tegmen mastoideum defects have to be repaired in a multilayered fashion, most often using a combination of autologous mastoid bone, temporalis fascia, and tissue sealant (Fig. 16.1). To address the tegmen defect, the dura is separated from the surrounding bone first. We have found that when multiple defects are present, it is easier to remove the intervening bone (if the defects are clustered in an area) and to make a larger defect that is easier to repair. A joint knife or an angled hook is used to distinguish the plain between the bone and the dura. Furthermore, a longer blunt hook (or whirlybird) is used to separate the dura from the tegmen. It is crucial to be mindful of the thin area surrounding a spontaneous defect because the dura is generally thin and the bone may further fracture, leading to a larger defect than is needed. The dura in patients with spontaneous CSF leak tends to be thinner and may be strongly adherent (especially in older patients) to the bone. To separate the dura from the bone, sharp dissection may possibly be required. Next, a piece of temporalis fascia is placed between the middle (or posterior) fossa floor and the dura, covering the surrounding bone by approximately 4–5 mm. The underlay fascia must be positioned so well so as to completely stop the CSF leak (Fig. 16.2). The surgeon should not rely on the fibrin glue to control the leak as the surgery will likely fail when the fibrin glue is broken down in approximately 8 weeks. Fibrin glue is then used to seal the fascia into place. Sometimes, a piece of DuraGen (Integra LifeSciences, Plainsboro, NJ) is used as an additional support for large tegmen

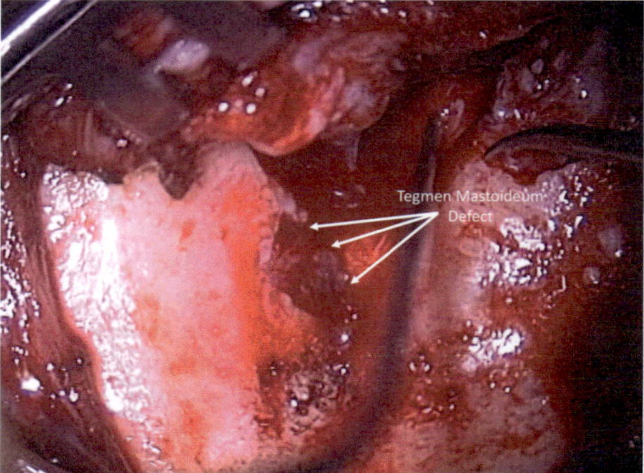

Fig. 16.1 Right tegmen mastoideum defect with active CSF leakage

Fig. 16.2 The underlay fascia graft is placed as an underlay with complete cessation of the CSF leak on its own

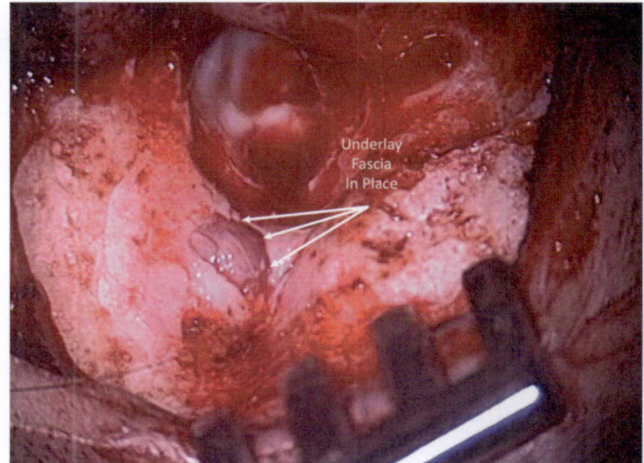

Fig. 16.3 A large fascia graft is placed to close off the attic and the rest of the mastoid air cells to prevent communication with the middle ear

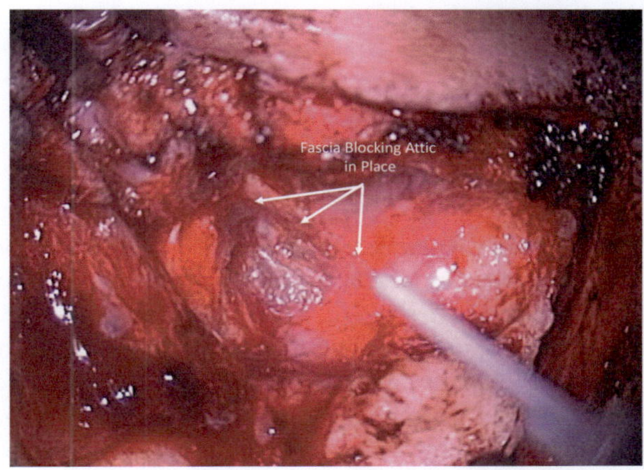

mastoideum defects (≥ 1 cm defects in elderly patients who are not MCF candidates). On the mastoid side, a second fascia layer is used as an onlay graft, it is packed tightly with abdominal fat, and a titanium mesh is used to close over the mastoid using three or four screws (Fig. 16.3). If the defect is >7 mm, we sometimes use an onlay cartilage graft or a mastoid cortex graft (obtained using osteotomes) on the onlay fascia graft. Compressing the titanium mesh in the middle creates better compression of the fat in the mastoid (Fig. 16.4). Placement of a postoperative lumbar drain is not required. Intraoperative antibiotics (vancomycin and ceftazidime) and mannitol (1 g/kg) are administered to the patient. A postoperative CT scan is usually done 6 h postoperatively to rule out any subdural or epidural hemorrhage triggered by the dissection of the dura. The patient is then observed for 24 h following the surgery in the hospital. The patient is started on acetazolamide 125 mg BID in the hospital, with escalation to 500 mg BID after several weeks based on the side effects, for a total of 6 weeks. All patients are monitored postoperatively for the

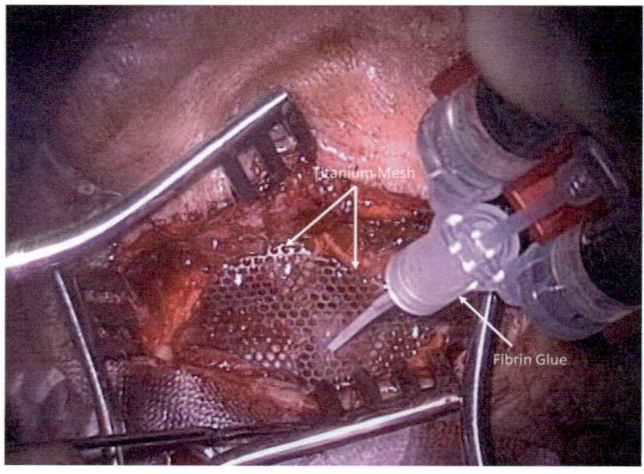

Fig. 16.4 A titanium mesh is used to compress the fat or muscle against the defect

development of benign intracranial hypertension every 3–6 months at an outpatient neuro-ophthalmology clinic.

Transcanal Approach

The transcanal approach is reserved for patients in poor medical state who are unable to undergo an extensive procedure or in cases where the patient does not have serviceable hearing (e.g., after a translabyrinthine approach). The purpose of this procedure is to isolate the CSF space from the nasopharynx to prevent meningitis. This procedure will cause a permanent conductive hearing loss from CSF in the middle ear. Therefore, it is reserved for those with no useful hearing or patients who cannot undergo general anesthesia but have an active CSF leak. This procedure can be performed under local anesthesia with monitored anesthesia care (MAC).

The procedure is performed transcanal but may require a secondary small incision in the temporalis area or post-auricularly to obtain fascia graft. Alternatively, a biomaterial such as DuraGen (Integra LifeSciences, Princeton, NJ), Biodesign Otologic Repair Graft (Cook Medical, Bloomington, IN), AlloDerm (Allergan Aesthetics, Irvine, CA), Surgicel (Ethicon, Raritan, NJ), etc may be employed. The middle ear is entered, and using an endoscope the Eustachian tube (ET) orifice is visualized. Alternatively, if possible, an anterior canal flap can be raised if the surgeon is comfortable with that approach and an anterior tympanomeatal flap is raised. Under direct visualization (or with an endoscope), using a Rosen needle the mucosa at the lateral most aspect of the ET orifice is gently lacerated. This will allow the grafts to become vascularized in the ET orifice and create a better seal. Next, fascia pieces that are cut in 2 mm strips are packed into the Eustachian tube using a blunt instrument (e.g., annulus elevator) one at a time. A sharp instrument should not be used to pack into the Eustachian tube as the carotid artery may be dehiscent and injury may occur. The fascia packing is placed one strip at a time and packed into place. It may be useful to cut the tensor tympani tendon to allow the malleus to be more mobile for manipulation. In cases of no serviceable hearing, the incus can be removed which will allow more flexibility in movement of the malleus to allow for better packing of the ET. The ET can accommodate a surprisingly large amount of fascia packing sometimes. Once the ET packing is no longer compressible, the incus (if available) can be used to wedge the fascia into place. If the incus is not available (e.g., patient in poor medical state with normal hearing), then the middle ear may be packed with muscle or fat, whichever is available. The tympanomeatal flap is replaced, and nonabsorbable packing is placed to hold the flap in place. The canal flap needs to be held tightly in place to prevent CSF leakage into the canal under the flap. The packing is left in place for 2 weeks and then removed. The authors use Xeroform packing for this dressing which can be layered and compressed in the medial canal.

Conclusion

The middle fossa craniotomy is the preferred surgical approach for the treatment of otogenic cerebrospinal fluid leaks from tegmen tympani and the petrous apex. It provides panoramic access to the tegmen tympani, tegmen mastoideum, and petrous apex, and both intradural and extradural repairs are possible. The transmastoid approach is used for posterior fossa defects or smaller or few tegmen mastoideum defects.

References

1. Kutz JW Jr, Husain IA, Isaacson B, Roland PS. Management of spontaneous cerebrospinal fluid otorrhea. Laryngoscope. 2008;118(12):2195–9. https://doi.org/10.1097/MLG.0b013e318182f833.
2. Hicks GW, Wright JW Jr, Wright JW III. Cerebrospinal fluid otorrhea. Laryngoscope. 1980;90(11 Pt 2 Suppl 25):1–25. https://doi.org/10.1288/00005537-198011001-00001.
3. Hernandez-Montero E, Caballero E, García-Ibanez L. Surgical management of middle cranial fossa bone defects: meningoencephalic herniation and cerebrospinal fluid leaks. Am J Otolaryngol. 2020;41(4):102560. https://doi.org/10.1016/j.amjoto.2020.102560.
4. Stevens SM, Rizk HG, McIlwain WR, Lambert PR, Meyer TA. Association between lateral skull base thickness and surgical outcomes in spontaneous CSF otorrhea. Otolaryngol Head Neck Surg. 2016;154(4):707–14. https://doi.org/10.1177/0194599816628528.
5. Eddelman DB, Munich S, Kochanski RB, Eggerstedt M, Kazan RP, Moftakhar R, et al. Repair of temporal bone defects via the middle cranial fossa approach: treatment of 2 pathologies with 1 operation. Neurosurgery. 2019;84(6):1290–5. https://doi.org/10.1093/neuros/nyy198.
6. LeVay AJ, Kveton JF. Relationship between obesity, obstructive sleep apnea, and spontaneous cerebrospinal fluid otorrhea. Laryngoscope. 2008;118(2):275–8. https://doi.org/10.1097/MLG.0b013e31815937a6.

7. Goddard JC, Meyer T, Nguyen S, Lambert PR. New considerations in the cause of spontaneous cerebrospinal fluid otorrhea. Otol Neurotol. 2010;31(6):940–5. https://doi.org/10.1097/mao.0b013e3181e8f36c.

8. Iurato S, Ettorre GC, Selvini C. Brain herniation into the middle ear: two idiopathic cases treated by a combined intracranial-mastoid approach. Laryngoscope. 1989;99(9):950–4. https://doi.org/10.1288/00005537-198909000-00008.

9. Nahas Z, Tatlipinar A, Limb CJ, Francis HW. Spontaneous meningoencephalocele of the temporal bone: clinical spectrum and presentation. Arch Otolaryngol Head Neck Surg. 2008;134(5):509–18. https://doi.org/10.1001/archotol.134.5.509.

10. Lim ZM, Friedland PL, Boeddinghaus R, Thompson A, Rodrigues SJ, Atlas M. Otitic meningitis, superior semicircular canal dehiscence, and encephalocele: a case series. Otol Neurotol. 2012;33(4):610–2. https://doi.org/10.1097/MAO.0b013e3182536de7.

11. Oh MS, Vivas EX, Hudgins PA, Mattox DE. The prevalence of superior semicircular canal dehiscence in patients with mastoid encephalocele or cerebrospinal fluid otorrhea. Otol Neurotol. 2019;40(4):485–90. https://doi.org/10.1097/mao.0000000000002155.

12. Garcia-Ibanez E, Garcia-Ibanez JL. Middle fossa vestibular neurectomy: a report of 373 cases. Otolaryngol Head Neck Surg. 1980;88(4):486–90.

13. House WF. Fatalities in acoustic tumor surgery. Arch Otolaryngol. 1968;88(6):687–99. https://doi.org/10.1001/archotol.1968.00770010689018.

14. Doig JA. Surgical treatment of acoustic neuroma. The translabyrinthine approach. Proc R Soc Med. 1970;63(8):775–7.

15. Cooper T, Choy MH, Gardner PA, Hirsch BE, McCall AA. Comparison of spontaneous temporal bone cerebrospinal fluid leaks from the middle and posterior fossa. Otol Neurotol. 2020;41(2):e232–7. https://doi.org/10.1097/mao.0000000000002473.

16. Wick CC, Killeen DE, Clark M, Kutz JW, Isaacson B. Posterior fossa spontaneous cerebrospinal fluid leaks. Otol Neurotol. 2017;38(1):66–72. https://doi.org/10.1097/mao.0000000000001261.

17. Nelson RA. Temporal bone surgical dissection manual. 3rd ed. Los Angeles: House Ear Institute; 2006.

18. Oliaei S, Mahboubi H, Djalilian HR. Transmastoid approach to temporal bone cerebrospinal fluid leaks. Am J Otolaryngol. 2012;33(5):556–61.

19. Pappas DG, Hoffmann RA, Holliday RA, et al. Evaluation and management of spontaneous temporal bone cerebrospinal fluid leaks. Skull Base Surg. 1995;5(1):1–7.

20. Rao AK, Merenda DM, Wetmore SJ. Diagnosis and management of spontaneous cerebrospinal fluid otorrhea. Otol Neurotol. 2005;26(6):1171–5.

21. Brown NE, Grundfast KM, Jabre A, et al. Diagnosis and management of cerebrospinal fluid-middle ear effusion and otorrhea. Laryngoscope. 2004;114(5):800–5.

22. Lundy LB, Graham MD, Kartush JM, LaRouere MJ. Temporal bone encephalocele and cerebrospinal fluid leaks. Am J Otol. 1996;17(3):461–9.

23. Patel RB, Kwatler JA, Hodosh RM, Baredes S. Spontaneous cerebrospinal fluid leakage and middle ear encephalocele in seven patients. Ear Nose Throat J. 2000;79(5):376–8.

Part IV
Anterior Skull Base Reconstruction

Chapter 17
Free Graft Techniques for Skull Base Reconstruction

John R. Craig (ID)

Introduction

Rhinologic surgeons reliably achieve >90% success when repairing nasal cerebrospinal fluid (CSF) leaks, whether free or vascularized tissue is used [1–5]. A wide variety of reconstructive techniques with free graft materials have been reported for CSF leak repair, and, generally speaking, all have been highly successful regardless of CSF leak etiology and location. The following sections will describe the terminology and physiology of skull base reconstruction, as well as the different free graft options used during nasal CSF leak repair.

Terminology for CSF Leak Repair

When discussing nasal CSF leak repair in both research and clinical environments, it is helpful to define certain terms so that readers or one's surgical colleagues share a common language. First, categorizing CSF leaks according to dural defect size can be helpful not only in understanding the literature but also in selecting reconstructive materials. While various terms exist in the literature, a common system categorizes CSF leaks as low-flow or high-flow, based mostly on dural defect size. Low-flow CSF leaks refer to <1 cm dural defects, and high-flow CSF leaks refer to >1 cm dural defects [6, 7].

Second, as multilayered closure of skull base defects is generally preferred for amenable defects, one must appreciate each of the possible reconstructive layers.

J. R. Craig (✉)
Department of Otolaryngology-Head and Neck Surgery, Henry Ford Health, Detroit, MI, USA
e-mail: Jcraig1@hfhs.org

© The Author(s), under exclusive license to Springer Nature Switzerland AG 2023
E. C. Kuan et al. (eds.), *Skull Base Reconstruction*,
https://doi.org/10.1007/978-3-031-27937-9_17

239

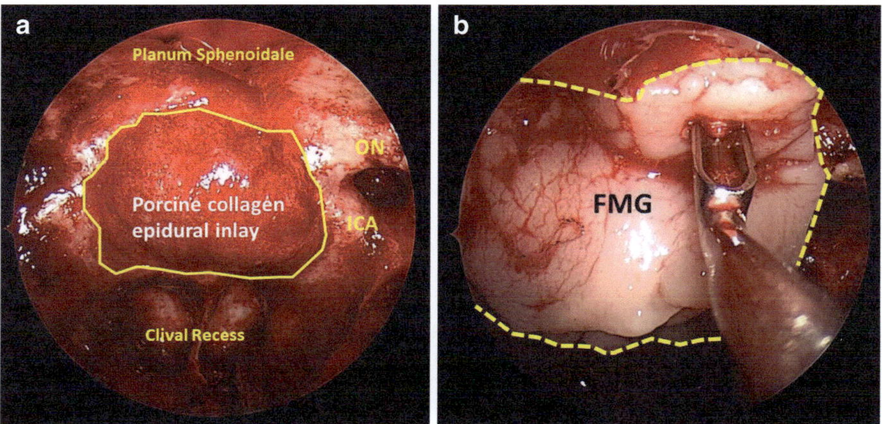

Fig. 17.1 Representative example of a two-layered closure of low-flow cerebrospinal fluid leak after pituitary adenoma resection, (**a**) using a porcine collagen inlay graft placed in the epidural space deep to the sellar bony defect (yellow outline) and (**b**) a free mucosal onlay graft placed over the edges of the bony sellar defect (yellow dashed outline). The mucosa was harvested from the nasal septum. *ON* optic nerve, *ICA* internal carotid artery, *FMG* free mucosal graft

First, one or more layers of autologous or synthetic grafts may be placed intracranially in an inlay or underlay fashion (subdural, epidural, or both) [8]. Autologous or synthetic grafts are then placed on the bone of the skull base surrounding the defect in an onlay or overlay fashion. For this chapter, "inlay" and "onlay" will be used to describe the layers of multilayered reconstructions. Figure 17.1 shows a representative two-layered closure of a low-flow sellar CSF leak after pituitary adenoma resection, with collagen epidural inlay and free septal mucosal onlay grafts. While multilayered closures are commonly performed, monolayer closures with inlay-only [9] and onlay-only [8, 10] layers have also been reportedly successful.

Free Graft Options and Physiology

There are a wide variety of graft materials that have been used to reconstruct skull base defects successfully. Free graft materials include temporalis fascia, fascia lata, abdominal or thigh fat, cartilage grafts (septum, auricular), bone grafts (septum, calvarium), acellular dermal allografts, and collagen xenografts. Interestingly, the literature has suggested that success rates are high regardless of the materials used [11, 12]. For multilayered closures, most studies report placing autologous or alloplastic/synthetic inlay grafts plus mucosal onlay grafts or flaps. However, reconstructions have often been heterogeneous with regard to materials used for each layer, how many layers are used, and the types of CSF leaks being repaired [1, 2, 5, 8, 13]. This makes it difficult to determine whether different materials are more successful as inlay or onlay grafts and whether CSF leak etiology or location affects the success of those layers. Amidst the conundrum of which layers and materials are most important for closing different types of CSF leaks, one must try to understand how these materials actually heal to seal off the skull base defects.

Free Graft Physiology

Regarding free graft wound healing physiology, there has been limited evidence to support how different free graft materials facilitate dural and bony defect closure after CSF leak repair. As free grafts have no direct vascular supply, they obtain nutrition initially through imbibition, but evidence for this comes mostly from skin graft literature [14]. Recent studies have shown synthetic allografts and xenografts becoming revascularized and integrated into the tissue of skull base defects [15, 16]. Interestingly, despite nasal mucosa being one of the most commonly used free graft materials for CSF leak repair, very few studies have explored the physiology of free mucosal graft healing.

Mahendran et al. harvested free mucosal grafts from lateral nasal walls and showed that 26/26 grafts healed successfully onto denuded bone after dacryocysto-rhinostomies. They also showed that grafts contracted by about 20% over 4 weeks [17]. Kim et al. showed that free mucosal grafts integrated into the bone around sellar defects, with mucosal enhancement on contrasted magnetic resonance imaging equivalent to surrounding mucosa at 3 months postoperatively [18]. Other than these few studies on free mucosal graft healing, the bulk of evidence on free mucosal graft healing is indirect through studies demonstrating high success rates with free mucosal grafts for CSF leak repair [1, 19, 20]. Together, these studies suggest that free mucosal grafts adhere to and integrate onto the skull base via blood supply from the adjacent sinus or intracranial tissue. However, it is also possible that free grafts could become nonviable in some cases, and underlying inlay layers allow for skull base defect closure, while the free onlay grafts become biologic dressings that eventually promote mucosalization.

Very little evidence exists with regard to wound healing of autologous fat, fascial, and bone grafts after skull base reconstruction, and further research is necessary to understand the healing process of these tissues. The remainder of this section will describe the differed graft types and how they are typically used.

Mucosal Grafts

Numerous materials have been used for CSF leak repair, but mucosal grafts or flaps are quintessential to most skull base reconstructions. While vascularized/pedicled mucosal flaps have gained in popularity for skull base reconstruction, especially for large dural defects [1, 2], free grafts still play an important role. Advantages of free grafts over pedicled flaps for CSF leak repair include shorter harvest time, custom

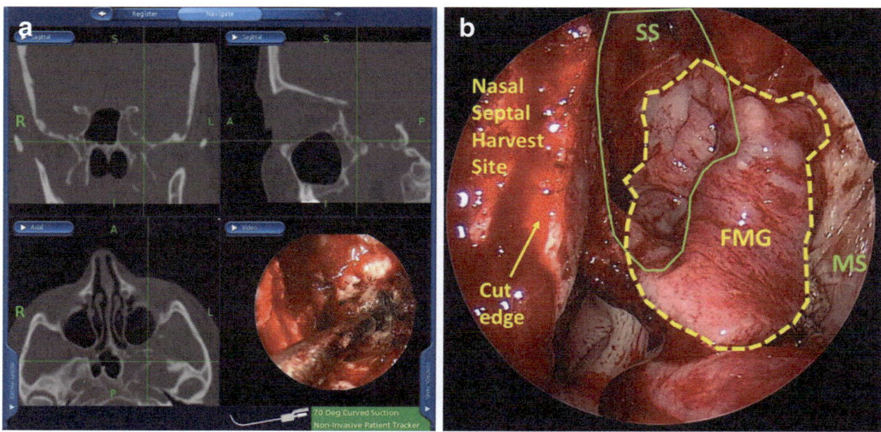

Fig. 17.2 Example of endoscopic repair of a skull base defect in the lateral recess of the left sphenoid sinus after removal of a meningoencephalocele in a patient with idiopathic intracranial hypertension. (**a**) Computed tomography image navigation with endoscopic correlation in the bottom right of the window, demonstrating the left lateral recess defect. (**b**) Free mucosal graft (FMG) reconstruction of the left sphenoid sinus (SS) lateral recess defect, after having been harvested from the left nasal septum. The graft also covered pterygopalatine fossa contents. A collagen epidural inlay graft had also been placed. The wide sphenoidotomy is represented by the green outline. *MS* maxillary sinus

shaping and sizing of grafts, and lack of pedicle tension that puts flaps at risk for retraction. Free grafts are therefore highly versatile and can be placed anywhere along the skull base that can be visualized and accessed with endoscopic instrumentation. Figures 17.2 and 17.3 illustrate the versatility of free mucosal grafts for difficult-to-reach areas of the skull base.

Free mucosal onlay grafts have been utilized to reconstruct a wide variety of skull base defects with excellent success, via both monolayer and multilayered reconstructions [1, 5, 8, 19, 20]. The graft is placed onto the bony edges of the skull base defect, with the graft's periosteal side contacting the bone. Mucosa should never be used as an intracranial inlay graft, as this can lead to an intracranial mucocele [21, 22]. One technical point is that due to free graft contraction [17], surgeons should harvest mucosal grafts at least 20% larger than what they feel to be an appropriately sized graft.

Free mucosal grafts also result in minimal morbidity. Free mucosa is most commonly harvested from the nasal septum, nasal floor, or middle turbinate [23], with no published differences in efficacy based on harvest site. Exposed bone or cartilage at harvest sites will cause nasal crusting that can last for 2–3 months postoperatively [8, 24], but patient sinonasal quality of life is typically minimally affected based on studies using both free grafts and mucosal flaps [8, 25].

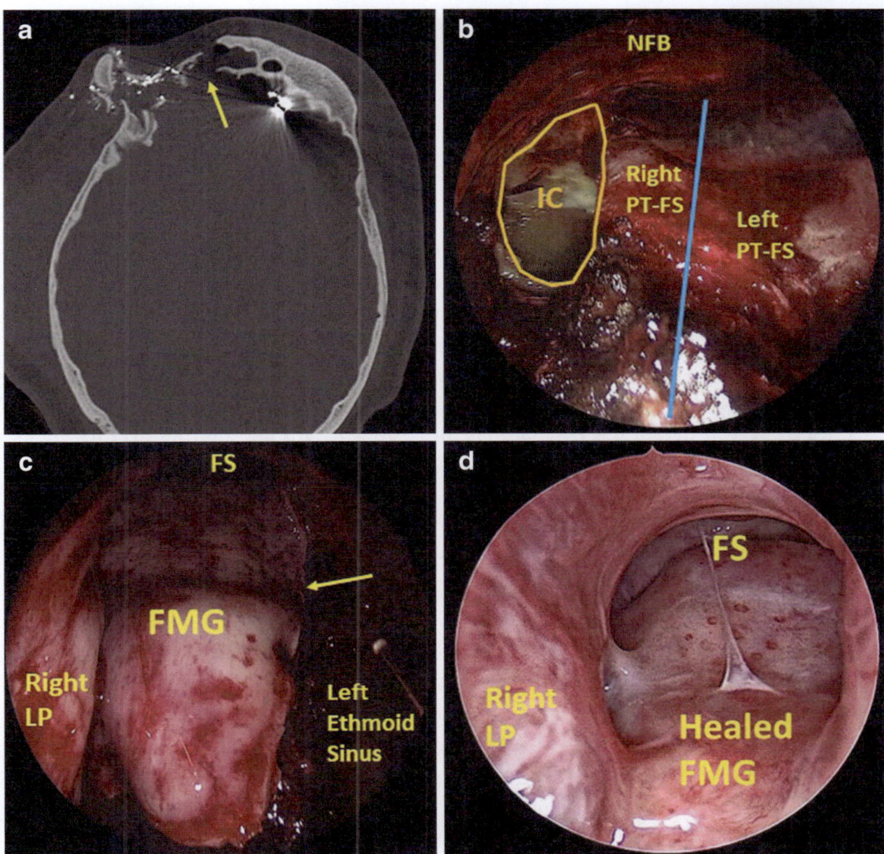

Fig. 17.3 Example of an endoscopic repair of a skull base defect in the posterior table of the right frontal sinus (PT-FS) after a shotgun wound to the face and head. (**a**) Axial computed tomography demonstrating the right-sided posterior table defect (yellow arrow). (**b**) Visualization with a 70° nasal endoscope after an endoscopic Draf III approach to repair the large right-sided posterior table defect (orange outline) that extended superiorly nearly to the roof of the frontal sinus. Nonviable intracranial (IC) contents are seen through the defect. The blue line represents the midline. (**c**) A nasoseptal flap had been harvested but could not adequately cover the superior-most aspect of the skull base defect, so the pedicle was transected, and the remaining large free mucosal graft (FMG) was then placed to cover the entirety of the bony defect. No intracranial inlay graft was placed due to the irregular geometry of the defect. One edge of the graft is highlighted with a yellow arrow. The graft extended laterally on the right side to cover the lamina papyracea (LP) as well. (**d**) Endoscopic result 10 months postoperatively, with a beautifully integrated free mucosal graft and a nicely patent, functional frontal sinus. *NFB* nasofrontal beak

Fat Grafts and Bath-Plug Technique

Autologous fat grafts can be used as stand-alone inlay or onlay grafts [26] or in combination with mucosal onlays [13, 27]. They are commonly harvested from the abdomen, thigh, or ear lobule. A number of different fat graft techniques have been described, and two common methods will be discussed here.

Wormald and McDonogh described a "bath plug" fat graft technique where a piece of abdominal fat is advanced intradurally, and a suture through the fat is used to pull the fat graft through the dural defect partially into the sinus cavity, until the fat seals off the leak [27]. This technique was utilized in 47/52 CSF leaks in a subsequent series with 90% primary success and 100% secondary success [28]. However, it is important to note that this technique also includes a concurrent free mucosal onlay graft.

Lam et al. published a retrospective series of 27 patients who had fat grafts for skull base repairs of various sizes, locations, and etiologies, 18 of whom also had onlay layers placed over the fat grafts. They used small 5 × 5 mm pieces of fat to facilitate sealing of irregularly shaped defects that were difficult to seal with other materials. They reported primary and secondary CSF closure rates of 92.6% and 96.3%, respectively, with two patients (7.4%) developing abdominal seromas or hematomas requiring drainage [13].

While complications from fat grafting are rare overall, harvest site hematomas, seromas, infections, and scars have been reported [13, 29]. Fat grafts have also caused lipoid meningitis [29] and can interfere with postoperative magnetic resonance imaging interpretation [30, 31]. Additionally, if too much fat is placed intracranially, it can have a compressive effect, such as optic apparatus compression [32].

Fascia

Fascia is another common autologous graft, typically harvested from tensor fascia lata or temporalis fascia. While fascia has been reported to be highly successful in skull base reconstruction, most fascial techniques have also included the use of free or vascularized mucosal onlays concurrently [1, 2, 11]. Additionally, similar to fat graft harvest, while the overall risks are low, there have been multiple reports of harvest site complications such as hematomas, seromas, pain, and scars and difficulty with ambulation [33, 34].

Bone

The bone has also been used successfully for nasal CSF leak repair as an inlay layer, in conjunction with mucosal onlays [1]. Bone grafts are typically harvested from tissue removed during the sinonasal surgery such as the nasal septum or turbinates to avoid extranasal harvest site morbidity [35]. While bone grafts have been described as providing a rigid layer of reconstruction that may be important for certain types of CSF leak repairs [11, 23], they have never been studied in a comparative manner with other graft materials for different CSF leak etiologies and locations. While bone grafts represent a viable inlay reconstructive material, they suffer from being dependent on the availability of bone that can be appropriately sized and contoured. Additionally, bone grafts can be technically difficult to place intracranially. Since most studies utilizing bony inlay grafts have reported heterogeneous repair techniques for various CSF leak etiologies [1, 10, 36], it is difficult to know when or whether they are beneficial compared to other graft materials.

Gasket-Seal Technique

Leng et al. described a gasket-seal technique where fascia or synthetic grafts are placed as onlays, followed by a rigid inlay layer of bone, titanium, or Porex (Porex Corp., Newnan, GA) countersunk into the epidural space [37]. The same group of surgeons then reported a 96% initial success rate of CSF leak repair in 46 consecutive patients with a variety of skull base defects after skull base tumor resections [38]. Note that they used nasoseptal flaps in 21/46 patients and, in a subsequent study, recommended nasoseptal flap use with these repairs [39]. Potential downsides to this technique include technical difficulty, as well as the potential issues with foreign body reactions or infections. For example, some authors have reported titanium sequestra after this technique, requiring removal during revision skull base reconstructions [35]. Very few other publications have corroborated the success of the gasket-seal technique, and it is difficult to know if it offers any advantage over technically easier and potentially less morbid reconstructive techniques.

Allografts and Xenografts

Allografts and xenografts grafts have been used successfully in many CSF leak repair studies. The most commonly reported grafts have been acellular cadaveric dermis (AlloDerm™, LifeCell Corp., Woodlands, TX), bovine collagen matrix (DuraGen™, Integra Neurosciences, Plainsboro, New Jersey, USA), and porcine collagen (Biodesign™, Cook Biomedical, West Lafayette, IN). Their main benefit is the avoidance of complications from extranasal tissue harvest like wound complications and external scars [5]. While they are commonly used as inlay grafts in multilayered reconstructions with free or pedicled mucosal onlays [8, 35, 40], they have also been used as the sole material for two-layered inlay and onlay reconstructions [20, 40]. They have also been used successfully in some series as single-layer inlay or onlay reconstructions [9, 10, 40].

Regarding allografts, Germani et al. showed a 97% success rate in 30 CSF leaks due to small/intermediate (<2 cm) and large skull base defects (>2 cm) by placing AlloDerm as an onlay or intracranial inlay [10]. Note that 50% of those repairs were multilayered with free mucosal graft onlays, and 50% were AlloDerm alone.

Collagen xenografts have also been used with excellent success. Oakley et al. showed high success rates in 120 CSF leak repairs with DuraGen used as the intracranial inlay layer of multilayered reconstructions, with low complication rates [35]. They placed nasoseptal flap onlays in 69% of those cases and free mucosal onlays in 31%. Illing et al. reviewed their results with Biodesign inlay grafts in 170 repairs of various CSF leak etiologies and demonstrated 95% success on first attempt and 100% eventual success. The collagen graft was applied as an inlay graft in 19 cases, onlay in 36, or as both inlay and onlay in 115 cases. Nasoseptal flaps were utilized in 122 of the cases, so 48 cases had only collagen grafts used [40]. However, they did not report the frequencies with which collagen grafts were inlay-only, onlay-only, or inlay + onlay in the 48 cases without nasoseptal flaps. While this study showed that Biodesign can be used successfully, it leaves open the question of whether collagen grafts improve CSF leak repair success more than nasoseptal mucosal flaps alone. Interestingly, Mueller et al. performed a preliminary sheep study to address this question. They repaired frontal dural defect repairs in sheep, with either a vascularized mucosal flap onlay or a combined Biodesign intracranial inlay and vascularized mucosal flap onlay. They showed histologically that repair with Biodesign resulted in a thicker repair, but both repair types (with or without the Biodesign) resulted in successful watertight sealing of defects by 7 days [16]. More studies are necessary to assess the utility of allografts and xenografts in CSF leak repair.

The main drawback to synthetic grafts is cost, although no studies have assessed whether their cost significantly impacts cost-effectiveness of CSF leak repair. Future well-designed studies are necessary to determine whether the cost of such grafts outweighs the potential morbidities of extranasal autografts. Until then, evidence supports that they are safe and highly effective in multilayered reconstructions with free or vascularized mucosal onlays. Larger studies are needed to corroborate the successes reported from small series regarding synthetic grafts being used as stand-alone reconstructions without mucosal onlays.

Adjunctive Techniques

After free graft reconstruction, are there additional techniques that can optimize graft adherence and integration, to improve reconstructive success rates? This question is not so simple to answer based on the literature, but this section will describe how surgeons may use the following techniques to improve adherence of the onlay portion of the reconstruction to underlying bone: sinonasal packing, lumbar drains, and tissue sealants.

Packing

Sinonasal packing is commonly used after CSF leak repair. Potential benefits include hemostasis, support to prevent migration of the reconstructive materials, stenting of sinus outflow tracts, and creation of an additional temporary barrier between the external environment and intracranial space [7]. However, very little evidence exists supporting the use of packing to improve CSF leak repair outcomes, and therefore practices have largely been guided by expert opinion [5, 7, 41].

A systematic review and meta-analysis in 2000 by Hegazy et al. reported nasal packing being used in 61% of the analyzed cases (125/204), but packing did not have a significant effect on surgical outcome [11]. Asmaro et al. recently published a prospective series of 76 CSF leaks of various etiologies repaired with monolayer or multilayered skull base reconstructions, 66% of which utilized free grafts. Sinonasal packing was never used. They achieved a 97.4% success rate, and the two postoperative CSF leaks were sealed with lumbar CSF diversion alone [8]. Of note, they had a low sample size of large clival defects, so whether packing could facilitate repairs in these types of cases could not be determined. Packing has also been shown to negatively impact patient quality of life after skull base surgery [42, 43]. While these studies require corroboration by other centers, they suggest that sinonasal packing may not be necessary for most CSF leak repairs.

Lumbar Drains

While opinions are mixed on the use of lumbar drains (LDs) for CSF leak repair, some studies have demonstrated higher success rates with LD use, especially for high-flow CSF leaks [6, 36, 44]. A recent large randomized controlled trial showed improved CSF leak repair outcomes with LD use for large dural defects [6]. Others have suggested that LDs may not impact success when repairing low- or high-flow CSF leaks [45–47]. However, the literature suffers from heterogeneous patient populations and mostly low evidence levels [48], so conclusions cannot be drawn definitively for when lumbar drains can be of utility. Until then, surgeons must use judgment as to the utility of LDs on a case-by-case basis.

Tissue Sealants

There has also been mixed evidence in the literature regarding tissue sealant use for CSF leak repair. Commonly reported sealants have been DuraSeal (Integra LifeSciences), Tisseel (Baxter Healthcare, Deerfield, IL), and Adherus AutoSpray (HyperBranch Medical Technology, Stryker, Durham, NC). Eloy et al. reported no benefit with Tisseel, DuraSeal, and Evicel (OMRIX Biopharmaceuticals Ltd.,

Ramat Gan, Israel) after repair of 42 high-flow CSF leaks compared to 32 high-flow leaks without sealant use in a retrospective case-control study [49]. However, there have been three porcine studies demonstrating improved biomechanical strength of CSF leak repairs with tissue sealants [50–52]. More human comparative studies are necessary to determine the utility of tissue sealants during CSF leak repair.

Overall Success Rates of Free Graft Techniques

While difficult to draw conclusions on optimal materials to use during CSF leak repair due to studies with small sample sizes or heterogeneous CSF leak etiologies and reconstructive techniques, consistently high success rates are seen in the literature with multilayered reconstruction.

There have been two large systematic reviews on CSF leak repair success. Soudry et al. reviewed 673 cases from 22 series and reported an overall CSF leak success rate of 92%. Of the reviewed cases, 292 were analyzed by low- or high-flow CSF leak status. For low-flow CSF leaks (5 studies, 74 patients), they showed that multilayered reconstructions with free grafts offered similar high success rates to vascularized flaps (92% for free grafts vs. 100% for nasoseptal flaps). For high-flow CSF leaks (6 studies, 218 patients), pedicled vascularized flaps were superior (82% for free grafts vs. 94% for flaps). They showed no significant differences between skull base defect sites [1]. Harvey et al. reviewed 38 studies that included 609 large dural defects and showed that 326 patients with free grafts had a 15.6% failure rate compared to 6.7% for 283 patients with vascularized reconstructions (p=0.001) [2].

To summarize, both free grafts and vascularized flaps are highly successful for low-flow CSF leaks, and vascularized reconstructions have been shown to be superior for high-flow CSF leaks. However, it is also important to appreciate from these review studies that free grafts are still successful for high-flow CSF leak repair in 80% or more of cases. Free mucosal grafts should therefore still be considered viable options for high-flow CSF leak repairs when vascularized reconstructions are not available or are felt to be unnecessarily morbid. Additionally, in some situations skull base defect location or geometry may not be favorable for pedicled flaps. It is also important to note that when free mucosal grafts have been used to repair high-flow CSF leaks, they have generally been used as onlays with multilayered reconstructions. Future studies would be needed to determine whether monolayered free mucosal graft reconstruction is successful for high-flow CSF leaks.

How Do You Choose?

The literature has been reviewed in this chapter, and despite a plethora of publications on nasal CSF leak repair, there is no "one-size-fits-all" approach. Surgeon judgment and preference will therefore guide many of the reconstructive decisions.

However, surgeons should be achieving >90% success in nasal CSF leak closure, and if not, they should consider other reliable published techniques outlined in this chapter. Based on the literature, a very reliable means to achieve high success rates with low morbidity is to perform multilayered closures when possible, with synthetic inlay grafts and mucosal onlay grafts or flaps. Other inlay materials are also viable options, but the benefits and risks should be considered. Deciding whether to use adjunctive measures such as sinonasal packing, lumbar drainage, and tissue sealants is largely up to the discretion of surgeons at this time, with more evidence mounting on these topics.

Conclusions

For endoscopic CSF leak repair, multilayered reconstructions with free nasal mucosal onlay grafts and a variety of inlay graft materials are highly successful for repairing the majority of nasal CSF leaks, including high-flow CSF leaks, when vascularized flaps are not available or applicable. For inlay grafts, a variety of graft materials are efficacious, but synthetic allografts or xenografts are effective and less morbid than extranasal autologous grafts. More research is needed to understand the wound healing physiology of free graft materials in skull base reconstruction, as well as the importance of each layer of multi layered closures for different CSF leak locations and etiologies.

References

1. Soudry E, Turner JH, Nayak JV, Hwang PH. Endoscopic reconstruction of surgically created skull base defects: a systematic review. Otolaryngol Head Neck Surg. 2014;150:730–8. https://doi.org/10.1177/0194599814520685.
2. Harvey RJ, Parmar P, Sacks R, Zanation AM. Endoscopic skull base reconstruction of large dural defects: a systematic review of published evidence. Laryngoscope. 2012;122:452–9. https://doi.org/10.1002/lary.22475.
3. Conger A, Zhao F, Wang X, Eisenberg A, Griffiths C, Esposito F, Carrau RL, Barkhoudarian G, Kelly DF. Evolution of the graded repair of CSF leaks and skull base defects in endonasal endoscopic tumor surgery: trends in repair failure and meningitis rates in 509 patients. J Neurosurg. 2018;130:861–75. https://doi.org/10.3171/2017.11.Jns172141.
4. Kassam AB, Prevedello DM, Carrau RL, Snyderman CH, Thomas A, Gardner P, Zanation A, Duz B, Stefko ST, Byers K, Horowitz MB. Endoscopic endonasal skull base surgery: analysis of complications in the authors' initial 800 patients. J Neurosurg. 2011;114:1544–68. https://doi.org/10.3171/2010.10.Jns09406.
5. Oakley GM, Orlandi RR, Woodworth BA, Batra PS, Alt JA. Management of cerebrospinal fluid rhinorrhea: an evidence-based review with recommendations. Int Forum Allergy Rhinol. 2016;6:17–24. https://doi.org/10.1002/alr.21627.
6. Zwagerman NT, Wang EW, Shin SS, Chang YF, Fernandez-Miranda JC, Snyderman CH, Gardner PA. Does lumbar drainage reduce postoperative cerebrospinal fluid leak after endo-

scopic endonasal skull base surgery? A prospective, randomized controlled trial. J Neurosurg. 2018;131:1172–8. https://doi.org/10.3171/2018.4.JNS172447.

7. Wang EW, Gardner PA, Zanation AM. International consensus statement on endoscopic skull-base surgery: executive summary. Int Forum Allergy Rhinol. 2019;9:S127–44. https://doi.org/10.1002/alr.22327.

8. Asmaro K, Yoo F, Yassin-Kassab A, Bazydlo M, Robin A, Rock JP, Craig JR. Sinonasal packing is not a requisite for successful cerebrospinal fluid leak repair. J Neuro Surg B Skull Base. 2021;83(5):476–84.

9. Yoo F, Wang MB, Bergsneider M, Suh JD. Single layer repair of large anterior skull base defects without vascularized mucosal flap. J Neurol Surg B Skull Base. 2017;78:139–44. https://doi.org/10.1055/s-0036-1593438.

10. Germani RM, Vivero R, Herzallah IR, Casiano RR. Endoscopic reconstruction of large anterior skull base defects using acellular dermal allograft. Am J Rhinol. 2007;21:615–8. https://doi.org/10.2500/ajr.2007.21.3080.

11. Hegazy HM, Carrau RL, Snyderman CH, Kassam A, Zweig J. Transnasal endoscopic repair of cerebrospinal fluid rhinorrhea: a meta-analysis. Laryngoscope. 2000;110:1166–72. https://doi.org/10.1097/00005537-200007000-00019.

12. Zweig JL, Carrau RL, Celin SE, Schaitkin BM, Pollice PA, Snyderman CH, Kassam A, Hegazy H. Endoscopic repair of cerebrospinal fluid leaks to the sinonasal tract: predictors of success. Otolaryngol Head Neck Surg. 2000;123:195–201. https://doi.org/10.1067/mhn.2000.107452.

13. Lam K, Luong AU, Yao WC, Citardi MJ. Use of autologous fat grafts for the endoscopic reconstruction of skull base defects: indications, outcomes, and complications. Am J Rhinol Allergy. 2018;32:310–7. https://doi.org/10.1177/1945892418773637.

14. Maeda M, Nakamura T, Fukui A, Koizumi M, Yamauchi T, Tamai S, Nagano-Tatsumi K, Haga S, Hashimoto K, Yamamoto H. The role of serum imbibition for skin grafts. Plast Reconstr Surg. 1999;104:2100–7. https://doi.org/10.1097/00006534-199912000-00023.

15. Taufique ZM, Bhatt N, Zagzag D, Lebowitz RA, Lieberman SM. Revascularization of AlloDerm used during endoscopic skull base surgery. J Neurol Surg B Skull Base. 2019;80:46–50. https://doi.org/10.1055/s-0038-1666851.

16. Mueller SK, Scangas G, Amiji MM, Bleier BS. Prospective transfrontal sheep model of skull-base reconstruction using vascularized mucosa. Int Forum Allergy Rhinol. 2018;8:614–9. https://doi.org/10.1002/alr.22058.

17. Mahendran S, Stevens-King A, Yung MW. How we do it: the viability of free mucosal grafts on exposed bone in lacrimal surgery—a prospective study. Clin Otolaryngol. 2006;31:324–7. https://doi.org/10.1111/j.1749-4486.2006.01170.x.

18. Kim CS, Patel U, Pastena G, Higgins M, Peris-Celda M, Kenning TJ, Pinheiro-Neto CD. The magnetic resonance imaging appearance of endoscopic endonasal skull base defect reconstruction using free mucosal graft. World Neurosurg. 2019;126:e165–72. https://doi.org/10.1016/j.wneu.2019.02.010.

19. Scagnelli RJ, Patel V, Peris-Celda M, Kenning TJ, Pinheiro-Neto CD. Implementation of free mucosal graft technique for sellar reconstruction after pituitary surgery: outcomes of 158 consecutive patients. World Neurosurg. 2019;122:e506–11. https://doi.org/10.1016/j.wneu.2018.10.090.

20. Roxbury CR, Saavedra T, Ramanathan M Jr, Lim M, Ishii M, Gallia GL, Reh DD. Layered sellar reconstruction with avascular free grafts: acceptable alternative to the nasoseptal flap for repair of low-volume intraoperative cerebrospinal fluid leak. Am J Rhinol Allergy. 2016;30:367–71. https://doi.org/10.2500/ajra.2016.30.4356.

21. Wang L, Kim J, Heilman CB. Intracranial mucocele as a complication of endoscopic repair of cerebrospinal fluid rhinorrhea: case report. Neurosurgery. 1999;45:1243–5.; ; discussion 1245–1246. https://doi.org/10.1097/00006123-199911000-00052.

22. Eloy JA, Fatterpekar GM, Bederson JB, Shohet MR. Intracranial mucocele: an unusual complication of cerebrospinal fluid leakage repair with middle turbinate mucosal graft. Otolaryngol Head Neck Surg. 2007;137:350–2. https://doi.org/10.1016/j.otohns.2007.02.039.

23. Ting JY, Metson R. Free graft techniques in skull base reconstruction. Adv Otorhinolaryngol. 2013;74:33–41. https://doi.org/10.1159/000342266.
24. de Almeida JR, Snyderman CH, Gardner PA, Carrau RL, Vescan AD. Nasal morbidity following endoscopic skull base surgery: a prospective cohort study. Head Neck. 2011;33:547–51. https://doi.org/10.1002/hed.21483.
25. Bhenswala PN, Schlosser RJ, Nguyen SA, Munawar S, Rowan NR. Sinonasal quality-of-life outcomes after endoscopic endonasal skull base surgery. Int Forum Allergy Rhinol. 2019;9:1105–18. https://doi.org/10.1002/alr.22398.
26. Bohoun CA, Goto T, Morisako H, Nagahama A, Tanoue Y, Ohata K. Skull base dural repair using autologous fat as a dural substitute: an efficient technique. World Neurosurg. 2019;127:e896–900. https://doi.org/10.1016/j.wneu.2019.03.293.
27. Wormald PJ, McDonogh M. 'Bath-plug' technique for the endoscopic management of cerebrospinal fluid leaks. J Laryngol Otol. 1997;111:1042–6. https://doi.org/10.1017/s0022215100139295.
28. Briggs RJ, Wormald PJ. Endoscopic transnasal intradural repair of anterior skull base cerebrospinal fluid fistulae. J Clin Neurosci. 2004;11:597–9. https://doi.org/10.1016/j.jocn.2003.09.011.
29. Taha AN, Almefty R, Pravdenkova S, Al-Mefty O. Sequelae of autologous fat graft used for reconstruction in skull base surgery. World Neurosurg. 2011;75:692–5. https://doi.org/10.1016/j.wneu.2011.01.023.
30. Sonnenburg RE, White D, Ewend MG, Senior B. Sellar reconstruction: is it necessary? Am J Rhinol. 2003;17:343–6.
31. Sade B, Mohr G, Frenkiel S. Management of intra-operative cerebrospinal fluid leak in transnasal transsphenoidal pituitary microsurgery: use of post-operative lumbar drain and sellar reconstruction without fat packing. Acta Neurochir. 2006;148:13–8; discussion 18–19. https://doi.org/10.1007/s00701-005-0664-6.
32. Slavin ML, Lam BL, Decker RE, Schatz NJ, Glaser JS, Reynolds MG. Chiasmal compression from fat packing after transsphenoidal resection of intrasellar tumor in two patients. Am J Ophthalmol. 1993;115:368–71. https://doi.org/10.1016/s0002-9394(14)73590-1.
33. Naugle TC Jr. Complications of fascia lata harvesting for ptosis surgery. Br J Ophthalmol. 1998;82:333–4. https://doi.org/10.1136/bjo.82.3.332c.
34. Vitali M, Canevari FR, Cattalani A, Grasso V, Somma T, Barbanera A. Direct fascia lata reconstruction to reduce donor site morbidity in endoscopic endonasal extended surgery: a pilot study. Clin Neurol Neurosurg. 2016;144:59–63. https://doi.org/10.1016/j.clineuro.2016.03.003.
35. Oakley GM, Christensen JM, Winder M, Jonker BP, Davidson A, Steel T, Teo C, Harvey RJ. Collagen matrix as an inlay in endoscopic skull base reconstruction. J Laryngol Otol. 2018;132:214–23. https://doi.org/10.1017/s0022215117001499.
36. Chaaban MR, Illing E, Riley KO, Woodworth BA. Spontaneous cerebrospinal fluid leak repair: a five-year prospective evaluation. Laryngoscope. 2014;124:70–5. https://doi.org/10.1002/lary.24160.
37. Leng LZ, Brown S, Anand VK, Schwartz TH. "Gasket-seal" watertight closure in minimal-access endoscopic cranial base surgery. Neurosurgery. 2008;62:ONSE342–3. ; discussion ONSE343. https://doi.org/10.1227/01.neu.0000326017.84315.1f.
38. Garcia-Navarro V, Anand VK, Schwartz TH. Gasket seal closure for extended endonasal endoscopic skull base surgery: efficacy in a large case series. World Neurosurg. 2013;80:563–8. https://doi.org/10.1016/j.wneu.2011.08.034.
39. McCoul ED, Anand VK, Singh A, Nyquist GG, Schaberg MR, Schwartz TH. Long-term effectiveness of a reconstructive protocol using the nasoseptal flap after endoscopic skull base surgery. World Neurosurg. 2014;81:136–43. https://doi.org/10.1016/j.wneu.2012.08.011.
40. Illing E, Chaaban MR, Riley KO, Woodworth BA. Porcine small intestine submucosal graft for endoscopic skull base reconstruction. Int Forum Allergy Rhinol. 2013;3:928–32. https://doi.org/10.1002/alr.21206.

41. Tien DA, Stokken JK, Recinos PF, Woodard TD, Sindwani R. Comprehensive postoperative management after endoscopic skull base surgery. Otolaryngol Clin N Am. 2016;49:253–63. https://doi.org/10.1016/j.otc.2015.09.015.
42. Little AS, Kelly D, Milligan J, Griffiths C, Prevedello DM, Carrau RL, Rosseau G, Barkhoudarian G, Otto BA, Jahnke H, Chaloner C, Jelinek KL, Chapple K, White WL. Predictors of sinonasal quality of life and nasal morbidity after fully endoscopic transsphenoidal surgery. J Neurosurg. 2015;122:1458–65. https://doi.org/10.3171/2014.10. Jns141624.
43. Lwu S, Edem I, Banton B, Bernstein M, Vescan A, Gentili F, Zadeh G. Quality of life after transsphenoidal pituitary surgery: a qualitative study. Acta Neurochir. 2012;154:1917–22. https://doi.org/10.1007/s00701-012-1455-5.
44. Zanation AM, Carrau RL, Snyderman CH, Germanwala AV, Gardner PA, Prevedello DM, Kassam AB. Nasoseptal flap reconstruction of high flow intraoperative cerebral spinal fluid leaks during endoscopic skull base surgery. Am J Rhinol Allergy. 2009;23:518–21. https://doi. org/10.2500/ajra.2009.23.3378.
45. Adams AS, Russell PT, Duncavage JA, Chandra RK, Turner JH. Outcomes of endoscopic repair of cerebrospinal fluid rhinorrhea without lumbar drains. Am J Rhinol Allergy. 2016;30:424–9. https://doi.org/10.2500/ajra.2016.30.4371.
46. Caballero N, Bhalla V, Stankiewicz JA, Welch KC. Effect of lumbar drain placement on recurrence of cerebrospinal rhinorrhea after endoscopic repair. Int Forum Allergy Rhinol. 2012;2:222–6. https://doi.org/10.1002/alr.21023.
47. Eloy JA, Kuperan AB, Choudhry OJ, Harirchian S, Liu JK. Efficacy of the pedicled nasoseptal flap without cerebrospinal fluid (CSF) diversion for repair of skull base defects: incidence of postoperative CSF leaks. Int Forum Allergy Rhinol. 2012;2:397–401. https://doi.org/10.1002/ alr.21040.
48. D'Anza B, Tien D, Stokken JK, Recinos PF, Woodard TR, Sindwani R. Role of lumbar drains in contemporary endonasal skull base surgery: meta-analysis and systematic review. Am J Rhinol Allergy. 2016;30:430–5. https://doi.org/10.2500/ajra.2016.30.4377.
49. Eloy JA, Choudhry OJ, Friedel ME, Kuperan AB, Liu JK. Endoscopic nasoseptal flap repair of skull base defects: is addition of a dural sealant necessary? Otolaryngol Head Neck Surg. 2012;147:161–6. https://doi.org/10.1177/0194599812437530.
50. Lin RP, Weitzel EK, Chen PG, McMains KC, Majors J, Bunegin L. Failure pressures of three rhinologic dural repairs in a porcine ex vivo model. Int Forum Allergy Rhinol. 2015;5:633–6. https://doi.org/10.1002/alr.21513.
51. Fandiño M, Macdonald K, Singh D, Whyne C, Witterick I. Determining the best graft-sealant combination for skull base repair using a soft tissue in vitro porcine model. Int Forum Allergy Rhinol. 2013;3:212–6. https://doi.org/10.1002/alr.21085.
52. de Almeida JR, Morris A, Whyne CM, James AL, Witterick IJ. Testing biomechanical strength of in vitro cerebrospinal fluid leak repairs. J Otolaryngol Head Neck Surg. 2009;38:106–11.

Chapter 18
Local Vascularized Pedicled Flaps for Skull Base Reconstruction

Ryan A. McMillan, Carlos Pinheiro-Neto, and Garret W. Choby

Introduction

As expanded endonasal approaches (EEA) have advanced, the need for more sophisticated skull base reconstructive techniques has also increased. Once the "Achilles heel" of EEA, the development of vascularized reconstructive options has allowed resection of more extensive intracranial tumors with minimal rates of post-operative CSF leak [1]. Local vascularized pedicle flaps provide robust and durable soft tissue coverage to the skull base and vital structures without the need for micro-vascular surgery or significant donor site morbidity. Local vascularized pedicle flaps represent a progression in the reconstructive ladder that takes advantage of the highly vascularized nature of the sinonasal cavity to provide soft tissue coverage to vital structures and prevent postoperative cerebrospinal fluid leaks [2–4].

Local vascularized pedicle flaps, typically based on a named artery, can be used in isolation or in tandem with other reconstructive principles to provide multilayer coverage of a defect. The flaps vary in their utility based on the size and location of

R. A. McMillan
Department of Otolaryngology – Head and Neck Surgery, Mayo Clinic, Rochester, MN, USA

C. Pinheiro-Neto
Department of Otolaryngology – Head and Neck Surgery, Mayo Clinic, Rochester, MN, USA

Department of Neurologic Surgery, Mayo Clinic, Rochester, MN, USA
e-mail: pinheironeto.carlos@mayo.edu

G. W. Choby (✉)
Department of Otolaryngology – Head and Neck Surgery, Mayo Clinic, Rochester, MN, USA

Rhinology and Skull Base Surgery, Mayo Clinic, Rochester, MN, USA

Department of Neurologic Surgery, Mayo Clinic, Rochester, MN, USA
e-mail: choby.garret@mayo.edu

© The Author(s), under exclusive license to Springer Nature Switzerland AG 2023
E. C. Kuan et al. (eds.), *Skull Base Reconstruction*,
https://doi.org/10.1007/978-3-031-27937-9_18

the defect. Having a thorough understanding of these options allows a skull base surgeon to navigate challenges such as prior surgery, radiation, or extensive tumor involvement [3–5]. The most utilized pedicled flap of endoscopic skull base reconstruction is the posteriorly pedicled nasoseptal flap (NSF); however, the inferior turbinate/lateral nasal wall, middle turbinate, facial artery buccinator, and palatal flaps deserve consideration and will be described in this chapter.

Evaluation

A detailed preoperative history and examination is critical for surgical planning. Pertinent elements of a patient's history include autoimmune disease, granulomatosis disease, diabetes mellitus, immunocompromised status, anticoagulation use, intranasal drug use, smoking status, and trauma. Previous procedural history should be fully elucidated including previous skull base surgery, septoplasty, endoscopic sinus surgery, and embolization. Rigid endoscopy should be performed to assess both ipsilateral and contralateral nasal cavities with a focus on the status of septum and turbinates. Reconstructive alternatives should always be assessed during clinical examination in preparation for unforeseen intraoperative findings.

Intraoperative Considerations

Pedicled flap harvest is typically performed at the beginning of an operation to ensure preservation of its pedicle and allow safe flap storage during skull base resection. However, if a flap is not initially raised and it is determined that a pedicled flap is required for skull base reconstruction, a delayed flap can be harvested without worsening CSF leak rates or complication [6]. If there is concern regarding the

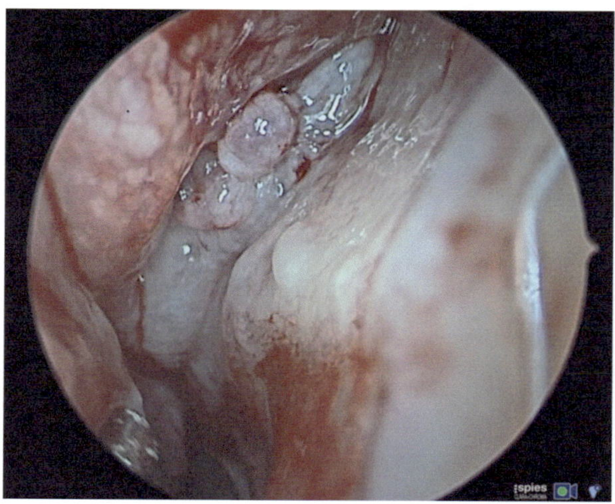

Fig. 18.1 Right NSF pedicle contaminated by chordoma

viability of a NSF after prior bilateral sphenoidotomy, acoustic Doppler sonography can be effectively used to assess the posterior septal artery. If there is concern regarding tumor extension into the proposed flap (Fig. 18.1), intraoperative frozen section pathology can be used to confirm that the flap is free from tumor [7].

Nasoseptal Flap

The posterior pedicled nasoseptal flap, or "Hadad-Bassagasteguy flap," was first described in 2006 as a novel endoscopic skull base reconstructive option [2]. Rotational flaps including the septal mucosa had been previously described as early as the 1950s; however, these were based on random blood supply and did not have the advantage of well vascularized tissue with an axial blood supply [2, 8]. Anatomically, the NSF is based off the posterior septal artery, a branch of the sphenopalatine artery, and includes the ipsilateral septal mucosa [2]. Prior to its description, large defects of the ventral skull base being approached by EEA were typically reconstructed with non-vascularized tissue such as fat grafts, muscle, or free mucosal grafts. Due to high rates of postoperative CSF leak with these techniques, some reconstruction was done via open approaches using regional vascularized flaps such as pericranium, galeal, or temporoparietal flaps or with microvascular free flap reconstruction [9, 10]. With advances in EEA, the NSF was designed to mitigate the need for an external approach and decrease morbidity of the procedure [2]. Indeed, shortly after its description, postoperative CSF leak rates for large high-flow defects were reduced to 5.7% [1].

The NSF can provide soft tissue coverage for defects from orbit to orbit and from the posterior table of the frontal sinus to the sella [2]. Additional surface area can be gained by extending the flap inferior onto the nasal floor or superiorly to the junction of the septum to the cribriform plate and inferiorly onto the floor of the nose and into the inferior meatus [11]. The NSF can be utilized as a single layer but is typically employed in large defects or high-flow leaks as an extracranial onlay flap in multilayered skull base reconstruction [3, 4]. Prior septoplasty is not an absolute contraindication to this flap; however, it can make harvesting this flap more technically difficult. In such cases, due to the absence of cartilage from a septoplasty, both subperichondrial surfaces of the septal mucosa are often healed to each other [12]. The elevation of the flap in those situations may require careful sharp dissection with microscissors to release the adherences between the mucosal layers and avoid laceration of the flap. Preoperative or intraoperative exam, potentially with Doppler, must ensure the posterior septal artery and the sphenopalatine artery are viable. Additional limitations include tumor involvement of the nasal septum. If past surgical history or tumor location necessitates, the contralateral NSF or an alternative local flap may be considered.

The surgical technique starts with infiltration of septum with local anesthetic and vasoconstrictor in a submucoperichondrial plane. A superior incision is made with a needle-tip electrocautery starting at the sphenoid os and moving anteriorly and parallel to the skull base approximately 1–2 cm below the cribriform plate to the level of the anterior axilla of the middle turbinate. At that level and depending on the size of the defect, the incision can be turned superiorly toward the nasal dorsum or in a more limited fashion continued at that level anteriorly toward the caudal border of the septum. If a larger flap was required, the superior incision along the nasal dorsum mucosa is also carried to the caudal border of the septum. The inferior incision starts at the lateral portion of the roof of the choana transitioning along the vomer and onto the nasal floor. Depending on the size of the defect, this incision can be extended laterally to include the nasal floor/inferior meatus mucosa or can be carried anteriorly to the nasal spine along the transition between the septum and nasal floor. Finally, the superior and inferior incisions are connected with an incision along the caudal border of the septum. The flap is then elevated in an anterior to posterior direction in a submucoperichondrial and submucoperiosteal plane (Fig. 18.2 medical illustration and Fig. 18.3 intraoperative endoscopic image). The flap can then be safely stored in the nasopharynx (for sellar or anterior skull base surgery) or maxillary sinus (for transclival or transodontoid surgery) during tumor resection [2, 3, 11].

Variations of the NSF have been described to increase the surface area of the flap and pedicle reach and provide rigid protection. The extended NSF which adds mucosa from the nasal floor and inferior meatus mucosa adds 20 mm of pedicle length and 774 mm^2 of surface area (Fig. 18.4) [11]. Additional descriptions have supported the ability to gain additional reach with mobilization of the sphenopalatine foramen and dissection of the sphenopalatine artery and internal maxillary artery [13, 14]. This provides an increase of 51% and 88% of anterior reach for dissection of the sphenopalatine and internal maxillary artery, respectively [14]. Studies have also described the incorporation of septal cartilage into a chondromucosal flap to provide rigidity and superior protection to skull base defects [15].

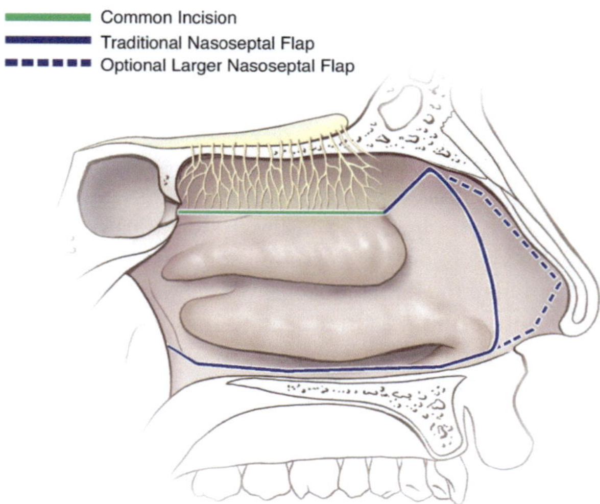

Fig. 18.2 Medical illustration demonstrating planned mucosal incision for the nasoseptal flap. (©MAYO CLINIC)

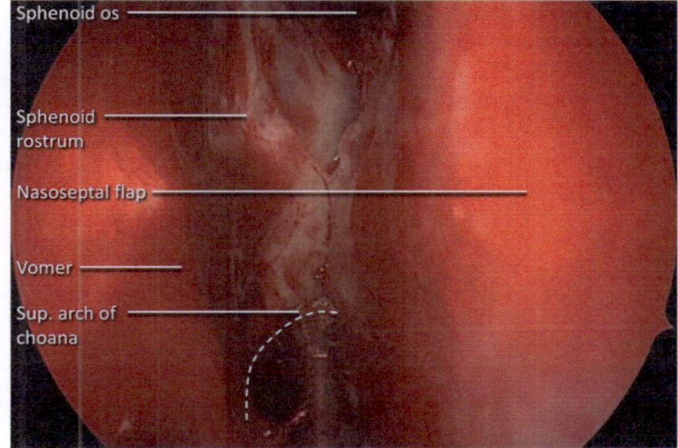

Fig. 18.3 Intraoperative endoscopic image of left-sided nasoseptal flap elevation off the sphenoid rostrum with view between the flap and the vomer and sphenoid rostrum

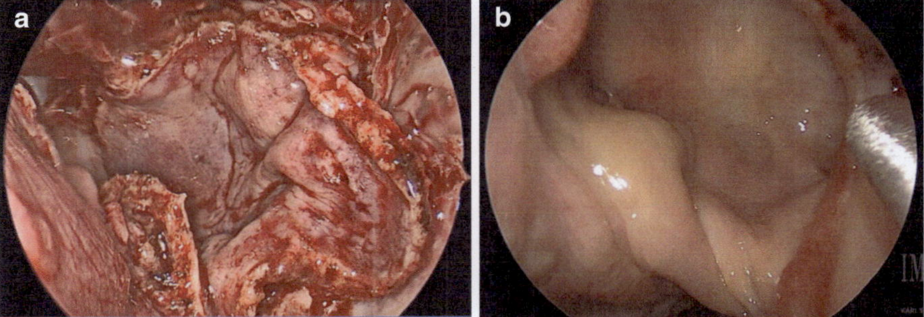

Fig. 18.4 Right extended nasoseptal flap for reconstruction of skull base defect after resection of left petroclival chondrosarcoma. (**a**) Intraoperative positioning of the nasoseptal flap prior to packing. (**b**) Well-healed nasoseptal flap at 8 week postoperative visit

Inferior Turbinate and Lateral Nasal Wall Flap

The inferior turbinate and lateral nasal wall flap was first described in 2007 as an alternative to the posterior-based septal flap [16]. Anatomically, this flap is based on the inferior turbinate artery, which is a branch of the posterior lateral nasal artery, a terminal branch of the sphenopalatine artery [16, 17]. Initially this flap was limited to provide vascularized coverage to small midclival defects due to its limited surface area and arc of rotation. However, extended variations including mucosa from the nasal floor and septum have expanded the flap's utility to larger clival defects [18, 19]. Limitations to this flap include difficult dissection secondary to adherent mucosa on inferior turbinate bone, small surface area for non-extended flaps, and potential for random blood supply for extended portions of the flap [16–19]. Additionally, without extending the dissection, these flaps have a limited reach to the anterior cranial fossa or sella [18].

Fig. 18.5 Medical illustration demonstrating planned mucosal incision for the inferior turbinate flap. (©MAYO CLINIC)

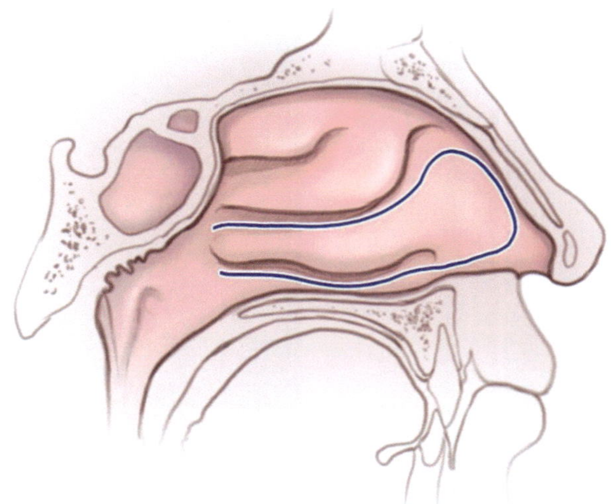

The dissection technique begins with a maxillary antrostomy followed by elevation of the mucosa over the vertical process of the palatine bone. A superior incision is made from the inferior aspect of the maxillary antrostomy toward the head of the inferior turbinate and can be extended high onto the lateral nasal wall. This incision is then carried inferiorly to the nasal floor. An additional horizontal incision is made at the head of the inferior turbinate to facilitate dissection of the mucosa in a subperiosteal plane off the turbinate. After the limits of subperiosteal dissection, the inferior turbinate bone can be resected, including the bone over the nasolacrimal duct. The dissection is carried on the lateral nasal wall down to the floor. At this point, the nasolacrimal duct is sharply transected with endoscopic microscissors to allow full elevation of the flap from the lateral wall (Fig. 18.5 medical illustration and Fig. 18.6 endoscopic images) [16, 17]. If a larger flap is required, mucosa of the lateral nasal wall anterior to the head of the inferior turbinate may be included [18, 19]. The inferior incision is continued posteriorly toward the tail of the inferior turbinate and the superior and lateral aspect of the arch of the choana. The flap can then be elevated in the anterior to posterior direction and stored in the nasopharynx or maxillary sinus to protect it during tumor resection.

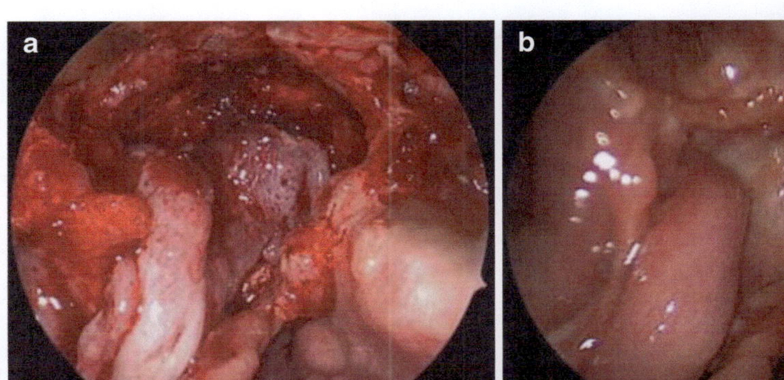

Fig. 18.6 Right inferior turbinate flap for reconstruction of skull base defect after revision resection of a recurrent clival chordoma. (**a**) Intraoperative position of inferior turbinate flap prior to packing. (**b**) Well-healed right inferior turbinate flap at 6 weeks postoperative

Middle Turbinate Flap

The middle turbinate flap (MTF) was first described in 2009 for reconstruction of small defects of the sella, tuberculum, planum, and fovea ethmoidalis [20]. Anatomically, the middle turbinate is supplied by the middle turbinate artery, which is a branch of the posterior lateral nasal artery of the sphenopalatine artery entering along its horizontal portion [20, 21]. The middle turbinate has an attachment anteriorly to the agger nasi and cribriform plate, an oblique attachment to the lamina papyracea forming the basal lamella, and a posterior attachment to the lateral nasal wall. The middle turbinate can be utilized in the absence of the NSF availability or for more limited defects to preserve the NSF for future considerations [20, 22, 23]. It has been described as yielding 5–6 cm^2 of mucosal coverage. The MTF is limited by the possible destabilization during previous operations and variable pneumatization pattern of the turbinate. Additionally, the MTF is limited by its reach and size and would not be suitable for many skull base defects, including clivus or odontoid reconstruction [20].

The dissection technique begins with a vertical incision with a needle-tip cautery anteriorly from the head of the middle turbinate superiorly toward the axilla. An additional horizontal incision can be made on the medial surface of the turbinate along the cribriform attachment. The mucosa is then elevated in a submucoperiosteal plane off the turbinate. The bony turbinate is then removed in a piecemeal fashion. An incision can then be made on the lateral surface of the turbinate starting at the axilla moving posteriorly toward its posterior attachment point, preserving the middle turbinate artery pedicle (Fig. 18.7 medical illustration). The elevated flap can then be stored in the nasopharynx or maxillary sinus to protect it during tumor resection [20–23].

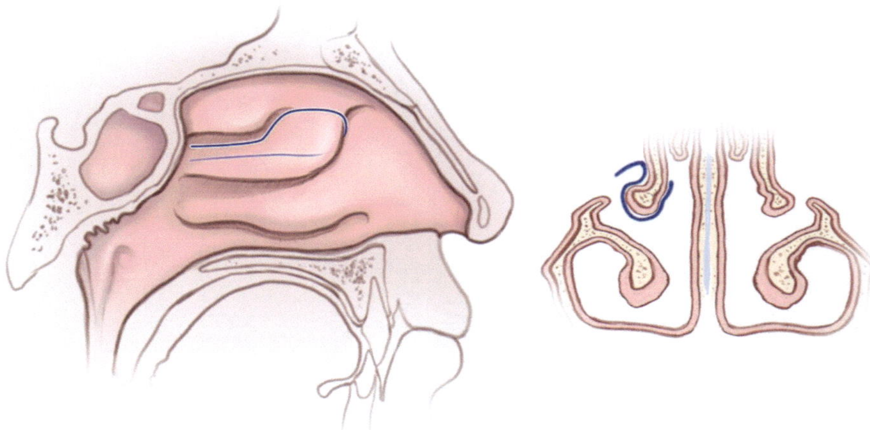

Fig. 18.7 Medical illustration demonstrating planned mucosal incision for the middle turbinate flap. (©MAYO CLINIC)

Extranasal Flaps

Extranasal vascularized pedicle flaps can be considered in cases where the more commonly utilized local flaps are unavailable due to previous surgical history or tumor involvement [24]. The facial artery buccinator (FAB) and palatal flap are two options that typically have different applications outside skull base reconstruction; however, due to their proximity and reach, these flaps can be considered in a surgeon's reconstruction algorithm [25, 26]. Pericranial flap and temporoparietal flap are more commonly used and are covered in another chapter.

For skull base reconstruction, the FAB flap is a superiorly based variation that can include mucosa and buccinator muscle or muscle alone and is dependent on retrograde arterial flow. Anatomic studies have demonstrated theoretical reach to the planum sphenoidale; however, tunneling necessitates a Caldwell-Luc osteotomy with a medial maxillectomy which in practice limits the posterior reach of flap [26]. At this juncture, the palatal flap is largely experimental for skull base reconstruction and involves harvesting the mucosa in a submucoperiosteal plane overlying the hard palate based off the greater palatine artery [24, 25]. The greater palatine foramen is then drilled transorally to allow transposition of the flap into the nasal cavity. This technique requires a medial maxillectomy and uncovering of the pterygopalatine foramen at the posterior maxillary sinus to tunnel the flap [25]. This flap can provide soft tissue coverage to the defects arising near the clivus or sella; however, the risk of postoperative oral-antral fistula makes this an unfavorable reconstructive option [24].

Outcomes

Extent of tumor resection, prevention of postoperative CSF leak, decreased morbidity, and acceptable quality of life are the main metrics for successful outcome in skull base reconstruction. A series has demonstrated postoperative leak rates of 0–5% for the nasoseptal flap when used for anterior skull base reconstruction [27]. Additionally, it has been shown that high-flow intraoperative CSF leaks have a 94% success rate with the nasoseptal flap [1]. A study by Zanation et al. demonstrated that obesity, large dural opening, tumor pathology, corridor of resection, and postoperative lumbar drain did not adversely correlate with postoperative flap failure [1]. However, other studies have shown previous radiation and flap utilization in pediatric population as being correlated with higher CSF leak rates after nasoseptal flap reconstruction [1, 28]. Institutional experience regarding outcomes for inferior turbinate, middle turbinate, and extranasal flaps is limited; however, Zanation et al. have previously reported successful repair utilizing inferior turbinate flap, facial artery buccinator flap, and lateral nasal wall flap [27]. The authors did have a failure utilizing the MTF and have limited its utilization in their reconstruction algorithm.

Short-term morbidity associated with intranasal pedicled flaps includes nasal obstruction, crusting, and hyposmia [29]. Studies have shown that there is a transient decrease in quality-of-life metrics in initial postoperative period that return to baseline by 3 months [30]. Other studies support that Sinonasal Outcome Test-22 (SNOT-22) surveys at 3 month postoperative visits are not worse compared to preoperative surveys [29]. However, it has been shown that up to 2 years postoperatively, Lund-Mackay scores show elevated scores indicating long-term mucosal inflammation [29]. Mucocele formation can occur due to incomplete removal of sinonasal mucosa at the reconstruction site. A series has demonstrated rates of postoperative mucocele formation at 0–3.6% [31].

NSF donor site morbidity can be associated with prolonged nasal crusting, septal perforation, and nasal deformity [31]. Reepithelialization of the exposed septal cartilage and bone is the proposed mechanism of significant crusting following surgery; however, studies have not demonstrated prolonged duration of crusting compared to endoscopic skull base patients without NSF. Additionally, when focusing on the crusting aspects of the SNOT-22 surveys, patients did not perceive worse symptoms after their 3 month follow-up [30]. Septal perforation rates have been shown to vary between 0.9% and 14.4%; however, it is important to note that more posterior perforations likely are asymptomatic in patients. Snyderman et al. have reported rates of nasal dorsum collapse of 5.8% [32].

Short-term and long-term olfactory outcomes must be considered after NSF harvest. Studies have shown that short-term (3 month) and long-term (1 year) postoperative University of Pennsylvania Smell Inventory Test was not significantly altered after nasoseptal flap harvest [33]. When testing the olfactory function of the ipsilateral side to NSF harvest, there was evidence of subclinical olfactory impairment [34]. Use of olfaction metrics on SNOT-22 scores suggests that patients experience a subjective decrease in sense of smell at 3 months postoperatively; however, long

Table 18.1 Summary of local vascularized pedicle flaps with named blood supply, length, and surface area

Flap	Blood supply	Length (cm)	Surface area (cm^2)	Extended length (cm)	Extended surface area (cm^2)	Locations used
Nasoseptal flap [11, 14, 35]	Posterior septal artery	9.4	25.0	32.7	13.4	S, P, FE, CP, C, O
Inferior turbinate flap [17, 18]	Inferior turbinate artery	5.4	2.4	5.0	27.3	S, C, O
Middle turbinate flap [20]	Middle turbinate artery	4.0	5.6	N/A	N/A	S, P, FE

S sella, *P* planum, *FE* fovea ethmoidalis, *CP* cribriform plate, *C* clivus, *O* odontoid

term these results returned to preoperative baseline [33]. Additionally, it has been shown that the use of cold knife versus monopolar cautery does not alter olfactory outcomes in these patients [33] (Table 18.1).

References

1. Zanation AM, et al. Nasoseptal flap reconstruction of high flow intraoperative cerebral spinal fluid leaks during endoscopic skull base surgery. Am J Rhinol Allergy. 2009;23(5):518–21.
2. Hadad G, et al. A novel reconstructive technique after endoscopic expanded endonasal approaches: vascular pedicle nasoseptal flap. Laryngoscope. 2006;116(10):1882–6.
3. Pinheiro-Neto CD, Snyderman CH. Nasoseptal flap. Adv Otorhinolaryngol. 2013;74:42–55.
4. Sigler AC, et al. Endoscopic skull base reconstruction: an evolution of materials and methods. Otolaryngol Clin N Am. 2017;50(3):643–53.
5. Reyes C, Mason E, Solares CA. Panorama of reconstruction of skull base defects: from traditional open to endonasal endoscopic approaches, from free grafts to microvascular flaps. Int Arch Otorhinolaryngol. 2014;18(Suppl 2):S179–86.
6. Choby GW, et al. Delayed nasoseptal flaps for endoscopic skull base reconstruction: proof of concept and evaluation of outcomes. Otolaryngol Head Neck Surg. 2015;152(2):255–9.
7. Pinheiro-Neto CD, et al. Use of acoustic Doppler sonography to ascertain the feasibility of the pedicled nasoseptal flap after prior bilateral sphenoidotomy. Laryngoscope. 2010;120(9):1798–801.
8. Hirsch O. Successful closure of cere brospinal fluid rhinorrhea by endonasal surgery. AMA Arch Otolaryngol. 1952;56(1):1–12.
9. Neligan PC, et al. Flap selection in cranial base reconstruction. Plast Reconstr Surg. 1996;98(7):1159–66; discussion 1167–8.
10. Snyderman CH, et al. Anterior cranial base reconstruction: role of galeal and pericranial flaps. Laryngoscope. 1990;100(6):607–14.
11. Peris-Celda M, et al. The extended nasoseptal flap for skull base reconstruction of the clival region: an anatomical and radiological study. J Neurol Surg B Skull Base. 2013;74(6):369–85.
12. Park W, et al. Nasoseptal flap elevation in patients with history of septal surgery: does it increase flap failure or cerebrospinal fluid leakage? World Neurosurg. 2016;93:164–7.

13. Pinheiro-Neto CD, Peris-Celda M, Kenning T. Extrapolating the limits of the nasoseptal flap with pedicle dissection to the internal maxillary artery. Oper Neurosurg (Hagerstown). 2019;16(1):37–44.
14. Shastri KS, et al. Lengthening the nasoseptal flap pedicle with extended dissection into the pterygopalatine fossa. Laryngoscope. 2020;130(1):18–24.
15. Ramsey T, et al. Composite chondromucosal nasoseptal flap for reconstruction of suprasellar defects. World Neurosurg. 2021;149:11–4.
16. Fortes FS, et al. The posterior pedicle inferior turbinate flap: a new vascularized flap for skull base reconstruction. Laryngoscope. 2007;117(8):1329–32.
17. Harvey RJ, Sheahan PO, Schlosser RJ. Inferior turbinate pedicle flap for endoscopic skull base defect repair. Am J Rhinol Allergy. 2009;23(5):522–6.
18. Choby GW, et al. Extended inferior turbinate flap for endoscopic reconstruction of skull base defects. J Neurol Surg B Skull Base. 2014;75(4):225–30.
19. Rivera-Serrano CM, et al. Posterior pedicle lateral nasal wall flap: new reconstructive technique for large defects of the skull base. Am J Rhinol Allergy. 2011;25(6):e212–6.
20. Prevedello DM, et al. Middle turbinate flap for skull base reconstruction: cadaveric feasibility study. Laryngoscope. 2009;119(11):2094–8.
21. Carnevale C, et al. Middle turbinate mucosal flap: a low-morbidity option in the management of skull base defects. Head Neck. 2021;43:1415.
22. Amin SM, Fawzy TO, Hegazy AA. Composite vascular pedicled middle turbinate flap for reconstruction of sellar defects. Ann Otol Rhinol Laryngol. 2016;125(9):770–4.
23. Simal Julian JA, et al. Middle turbinate vascularized flap for skull base reconstruction after an expanded endonasal approach. Acta Neurochir. 2011;153(9):1827–32.
24. Kim GG, et al. Pedicled extranasal flaps in skull base reconstruction. Adv Otorhinolaryngol. 2013;74:71–80.
25. Oliver CL, et al. Palatal flap modifications allow pedicled reconstruction of the skull base. Laryngoscope. 2008;118(12):2102–6.
26. Rivera-Serrano CM, et al. Pedicled facial buccinator (FAB) flap: a new flap for reconstruction of skull base defects. Laryngoscope. 2010;120(10):1922–30.
27. Patel MR, et al. Beyond the nasoseptal flap: outcomes and pearls with secondary flaps in endoscopic endonasal skull base reconstruction. Laryngoscope. 2014;124(4):846–52.
28. Harvey RJ, et al. Intracranial complications before and after endoscopic skull base reconstruction. Am J Rhinol. 2008;22(5):516–21.
29. Riley CA, et al. Long-term sinonasal outcomes after endoscopic skull base surgery with nasoseptal flap reconstruction. Laryngoscope. 2019;129(5):1035–40.
30. Jalessi M, et al. Impact of nasoseptal flap elevation on sinonasal quality of life in endoscopic endonasal approach to pituitary adenomas. Eur Arch Otorhinolaryngol. 2016;273(5):1199–205.
31. Lavigne P, et al. Complications of nasoseptal flap reconstruction: a systematic review. J Neurol Surg B Skull Base. 2018;79(Suppl 4):S291–9.
32. Rowan NR, et al. Nasal deformities following nasoseptal flap reconstruction of skull base defects. J Neurol Surg B Skull Base. 2016;77(1):14–8.
33. Puccinelli CL, et al. Long-term olfaction outcomes in transnasal endoscopic skull-base surgery: a prospective cohort study comparing electrocautery and cold knife upper septal limb incision techniques. Int Forum Allergy Rhinol. 2019;9(5):493–500.
34. Soyka MB, et al. Long-term olfactory outcome after nasoseptal flap reconstructions in midline skull base surgery. Am J Rhinol Allergy. 2017;31(5):334–7.
35. Pinheiro-Neto CD, et al. Study of the nasoseptal flap for endoscopic anterior cranial base reconstruction. Laryngoscope. 2011;121(12):2514–20.

Chapter 19
Extracranial Flaps for Skull Base Reconstruction

Daniel A. Alicea and Patrick Colley

Pericranial Flap

History

The pericranial flap was first introduced in 1978 by Wolfe [1]. Since that time, it has become a workhorse vascular flap for open anterior skull base reconstruction. In regard to endoscopic surgery, the pericranial flap is typically used for reconstruction when the nasal septal flap is unavailable or compromised due to surgical pathology or previous treatment. In order to use the pericranial flap, a point of entry needs to be made into the sinuses or nasal cavity. The details of this will be discussed later in this section.

Anatomy

The scalp consists of five discrete tissue layers: skin, subcutaneous tissue, galea aponeurotica, subgaleal loose connective tissue, and pericranium (Fig. 19.1). The galea aponeurotica is continuous with the frontalis muscle anteriorly, the occipitalis muscle posteriorly, and the temporoparietal fascia laterally at the superior temporal line. The subgaleal loose connective tissue provides a reliable plane for easy

D. A. Alicea
Icahn School of Medicine at Mount Sinai, New York, NY, USA

P. Colley (✉)
Montefiore Medical Center, Bronx, NY, USA
e-mail: pcolley@montefiore.org

E. C. Kuan et al. (eds.), *Skull Base Reconstruction*,
https://doi.org/10.1007/978-3-031-27937-9_19

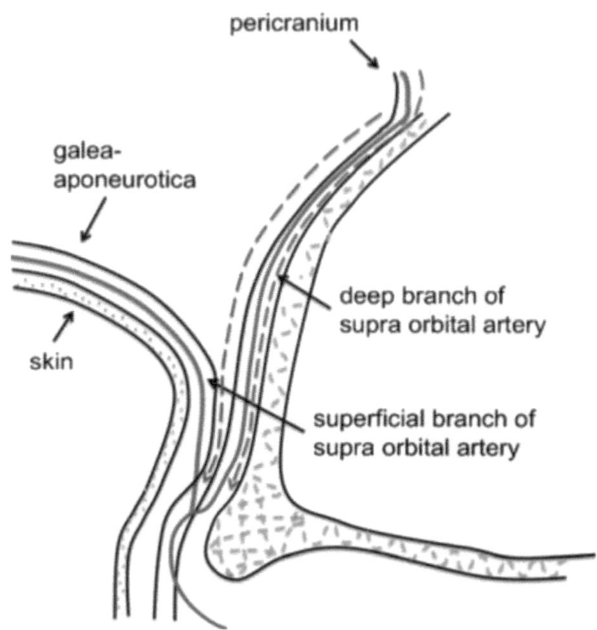

Fig. 19.1 Vascular supply of the pericranial flap. (Figure adapted from Yano, T. Reliability of and Indications for Pericranial Flaps in Anterior Skull Base Reconstruction. J Craniofacial Surg. 2011. 22;2: 482–485)

dissection just superior to the pericranium. The pericranium is the outermost layer of the skull bones and is therefore adherent to these underlying structures. Laterally, the pericranium is continuous with the deep temporal fascia of the temporalis muscle. The temporal line is the lateral point where these two structures meet and marks the lateral border of the anteriorly based pericranial flap.

The pericranium has a robust blood supply that comes from multiple axial vessels as well as connections to perforators from the underlying calvaria. These axial vessels include the supratrochlear, supraorbital, superficial temporal, greater auricular, and occipital arteries [2]. Due to this rich blood supply, the pericranial flap can be used as an anteriorly or laterally based flap. For the purposes of this chapter, the anteriorly based flap will be discussed as the lateral based flaps are typically reserved for open skull base reconstruction and lateral skull base defects. In addition, these laterally based flaps have a less consistent blood supply pattern. The anterior vessels that supply the pericranium are the supraorbital and supratrochlear arteries. These vessels divide into superficial and deep branches within a centimeter after exiting their respective foramina [2, 3]. The superficial branches supply the galea and the overlying skin, while the deep arteries travel within the pericranium and provide the blood supply to this flap. This bilateral perfusion pattern allows the pericranial flap to be harvested in a unilateral or bilateral fashion. The average width of the bilateral flap is 10 cm, while the unilateral flap is 5 cm [3]. Based on these distances, the width of the unilateral flap is likely to be adequate for coverage of the entire anterior skull base extending from orbit to orbit [4].

The length of the pericranial flap is also of significant importance. Robust perfusion has been demonstrated in the pericranium to an average of 17 cm from the orbital rim [3]. Recommended pericranial flap lengths have been published based on the radiographic length of the anterior skull base. The sella is the most posterior portion of the anterior skull base, and the length of pericranial flap required to cover this area is typically between 14 and 17 cm. Other reports have been published discussing the use of the pericranial flap to repair posterior skull base defects, mostly involving the clivus. The average length of a pericranial flap required to repair a defect in this location is 18–21 cm [4]. At this length, the blood supply of the pericranial flap is questionable, but the pericranial flap was still shown to be an effective means of repairing skull base defects in this area [3, 5].

Skull base location	Length of PCF—measured from brow (cm)
Anterior skull base	12–14
Sella	14–17
Clivus	18–21

Based on data from Patel, MR, Shah RV, Snyderman CH et al. Pericranial flap for endoscopic skull-base reconstruction: clinical outcomes and radioanatomic analysis of preoperative planning

Surgical Steps

Harvesting the pericranial flap starts with an external incision. The forehead and face should be prepped and draped in a sterile fashion. The required flap length should be calculated based on the anticipated site of repair and marked for identification during the surgery. This can be performed by measuring from the orbital rim posteriorly and using staples or a clamp on the drapes. The type of incision is determined primarily based on whether the flap is harvested via an endoscopic technique or open technique (Fig. 19.2). Classically, an open technique has been used to harvest the pericranial flap. This involves a coronal incision posterior to the hairline that is carried down to the level of the loose connective tissue just superficial to the pericranium. This tissue layer allows for an easily identifiable dissection plane that can be used to dissect the superficial tissue layers of the scalp from the pericranium. Dissection within the loose connective tissue should continue from the temporal line laterally to a point approximately 1 cm superior to the orbital rim. Care should be taken at this point in the dissection as it is possible to damage the deep branches of the supratrochlear and supraorbital arteries as they course to the pericranium within a centimeter of the orbital rim. Depending on the length of the flap that is required, dissection posterior to the skin incision may be required. This should proceed in the same loose connective tissue layer as the anterior dissection until the appropriate length of pericranial flap can be harvested.

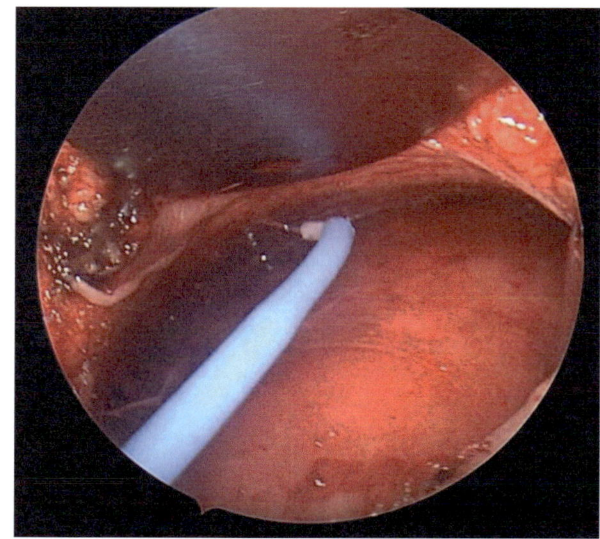

Fig. 19.2 PCF incisions. Lighted retractors and endoscopic brow lift instruments can be used for dissection of the subgaleal plane. A long needle tip bovie can be used to make the pericranial flap incisions to allow for dissection of the flap from the underlying calvaria

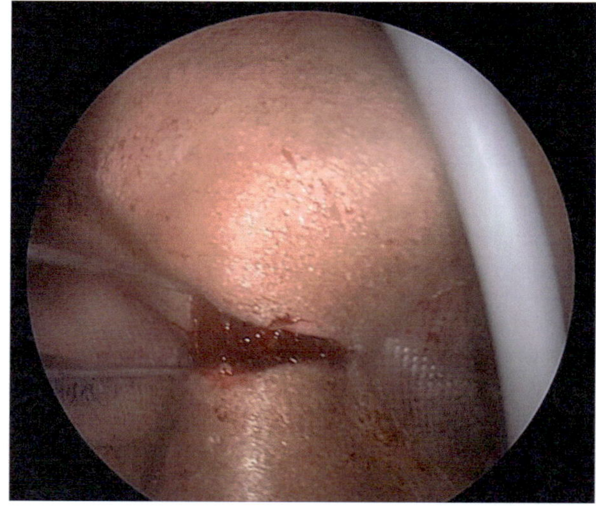

Fig. 19.3 Nasionectomy with PCF. The nasion skin incision should be made in any available skin creases and should extend as wide as possible without disrupting the medial canthal tendon. The bony opening should extend the same width and should be at least 5 mm in superior-inferior dimension

The endoscopic harvest of the pericranial flap was originally described by Zanation et al. and involves a different incision than the open flap [6]. Three vertical 2 cm incisions can be made within the hairline, or a 3 cm pretrichial incision can be used to allow for instrument and endoscope access (Fig. 19.3). The endoscopic pericranial flap typically involves a unilateral pericranial flap, so the pretrichial incision should be marked just lateral to the midline. Regardless of the incision used, dissection is performed using typical open surgical techniques until the loose connective tissue layer is identified. A pocket is dissected within this layer to allow for placement of the endoscope and instrument. Further dissection is performed using endoscopic techniques and typically involves a suction Freer and Cottle elevator. A 0° or 30° endoscope can be used, and endoscopic brow equipment such as optical dissectors with distal suction may also be helpful but is not required. The same surgical borders are used in the endoscopic pericranial flap including the temporal lines laterally and orbital rim inferiorly. Dissection generally crosses the midline by approximately 1 cm at most to allow for preservation of the contralateral pericranial flap and to decrease postoperative edema.

Once the superficial dissection is complete, the flap incisions are made. These can be completed using a long needle tip bovie if the endoscopic technique is used (Fig. 19.4). Blunt dissection is then used to carefully dissect the flap from the underlying calvarial bone. Dissection deep to the flap should be continued inferiorly to the orbital rim taking care not to damage the supratrochlear or supraorbital vessels as they exit their foramina. The inferior lateral portion of the flap often requires a small horizontal releasing incision along the lateral orbital rim to allow for the flap to be properly rotated. To protect the supraorbital artery, palpation or a Doppler can be used to identify the foramina, and the releasing incision should remain lateral to this point. The supraorbital foramen is typically 2.75 cm from the nasal midline [6].

In open skull base surgery, a craniotomy is performed, and the pericranial flap can be rotated over the anterior portion of the craniotomy in an epidural plane to allow for skull base repair. In endoscopic surgery, an entry point into the frontal sinus must be made in order to pass the pericranial flap from its extranasal location to the intranasal area for use in skull base repair. In addition, a modified Lothrop frontal sinusotomy must also be performed in order to allow for passage of the flap during surgery and proper frontal sinus drainage after surgery. The external frontal osteotomy can be accomplished via two methods. The first method involves an

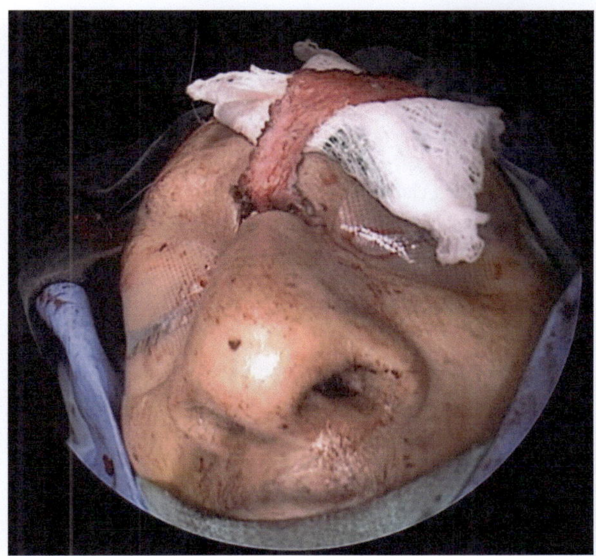

Fig. 19.4 Endoscopic harvest of PCF. The unilateral pericranial flap should be rotated and advanced through the nasion skin incision to ensure full rotation without compromising the pedicle vasculature

osteotomy made through the superior portion of the anterior table of the frontal sinus via the same skin incision used to harvest the flap. The incision should be made approximately 2 cm in medial to lateral dimension and 5 mm in vertical dimension. This has been described as the letterbox technique. The pericranial flap is typically inserted superiorly in the frontal sinus which would allow for coverage of the posterior table of the sinus in addition to the ethmoid and cribriform skull base [7]. The second method of insertion involves a nasion skin incision. The skin incision should be made in a natural crease if possible and should allow for easy access to the underlying frontal bone. Via this second incision, a bony osteotomy is made of a similar dimension to the letterbox technique. The pericranial flap is then carefully rotated to allow for passage through this osteotomy into the frontal sinus (Fig. 19.4). This osteotomy is typically performed more inferiorly than the letterbox technique and allows for a more direct application of the flap to the anterior skull base and therefore requires a slightly shorter flap length than the letterbox technique. Regardless of which technique is chosen, care should be taken not to rotate the flap in a manner that compresses the flap pedicle and causes decreased perfusion. A third, transorbital method of insertion has been described in cadavers but has not been used in the clinical setting at this time.

Once the flap is present in the nose, it can be used as an onlay in a multilayer technique to repair areas of the skull base extending from the most inferior portion of the posterior table to the sella. Dural substitutes or autologous materials such as fascia lata should be placed as an inlay with the edges tucked behind the bony margins of the endonasal craniotomy. The pericranial flap can then be placed over the top of this graft and secured in place using Surgicel, NasoPore, or whichever packing material is preferred (Fig. 19.5). Care should be taken to ensure that the edges of the pericranial flap sit directly on the bony edges of the craniotomy and no

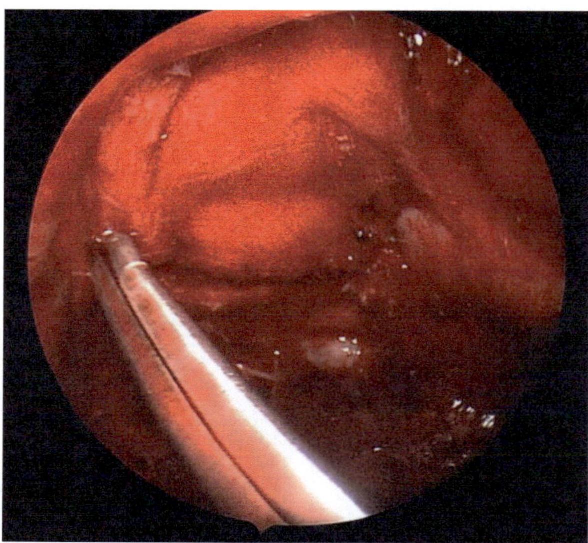

Fig. 19.5 Inlay present w/o PCF/PCF covering inlay. After placement of an inlay graft, the pericranial flap is advanced through the nasionectomy bony opening and carefully pulled to cover the skull base opening to form a watertight seal

mucosa is left between the bone and the flap. If the frontal sinuses are narrow and the flap appears to completely obstruct these outflow tracts, packing or stents can be placed into the lateral portions of the frontal sinuses to allow them to remain patent in the postoperative setting.

The skin incisions should be closed using fine suture material in a multilayer technique. Subgaleal edema in the area of the pericranial flap harvest is often seen in the first 24–72 h after surgery. A head wrap can be placed over this area to help prevent a hematoma or decrease edema once it is present. Care should be taken to avoid placing pressure on the supraorbital rim with any head wraps that are placed to avoid compressing the flap pedicle. Placement of drains into this space is not typically necessary.

Outcomes

As stated previously, the pericranial flap has been used routinely for open skull base surgery for over 30 years with a significant rate of success. Since the introduction of endoscopic skull base reconstruction with the pericranial flap in 2010, multiple case series have demonstrated a similarly high success rate for this technique [4, 5, 8]. Patel et al. published a series of 16 endoscopic skull base reconstructions with pericranial flaps in 2014 with a 100% success rate. The pericranial flap has even been used as a rescue flap in secondary posterior fossa reconstructions. Gode et al. also published a series using the endoscopic pericranial flap for secondary reconstruction of posterior fossa defects and found a similarly high success rate although multiple patients needed augmentation in the post-op period with further tissue grafts. It should be noted that many of these series used pericranial flaps as a secondary reconstructive means after failure of the initial repair.

Conclusion

The pericranial flap is a reliable vascular flap that can be used for primary and secondary reconstruction of the anterior skull base after endoscopic surgery. It does require an external frontal sinusotomy to passage into the nasal cavity as well as a skin incision. However, the high success rate of skull base repair should make this flap a valuable tool in complex endoscopic skull base surgery.

Temporoparietal Fascia Flap

The temporoparietal fascia flap (TPFF) is an extracranial pedicled flap used for anterior skull base reconstruction that is based on the superficial temporal artery, a terminal branch of the external carotid artery. The anatomy of the temporoparietal

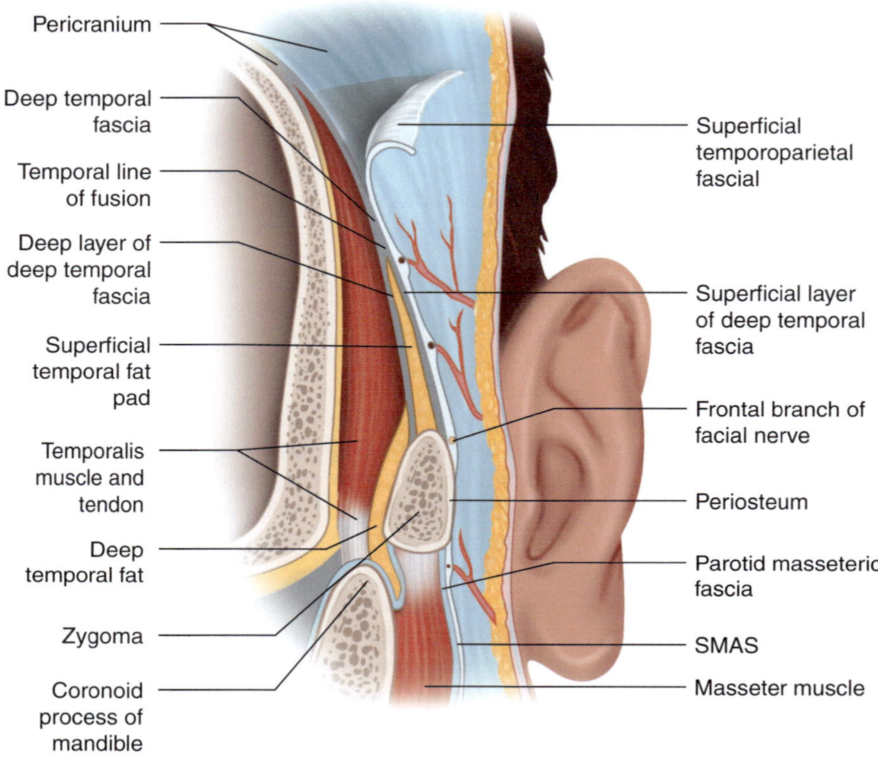

Fig. 19.6 Anatomy of the temporal region. *SMAS* superficial musculoaponeurotic system (Baker, SR. Local Flaps in Facial Reconstruction; Fourth Edition, 2022)

region is comprised of several soft tissue layers: skin, subcutaneous tissue, temporoparietal fascia, loose areolar tissue, temporalis fascia, temporalis muscle, and pericranium (Fig. 19.6). The temporoparietal fascia is continuous with the superficial musculoaponeurotic system (SMAS) inferiorly, the orbicularis oculi and frontalis muscles anteriorly, the galea aponeurotica superiorly, and the occipitalis muscle posteriorly [9, 10]. The superficial temporal artery runs within the temporoparietal fascia and provides its blood supply. It divides into an anterior and a posterior branch roughly at the level of the zygomatic arch. The TPFF is based on the anterior branch of the superficial temporal artery [10]. Deep to the temporoparietal fascia runs the frontal branch of the facial nerve after it crosses the superficial surface of the zygomatic arch. The nerve generally runs along Pitanguy's Line, an imaginary line starting from 0.5 cm below the tragus to 1.5 cm above the lateral eyebrow.

The pedicled TPFF is a versatile flap that has been used for the reconstruction of a variety of head and neck defects (e.g., intraoral, oronasal, nasocutaneous, auricular). It has also been described as a free microvascular flap [9, 10]. Traditionally, it has been used for skull base reconstruction after open craniofacial resections. Recently, the use of the TPFF in the reconstruction of anterior and central skull base defects has been described [9–13]. Some authors have also described its use for the reconstruction of lateral skull base defects [12]. Its rich vascularity makes it a robust flap and an ideal option for patients who have undergone prior radiation therapy to the surgical site. At its largest dimension, the fan-shaped flap is 2–3 mm in thickness and can reach up to 17 cm × 14 cm in size [10, 14]. It is thin and pliable which makes it a favorable reconstructive option for skull base defects with complex irregular surfaces.

Once the defect size and site are determined, the flap may be harvested from either side of the scalp [10] (Fig. 19.7). Several surgical techniques have been described in the literature. There are four surgical "corridors" to transpose the TPFF into the nasal cavity: (1) infratemporal/transpterygoid pathway (traditional, Fig. 19.8); (2) anterior cranial fossa pathway via a pterional frontoparietal craniotomy; (3) orbital pathway via a window in the lateral orbital wall; and (4) middle cranial fossa pathway via a temporoparietal craniotomy [9]. To harvest the TPFF, a hemicoronal incision is made down to the level of the hair follicles. Care is taken not to injure the vascular pedicle during this step. The skin and subcutaneous tissues are then elevated off the temporoparietal fascia until an adequate surface area is exposed. The dimensions of the flap are designed, and the temporoparietal fascia is incised and elevated off the cranium and deep temporal fascia down to its vascular

Fig. 19.7 Planned left hemicoronal incision for the harvest of the temporoparietal flap [10]

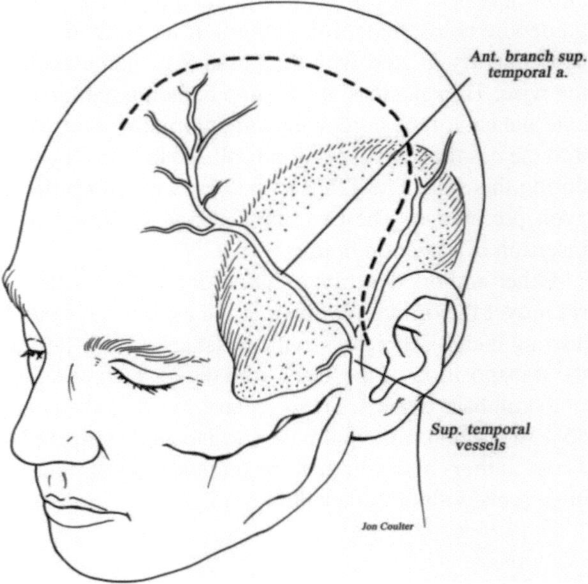

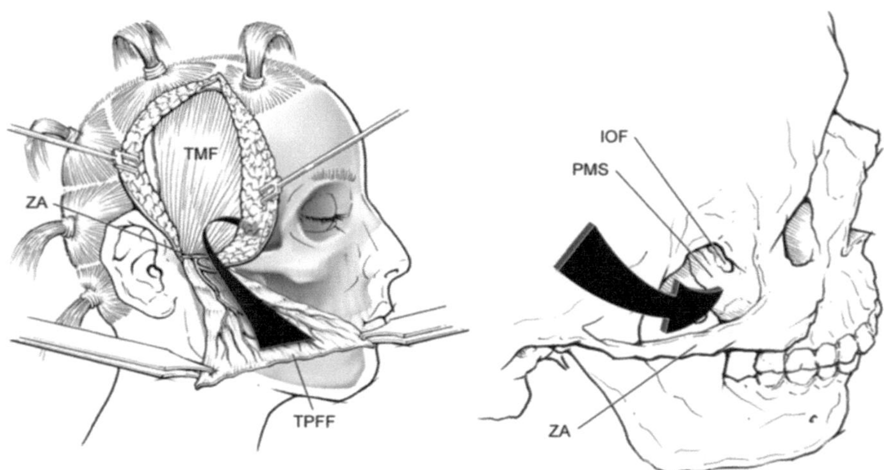

Fig. 19.8 Transposition of the temporoparietal fascia flap through the infratemporal/transpterygoid pathway [15]. *ZA* zygomatic arch, *TMF* temporalis muscle fascia, *TPFF* temporoparietal fascia flap, *PMS* posterior maxillary sinus, *IOF* inferior orbital fissure

pedicle. At this point, a surgical corridor is chosen to transpose the TPFF into the nasal cavity. The traditional approach involves the transposition of the flap through the pterygopalatine fossa. This space is first exposed endoscopically prior to harvesting the TPFF. Then, after harvesting the TPFF, a wide subperiosteal tunnel is then made over the surface of the zygomatic arch to allow passage of the flap without compression of the pedicle. The temporalis muscle is elevated posteriorly to allow access to the temporal, infratemporal, and pterygopalatine fossae [10, 11]. A guidewire is inserted through this soft tissue tunnel into the nasal cavity and is then subsequently dilated with the passage of percutaneous tracheostomy dilators over the wire. Transposition of the flap is facilitated by suturing its distal portion to the external end of the guidewire and pulling the wire through the transpterygoid tunnel into the nasal cavity. Attention is placed to avoid any twisting of the vascular pedicle during this step. The TPFF is then used to reconstruct the skull base defect per surgeon preference. The external incision is closed in a multilayered fashion after insertion of a suction drain.

Other authors describe a "side-door TPFF" with the creation of an epidural corridor over the orbital roof by making a pterional frontoparietal craniotomy and connecting it endoscopically to the nasal cavity [9]. This allows a straight trajectory for the transposition of the TPFF into the nasal cavity for reconstruction of large anterior skull base defects. In this cadaveric study, the authors found that the TPFF lined 85% of the anterior skull base surface area compared to the pericranial flap (65%). These authors also comment on a theoretical orbital pathway which could be useful in patients with orbital exenteration.

Special considerations when harvesting the TPFF include reducing the incidence of facial nerve injury and alopecia. Since the frontal branch of the facial nerve runs along Pitanguy's Line, dissection past this imaginary line between the tragus and the lateral eyebrow is discouraged. Also, careful dissection in the plane between the subcutaneous tissue and the temporoparietal fascia will reduce the incidence of alopecia [10].

Other Experimental Flaps

Pedicled Palatal Flap

The pedicled palatal flap is an experimental flap based on the greater palatine artery, a branch of the internal maxillary artery. It involves harvesting the mucosa from the hard palate and transposing it into the nasal cavity through the greater palatine foramen [16] (Fig. 19.9). The authors describe using a high-speed drill to enlarge the greater palatine foramen to create a corridor into the nasal cavity for the palatal flap. To allow for a greater arc of rotation, the descending palatine artery is carefully dissected and mobilized from the pterygopalatine canal. Once the palatal flap is inside the nasal cavity, the bony palatal defect is covered with the mucosa of the nasal floor and inferior turbinate. The pedicled flap is then used to reconstruct the skull base defect per surgeon preference.

In the cadaveric study, the flap was noted to have a pedicle roughly 3 cm in length and a surface area of 12–18 cm^2. Given this configuration, the authors found the palatal flap amenable to reconstruction of planum, sellar, and clival defects. The bony palatal defect was noted not to exceed 1.5 cm^2 in surface area. Nevertheless, the most dreaded morbidity is a persistent oronasal fistula. To date, there has been no clinical application of the palatal flap in the literature. As a result, the palatal flap remains an option of last resort in endoscopic skull base reconstruction.

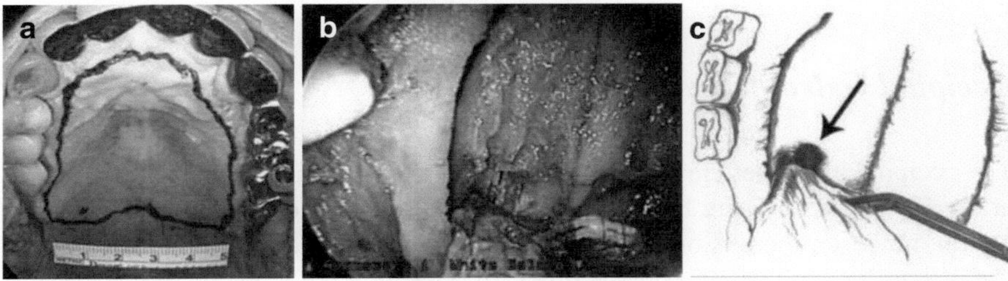

Fig. 19.9 Illustration of the pedicled palatal flap [16]. (**a**) Outline of the palatal flap; (**b, c**) harvest of the palatal flap with preservation of the greater palatine pedicle

Facial Artery Buccinator Flap

The facial artery buccinator flap (FABF) is a well-described pedicled flap for the reconstruction of oral cavity and other head and neck defects; however, it has recently been proposed as a reconstructive option for the anterior skull base [17, 18]. As its name implies, this flap is based on the facial artery, and it can be harvested as either a muscular or a myomucosal flap. In the application for anterior skull base reconstruction, the FABF is designed as a superiorly based flap with retrograde flow through the facial/angular artery. Venous outflow is primarily via the buccal plexus rather than named veins; hence, maximizing pedicle width is important to minimizing venous congestion. A cadaveric study demonstrated that the FABF, transposed through an anterior maxillary corridor, can reliably reach the anterior skull base and planum sphenoidale [17]. Flap dimensions were described as >10 cm^2 and a length of 7–8 cm.

To harvest the flap, incisions are made in the buccal mucosa taking care to preserve Stensen's duct postero-superiorly. The facial artery is identified inferiorly, transected, and ligated to allow a greater arc of rotation superiorly for the transposition of the flap. After the flap is raised, the anterior wall of the maxilla is exposed, and a generous maxillary osteotomy is created with the superior limit at the level of the infraorbital foramen. The flap is then transposed into the previously dissected sinonasal cavity and placed accordingly to cover the skull base defect (Fig. 19.10). If harvesting a myomucosal flap, a 180-degree rotation of the flap is necessary to keep the mucosa facing the sinonasal cavity, increasing the risk of venous congestion. The buccal defect, when present, is closed primarily or with AlloDerm [17, 18].

Complications include facial and/or dental paresthesias and persistent epiphora due to nasolacrimal duct injury. Facial nerve injury is unlikely given that the plane of dissection is deep to the facial nerve branches. Multiple publications have reported no long-term facial nerve complications with FABF harvest [17, 18]. Special considerations for the oral cavity donor site include the development of trismus and the transfer of oral cavity flora to the skull base.

Occipital Galeo-pericranial Flap

The occipital galeo-pericranial flap (OGPF) is a pedicled flap based on the occipital artery [13, 14, 19]. There have been several uses of this flap in the head and neck region; however, there is only one cadaveric study reported in the literature for its use in anterior skull base reconstruction [20]. The authors found that the OGPF was able to provide complete coverage of the anterior skull base in all the specimens. The mean pedicle length was found to be 8 cm, and surface areas up to 44 cm^2 (11 cm long × 4 cm wide) were harvested.

Fig. 19.10 Transposition of the facial artery buccinator flap onto the anterior skull base [17]. Black arrows, facial artery; white arrows, flap inset on the anterior skull base; white circle, sphenoid sinus; black square, nasopharynx; black diamond, frontal sinus

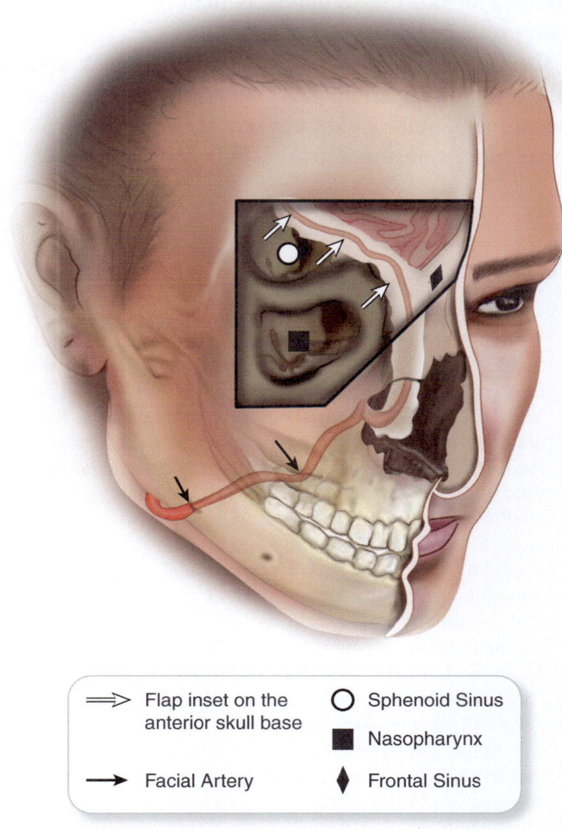

An incision is made along the anterior border of the sternocleidomastoid (SCM) muscle and then continued postero-superiorly to the midportion of the ipsilateral occipital scalp. The attachment of several neck muscles (SCM, splenius capitis, longissimus capitis) is transected just below the mastoid process. This exposes the vascular pedicle which is then dissected postero-superiorly until the occipital scalp is reached. The galea is then exposed by raising subcutaneous (supragaleal) skin flaps until adequate surface area is obtained. The flap design is centered on the vascular pedicle and the galeoperiosteum incised and elevated in a subperiosteal plane. Once the flap is elevated, transposition occurs through a transparapharyngeal/transpterygoid tunnel. This tunnel is bluntly dissected in the neck and then connected to the sinonasal cavity by performing a wide maxillary antrostomy with posterior medial maxillectomy. Ligation of the vascular structures in the pterygopalatine fossa and the removal of the inferior aspect of the pterygoid plates are necessary to open the corridor to the sinonasal cavity. Percutaneous tracheostomy dilators are then used from the neck into the nasal cavity to dilate this tunnel until the flap can be delivered into the nasal cavity. The skull base defect is then repaired and the donor site closed per surgeon preference.

Complications include injury to critical neck structures (e.g., cranial nerves, vascular injury, inadvertent pharyngeal entry), as well as flap compromise. Even though several neck muscles are transected, some authors have noted no significant functional deficits postoperatively [20].

References

1. Wolfe SA. The utility of pericranial flaps. Ann Plast Surg. 1978;1:147–53.
2. Safavi-Abbasi S, Komune N, Archer JB, et al. Surgical anatomy and utility of pedicled vascularized tissue flaps for multilayered repair of skull base defects. J Neurosurg. 2016;125(2):419–30.
3. Yano T, Tanaka K, Kishimoto S, Iida H, Okazaki M. Reliability of and indications for pericranial flaps in anterior skull base reconstruction. J Craniofac Surg. 2011;22(2):482–5.
4. Patel MR, Shah RV, Snyderman CH, et al. Pericranial flap for endoscopic skull-base reconstruction: clinical outcomes and radioanatomic analysis of preoperative planning. Neurosurgery. 2010;66(3):506–12.
5. Gode S, Lieber S, Nakassa AC, et al. Clinical experience with secondary endoscopic reconstruction of clival defects with extracranial pericranial flaps. J Neuro Surg B. 2019;80:276–82.
6. Zanation AM, Snyderman CH, Carrau RL, Kassam AB, Gardner PA, Prevedello DM. Minimally invasive endoscopic pericranial flap: a new method for endonasal skull base reconstruction. Laryngoscope. 2009;119(01):13–8.
7. Majer J, Herman P, Verillaud B. "Mailbox Slot" pericranial flap for endoscopic skull base reconstruction. Laryngoscope. 2016;126(8):1736–8.
8. Patel MR, Stadler ME, Snyderman CH, et al. How to choose? Endoscopic skull base reconstruction options and limitations. Skull Base. 2010;20(6):397–404.
9. Ferrari M, Vural A, Schreiber A, Mattavelli D, Gualtieri T, Taboni S, Bertazzoni G, Rampinelli V, Tomasoni M, Buffoli B, Doglietto F, Rodella LF, Deganello A, Nicolai P. Side-door temporoparietal fascia flap: a novel strategy for anterior skull base reconstruction. World Neurosurg. 2019;126:e360–70. https://doi.org/10.1016/j.wneu.2019.02.056. Epub 2019 Feb 27. PMID: 30822581.
10. Fortes FS, Carrau RL, Snyderman CH, Kassam A, Prevedello D, Vescan A, Mintz A, Gardner P. Transpterygoid transposition of a temporoparietal fascia flap: a new method for skull base reconstruction after endoscopic expanded endonasal approaches. Laryngoscope. 2007;117(6):970–6. https://doi.org/10.1097/MLG.0b013e3180471482. PMID: 17417106.
11. Bolzoni Villaret A, Nicolai P, Schreiber A, Bizzoni A, Farina D, Tschabitscher M. The temporo-parietal fascial flap in extended transnasal endoscopic procedures: cadaver dissection and personal clinical experience. Eur Arch Otorhinolaryngol. 2013;270(4):1473–9. https://doi.org/10.1007/s00405-012-2187-0. Epub 2012 Sep 21. PMID: 22996083.
12. Patel R, Buchmann LO, Hunt J. The use of the temporoparietal fascial flap in preventing CSF leak after lateral skull base surgery. J Neurol Surg B Skull Base. 2013;74(5):311–6. https://doi.org/10.1055/s-0033-1349059. Epub 2013 Jun 24. PMID: 24436930; PMCID: PMC3774827.
13. Clavenna MJ, Turner JH, Chandra RK. Pedicled flaps in endoscopic skull base reconstruction: review of current techniques. Curr Opin Otolaryngol Head Neck Surg. 2015;23(1):71–7. https://doi.org/10.1097/MOO.0000000000000115. PMID: 25415749.
14. Kim GG, Hang AX, Mitchell CA, Zanation AM. Pedicled extranasal flaps in skull base reconstruction. Adv Otorhinolaryngol. 2013;74:71–80. https://doi.org/10.1159/000342282. Epub 2012 Dec 18. PMID: 23257554; PMCID: PMC3568756.

15. Rastatter JC, Walz PC, Alden TD. Pediatric skull base reconstruction: case report of a tunneled temporoparietal fascia flap. J Neurosurg Pediatr PED. 2016;17(3):371–7. Retrieved Jan 29, 2022.
16. Oliver CL, Hackman TG, Carrau RL, Snyderman CH, Kassam AB, Prevedello DM, Gardner P. Palatal flap modifications allow pedicled reconstruction of the skull base. Laryngoscope. 2008;118(12):2102–6. https://doi.org/10.1097/MLG.0b013e318184e719. PMID: 19029856.
17. Rivera-Serrano CM, Oliver CL, Sok J, Prevedello DM, Gardner P, Snyderman CH, Kassam AB, Carrau RL. Pedicled facial buccinator (FAB) flap: a new flap for reconstruction of skull base defects. Laryngoscope. 2010;120(10):1922–30. https://doi.org/10.1002/lary.21049. PMID: 20824643.
18. Farzal Z, Lemos-Rodriguez AM, Rawal RB, Overton LJ, Sreenath SB, Patel MR, Zanation AM. The reverse-flow facial artery buccinator flap for skull base reconstruction: key anatomical and technical considerations. J Neurol Surg B Skull Base. 2015;76(6):432–9. https://doi.org/10.1055/s-0035-1551669. Epub 2015 Jun 1. PMID: 26682122; PMCID: PMC4671905.
19. Patel MR, Taylor RJ, Hackman TG, Germanwala AV, Sasaki-Adams D, Ewend MG, Zanation AM. Beyond the nasoseptal flap: outcomes and pearls with secondary flaps in endoscopic endonasal skull base reconstruction. Laryngoscope. 2014;124(4):846–52. https://doi.org/10.1002/lary.24319. Epub 2014 Jan 15. PMID: 23877996.
20. Rivera-Serrano CM, Snyderman CH, Carrau RL, Durmaz A, Gardner PA. Transparapharyngeal and transpterygoid transposition of a pedicled occipital galeopericranial flap: a new flap for skull base reconstruction. Laryngoscope. 2011;121(5):914–22. https://doi.org/10.1002/lary.21376. PMID: 21520102.

Chapter 20
Free Flap Reconstruction of Anterior Skull Base Defects

Ashley Lonergan and Tjoson Tjoa

Anterior skull base surgery can present challenges to both ablative and reconstructive surgeons due to the complex regional anatomy and lack of surgical space. Historically, open approaches to the anterior skull base often resulted in high rates of morbidity and mortality [1]. Over the past two decades, technological advances in preoperative imaging and intraoperative monitoring have increased the safety and efficacy of these surgeries. Additionally, with improved collaboration and innovation within the fields of both neurosurgery and otolaryngology, more aggressive approaches via minimally invasive endoscopic endonasal surgery have broadened the indications for anterior skull base procedures [2]. As these indications have expanded, ablative surgery of the anterior skull base has allowed for more radical tumor extirpation, resulting in increasingly larger and more complex defects.

A combination of noncellular materials and local flaps are standardly used in anterior skull base surgery and are very effective for limited skull base resections. These include manufactured alloplastic materials and avascular grafts such as fascia lata grafts, in addition to local and regional pedicled flaps such as turbinate flaps, temporalis flaps, nasoseptal pedicled flaps, and pericranial flaps—the latter two being the accepted standard for the majority of such defects [3, 4]. However, many ablative procedures for the anterior skull base involve structures outside of the sinonasal cavity and include large volumes of tissue loss requiring reconstruction, often with a variety of tissue types. Open skull base reconstruction with free tissue transfer continues to be performed, particularly for larger malignant tumors and composite defects, as well as for major craniofacial trauma, osteoradionecrosis, and failed prior endoscopic reconstruction [4]. Additionally, in patients with prior radiation or expected postoperative radiation, there is significant fibrosis and decreased vascularization of the area [5]. Free tissue transfer has been shown to more effectively

A. Lonergan · T. Tjoa (✉)
University of California Irvine Medical Center, Orange, CA, USA
e-mail: tjoat@hs.uci.edu

E. C. Kuan et al. (eds.), *Skull Base Reconstruction*,
https://doi.org/10.1007/978-3-031-27937-9_20

prevent intracranial complications than local and regional flaps, which may be due to the fact that the distal portion of pedicled flaps with the most precarious blood supply is often placed at the most critical portion of the reconstruction site [6]. When indicated free tissue transfer is uniquely suited for composite and extensive reconstruction of the anterior skull base, particularly in the case of the irradiated field [7].

This chapter discusses the use of free tissue transfer in the reconstruction of anterior skull base defects. Critical to this is an understanding of the goals of reconstruction, the relevant regional anatomy, and the techniques to limit complications.

Anatomic Considerations and Defect Classification

The anterior skull base comprises the base of the anterior cranial fossa. By definition, ablative defects in this region allow for communication between the sterile intracranial space and the inherently contaminated mucosal spaces of the nasal cavity, paranasal sinuses, and nasopharynx. The anterior skull base is a narrow and deep space with the thin basal dura tightly attached to the bone superiorly and the sinonasal mucosa closely adherent inferiorly. The frontal and ethmoid sinuses as well as the cribriform plate, olfactory nerve, and orbital roof are adjacent. These factors make reconstruction of the skull base both critical and challenging.

There are also several neurovascular structures that traverse the bony skeleton of the anterior cranial fossa. The foramen cecum anteriorly transmits venous drainage from the nose to the superior sagittal sinus, and the anterior and posterior ethmoid arteries are often included in the ablative defect. The orbital contents lead into the optic canal and superior and inferior orbital fissures, transmitting cranial nerves II, III, IV, VI, VI, and the ophthalmic artery and vein towards the cavernous sinus [4]. The involvement of these structures as they traverse into the middle cranial fossa often defines the limit of the anterior cranial base resections.

Prior to pr oceeding with reconstruction, it can be helpful to characterize the type and extent of the defect in order to guide flap selection. There have been several defect classification schemes proposed for the anterior skull base. The earliest attempt at classifying skull base defects was by Urken et al. in 1993, who described 26 patients who underwent skull base reconstruction [8]. They described seven major defect categories to consider in reconstruction, including (1) dura, (2) bone, (3) cutaneous, (4) mucosal, (5) cavity, (6) neurologic, and (7) carotid artery. Consideration of each of these categories was critical in planning reconstruction and limiting complications. In 1994, Irish et al. proposed three anatomical regions of the skull base according to common tumor growth patterns and surgical approaches for resection, primarily to provide direction regarding the surgical approach required for tumor resection. The first of these regions was the area from the clivus to the foramen magnum, defined as the anterior skull base [9]. This area includes the frontal bone, ethmoid bone, and the planum sphenoidale and anterior clinoid process of the sphenoid bone.

Califano et al. divided anterior skull base resections into simple, complex, and other as an indicator of anatomic complexity and corresponding need for more complex reconstruction [10]. Simple resections included the local area of skull base adjacent to tumor with partial palatectomy *or* partial resection of orbital contents. Complex resections encompassed those that (1) included the local area of skull base adjacent to the tumor and dura and/or brain; (2) resections that included local skull base, orbital contents, *and* the palate together; and (3) those resections that included the local area of skull base, the orbital contents, and another major anatomic structure together. Other types of anterior cranial fossa resections include the skull base as well as a single additional major structure other than the dura, brain, palate, or orbital contents. Free tissue transfer reconstruction was significantly associated with complex defects such as these. Another way to categorize these defects requiring free tissue transfer is based on anatomic location and loss of volume, support, and skin coverage. Resected structures are further subdivided into central and/or lateral components, which can involve any combination of the dura, brain, orbital contents, nasal cavity, palate, and frontal tables (Fig. 20.1) [11]. Reconstructive soft tissue requirements for these structures can be bony, cutaneous, and mucosal, or any combination of the three.

Due to the complex three-dimensional anatomy of the anterior skull base and varied nature of the defects, it has been difficult to translate any of these classification schemes directly into an algorithmic approach to reconstruction. However,

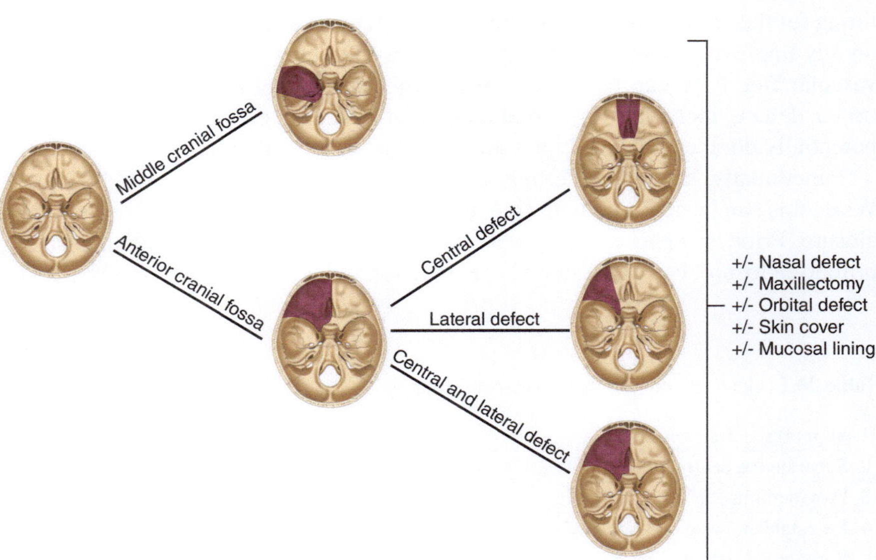

Fig. 20.1 Classification of skull base defects (adapted from Pusic et al. [11]). Categorizing anterior skull base defects based on anatomic location (central versus lateral) and loss of volume, support, and skin coverage can help determine reconstructive requirements

consideration of the regional anatomy and complexity of structures resected can help guide the soft tissue requirements and geometric needs of the reconstruction.

Goals of Reconstruction

The most critical goal of anterior skull base reconstruction following ablative surgery is the durable and vital separation of intracranial from extracranial contents. As Urken stated [8]:

> The protection afforded to the central nervous system is unique in the human body. It is the surgeon's responsibility to duplicate the protection afforded by natural evolution when it has been violated by trauma or an ablative procedure.

This protection is the primary reason why free tissue transfer was initially used in anterior skull base reconstruction and why it provides an advantage over local and pedicled flaps in certain patients. Successful separation of the central nervous system from the sinonasal cavity results in sealing off cerebrospinal fluid (CSF) from the upper aerodigestive tract, preventing pneumocephalus and ascending infections such as meningitis, encephalitis, or abscesses [3]. Additional aims of skull base reconstruction include support for intracranial contents and orbit when inferior bony support has been resected; reduction in dead space; and restoration of craniofacial contour and function [6]. Functionally, re-establishing and providing lining for the nasal cavity and separating it from the oral cavity and oropharynx can greatly improve patients' quality of life postoperatively (Table 20.1). While microvascular free flaps can be used to reconstruct nearly any anterior skull base soft tissue defect, including any combination of mucosa, cartilage, calvarium, and potentially dura, certain principles are important to keep in mind.

Functionally, layered, watertight closures are paramount to seal off CSF leaks. While this can be achieved with free tissue alone, it is often aided with a multilayer closure. Prior to repair with any vascularized flaps, dural defects not amenable to primary closure can and should be repaired with free fascial grafts, bovine

Table 20.1 Goals of anterior skull base reconstruction

1. Support the brain and orbit
2. Separate the central nervous system from the upper aerodigestive tract
3. Provide lining for the nasal cavity
4. Re-establish nasal and oral cavities
5. Provide volume to eliminate dead space
6. Restore the three-dimensional contour of the maxillofacial bony and soft tissue structures

pericardium, or allograft materials such as DuraGen (Integra LifeSciences), AlloDerm (Allergan), and DuraSeal (Integra LifeSciences) [4, 12]. Bony defects that could predispose the brain to herniation can be grafted with split calvarial bone grafts or free rib grafts [13]. Additionally, pedicled turbinate and nasoseptal flaps—as well as regional pedicled flaps such as the galeal or pericranial flap and temporo-parietal fascial flap—can be used as a second layer and are effective for many skull base reconstructions [4]. In fact, in one series, vascularized free tissue transfer reconstruction was used in combination with pedicled flaps in almost half (48%) of the patients [10]. This highlights the critical need for a safe reconstruction related to compromise of the intracranial space, with a "belt and suspenders" approach to minimizing complications in these patients.

Additional reconstructive techniques can also assist in restoring contour and morphology to structures of the face. Once the dura is sealed, small bony defects can be repaired using either a split calvarial bone graft or the inner table of the frontal sinus, if uninvolved with tumor or previously radiated [14]. Septal bone and rib grafts have also been described [12]. For defects of the orbital rim or other structurally supportive areas, titanium mesh is well suited. It can be shaped to restore contour and can help provide support to prevent meningoencephalocele. In rare cases where orbital floor is resected, but the globe and extraocular muscles are spared, a tensor fascia lata sling can be harvested from the thigh and used to support the orbital contents. For patients who have been radiated or are planned for radiation postoperatively, it is critical that these non-vascularized reconstructive options (like bone grafts and titanium) are covered with abundant tissue when the free flap is inset to avoid extrusion and infection.

Reconstructive Technique and Tissue Selection

With most major anterior skull base resections requiring free tissue transfer reconstruction, a multiple-team approach is utilized. Whenever possible, simultaneous harvesting of the free flap during the extirpation and preparation of the wound bed is recommended. After ablation, the neurosurgical team often repairs the dural defect, and the ablative team creates a subcutaneous tunnel for the flap vessels. The margins of the bony defect can be trimmed with a rongeur or Kerrison or drilled down to avoid bony spurs that can irritate or kink the flap pedicle. Copious irrigation with sterile saline should be performed to limit the chance of infection.

As with any microvascular flap, a well-supported blood supply is of utmost importance at the level of the anterior skull base. Several case series describe the superficial temporal vessels as preferred donor vessels [15–18]. These have the advantage of being close to the soft tissue inset, which can be three-dimensionally complex, allowing for a shorter pedicle length for the free flap. They can also be readily accessed through a small preauricular incision or an inferior extension of the coronal incision in cases that require an open approach. The superficial temporal artery lies between the galea and subcutaneous layers, so careful dissection is required during coronal flap elevation to avoid vessel injury. The disadvantage of the superficial temporal vessels is that where they are most easily accessible, their diameter is often smaller than that of branches of other donor vessels in the neck. Thus, they must often be dissected proximally, frequently inferior to the zygomatic arch where they course deeper into the substance of the parotid gland. Other institutions often extend the preauricular incision into a skin crease in the neck or make a separate neck incision to access the cervical branches of the external carotid artery [19]. These vessels include the facial artery and vein, the lingual artery, the superior thyroid artery, and the external jugular vein. These vessels are often used as donor vessels in the microvascular reconstruction of other head and neck ablative defects, so the reconstructive team may be more familiar with their dissection. They are also typically larger caliber than the distal superficial temporal vessels. Using the internal jugular vein has the added benefit of providing a means for side-to-side rather than the end-to-end anastomosis required of the other venous options. It is important to keep donor vessel availability in mind when designing the free flap skin paddle, as the placement of the skin paddle relative to the flap vessels during harvest can affect vessel length and ultimately flap maneuverability and survival.

Radial Forearm Free Flap

A commonly performed flap in head and neck reconstruction, the radial forearm free flap (RFFF), receives its blood supply from the radial artery (with its fasciocutaneous perforators) and venae comitantes draining into the cephalic vein [8]. It is most commonly harvested as a thin fasciocutaneous flap but has also been described as an adipofascial flap in anterior skull base reconstruction [19]. It can additionally be raised to include about one-third of the diameter of the radius as an osseocutaneous flap. The benefit of the RFFF in anterior skull base reconstruction lies in its thinness, pliability, and long vessel length, which make it a very versatile flap for geometrically complex defects. It has been particularly useful as a substitute for the pericranial flap in patients who have had prior surgery or radiation and is the preferred flap for closing isolated recalcitrant CSF leaks [12, 20]. For those defects, a portion of the skin paddle can be de-epithelialized and folded upon itself to help decrease the dead space above the flap. If accessible, several drill holes can be placed circumferentially around the bony skull base defect in order to suspend the flap with sutures. However, even when access is limited, the radial forearm free flap is often thin enough to be inset endoscopically, which has been described in isolated case series, particularly when raised as an adipofascial flap [19]. When harvested as a large fasciocutaneous flap, the skin paddle can be used to both reconstruct the skull base and be folded to line an orbital exenteration cavity, which make it an ideal reconstructive option for patients considering prosthetic rehabilitation in the future.

The biggest limitation of the RFFF is the limited surface area and volume of the flap, making it unsuitable for resurfacing larger defects. Postoperative hand ischemia is a well-known but rare postoperative complication of this flap. A preoperative Allen's test to confirm adequate collateral supply from the ipsilateral ulnar artery can often but not entirely rule out future compromise after radial artery resection. Nonetheless, postoperative functional deficits are typically minor, particularly when the nondominant arm is selected [21].

Anterolateral Thigh Free Flap

The anterolateral thigh (ALT) free flap is a perforator flap that can supply a larger skin paddle than the radial forearm free flap, deriving its vascular supply from the lateral femoral circumflex artery. Typically, this artery is accompanied by a pair of venae comitantes which coalesce at the level of the profunda femoral vein. Additionally, the flap can be harvested with tensor fascia lata for morphologic reconstruction and vascularized vastus lateralis muscle to help fill dead space and seal leaks [9, 11]. The ALT skin paddle typically has a thicker layer of subcutaneous fat than the RFFF, which can help fill contour in larger-volume defects like those seen with maxillectomies. The trade-off, however, is that the ALT vascular pedicle in its entirety can only be as long as 7–8 cm depending on patient anatomy, which is slightly shorter than the radial forearm free flap pedicle. This can be a problem in the vessel-depleted patient.

Limitations of the ALT flap include minimal donor site dysfunction, which has been correlated to the amount of damage suffered by the vastus lateralis. Removal of large portions of musculocutaneous tissue can limit range of motion at the hip and knee. The rectus femoris muscle's blood supply can also become compromised by vessel harvest, adding to reduction in mobility and increasing morbidity [12]. Overall, however, the ALT donor site morbidity is very low, and early ambulation is well tolerated [22].

Rectus Abdominis Free Flap

For the most significant complex defects of the anterior skull base, bulky soft tissue is often required to create contour and fill dead space. The rectus abdominis myocutaneous free flap can provide both adequate skin coverage and nasal lining as well as the requisite bulk needed for these extensive defects. It is an excellent option for defects involving both orbital and palatal tissue, as a large skin paddle can be reliably harvested and placed vertically into the orbit and de-epithelialized and folded into the mouth for palatal reconstruction. Its robust blood supply can be a boon in the case of irradiated patients who rely heavily on revascularization [13]. The loss of innervation of the muscle itself will cause the flap to reduce in size, but the frequently thick subcutaneous adipose tissue will allow the flap to retain much of its bulk.

Like the RFFF and the ALT flaps, this flap can be harvested simultaneously to the ablative portion of the procedure. It can be harvested with or without an overlying skin paddle. The vascular pedicle consists of the deep inferior epigastric artery and vein with musculocutaneous perforators; these perforators are found within the anterior rectus sheath, and thus this must be included as the flap is lifted. The tendinous attachments and inscriptions are useful for suture placement during insetting [10].

The disadvantages of the rectus abdominus flap include the possibility of abdominal wall hernia, wound dehiscence, and seroma or hematoma after closure. This can be minimized using meticulous donor site closure, including closure of both the internal and external oblique aponeurosis as well as tacking the undermined skin flaps down to the rectus aponeurosis to close off dead space. Postoperative pain can be increased with this donor site relative to others as well.

Latissimus Dorsi Free Flap

Similar to the rectus abdominus flap, the latissimus dorsi flap is a myocutaneous flap best suited for large defects including complex orbito-palatal defects. Its blood supply arises from the thoracodorsal artery and vein [14]. In certain cases, this flap can be used in a pedicled fashion; however, the distance to the recipient defect in anterior skull base cases poses a challenge for both pedicle length and avoidance of vascular congestion. Therefore, the latissimus is more commonly used for free tissue transfer. It has typically a straightforward harvest with large-caliber vessels and up to 16 cm of vessel length [23]. Loss of shoulder mobility on the donor side must be weighed with the reconstructive need [15]. Unlike the RFFF, ALT, and rectus flaps, the latissimus flap is raised in the lateral decubitus position and cannot be raised simultaneously to the ablation. The back also tends to have a smaller volume of subcutaneous fat than the abdomen, so much of the bulk of the latissimus flap is contributed by the muscle, which undergoes atrophy and can lead to dead space and poor contour in the long term [12].

Subscapular System

Upfront osseocutaneous free flap reconstruction is rarely reported in the literature for reconstruction of anterior skull base defects [8, 9, 11]. Soft tissue flaps lend themselves to various geometries with their ease of configuration. When the bone is required for reconstruction, often secondary bone grafting of the facial skeleton is performed in a delayed fashion. However, as stated in the goals of reconstruction, the most critical aim of anterior skull base reconstruction is separation of the intracranial space from the extracranial space with a watertight seal. Due to the frequent complexity of the relationships between bony defects and epithelial surfaces required for reconstruction, the ideal bony reconstruction is often not possible when the primary goal is to seal off the intracranial space.

In rare instances, however, where a bone defect is required with little need for a complicated soft tissue inset, the subscapular system and the scapular bone provide a good option. This system allows for a variety of chimeric tissue options, including the scapula bone, latissimus muscle, serratus muscle, and skin. Additionally, due to separate pedicles, the flap offers the greatest freedom of movement between the soft tissue and bony components, which allows it to be more flexible in its geometry relative to the fibula free flap. One of the downsides of this system is the short pedicle length that results when the bone is harvested based on the circumflex scapular branch of the subscapular artery. This can be circumvented by harvesting the scapular tip bone based off the angular artery, which provides several centimeters of additional pedicle length. However, in the vast majority of cases, it is prudent to prioritize the primary life-threatening goal of protecting the central nervous system from leak and contamination over the secondary goals of morphology and contour. This results in staged reconstructions of the bone rather than composite reconstructions.

Postoperative Considerations

In cases where anti-gravity support is required, resorbable nasal packing placed lightly into the nasal cavity is sufficient. For bulkier reconstructions, a shortened nasal trumpet can be placed to stent the nasal cavity open. For postoperative monitoring of free flaps, if a skin paddle is easily accessible, pinpricking with a 25-gauge needle or transcutaneous Doppler of perforator vessels is used to ascertain viability. For isolated cribriform plate reconstructions without a visible skin paddle, an implantable Doppler can be used for continuous monitoring. For infection prevention, many institutions utilize standard postoperative antibiotics and continuous nasal irrigation with a suction system for several days postoperatively. A lumbar drain can keep intracranial pressure from exerting force on the suture line, and elevation of the head of bed at 30° can be helpful.

Outcomes and Limitations

The incidence of major local and/or systemic postoperative complications following microvascular free flap reconstruction of the skull base ranges from 30 to 60% in most large published series [8, 10, 16]. Early complications (occurring <28 days postoperatively) include partial or total flap loss, CSF leak, hematoma, myocardial infarction, and deep vein thrombosis. Late complications (>28 days) consist of palatal fistula, delayed wound healing or wound infection, meningitis, intracranial abscess, infected hardware, ectropion, enophthalmos, and persistent diplopia [21]. As with any major head and neck reconstruction, free flap reconstruction at the anterior skull base has risks associated with continuity with the intracranial and oral cavities. CSF leak, pneumocephalus, stroke, intracranial abscess, and vascular compromise comprise the most significant challenges in the immediate postoperative period. Wound complications and delayed infection can occur late. Medical comorbidities and prior treatment with radiation therapy are statistically significant predictors of wound complications. Significant risk factors for CNS complications include prior radiation therapy, dural invasion of the tumor, and brain invasion [1]. Infection prevention can be effectively achieved with perioperative antibiotics and should be employed for all patients with gauze packing or implantable hardware. Mortality has been estimated at roughly 5%, with increased risk seen in patients above 50 years of age—with multiple medical comorbidities being an independent factor [16].

Despite advances in technique, the mortality risk and complication rate have remained stable in light of the ability to perform more aggressive resections [17, 24]. Free flap reconstruction, however, remains the best option for large craniofacial defects in the appropriate patient and provides the microvascular surgeon a greater versatility in flap selection and reconstructive outcome.

References

1. Ganly I, Patel SG, Singh B, et al. Complications of craniofacial resection for malignant tumors of the skull base: report of an international collaborative study. Head Neck. 2005;27:445–51.
2. Bell EB, Cohen ER, Sargi Z, Leibowitz J. Free tissue reconstruction of the anterior skull base: a review. World J Otorhinolaryngol Head Neck Surg. 2020;6(2):132–6.
3. Patel MR, Stadler ME, Snyderman CH, Carrau RL, Kassam AB, Germanwala AV, Gardner P, Zanation AM. How to choose? Endoscopic skull base reconstructive options and limitations. Skull Base. 2010;20(6):397–404.
4. Kwon D, Iloreta A, Miles B, Inman J. Open anterior skull base reconstruction: a contemporary review. Semin Plast Surg. 2017;31(4):189–96.
5. Chang DW, Langstein HN, Gupta A, De Monte F, Do KA, Wang X, Robb G. Reconstructive management of cranial base defects after tumor ablation. Plast Reconstr Surg. 2001;107(6):1346–55; discussion 1356–7.
6. Neligan PC, Mulholland S, Irish J, et al. Flap selection in cranial base reconstruction. Plast Reconstr Surg. 1996;98:1159–66; discussion 1167–8.
7. Luu Q, Farwell D. Microvascular free flap reconstruction of anterior skull base defects. Oper Tech Otolaryngol Head Neck Surg. 2010;21:91–5.
8. Urken ML, Catalano PJ, Sen C, Post K, Futran N, Biller HF. Free tissue transfer for skull base reconstruction analysis of complications and a classification scheme for defining skull base defects. Arch Otolaryngol Head Neck Surg. 1993;119(12):1318–25.
9. Irish JC, Gullane PJ, Gentili F, et al. Tumors of the skull base: outcome and survival analysis of 77 cases. Head Neck. 1994;16(1):3–10.
10. Califano J, Cordeiro PG, Disa JJ, Hidalgo DA, DuMornay W, Bilsky MH, Gutin PH, Shah JP, Kraus DH. Anterior cranial base reconstruction using free tissue transfer: changing trends. Head Neck. 2003;25(2):89–96.
11. Pusic AL, Chen CM, Patel S, Cordeiro PG, Shah JP. Microvascular reconstruction of the skull base: a clinical approach to surgical defect classification and flap selection. Skull Base. 2007;17(1):5–15.

12. Schmalbach CE, Webb DE, Weitzel EK. Anterior skull base reconstruction: a review of current techniques. Curr Opin Otolaryngol Head Neck Surg. 2010;18:238–43.
13. Cantù G, Solero CL, Pizzi N, Nardo L, Mattavelli F. Skull base reconstruction after anterior craniofacial resection. J Craniomaxillofac Surg. 1999;27(4):228–34.
14. Gil Z, Abergel A, Leider-Trejo L, Khafif A, Margalit N, Amir A, Gur E, Fliss DM. A comprehensive algorithm for anterior skull base reconstruction after oncological resections. Skull Base. 2007;17(1):25–37.
15. Georgantopoulou A, Hodgkinson PD, Gerber CJ. Cranial-base surgery: a reconstructive algorithm. Br J Plast Surg. 2003;56:10–3.
16. Hanasono MM, Silva A, Skoracki RJ, Gidley PW, DeMonte F, Hanna EY, et al. Skull base reconstruction: an updated approach. Plast Reconstr Surg. 2011;128:675–86.
17. Kim SH, Lee WJ, Chang JH, Moon JH, Kang SG, Kim CH, Hong JW. Anterior skull base reconstruction using an anterolateral thigh free flap. Arch Craniofac Surg. 2021;22(5):232–8.
18. Chiu ES, Kraus D, Bui DT, Mehrara BJ, Disa JJ, Bilsky M, Shah JP, Cordeiro PG. Anterior and middle cranial fossa skull base reconstruction using microvascular free tissue techniques: surgical complications and functional outcomes. Ann Plast Surg. 2008;60(5):514–20.
19. Dang RP, Ettyreddy AR, Rizvi Z, Doering M, Mazul AL, Zenga J, Jackson RS, Pipkorn P. Free Flap Reconstruction of the Anterior Skull Base: A Systematic Review. Journal of Neurological Surgery, Part B: Skull Base, 2022;83(2):125–32.
20. Weber SM, Kim J, Delashaw JB, Wax MK. Radial forearm free tissue transfer in the management of persistent cerebrospinal fluid leaks. Laryngoscope. 2005;115(6):968–72.
21. Herr MW, Lin DT. Microvascular free flaps in skull base reconstruction. Adv Otorhinolaryngol. 2013;74:81–91.
22. Hanasono MM, Skoracki RJ, Yu P. Donor-site morbidity after anterolateral thigh fasciocutaneous and myocutaneous free flap harvest in 220 patients. Plast Reconstr Surg. 2010;125:209–14.
23. Valentini V, Fabiani F, Nicolai G, Torroni A, Gennaro P, Marianetti TM, Iannetti G. Use of microvascular free flaps in the reconstruction of the anterior and middle skull base. J Craniofac Surg. 2006;17(4):790–6.
24. Teknos TN, Smith JC, Day TA, et al. Microvascular free tissue transfer in reconstructing skull base defects: lessons learned. Laryngoscope. 2002;112:1871–6.

Chapter 21
Reconstruction of Frontal and Ethmoid Defects

Mark A. Arnold, Emily M. Barrow, and Joshua M. Levy

Introduction

Anterior skull base reconstruction has undergone significant development over the past few decades. Today, skull base reconstruction is an interdisciplinary specialty, and a variety of approaches are available to the skull base team. While many defects of the frontal and ethmoid region can be addressed by transnasal endoscopic approaches, challenging cases may require endoscopic-assisted or traditional external approaches. The anatomy and pathology of this region are variable and complex, necessitating individualized surgical plans.

Obliteration

Prior to the advent of endoscopic techniques, chronic frontal sinusitis was a difficult-to-treat disease. As surgeons were unable to maintain patency of the frontal sinus outflow tract, most frontal sinus procedures carried a high complication rate of infection. Montgomery popularized obliteration in the 1960s to treat recalcitrant frontal sinusitis [1]. Frontal sinus obliteration is defined by eliminating the frontal sinus cavity while maintaining the anterior and posterior tables. Obliteration is usually accomplished by raising an osteoplastic flap consisting of the anterior table. Following this, all frontal sinus mucosa is meticulously removed, and the dead space is replaced with filler material. The shape of the frontal sinus is maintained,

M. A. Arnold (✉) · E. M. Barrow · J. M. Levy
Department of Otolaryngology-Head and Neck Surgery, Emory University School of Medicine, Atlanta, GA, USA
e-mail: Emily.barrow@emory.edu; joshua.levy2@emory.edu

E. C. Kuan et al. (eds.), *Skull Base Reconstruction*,
https://doi.org/10.1007/978-3-031-27937-9_21

while the function is lost. The removal of mucosa aims to prevent future mucocele formation and chronic frontal sinusitis.

Presently, obliteration is less commonly performed for inflammatory conditions. However, there is still a role for obliteration in the setting of endoscopic failure [2]. In addition, patients who have had a previous obliteration may develop mucoceles or chronic sinusitis, necessitating re-obliteration or unobliteration [3]. Occasionally, obliteration may be performed in the setting of traumatic or iatrogenic cerebrospinal fluid (CSF) leaks. However, it is known that most traumatic CSF leaks resolve with conservative management [4]. With persistent posterior table CSF leaks, obliteration is necessary if patency of the frontal outflow tract cannot be maintained. Furthermore, if there is a significant comminution of the posterior table, cranialization is preferable to obliteration.

While spontaneous leaks secondary to idiopathic intracranial hypertension tend to be in the ethmoid cribriform area or lateral recess of the sphenoid sinus, spontaneous leaks of the posterior table are not uncommon [5]. In a 5-year review of 46 CSF leaks, Chabaan et al. noted that 20 patients had spontaneous posterior table leaks. Importantly however, none required frontal sinus obliteration [5]. Today, endoscopic techniques are preferred over obliteration, as they have shown excellent success rates in closing posterior table CSF leaks while maintaining frontal sinus patency [6].

The standard approach for frontal sinus obliteration is the coronal incision, hidden posterior to the hairline of non-balding individuals. A pericranial flap is often raised simultaneously and preserved with the skin flap for later use in reconstruction. Otherwise, pericranium may be left attached to the osteoplastic flap, pedicled inferiorly with a robust blood supply from the supratrochlear and supraorbital arteries. Next, an outline of the limits of the frontal sinus is determined for raising an osteoplastic flap. The margins of the frontal sinus can be judged with a sterile 6-foot Caldwell radiograph, palpation by a wire brought in and out of a frontal sinus trephination, or intraoperative navigation. During bony flap elevation, the frontal intersinus septum is divided, allowing for down fracture of the osteoplastic flap. Removal of the anterior table via osteoplastic flap allows for direct access and removal of mucosa. Drilling is usually necessary for adequate removal of mucosa and creation of a single, smooth frontal cavity [7]. Removing the outer cortex of the bone also provides a bleeding surface necessary for graft revascularization [8, 9].

A variety of materials have been utilized for obliterating the frontal sinus, with varying success. Autologous fat has a long history of use but may risk infection and chronic frontal sinusitis [10]. In addition, surveillance for mucocele formation is more difficult after the frontal sinus has been filled with fat, as they may have similar imaging characteristics (Fig. 21.1). Grafting with bone from the iliac crest had a high 50% complication rate in a series of eight cases [8]. Hydroxyapatite is also commonly used, and placement of the pericranial flap along the floor of the frontal sinus provides an additional barrier to the ethmoid sinuses below [11]. It should be noted, however, that any obliteration has the chance for failure and may occur years

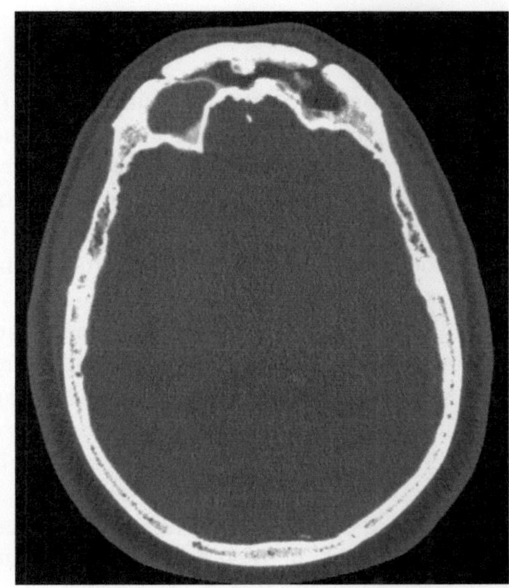

Fig. 21.1 Computed tomography of a 64-year-old male with a history of frontal sinus osteoplastic flap obliteration with autologous fat for trauma 30 years prior. He presented with right forehead pain and mucocele formation posterior to the autologous fat graft. Unobliteration was performed endoscopically via Draf 3

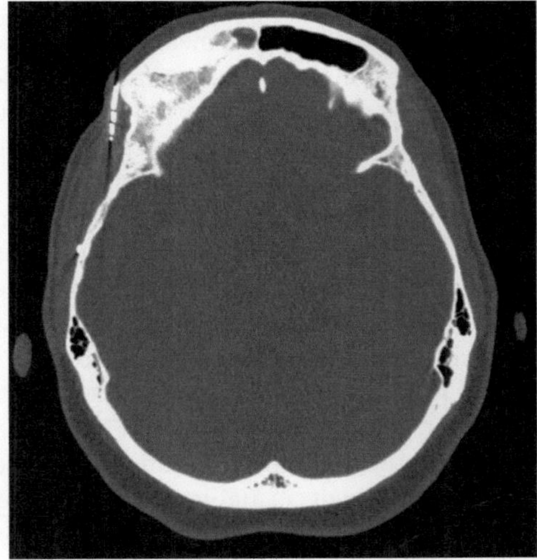

Fig. 21.2 Computed tomography of a right frontal sinus obliteration with calcium hydroxyapatite, presenting with pain and mucocele formation 12 years later. Unobliteration was performed endoscopically via Draf 3, with free mucosal grafting of the frontal sinus anterior table

later to require unobliteration or re-obliteration (Fig. 21.2). Hydroxyapatite, while having a similar complication rate as other materials, carries a higher re-revision rate after initial revision [3]. While obliteration is infrequently performed, for certain patients, it may be the only remaining option. Fortunately, complications from osteoplastic flaps are less common for non-inflammatory pathologies, such as CSF leaks [3].

Cranialization

Cranialization of the frontal sinuses was originally described in 1978 by Donald and Bernstein as a technique to manage traumatic injuries of the posterior table [12]. By removing all sinonasal mucosa, bony overhangs, and the posterior table of the frontal sinus, cranialization allows the frontal lobe to fill in the dead space over the next weeks to months. The frontal sinus is effectively removed, and the frontal sinus outflow tract is sealed off to separate the intracranial space from the nasal cavity.

Although a historic technique, cranialization still has a role in addressing certain frontal and ethmoid defects [13]. Whether from trauma or malignant tumor resection, some defects may be better suited for cranialization. With larger defects involving the posterior table and corresponding dura, conservative management and endoscopic approaches become less reliable in repairing a CSF leak.

Cranialization is usually approached via coronal incision, but existing lacerations may be utilized when present. The posterior table is accessed via craniotomy or osteoplastic flap. With significantly comminuted fractures, large dural defects may also be present, which can be repaired with a pericranial flap, harvested at the time of fracture repair [14]. Bilateral frontal sinus cranialization is recommended over unilateral, as this better allows the brain to fill the dead space [15]. Similarly, any bony ledges should be meticulously drilled smooth with the calvarium. In addition, the frontal sinus outflow tract must be separated from the neo-intracranial space, previously occupied by the frontal sinus. Plugging of the outflow tract can be accomplished with autologous muscle, fascia, fat, or collagen matrices [16]. Failure to completely cranialize the frontal sinuses or adequately plug the outflow tracks may result in persistent pneumocephalus and/or CSF leak (Fig. 21.3). Fortunately, these complications can be successfully managed endoscopically "from below" (Fig. 21.4), avoiding open revision. In three patients with pneumocephalus after cranialization, Soler et al. described the harvesting of the lateral portion of middle turbinate mucosa. The flap was then rotated to cover an autologous fat graft at the frontal recess [17]. Alternatively, if available, a nasoseptal flap can provide generous coverage of the outflow tract (Fig. 21.4).

The complication rate of cranialization has decreased over time; however, they may be significant, including meningitis, persistent CSF leak, osteomyelitis, and mucocele formation [18]. Early in the literature, the rate of meningitis approached 50%, but this has improved to presently around just 2% [19, 20]. These reduced rates stem from many factors, including improved surgical techniques, antibiotic use, and decreasing severity of fractures over time related to seat belt laws and air bags [19].

The decision to proceed with cranialization versus obliteration is multifactorial. Cranialization avoids implanting material that may cause future complications yet requires a craniotomy. In one of the largest retrospective reviews on the topic, a

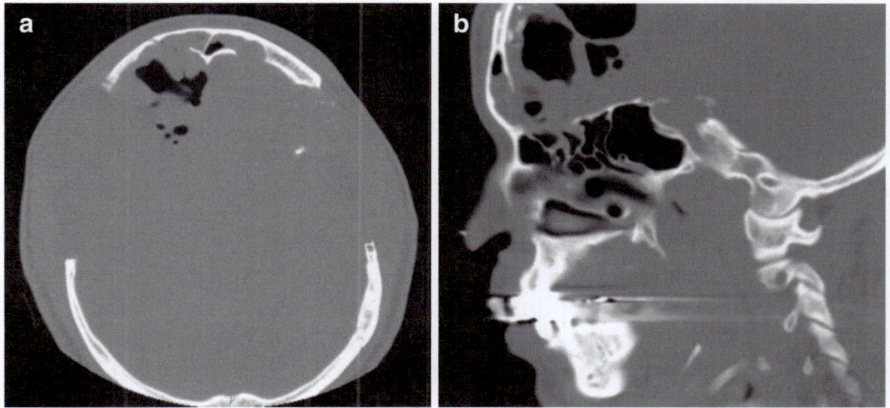

Fig. 21.3 Computed tomography in the axial (**a**) and sagittal (**b**) planes of a 46-year-old male presenting with pneumocephalus after bifrontal craniotomy for a gunshot wound a month prior. The frontal sinuses are partially cranialized, with persistent posterior tables and intersinus septum

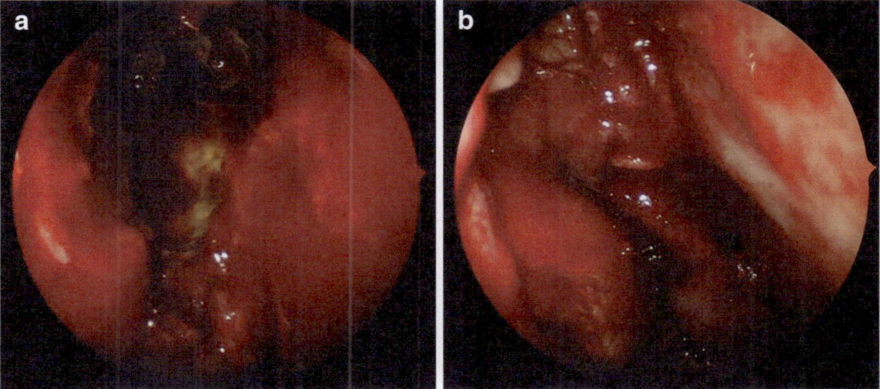

Fig. 21.4 Intraoperative views of patient described in Fig. 21.3. (**a**) Partially cranialized frontal sinus, with posterior table defect with intracranial communication. (**b**) Posterior table defect repaired with autologous abdominal fat graft filling frontal sinus, to be covered by nasoseptal flap

review of 857 patients over a 26-year period by Rodriguez et al. in 2008 found that the rate of significant complications of obliteration with autologous fat was higher at 22% in comparison with cranialization at just 8.4% [18]. However, other studies have demonstrated comparable complication rates of obliteration at 10% [19, 21, 22]. It is important to recognize that these complications also occur with conservative management. Both obliteration and cranialization are performed to reduce the risk of infection and persistent CSF leak.

Direct Repair for Frontal Sinus Posterior Table Defects

Pathology of the posterior table represents one of the most difficult areas for the surgeon to reach. With highly variable frontal sinus pneumatization, certain defects may be unable to be addressed endoscopically. Although one might be able to visualize the defect with an angled endoscope, those that are far superior and lateral within a narrow frontal recess may be impossible to address even with the appropriate angled instrumentation. Furthermore, defects that lie medial and within the narrower portion of the frontal recess also pose a challenge, as repair may compromise the frontal sinus outflow tract. In these cases, obliteration is recommended [23]. While obliteration is possible via trephination, open approaches may result in less mucocele or infectious complications depending on surgeon experience [24].

In these cases, direct repair of the posterior table may be the most appropriate. The approach via coronal incision and raising an osteoplastic flap was previously described in this chapter. Alternatively, the frontal sinus may be approached directly via preexisting lacerations or by concealing the incision within a thick rhytid of a balding male. Furthermore, extensive trauma or prior surgery may preclude the raising of a pericranial flap from a coronal incision, necessitating a direct approach.

Frontal defects arise from various etiologies, including trauma, meningoencephaloceles, dural resection secondary to tumor removal, and iatrogenic injuries. However, it is important to note that they are not managed equally. The management of CSF leaks in posterior table trauma, for example, remains controversial. Historically, these were managed aggressively due to high rates of meningitis. Yet today, with conservative measures including prophylactic antibiotics, head-of-bed elevation, antiemetics, and sinus precautions, most traumatic leaks will resolve. In one series, 85% of 34 patients had resolution of anterior skull base leaks after 1 week [25]. However, there is some retrospective evidence that resolution of posterior table leaks is less successful with conservative management. Chen et al. in 2006 noted that only CSF leakage resolved in only 35% of 26 posterior table fractures [21]. Similarly, Choi et al. in 2012 found that only 6 of 11 patients with posterior table leaks resolved with conservative management [26]. However, the other five were successfully managed with direct repair without obliteration nor cranialization.

Management of the Frontal Recess

For frontal and ethmoid roof defects, the surgeon contends not only with repairing the CSF leak but also with maintaining the patency of the frontal sinus outflow tract. Certainly, this is less important for posterior table defects or other reconstructions that do not overlap with the frontal recess. Fractures of the posterior table rarely occur in isolation, at 1–7%, but are more likely to have a concomitant injury of the frontal recess [19, 27]. Therefore, historically injuries were managed aggressively with cranialization or obliteration to prevent infectious sequelae. Nevertheless, there has been a trend towards managing these injuries conservatively with follow-up imaging to confirm frontal sinus patency [27].

During repair, the frontal recess should be opened as widely as the patient's anatomy allows, ideally greater than 4 mm. A Draf 2B exposes the frontal sinus from the posterior to the anterior table and from the lamina of the orbit to the nasal septum by removing the attachment of the anterior portion of the middle turbinate. This approach provides excellent exposure while minimizing mucosal disruption and postoperative scarring that can occur after frontal drill-out or Draf 3. If there is significant bony exposure, grafting the frontal recess with free mucosal grafts or collagen matrices may reduce postoperative stenosis [28]. However, in patients without preexisting sinus disease, grafting is usually unnecessary.

Stents including Rains self-retaining silicone tube or thin (~1 mm) Silastic sheeting aid in maintaining patency of the frontal sinus while bolstering the reconstruction [29, 30]. Steroid eluting stents may also be considered [31]. Significant packing of the frontal sinus, such as with GelFoam, should be avoided.

After repair, the frontal recess should be monitored closely. Stents are left in place for 4–6 weeks. Intraoperatively, a wide frontal sinusotomy facilitates endoscopic postoperative surveillance. If the frontal recess cannot be visualized or the patient is symptomatic with pressure, pain, or nasal drainage, CT imaging should be performed at 6 weeks to confirm frontal sinus patency.

If a frontal recess injury is managed conservatively or by an open approach, the patency of the outflow tract may not be visualized endoscopically. In the setting of a frontal recess injury managed non-operatively, a 3-month CT is appropriate to confirm frontal sinus patency [32]. Most, over 85%, of frontal recess injuries will undergo spontaneous ventilation [32]. Similarly, imaging should be performed post-craniotomy to surveil for mucocele formation [33].

Endoscopic Approaches

For frontal defects, open approaches with cranialization represent the gold standard in management. Most ethmoid defects, however, including difficult "excavating" meningoencephaloceles, are best suited for endoscopic management [34]. The roughly horizontal plane of the ethmoid anterior skull base is easier to approach endoscopically, while they present a challenge to access via an open approach. Conversely, the transition of the anterior skull base from horizontal to vertical at the posterior table of the frontal sinus may be better addressed "head-on" via an open approach.

Yet, there is emerging evidence that posterior table defects can be managed endoscopically [29]. Purely endoscopic approaches offer significantly less morbidity while maintaining the frontal sinus outflow tract. In 2014, Chaaban et al. reported a 93% success rate in repairing 46 spontaneous CSF leaks, with 20 of these patients having posterior table defects. Bozkurt et al. in 2019 noted that 17 of 54 patients with frontal sinus CSF leaks were repaired with a purely endoscopic approach [35].

Furthermore, the endoscope is poised to manage complications of open approaches. Previously obliterated sinuses may be unobliterated endoscopically [36]. Similarly, a case series of 22 patients with frontal sinus disease after craniotomy were successfully managed endoscopically.

Endoscopic-Assisted Techniques

Despite advances in instrumentation and techniques, certain frontal defects remain difficult to address with a purely endoscopic transnasal approach. In these cases, endoscopic-assisted approaches may improve both visualization and may obviate the need for both a large coronal incision and osteoplastic flap [37]. A brow incision with frontal sinus trephination allows for placement of either instruments or endoscopes to access the far reaches of the frontal sinus [38]. A trephination of 8 mm allows for both a 4 mm endoscope and instrument, termed a "mega-trephination" [39]. Geltzeiler et al. reviewed 64 patients who underwent a mega-trephination. They noted scarring was minimal, and the most common was self-limited paresthesia at 11% [39].

Transorbital neuroendoscopic surgery (TONES) is a relatively novel technique originally described by Moe et al. in 2010 [40]. As the frontal and ethmoid regions comprise only a small portion of the anterior cranial fossa, transorbital endoscopic techniques allow for multi-portal, multi-angled approaches that are complementary to traditional transnasal techniques. In dividing the orbit into quadrants, a superior eyelid crease incision allows access to the anterior cranial fossa and orbital roof, while a precaruncular approach also gives access to the anterior cranial fossa, lateral nasal cavity, frontal recess, and optic nerve [40]. While these areas are accessible by transnasal transethmoid techniques, complementing access with a transorbital portal may provide direct access with less instrument collisions. In their single-institution experience, Ramakrishna et al. in 2016 reported success in treating 40 patients with a variety of highly selected pathology, including CSF leaks, meningo-encephaloceles, trauma, and tumors [41]. Although nearly all patients had postoperative ocular dysfunction, no vision loss occurred, and long-term complication rates were low.

As a corollary, a transorbital corridor may provide wide access to the frontal sinus. In a cadaveric study, Husain et al. compared Lynch incisions to transcaruncular approaches, both combined with a Draf 3 [42]. The transorbital portal through the superior nasal septum allows for access to the lateral frontal sinus. The authors found that these two approaches fared similarly with 0-degree endoscopes and straight instrumentation. However, with 30-degree endoscopes and curved instruments, the transcaruncular approach placed instruments inferior to the frontal recess, and it was difficult to work around the contralateral orbital roof with curved instruments. While a frontal sinus trephination allows for direct access to most frontal sinus pathology and allows for placement of two working instruments, these transorbital approaches may provide an alternative approach to lesions that would otherwise obstruct a frontal sinus trephination. At this time, evidence for these techniques are limited with single-institution experiences and cadaveric studies. As familiarity with transorbital techniques increases across multiple institutions, direct comparisons can be made to other endoscopic and open techniques.

Supraorbital Ethmoid Pathology

Successful frontal and ethmoid sinus surgery depends upon the integration of CT imaging into the surgical plan. Supraorbital ethmoid cells are an anterior ethmoid cell that is superiorly based above the ethmoid bulla, pneumatizing around the anterior ethmoid artery and over the orbit [43]. These cells create a cleft between the anterior cranial fossa and orbit and are present in over 50% of Western populations [44]. Consequently, they may be difficult to access, yet contain a variety of pathology, including meningoencephaloceles and inverted papillomas [45, 46]. Most commonly, the supraorbital ethmoid cells are approached transnasally. Often, they form the posterior border of a well-pneumatized frontal sinus, and removal of this partition improves access. However, a narrow anterior-posterior diameter of the frontal recess combined with a supraorbital ethmoid extending far laterally over the orbit is especially challenging and may require endoscopic-assisted or open techniques [45].

Reconstructive Ladder

The nasoseptal flap, based on the posterior septal artery, is the workhorse flap of closing frontal and ethmoid defects [47]. Under normal circumstances, the nasoseptal flap reaches the entire ethmoid roof. If necessary, extending dissection of the pedicle along the lateral nasal wall and into the pterygopalatine fossa increases pedicle length for coverage of most frontal defects [48].

However, many leaks do not require vascularized reconstruction. With all leaks, adherence to a few principles maximizes success as a surgeon gains experience [49]. First, meticulous resection of surrounding mucosa not only allows for better visualization of the defect itself but also facilitates revascularization of the overlay graft with the exposed bone. Second, intracranial inlay grafts, either intradural or extradural, should be utilized when possible (Fig. 21.5). Mucosa should not be placed intracranially. Closure in multiple layers is preferable. Finally, frontal sinus patency should be maintained (Fig. 21.6).

There are several factors to consider in reconstruction. The defect size, location, presence, or absence of intraoperative CSF leak, CSF leak quality (high flow vs. low

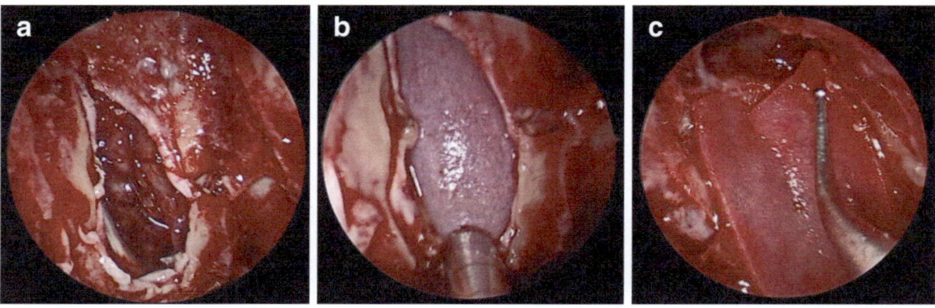

Fig. 21.5 Unilateral resection for olfactory neuroblastoma. (**a**) Dural defect with active CSF leak. (**b**) Durepair inlay with cessation of CSF leak. (**c**) Generous Durepair onlay, supported with dissolvable packing and tissue sealant

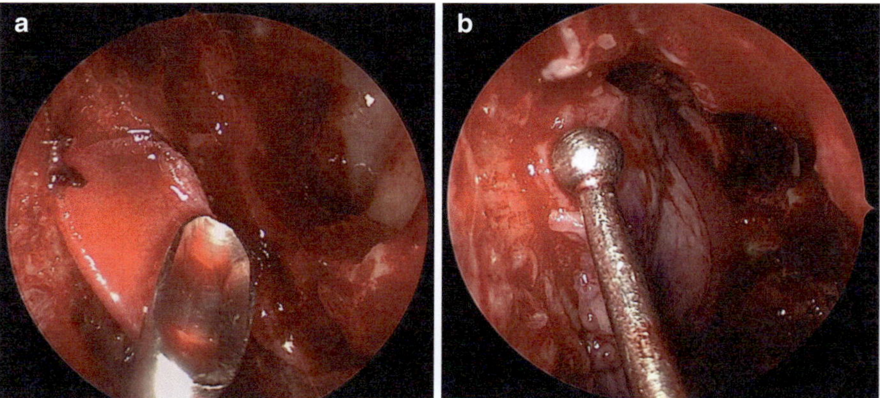

Fig. 21.6 Cribriform encephalocele. (**a**) Partial inlay with collagen matrix Durepair. (**b**) Overlay with collagen matrix Durepair followed by middle turbinate free mucosa graft. Draf 2B allows for widely patent frontal sinus without stenting after dissolvable packing placed over reconstruction

flow), pathology, patient risk factors, presence of a bony rim around the defect, and need for postoperative radiation all influence the choice of reconstruction [50].

Autologous fat has a long history of use in skull base reconstruction. Fat excels at filling dead space, such as an obliterated frontal sinus or within the sphenoid sinus. However, this property makes tissue handling difficult at the frontoethmoid junction. Consequently, it may be challenging to maintain patency of the frontal sinus around a plug of fat. Autologous cartilage and bone provides rigid support and can be fashioned as a "gasket seal" surrounded by a plug of fascia [51]. Yet, whether or not this rigid support is necessary is unknown.

Free grafts have been successful in repair of even large anterior skull base defects (Fig. 21.7). In a 2007 review by Germani et al. of 55 CSF leaks, 30 were repaired with AlloDerm, an acellular dermal allograft. Despite 16 of the leaks being greater than 2 cm, they noted a 97% success rate by placing the graft as an inlay

Fig. 21.7 Collagen matrix DuraGen inlay for bilateral anterior cranial fossa resection for olfactory neuroblastoma. Next, a second, larger onlay of collagen matrix was positioned over the exposed bone, followed by dissolvable packing and tissue sealant to support the reconstruction

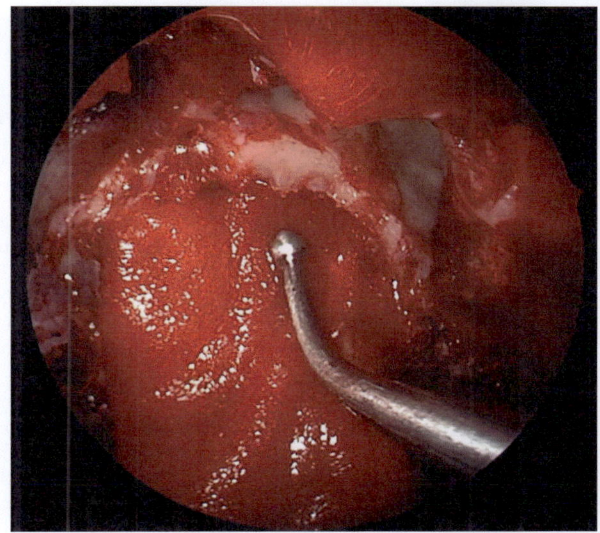

intracranially yet extending the margins of the graft intranasally to overlay the bone surrounding the defect. Similarly, in a review of 120 patients requiring skull base reconstruction by Oakley et al., an inlay was performed with DuraGen, a collagen-based dural replacement. An onlay nasoseptal flap was placed in the majority (70%) of patients, while the free mucosal grafts were otherwise used. The use of a nasoseptal did not impact CSF leak rates or any other perioperative complication. At the authors' institution, collagen matrix allografts are routinely utilized given their high success rate without any donor site morbidity. In the event of failure, vascularized pedicled flaps remain as a backup.

Following a multilayer closure, tissue sealants are an option as a final step in reconstruction. There are several commercially available tissue sealants. While there have been several studies suggesting tissue sealants can withstand pressure in vivo and in vitro, the evidence for their use in endoscopic skull base surgery remains limited [50].

Conclusion

Reconstruction of frontal and ethmoid defects is challenging to manage. Fortunately, there have been significant advances in instrumentation and reconstructive options. If feasible, endoscopic approaches offer the least morbidity while maintaining sinus patency. However, experience with the variety of approaches and reconstructive techniques allows one to individualize a surgical plan to yield the best possible result.

References

1. Anterior osteoplastic frontal sinus operation. Five years' experience. https://pubmed.ncbi.nlm.nih.gov/13900256/. Accessed 25 May 2021.
2. Silverman JB, Gray ST, Busaba NY. Role of osteoplastic frontal sinus obliteration in the era of endoscopic sinus surgery. Int J Otolaryngol. 2012;2012:501896. https://doi.org/10.1155/2012/501896.
3. Ochsner MC, Delgaudio JM. The place of the osteoplastic flap in the endoscopic era: indications and pitfalls. Laryngoscope. 2015;125(4):801–6. https://doi.org/10.1002/lary.25014.
4. Schultz JJ, Chen J, Sabharwal S, et al. Management of frontal bone fractures. J Craniofac Surg. 2019;30(7):2026–9. https://doi.org/10.1097/SCS.0000000000005720.
5. Chaaban MR, Illing E, Riley KO, Woodworth BA. Spontaneous cerebrospinal fluid leak repair: a five-year prospective evaluation. Laryngoscope. 2014;124:70–5. https://doi.org/10.1002/lary.24160.
6. Woodworth BA, Schlosser RJ, Palmer JN. Endoscopic repair of frontal sinus cerebrospinal fluid leaks. J Laryngol Otol. 2005;119(9):709–13. https://doi.org/10.1258/0022215054797961.
7. Strong EB. Frontal sinus fractures: current concepts. Craniomaxillofac Trauma Reconstr. 2009;2(3–4):161–75. https://doi.org/10.1055/s-0029-1234020.
8. Monnazzi M, Gabrielli M, Pereira-Filho V, Hochuli-Vieira E, De Oliveira H, Gabrielli M. Frontal sinus obliteration with iliac crest bone grafts. Review of 8 cases. Craniomaxillofac Trauma Reconstr. 2014;7(4):263–70. https://doi.org/10.1055/s-0034-1382776.
9. Rice DH. Management of frontal sinus fractures. Curr Opin Otolaryngol Head Neck Surg. 2004;12(1):46–8. https://doi.org/10.1097/00020840-200402000-00013.
10. Sessions RB, Alford BR, Stratton C, Ainsworth JZ, Roswell NM, Shill O. Current concepts of frontal sinus surgery: an appraisal of the osteoplastic flap-fat obliteration operation. Laryngoscope. 1972;82(5):918–30. https://doi.org/10.1288/00005537-197205000-00021.
11. Petruzzelli GJ, Stankiewicz JA. Frontal sinus obliteration with hydroxyapatite cement. Laryngoscope. 2002;112(1):32–6. https://doi.org/10.1097/00005537-200201000-00006.
12. Donald PJ, Bernstein L. Compound frontal sinus injuries with intracranial penetration. Laryngoscope. 1978;88(2 Pt 1):225–32. https://doi.org/10.1288/00005537-197802000-00002.
13. Morse JC, Chandra RK. Is there still a role for cranialization in modern sinus surgery? Curr Opin Otolaryngol Head Neck Surg. 2021;29(1):53–8. https://doi.org/10.1097/MOO.0000000000000691.
14. Arnold MA, Tatum SA. Frontal sinus fractures: evolving clinical considerations and surgical approaches. Craniomaxillofac Trauma Reconstr. 2019;12(2):85–94. https://doi.org/10.1055/s-0039-1678660.
15. Belzberg M, Shalom NB, Wolff A, Huang J, Gordon C. Bilateral versus unilateral cranialization in the management of a breached frontal sinus. J Craniofac Surg. 2020;31(1):261–4. https://doi.org/10.1097/SCS.0000000000006023.
16. Oakley GM, Christensen JM, Winder M, et al. Collagen matrix as an inlay in endoscopic skull base reconstruction. J Laryngol Otol. 2018;132(3):214–23. https://doi.org/10.1017/S0022215117001499.
17. Soler ZM, Khalid AN, Smith TL. Middle turbinate hinge flap for frontal recess obliteration following prior cranialization. Laryngoscope. 2009;119(7):1403–5. https://doi.org/10.1002/lary.20482.
18. Rodriguez ED, Stanwix MG, Nam AJ, et al. Twenty-six-year experience treating frontal sinus fractures: a novel algorithm based on anatomical fracture pattern and failure of conventional techniques. Plast Reconstr Surg. 2008;122(6):1850–66. https://doi.org/10.1097/PRS.0b013e31818d58ba.
19. Strong EB, Pahlavan N, Saito D. Frontal sinus fractures: a 28-year retrospective review. Otolaryngol Head Neck Surg. 2006;135(5):774–9. https://doi.org/10.1016/j.otohns.2006.03.043.

20. Wallis A, Donald PJ. Frontal sinus fractures. Laryngoscope. 1988;98(6):593–8. https://doi.org/10.1288/00005537-198806000-00002.
21. Chen KT, Chen CT, Mardini S, Tsay PK, Chen YR. Frontal sinus fractures: a treatment algorithm and assessment of outcomes based on 78 clinical cases. Plast Reconstr Surg. 2006;118(2):457–68. https://doi.org/10.1097/01.prs.0000227738.42077.2d.
22. Zubillaga Rodríguez I, Lora Pablos D, Falguera Uceda MI, Díez Lobato R, Sánchez AG. Frontal sinus obliteration after trauma: analysis of bone regeneration for two selected methods. Int J Oral Maxillofac Surg. 2014;43(7):827–33. https://doi.org/10.1016/j.ijom.2014.02.012.
23. Woodworth BA, Schlosser RJ. Frontal sinus cerebrospinal fluid leaks. In: Kountakis SE, Senior, BA, Draf, W. (eds) The Frontal Sinus. Springer, Berlin, Heidelberg. 2005. https://doi.org/10.1007/3-540-27607-6_1.
24. Zacharek MA, Fong KJ, Hwang PH. Image-guided frontal trephination: a minimally invasive approach for hard-to-reach frontal sinus disease. Otolaryngol Head Neck Surg. 2006;135(4):518–22. https://doi.org/10.1016/j.otohns.2006.05.033.
25. Bell RB, Dierks EJ, Homer L, Potter BE. Management of cerebrospinal fluid leak associated with craniomaxillofacial trauma. J Oral Maxillofac Surg. 2004;62(6):676–84. https://doi.org/10.1016/j.joms.2003.08.032.
26. Choi M, Li Y, Shapiro SA, Havlik RJ, Flores RL. A 10-year review of frontal sinus fractures: clinical outcomes of conservative management of posterior table fractures. Plast Reconstr Surg. 2012;130(2):399–406. https://doi.org/10.1097/PRS.0b013e3182589d91.
27. Fox PM, Garza R, Dusch M, Hwang PH, Girod S. Management of frontal sinus fractures: treatment modality changes at a Level I Trauma Center. J Craniofac Surg. 2014;25(6):2038–42. https://doi.org/10.1097/SCS.0000000000001105.
28. Conger BT, Riley K, Woodworth BA. The draf III mucosal grafting technique: a prospective study. Otolaryngol Head Neck Surg. 2012;146(4):664–8. https://doi.org/10.1177/0194599811432423.
29. Grayson JW, Jeyarajan H, Illing EA, Cho DY, Riley KO, Woodworth BA. Changing the surgical dogma in frontal sinus trauma: transnasal endoscopic repair. Int Forum Allergy Rhinol. 2017;7(5):441–9. https://doi.org/10.1002/alr.21897.
30. Rains BM. Frontal sinus stenting. Otolaryngol Clin N Am. 2001;34(1):101–10. https://doi.org/10.1016/s0030-6665(05)70298-x.
31. Ackall FY, Issa K, Jang D, Hachem RA. Steroid-eluting stent bolster for CSF leak reconstruction during endoscopic endonasal repair. J Neurol Surg B Skull Base. 2021;82:P001. https://doi.org/10.1055/s-0041-1725398.
32. Patel SA, Berens AM, Devarajan K, Whipple ME, Moe KS. Evaluation of a minimally disruptive treatment protocol for frontal sinus fractures. JAMA Facial Plast Surg. 2017;19(3):225–31. https://doi.org/10.1001/jamafacial.2016.1769.
33. Farag A, Rosen MR, Ziegler N, et al. Management and surveillance of frontal sinus violation following craniotomy. J Neurol Surg Part B Skull Base. 2020;81(1):1–7. https://doi.org/10.1055/s-0038-1676826.
34. Loftus PA, Wise SK, Daraei P, Baugnon K, DelGaudio JM. Excavating meningoencephaloceles: a newly recognized entity. Am J Rhinol Allergy. 2017;31(2):127–34. https://doi.org/10.2500/ajra.2017.31.4413.
35. Bozkurt G, Zocchi J, Russo F, et al. Frontal sinus preservation during cerebrospinal fluid leak repair. J Craniofac Surg. 2019;30(8):e763–8. https://doi.org/10.1097/SCS.0000000000005764.
36. Kanowitz SJ, Batra PS, Citardi MJ. Comprehensive management of failed frontal sinus obliteration. Am J Rhinol. 2008;22(3):263–70. https://doi.org/10.2500/ajr.2008.22.3164.
37. Jaźwiec AM, Rechner B, Komorowska-Timek E. Endoscopy-assisted frontal sinus obliteration. J Craniofac Surg. 2018;29(5):e513–5. https://doi.org/10.1097/SCS.0000000000004562.
38. Ung F, Sindwani R, Metson R. Endoscopic frontal sinus obliteration: a new technique for the treatment of chronic frontal sinusitis. Otolaryngol Head Neck Surg. 2005;133(4):551–5. https://doi.org/10.1016/j.otohns.2005.06.014.

39. Geltzeiler M, Mowery A, Detwiller KY, Mace JC, Smith TL. Frontal sinus "mega-trephination" in a tertiary rhinology practice. Int Forum Allergy Rhinol. 2019;9(10):1189–95. https://doi.org/10.1002/alr.22405.
40. Moe KS, Bergeron CM, Ellenbogen RG. Transorbital neuroendoscopic surgery. Neurosurgery. 2010;67(3 Suppl Operative):ons16–28. https://doi.org/10.1227/01.NEU.0000373431.08464.43.
41. Ramakrishna R, Kim LJ, Bly RA, Moe K, Ferreira M. Transorbital neuroendoscopic surgery for the treatment of skull base lesions. J Clin Neurosci. 2016;24:99–104. https://doi.org/10.1016/j.jocn.2015.07.021.
42. Husain Q, Banks C, Bleier BS. Lynch vs transcaruncular approach: optimizing access to the lateral frontal sinus. Int Forum Allergy Rhinol. 2020;10(8):991–5. https://doi.org/10.1002/alr.22560.
43. Wormald PJ, Hoseman W, Callejas C, et al. The International Frontal Sinus Anatomy Classification (IFAC) and classification of the extent of endoscopic frontal sinus surgery (EFSS). Int Forum Allergy Rhinol. 2016;6(7):677–96. https://doi.org/10.1002/alr.21738.
44. Jang DW, Lachanas VA, White LC, Kountakis SE. Supraorbital ethmoid cell: a consistent landmark for endoscopic identification of the anterior ethmoidal artery. Otolaryngol Head Neck Surg. 2014;151(6):1073–7. https://doi.org/10.1177/0194599814551124.
45. Purkey MT, Woodworth BA, Hahn S, Palmer JN, Chiu AG. Endoscopic repair of supraorbital ethmoid cerebrospinal fluid leaks. ORL J Otorhinolaryngol Relat Spec. 2009;71(2):93–8. https://doi.org/10.1159/000193219.
46. Adriaensen GFJPM, van der Hout MW, Reinartz SM, Georgalas C, Fokkens WJ. Endoscopic treatment of inverted papilloma attached in the frontal sinus/recess. Rhinology. 2015;53(4):317–24. https://doi.org/10.4193/Rhin14.177.
47. Hadad G, Bassagasteguy L, Carrau RL, et al. A novel reconstructive technique after endoscopic expanded endonasal approaches: vascular pedicle nasoseptal flap. Laryngoscope. 2006;116(10):1882–6. https://doi.org/10.1097/01.mlg.0000234933.37779.e4.
48. Shastri KS, Leonel LCPC, Patel V, et al. Lengthening the nasoseptal flap pedicle with extended dissection into the pterygopalatine fossa. Laryngoscope. 2020;130(1):18–24. https://doi.org/10.1002/lary.27984.
49. Patron V, Roger V, Moreau S, Babin E, Hitier M. State of the art of endoscopic frontal sinus cerebrospinal fluid leak repair. Eur Ann Otorhinolaryngol Head Neck Dis. 2015;132(6):347–52. https://doi.org/10.1016/j.anorl.2015.08.031.
50. Wang EW, Zanation AM, Gardner PA, et al. ICAR: endoscopic skull-base surgery. Int Forum Allergy Rhinol. 2019;9(S3):S145–365. https://doi.org/10.1002/alr.22326.
51. Leng LZ, Brown S, Anand VK, Schwartz TH. "Gasket-seal" watertight closure in minimal-access endoscopic cranial base surgery. Neurosurgery. 2008;62(5 Suppl 2):ONSE342–3; discussion ONSE343. https://doi.org/10.1227/01.neu.0000326017.84315.1f.

Chapter 22
Reconstruction of Sphenoid Defects: Lateral Recess, Sellar, Tuberculum, and Planum Defects

Tapan D. Patel, Daniel Yoshor, and Nithin D. Adappa

Introduction

Over the past two decades, advances in endoscopic techniques have revolutionized the surgical management of sinonasal and skull base pathology. As increasingly complex intradural and extradural pathologies have been managed endoscopically, the difficulty of associated skull base reconstruction has also increased. Extended endoscopic transsphenoidal approaches have provided improved surgical access to numerous tumors in the sagittal plane. Historically, smaller skull base defects were most commonly reconstructed with free tissue grafts. Although these forms of repair have exhibited high success rates in the repair of smaller defects, skull base pathology requiring extensive resection with large skull base defects demonstrated the need for more robust forms of repair, which led to the introduction of pedicled, vascularized flaps. These techniques were adapted from experience accumulated with the endoscopic repair of CSF leaks associated with endoscopic sinus surgery and trauma and then expanded to repair larger dural defects as well as defects over

T. D. Patel
Division of Otolaryngology, Yale New Haven Health, Yale School of Medicine, New Haven, USA
e-mail: tapan.patel@ynhh.org

D. Yoshor
Department of Neurosurgery, University of Pennsylvania, Philadelphia, PA, USA
e-mail: Daniel.yoshor@pennmedicine.upenn.edu

N. D. Adappa (✉)
Department of Otorhinolaryngology, University of Pennsylvania, Philadelphia, PA, USA

Penn AERD Center, University of Pennsylvania, Philadelphia, PA, USA

Division of Rhinology and Skull Base Surgery, Hospital of the University of Pennsylvania, Philadelphia, PA, USA
e-mail: nithin.adappa@pennmedicine.upenn.edu

© The Author(s), under exclusive license to Springer Nature Switzerland AG 2023
E. C. Kuan et al. (eds.), *Skull Base Reconstruction*,
https://doi.org/10.1007/978-3-031-27937-9_22

high-flow intraoperative CSF leaks [1]. As the field of endoscopic skull base surgery evolved, overall CSF leak rates have decreased as a result of improvements in reconstruction techniques utilizing multilayer closure with vascularized local tissue flaps. Reconstructive strategies must be modified based on the size and location of the skull base defect, the extent of dural resection, whether the arachnoid is violated, the nature of the patient's CSF pressure, states of poor wound healing such as Cushing's disease and prior irradiation, and whether the patient has had previous surgery or treatment that would preclude use of vascularized local tissue flaps. This chapter will review the techniques involved in the reconstruction of sphenoid defects.

When considering reconstruction of the sphenoid defects, a multilayer approach should be used to reconstruct the layers that have been breached (i.e., mucosa, bone, dura) in order to get access to the skull base lesion. Three layers separate the sphenoid cavity from the intracranial compartment: (1) sphenoid mucosa, (2) bone of the posterior sphenoid wall, and (3) dura mater. When reconstructing a sphenoid defect, at least two out of the three of these layers should be addressed. When two of the three layers are adequately reconstructed, resulting in a watertight closure, there is generally minimal reconstructive failure.

Materials for Skull Base Repair (Divided by Reconstruction Layer)

Dural Reconstruction

The sellar dura separates the sphenoid cavity from intracranial components of the middle cranial fossa. This is the first layer that should be reconstructed when closing sphenoid defects. Adequate watertight closure of this layer will ensure a reconstructive success. Multiple autologous and heterologous materials are available for closure of this layer. Autologous grafts include abdominal fat and fascia lata. Fat is typically used in a "plug" fashion to fill the dead space created after removal of the skull base lesion. It can also be used in conjunction with fascia lata to create a "button graft," where a layer of fat is placed between two layers of fascia lata. This multilayered graft has proven to be especially effective in the management of high-flow CSF leaks [2].

There are also a wide variety of heterologous materials available for dural reconstruction. Acellular human dermis (AlloDerm, LifeCell Corporation, Branchburg, NJ, USA) has been used in many areas of head and neck surgery and has gained popularity for the reconstruction of anterior and middle cranial fossa skull base defects over the past decade. Advances in tissue engineering have also led to proliferation of collagen-based dural replacement products. These products consist of collagen-rich animal tissues that have been processed to remove all cells and antigens. They are designed to fully incorporate into native tissues via collagen remodeling while minimizing the inflammatory response. Several collagen-based dural substitutes are available which include TissuDura (Baxter Biomedical, Vienna, Austria), Durafoam (Codman & Shurtleff, Inc., Raynham, MA, USA), DuraGen (Integra Neurosciences, Plainsboro, NJ, USA), and Durepair (Medtronic, Minneapolis, MN, USA). These are sterile, absorbable implants intended for the repair of the dura as a sutureless onlay grafts.

Bone Reconstruction

The next layer that should be considered after the reconstruction of the dural layer is the bony posterior sphenoid wall. This layer is often either removed in order to gain access to the sellar lesion or is dehiscent in the case of a sphenoid encephalocele. Autologous bone can be utilized for rigid reconstruction of this layer. Fragments of autologous bone can be obtained from the middle turbinate, nasal septum, and anterior sphenoid wall. It can be used to buttress the brain and minimize the effect of dural pulsations. The advantages of autologous bone materials are their absent cost and biocompatibility. However, the amount of useful bone is often unpredictable. Bone fragments have variable and irregular sizes, shapes, and thicknesses and often require the use of more than one fragment which makes the repair cumbersome and unwieldy. Synthetic options for bony reconstruction include absorbable and nonabsorbable miniplates that may be placed as onlay or underlay grafts. Although available without additional harvesting, the potential for infection and scatter on imaging are distinct disadvantages to using synthetic materials.

Mucosal Reconstruction

The final layer in the reconstructive algorithm is the mucosal layer. The mucosal layer of small defects with low-flow CSF leaks can be reconstructed with free mucosal grafts. These can be harvested from the septum and turbinates, as well as the nasal floor. Septal mucosa harvest results in exposed cartilage that may take longer to heal, increases the risk of a septal perforation, and could potentially compromise the future use of a nasoseptal flap [3]. If the middle turbinate is resected for exposure, harvest of the middle turbinate mucosal graft on the back table has no additional morbidity. Resection of the middle turbinate does however increase the risk of bleeding from branches of the sphenopalatine artery supplying the middle turbinate. Mucosa of the inferior turbinate can also be harvested, which tends to be thicker than the mucosa harvested from the middle turbinate. The nasal floor is an ideal site for free mucosal graft harvest as it provides a large graft size and has little donor site morbidity with complete remucosalization that is typically achieved quickly [4].

When there is a large defect with a high-flow CSF leak, the mucosal layer should be reconstructed with a pedicled, vascularized flap. The cornerstone of endonasal reconstruction is the nasoseptal flap [5]. Prior to adaptation of the nasoseptal flap for skull base reconstruction, dural defects were repaired with multiple layers of non-vascularized tissues. With high-flow CSF leaks, the incidence of postoperative CSF leaks was too high (20–30%) and a valid constraint to the propagation of endonasal skull base surgery. With the advent of vascularized mucosal nasoseptal flap, the postoperative CSF leak rate dramatically decreased to less than 5% [5–7]. In the last decade, alternatives to the nasoseptal flap have been described, consisting of vascularized local and regional flaps. Local flaps are harvested from the mucosa of the nasal cavity, including the middle turbinate and inferior turbinate. Regional flaps are harvested from areas adjacent to the nasal cavity and include extracranial pericranium and temporoparietal fascia. Despite these alternatives, the nasoseptal flap remains the first choice for the reconstruction of the mucosal layer.

Tissue Glues

Several surgical glues are described in the literature for use during endoscopic skull base surgery. These include Tisseel/Tissucol (Baxter BioSciences, Deerfield, IL, USA), BioGlue (CryoLife, Kennesaw, GA, USA), and DuraSeal (Covidien, Waltham, MA, USA). BioGlue is a semisynthetic glue composed of purified bovine serum albumin and glutaraldehyde. While supraphysiologic burst strengths have been reported with BioGlue, glutaraldehyde is associated with some degree of tissue toxicity, and application to adjacent critical neurovascular structures should be performed with caution. Tisseel is a two-component biologic system made from pooled human plasma, consisting of fibrinogen solution and thrombin, with a calcium cofactor promoting the final stage of coagulation [8]. DuraSeal is a polyethylene glycol hydrogel sealant used for watertight closure of the dura. While DuraSeal is FDA-approved for use in dural closure, it may expand significantly following application, and placement in a subdural plane may result in the compression of adjacent structures or in the displacement of an overlay graft.

Surgical Reconstruction (Divided by Location)

Reconstruction of Sellar Defects

In pituitary surgery, we typically create pedicle-sparing "rescue flaps," whereby limited posterior septal incisions are made, which allow the nasoseptal flap pedicles to be protected bilaterally and the sella to be approached via a posterior septectomy. In this approach, small incisions are made at the level of the sphenoid ostia bilaterally and carried anteriorly onto the superior nasal septum with electrocautery. The mucosa is then elevated inferiorly from the sphenoid ostium, thereby preserving the posterior septal branch of the sphenopalatine artery, which serves as the blood supply to the nasoseptal flap [9]. This is performed bilaterally to ensure that both the nasoseptal flap vascular pedicles are preserved, if needed for the reconstruction of the sellar defect.

Once the sellar lesion has been removed, the resulting defect should be reconstructed. With pituitary surgery, an intraoperative CSF leak is not always encountered. Some have argued that without an active CSF leak, this region does not need to be reconstructed, but in our experience, a mucosal layer reconstruction provides much quicker healing of the skull base. We typically will perform a posterior nasoseptal flap, i.e., "mini-nasoseptal flap," as this provides vascularized mucosal coverage over the exposed bone and dura without the donor site morbidity of traditionally described nasoseptal flap [10]. In the event of an intraoperative CSF leak which indicates a violation of the arachnoid membrane, the resulting CSF leak must be addressed, and a reconstruction of the sellar defect should be performed to prevent a postoperative CSF leak. Reconstruction can be performed with a variety of autologous materials, including abdominal fat, cartilage, or fascia lata. A variety of rigid materials, including cartilage or bone fragments, alumina ceramic, silicone, or titanium plates, have been used to reconstruct the sellar floor [11]. The advantages of autologous materials include biocompatibility and absent cost; however, the disadvantages include prolonged operative time, the need for a separate incision, donor site pain, infection, and hematoma formation. This has driven the transition to heterologous materials for sellar repair [12].

Our protocol for sellar reconstruction addresses both the dural layer and mucosal layer keeping with reconstruction of two of the three involved skull base layers (Fig. 22.1). If there is a low-flow CSF leak, our multilayer reconstruction consists of a synthetic dural substitute and a vascularized mini-nasoseptal flap. A collagen matrix is placed to reduce the sellar dead space (Fig. 22.1b). The dura is then separated from the bony sellar floor using a round knife. Durepair (Medtronic, Minneapolis, MN, USA), a type I and type III collagen matrix from acellular fetal bovine skin, is then placed in the epidural space in an underlay fashion (Fig. 22.1c). A small amount of fibrin glue (Tisseel, Baxter BioSciences, Deerfield, IL, USA) is then placed over the Durepair to secure it into position. The vascularized mini-nasoseptal flap is then harvested from the prior rescue flap by completing the septal mucosal incisions with electrocautery. This flap is then laid over the sellar defect in the sphenoid sinus ensuring that there is maximal bony contact with flap and complete coverage of the defect (Fig. 22.1d). Additional fibrin glue is then placed over the flap to secure it into position and to facilitate adherence of the flap to the skull base. If a high-flow CSF leak of the sella is identified, it should be reconstructed in a similar fashion to the reconstruction of the tuberculum and planum defects described below.

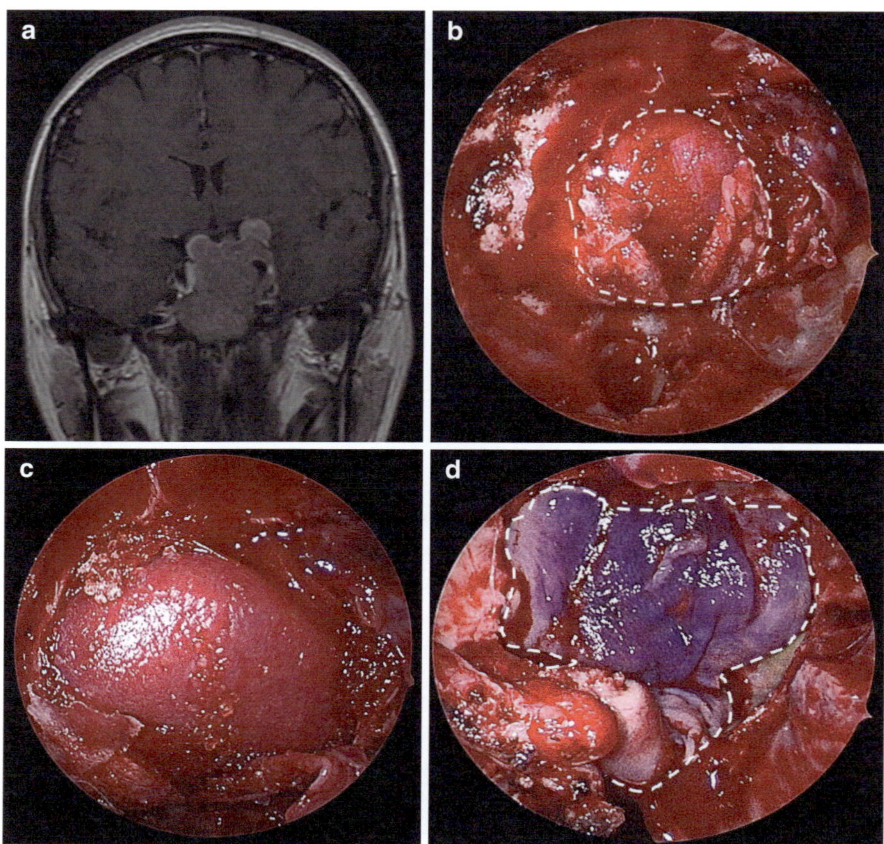

Fig. 22.1 Reconstruction of a sellar defect. (**a**) Preoperative coronal MRI showing a pituitary macroadenoma with suprasellar extension. (**b**) Resulting defect (dotted white circle) of the sella after removal of the lesion. Collagen sponge is placed in the sellar cavity to reduce the dead space. (**c**) Durepair, a collagen matrix, placed in the epidural space in an underlay fashion to reconstruct the dural layer. (**d**) Posterior nasoseptal flap, or mini-nasoseptal flap (dotted line), placed over the sellar defect to reconstruct the mucosal layer

Reconstruction of Tuberculum and Planum Defects

Tumors of the tuberculum sellae and planum sphenoidale can be approached through an extended transsphenoidal approach. This approach expands the operative exposure beyond the sella by removing the bone in the region of the tuberculum sellae and planum sphenoidale [13]. Tumors in this region include suprasellar pituitary tumors, tuberculum sella meningiomas, Rathke's cleft cysts, optic nerve gliomas, and craniopharyngiomas. Removal of these tumors often leads to a large arachnoid membrane defect with a high-flow CSF leak. Often the arachnoid membrane is intentionally opened to get access to the tumor. Traditional sellar floor reconstruction techniques are insufficient for the defects that results from this extended approach [14]. Closure techniques that can withstand the increased CSF flow are required. In contrast to the repair of the sella, it is often difficult to detach the dura from the skull base bone in the region of planum and tuberculum during extended approaches, preventing a watertight extradural closure. In designing the skull base repair for extended approaches, multiple factors should be considered including the size of the tumor, adequacy and geometry of the remaining dural and bone margins, and previous intranasal surgery.

Different reconstructive techniques continue to evolve for the reconstruction of planum and tuberculum defects depending on the dimension and location of the defects. These reconstructive techniques utilize a multilayer combination of bone and dural substitutes placed in an inlay and onlay fashion in the intradural, extradural (i.e., epidural), and extracranial spaces. Vascularized local and regional tissue flaps have increasingly been used to repair planum and tuberculum skull base defects. Vascularized tissue is used to complete the reconstruction, to increase the effectiveness of the reconstruction, and to facilitate wound healing. The most commonly used vascularized flap is the nasoseptal flap. The large surface area of the nasoseptal flap allows great versatility of movement. It is capable of reaching most regions of the ventral skull base, including the sella turcica, planum sphenoidale, clivus, or cribriform plate [5, 15]. For large defects like these, we utilize an extended nasoseptal flap that includes mucosa from the nasal floor and the lateral nasal wall to increase the width and bring the incision anteriorly to the junction of the mucosa and vestibular skin to maximize its length for maximal flap on bone adherence. We minimize donor site morbidity of the anterior cartilage by harvesting and placing a reverse rotation flap [16].

Our protocol for the reconstruction of tuberculum and planum defects addresses the dural layer and the mucosal layer (i.e., two out of the three layers). Reconstruction begins with the obliteration of the dead space with fat to prevent pooling of CSF at the bony defect (Fig. 22.2). Fat and fascia lata are harvested from the thigh and used to create a "button graft." The button graft consists of fat placed between two layers of fascia lata sutured together to form an inlay and onlay component (Fig. 22.2c). The inlay portion sits within the subdural space, while the onlay portion covers the epidural space to create a tight primary dural closure (Fig. 22.2d). A small amount of fibrin glue is then placed over the graft to secure it into position. A nasoseptal flap is then rotated to cover the defect (Fig. 22.2e), and more fibrin glue is used to secure the graft in place [13].

The use of lumbar drains for extended transplanum and transtubercular approaches is institution dependent. Some institutions routinely use lumbar drains for extended approaches, while others use them on a more selective basis. For patients without elevated intracranial pressures (ICPs), the authors do not typically use a lumbar drain.

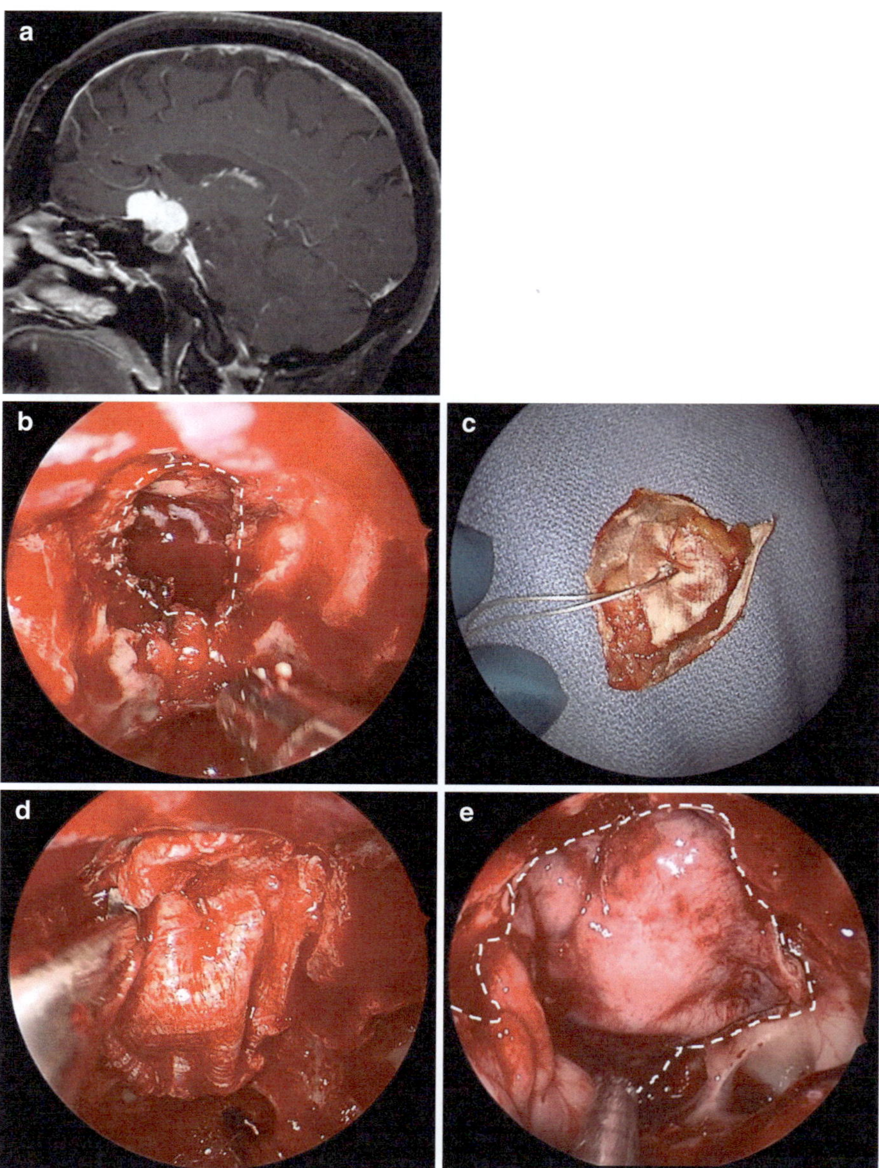

Fig. 22.2 Reconstruction of a tuberculum and planum defect. (**a**) Preoperative sagittal MRI showing a tuberculum meningioma with extension to the planum sphenoidale. (**b**) Resulting defect (dotted white line) after removal of the lesion. (**c**) A button graft consisting of fat placed between two layers of fascia lata sutured together will serve as a reconstruction of the dural layer. (**d**) Button graft positioned over the defect with one layer placed in the subdural space and the other layer placed in the epidural space. (**e**) Extended nasoseptal flap (dotted line) placed over the defect to reconstruct the mucosal layer

Reconstruction of Lateral Recess Defects

Spontaneous CSF leaks are thought to occur due to elevated intracranial pressures. The lateral recess of the sphenoid sinus is a common location for spontaneous CSF leaks. Leaks in this region generally are associated with a hyperpneumatized sinus, extending lateral to the vidian canal and foramen rotundum [17, 18]. Skull base defects in this region can be large, and encephaloceles represent herniation of the temporal lobe into the sphenoid sinus, often in close proximity to the optic nerve and carotid artery. Given the lateral location of these defects, a standard transnasal sphenoidotomy usually provides insufficient access, even with angled scopes and instruments. The transpterygoid approach typically provides superior visualization and access for reconstruction.

Our surgical management of this defect begins with placement of a lumbar drain, which allows fluorescein to be used to localize the leak intraoperatively and ensure a watertight seal following repair. Of note, intrathecal fluorescein is an off-label usage and must be discussed with the patient prior to utilization. The lumbar drain is left open to drain following surgery, reducing the intracranial pressure and diverting the flow of CSF away from the repair site during the early phase of healing. Use of lumbar drain is based on theoretical premises, and clinical trials are not available to evaluate their effectiveness. The use of lumbar drains should be considered on an individual basis as they may result in complications.

The transpterygoid approach begins with a wide maxillary antrostomy and trans-ethmoid sphenoidotomy (Fig. 22.3). The sphenoid sinus is opened widely and extended as far lateral as possible. The maxillary antrostomy is widened posteriorly to the posterior wall of the sinus until the hard palatine bone is encountered (Fig. 22.3b). The crista ethmoidalis is then identified, which marks the location of the sphenopalatine artery. High-speed diamond drill and Kerrison rongeurs are then used to remove the posterior wall of the maxillary sinus from medial to lateral beginning with the crista ethmoidalis. The periosteum of the pterygopalatine fossa (PPF) is then cauterized with bipolar electrocautery and incised horizontally along the course of the internal maxillary artery (IMA) (Fig. 22.3c). Using blunt dissection, the IMA can be identified and retracted. Vessel clips or bipolar electrocautery can then be used to ligate and divide the IMA. This allows access to the posterior wall of the PPF, which is also the anterior wall of the lateral sphenoid recess. At this point, it is helpful to confirm the anatomical location with image guidance. A curette or high-speed diamond drill is then used to enter through the anterior wall of the lateral sphenoid recess, with the opening expanded circumferentially using Kerrison rongeurs (Fig. 22.3d). The skull base defect and encephalocele should then be directly visible. A bipolar electrocautery or coblator is used to reduce the encepha-locele, if present (Fig. 22.3e). After exposing the skull base defect, we begin the reconstruction.

At our institution, we lean towards reconstructing the bone and the mucosal layer (i.e., two of the three involved layers) in the case of spontaneous CSF leaks of the lateral recess due to the increased intracranial pressures. Ideally, the bone or

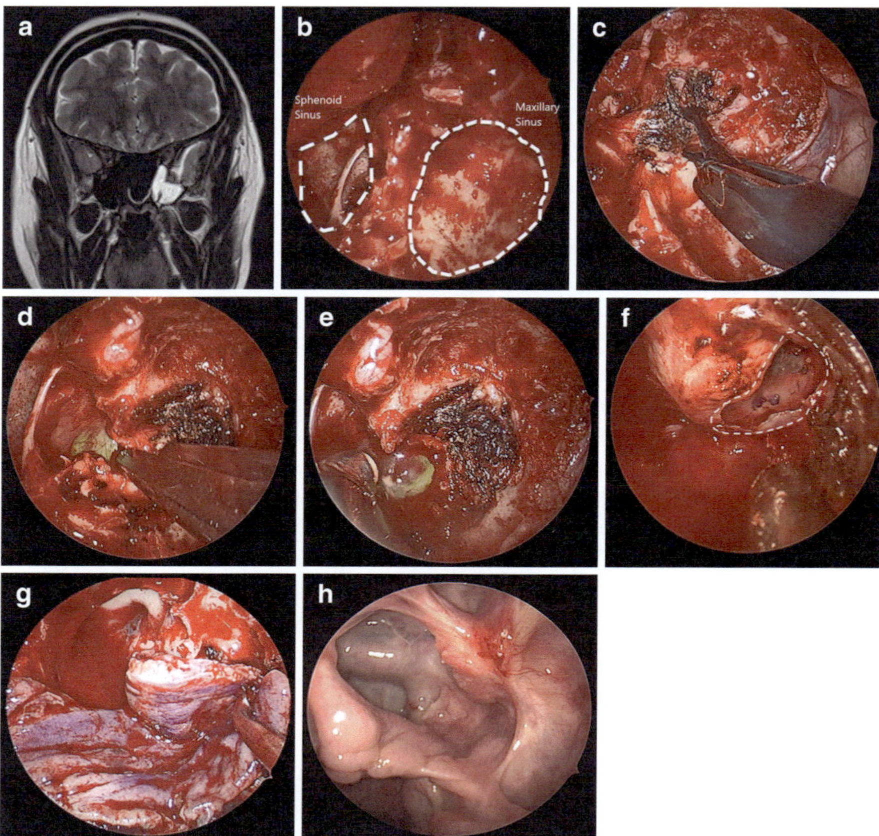

Fig. 22.3 Reconstruction of lateral recess defect. (**a**) Preoperative coronal MRI showing a left lateral sphenoid recess encephalocele. (**b**) Transpterygoid approach, which is needed for adequate exposure of lateral recess defect, begins with a wide maxillary antrostomy and sphenoidotomy (dotted lines). (**c**) Bipolar electrocautery is used to cauterize the periosteum of pterygopalatine fossa (PPF) after removal of the posterior maxillary wall. (**d**) After ligation of the internal maxillary artery, the posterior wall of PPF (i.e., anterior wall of the lateral sphenoid recess) is removed with Kerrison punch, thereby exposing the lesion. (**e**) Coblator is used to reduce the lateral recess encephalocele. (**f**) Autologous bone harvested from septum is placed over the defect in an underlay fashion (dotted circle) to reconstruct the bony layer. (**g**) Contralateral nasoseptal flap is then placed over the defect to reconstruct the mucosal layer. (**h**) Postoperative endoscopic view of a well healed lateral recess defect

cartilage harvested from the septum can be shaped to span the defect and placed in an underlay fashion (Fig. 22.3f). The purpose of this rigid or semirigid reconstruction is to buttress the brain and meninges, which minimizes the effect of dural pulsations and overall increased ICPs. In very narrow defects (<2 mm), a rigid underlay may not be possible, and a wedge-shaped graft may be placed in an overlay fashion. At this stage, there should be a watertight closure of the defect, which can be confirmed by the absence of any fluorescein leaking through the defect. A very small amount of absorbable fibrin glue (Tisseel, Baxter BioSciences, Deerfield, IL, USA) is then placed over the rigid material to secure it into position. Mucosal overlay grafts are then placed over the defect, and these can be free or pedicled. We prefer to use the contralateral pedicled nasoseptal flap for an additional multilayer closure of the defect (Fig. 22.3g). The graft is then secured into position with additional fibrin glue. The lumbar drain is opened at the time of repair and is used to remove 10 mL CSF/h for the first 48 h. Postoperative nasal endoscopy at 6 months shows a well healed nasoseptal flap with minimal crusting (Fig. 22.3h).

Conclusion

With the advances in endoscopic techniques, the reconstruction of sphenoid defects has evolved utilizing the principles of a meticulous multilayer closure employing closure of two of the three natural tissue planes. While the basic tenets stay the same, the tissue materials including fashioning of the nasoseptal flap differ based on location and pathology.

References

1. Zanation AM, et al. Reconstructive options for endoscopic skull base surgery. Otolaryngol Clin North Am. 2011;44(5):1201–22.
2. Luginbuhl AJ, et al. Endoscopic repair of high-flow cranial base defects using a bilayer button. Laryngoscope. 2010;120(5):876–80.
3. Suh JD, Ramakrishnan VR, DeConde AS. Nasal floor free mucosal graft for skull base reconstruction and cerebrospinal fluid leak repair. Ann Otol Rhinol Laryngol. 2012;121(2):91–5.
4. de Almeida JR, et al. Nasal morbidity following endoscopic skull base surgery: a prospective cohort study. Head Neck. 2011;33(4):547–51.
5. Hadad G, et al. A novel reconstructive technique after endoscopic expanded endonasal approaches: vascular pedicle nasoseptal flap. Laryngoscope. 2006;116(10):1882–6.
6. Harvey RJ, et al. Endoscopic skull base reconstruction of large dural defects: a systematic review of published evidence. Laryngoscope. 2012;122(2):452–9.
7. Zanation AM, et al. Nasoseptal flap reconstruction of high flow intraoperative cerebral spinal fluid leaks during endoscopic skull base surgery. Am J Rhinol Allergy. 2009;23(5):518–21.
8. Menovsky T, de Vries J, Bloss HG. Treatment of postoperative subgaleal cerebrospinal fluid fistulas by using fibrin sealant. Technical note. J Neurosurg. 1999;90(6):1143–5.
9. Rivera-Serrano CM, et al. Nasoseptal "rescue" flap: a novel modification of the nasoseptal flap technique for pituitary surgery. Laryngoscope. 2011;121(5):990–3.
10. Barger J, et al. The posterior nasoseptal flap: a novel technique for closure after endoscopic transsphenoidal resection of pituitary adenomas. Surg Neurol Int. 2018;9:32.
11. Seiler RW, Mariani L. Sellar reconstruction with resorbable vicryl patches, gelatin foam, and fibrin glue in transsphenoidal surgery: a 10-year experience with 376 patients. J Neurosurg. 2000;93(5):762–5.
12. Cappabianca P, et al. Sellar repair with fibrin sealant and collagen fleece after endoscopic endonasal transsphenoidal surgery. Surg Neurol. 2004;62(3):227–33; discussion 233.

13. Laufer I, Anand VK, Schwartz TH. Endoscopic, endonasal extended transsphenoidal, transplanum transtuberculum approach for resection of suprasellar lesions. J Neurosurg. 2007;106(3):400–6.
14. Cavallo LM, et al. Skull base reconstruction in the extended endoscopic transsphenoidal approach for suprasellar lesions. J Neurosurg. 2007;107(4):713–20.
15. Bhatki AM, et al. Reconstruction of the cranial base after endonasal skull base surgery: local tissue flaps. Oper Tech Otolaryngol Head Neck Surg. 2010;21(1):74–82.
16. Caicedo-Granados E, et al. Reverse rotation flap for reconstruction of donor site after vascular pedicled nasoseptal flap in skull base surgery. Laryngoscope. 2010;120(8):1550–2.
17. Illing E, et al. Spontaneous sphenoid lateral recess cerebrospinal fluid leaks arise from intracranial hypertension, not Sternberg's canal. Int Forum Allergy Rhinol. 2014;4(3):246–50.
18. Woodworth BA, Palmer JN. Spontaneous cerebrospinal fluid leaks. Curr Opin Otolaryngol Head Neck Surg. 2009;17(1):59–65.

Chapter 23
Reconstruction of Clival and Craniocervical Junction Defects

Neal R. Godse, Vijay A. Patel, and Eric W. Wang

Introduction

Endoscopic endonasal approaches have been employed to address an ever-growing number of pathologies of the skull base including sellar, anterior cranial fossa, petrous apex, clival, and craniocervical junction pathologies. A key step in the widespread adoption of endoscopic endonasal surgery has been the ability to reliably reconstruct the resultant cranial base defect. The goals of reconstruction, regardless of location, are to create a barrier between the intra- and extracranial spaces, mitigate cerebrospinal fluid (CSF) leak, and provide soft tissue coverage of key neurovascular structures.

Endoscopic endonasal approaches to the nasopharynx, clivus, and craniocervical junction are used for a variety of conditions including benign cervical lesions, like rheumatoid pannus, to skull base malignancies, such as chordoma, chondrosarcoma, and nasopharyngeal carcinoma. The primary goal of this section is to provide a comprehensive review of skull base reconstruction with a particular focus on the nuances of clival and craniocervical junction defect management.

N. R. Godse · V. A. Patel · E. W. Wang (✉)
Department of Otolaryngology, University of Pittsburgh School of Medicine, Pittsburgh, PA, USA
e-mail: patelva@upmc.edu; wangew@upmc.edu

© The Author(s), under exclusive license to Springer Nature Switzerland AG 2023
E. C. Kuan et al. (eds.), *Skull Base Reconstruction*,
https://doi.org/10.1007/978-3-031-27937-9_23

Applied Anatomy and Reconstructive Goals

Key Surgical Anatomy

The nasopharynx is a space of the upper aerodigestive tract bounded by the nasal choanae and posterior septum anteriorly, the floor of the sphenoid sinus superiorly, the eustachian tubes laterally, and the soft palate inferiorly. The clivus is a sloping bony structure posteroinferior to the dorsum sellae formed by the fusion of the sphenoid body (upper one-third of the clivus) and the occipital bone (lower two-thirds of the clivus). The posterior boundaries of the nasopharynx are the first and second cervical vertebrae (C1 and C2), which, along with an array of complex fibroligamentous attachments and articulations, form the fibro-osseous craniocervical junction (Fig. 23.1).

There are many critical anatomic structures in this region when considering surgical intervention and reconstruction; of particular importance are the paraclival carotid arteries that run lateral to the clivus; the sella turcica; the cavernous sinus; cranial nerves III, IV, V, and VI that course through the sinus; and the optic chiasm. The basilar artery courses in the posterior cranial fossa, posterior to C1 and C2 within the craniocervical junction. Laterally, the prominence of the jugular tubercle can define the position of cranial nerve XII as it enters the hypoglossal canal. The prepontine cistern is the CSF-filled subarachnoid cistern immediately posterior to the clivus and craniocervical junction. Entry into this cistern results in a high-flow CSF leak, posterior to the paraclival internal carotid arteries. The abducens nerve (cranial nerve VI) is the most medial of the three cranial nerves that exit the

Fig. 23.1 Anatomic schematic of clivus, nasopharynx, and craniocervical junction. *C* clivus, *ICA* internal carotid artery, *PG* pituitary gland, *SSF* sphenoid sinus floor, *C1* first cervical vertebrae, *C2* second cervical vertebrae, *D* dens, *SP* soft palate, *ETO* eustachian tube orifice, *TT* torus tubarius, *MT* middle turbinate, *IT* inferior turbinate

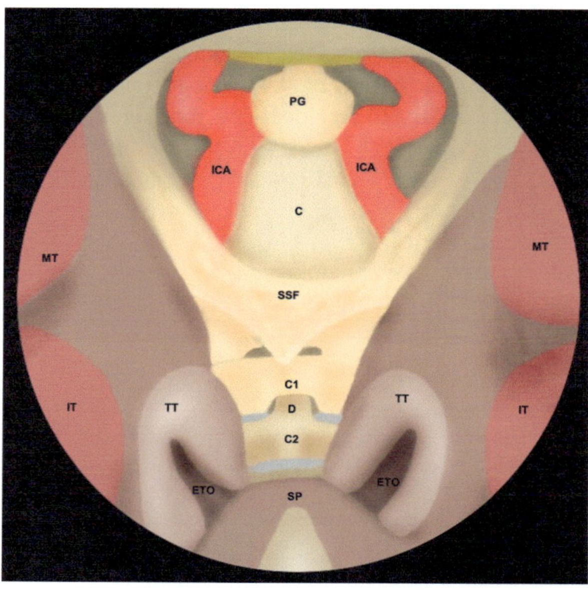

pontomedullary junction (facial nerve, vestibulocochlear nerve, and abducens nerve). After exiting the pontomedullary junction, the nerve courses anteriorly, superiorly, and laterally and enters Dorello's canal—a fibro-osseous channel bounded superiorly by the petrosphenoidal ligament and inferiorly by the bone of the petrous apex and the superolateral clivus. It pierces the dura and turns forward to project into the cavernous sinus. The medial position at the pontomedullary junction, medial position in the cavernous sinus, relative fixation within Dorello's canal, and long course put the nerve at a high risk for injury from surgical manipulation (particularly from transclival work and transclival approaches to the petrous apex) and elevated intracranial pressure leading to stretch injury.

Principles and Challenges of Clival and Craniocervical Junction Reconstruction

Common clinical pathologies involving the nasopharynx, clivus, and craniocervical junction include nasopharyngeal carcinoma, clival chordoma, petroclival chondrosarcoma, and rheumatoid pannus of the odontoid process of C2. Surgical intervention often results in a mucosal defect (from mucosal elevation and/or resection in the setting of tumor involvement), a bone defect (from bone removal and/or resection given tumor involvement), and/or a dural defect (from intradural access and/or dural resection given tumor involvement). Within this framework, the goals of reconstruction are to separate the intracranial and extracranial compartments to prevent complications like meningoencephalitis, pneumocephalus, and CSF leak, provide soft tissue coverage of the key neurovascular structures (cranial nerves, paraclival carotids, and basilar artery), minimize risk of pontine encephalocele, and potentially accelerate wound healing.

An overarching, specific challenge of clival and craniocervical junction defect reconstruction is their orientation—the clivus slopes inferiorly as it progresses posteriorly, and the craniocervical junction is essentially vertically oriented. Typically, the floor of the sphenoid sinus is removed to facilitate access to the mid and lower clivus and upper craniocervical junction. As such, when graft materials are inset into a skull base defect, there is not a stable "floor" to build off of to support the proposed reconstruction. This issue is surpassed by careful placement of the graft materials and the strategic use of resorbable and permanent nasal packing to create a bolster to hold the grafts in position. However, aggressive packing to overcome this issue can lead to compression of critical brainstem neurovascular with significant risk of resultant morbidity or mortality. Additionally, inferiorly based flaps of the nasopharyngeal mucosa and pharyngobasilar fascia may help to provide inferior support to the reconstruction.

In their study evaluating lumbar drains after endoscopic skull base surgery, Zwagerman et al. found that the size of clival dural defects tended to be larger than dural defects following suprasellar surgery [1]. Moreover, the size of the dural defect was significantly, positively associated with the risk of post-operative CSF leak—patients with CSF leaks had an average dural defect of 6.2 cm^2 compared to 2.9 cm^2 for patients who did not have CSF leaks ($p = 0.03$). As such, the size of the dural defect following clival or craniocervical junction surgery is a key issue for clival and craniocervical junction defect reconstruction.

The depression created by the removal of the bone of the clivus while maintaining the superficial position of the paraclival carotids and the pituitary gland offers another challenge to the reconstructive surgeon. If left unaddressed, this depth discrepancy increases the surface area of reconstruction required and creates a complex contour that can create gaps within the reconstruction, allowing for fistula formation.

The proximity of the prepontine cistern and the frequency of intradural extension of common clival pathology create the potential for high-flow CSF leaks either during tumor ablation or if inadvertently opened. The severity of the leak, if present, is exacerbated by the dependent position of the cistern. In this scenario, reconstruction often requires multilayered closure with vascularized tissue coverage as well as lumbar drain placement.

Finally, a number of malignant skull base pathologies can be managed either primarily or in the adjuvant setting with radiation therapy. A history of radiation exposure (e.g., for nasopharyngeal carcinoma treated primarily with chemoradiation) reduces the availability of local, robustly vascularized tissue. Should salvage surgery be deemed necessary, regional vascularized flap reconstruction of the defect is recommended to mitigate radiation-induced breakdown and treatment-related complications (e.g., osteoradionecrosis of the skull base).

The complexity of posterior cranial fossa is underscored by prior research efforts to understand the incidence of complication rates noted in the skull base literature: in an aggregate population of 299 patients who underwent skull base surgery of the clivus from 7 systematic and retrospective studies, Wang et al. noted a 19.1% reconstructive failure rate; by contrast there was a 4.2% reconstructive failure rate of 140 patients who underwent surgery of the craniocervical junction [2]. A general reconstructive algorithm is presented in Fig. 23.2.

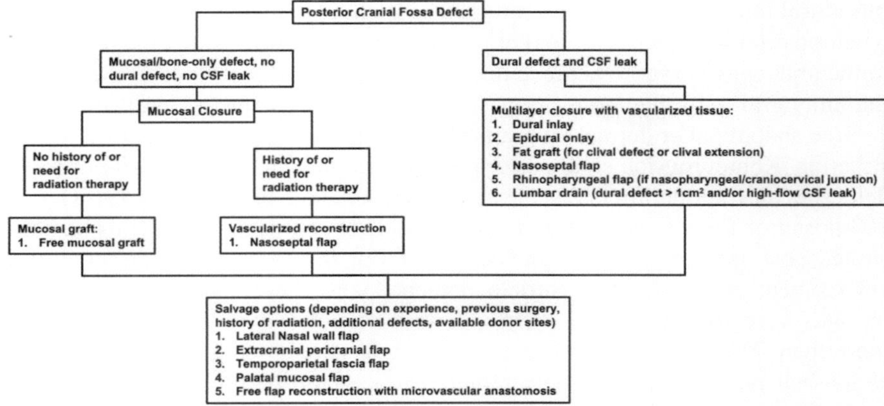

Fig. 23.2 General reconstructive algorithm. Assessment of tissue defect, size of the defect, presence of a cerebrospinal fluid (CSF) leak, history of radiation therapy or need for adjuvant radiation therapy, and degree of clival and/or craniocervical junction involvement in the defect are key factors in considering reconstructive options. The final reconstructive strategy, use of antibiotics, endonasal packing, and lumbar drain are influenced by surgeon experience and preference as well

Review of Reconstructive Techniques

Multilayered Reconstruction Paradigm

The techniques available for skull base defect reconstruction can be largely divided into free mucosal grafts, local pedicled flaps, regional flaps, and microvascular free tissue transfer. Regardless of the final choice of tissue, multilayered closure is recommended when reconstructing complex defects of the clivus and craniocervical junction with an intraoperative CSF leak. While there are no studies directly comparing single-layer and multilayer closures, expert opinion does favor multilayer closure for complex defects that result in a high-flow CSF leak, as is often the case with clival dissection [2].

When the mucosa, periosteum, bone, and dura are resected, multilayer reconstruction is typically composed of an inlay intradural graft (between the brainstem and dura) and a composite extradural onlay (overexposed dura and bone) comprised of a combination of materials including fascia lata free graft, fat graft (either abdominal or dermal), and/or vascularized mucoperiosteal flaps (nasoseptal flap, lateral nasal wall flap, etc.). Several materials have been utilized for the dural inlay and extradural onlay grafts, including fascia lata and allograft materials such as acellular cadaveric human dermis (AlloDerm, LifeCell Corporation, Branchburg, NJ) and collagen matrix grafts (DuraGen, Integra LifeSciences Corporation, Plainsboro, NJ; DuraMatrix, Stryker Corporation, Oakland, NJ). The choice between graft types is classically based on surgeon experience and preference; the authors prefer a collagen graft intradural inlay and fascia lata graft onlay for clival defects. Care must be taken when positioning the lateral extent of the intradural inlay graft to avoid injury to the abducens nerve; to achieve this, a slit can be cut into the lateral edges of the inlay graft that the nerve can pass through as it courses to Dorello's canal.

Free abdominal or dermal fat grafts also play an important role in clival reconstruction. Koutourousiou et al. performed radiographic analysis of posterior fossa defect reconstruction after transclival endoscopic skull base surgery [3]. Out of 103 posterior fossa tumors treated via a transclival approach, 14 patients demonstrated post-operative changes including anterior displacement of the pons and enlargement of the fourth ventricle. Patients with these specific radiographic changes were noted to have extensive clival dissection (>50% bone removal), and more than 50% of the patients were overweight (BMI > 25). The use of a free abdominal fat graft was the only protective factor in the prevention of pontine herniation, associated with 91% lower odds of developing pontine herniation/ encephalocele.

The use of abdominal fat in multilayer reconstruction of clival defects has the added benefit of reducing the distance created by the removal of the clivus when contouring a locoregional flap over the paraclival carotid arteries. Filling this space reduces the required surface area of mucosal graft and provides a level contour that improves the contact between the layers of the reconstruction and the surgical defect. An overview of the steps of reconstruction from the preoperative evaluation to the post-operative setting is presented in Fig. 23.3.

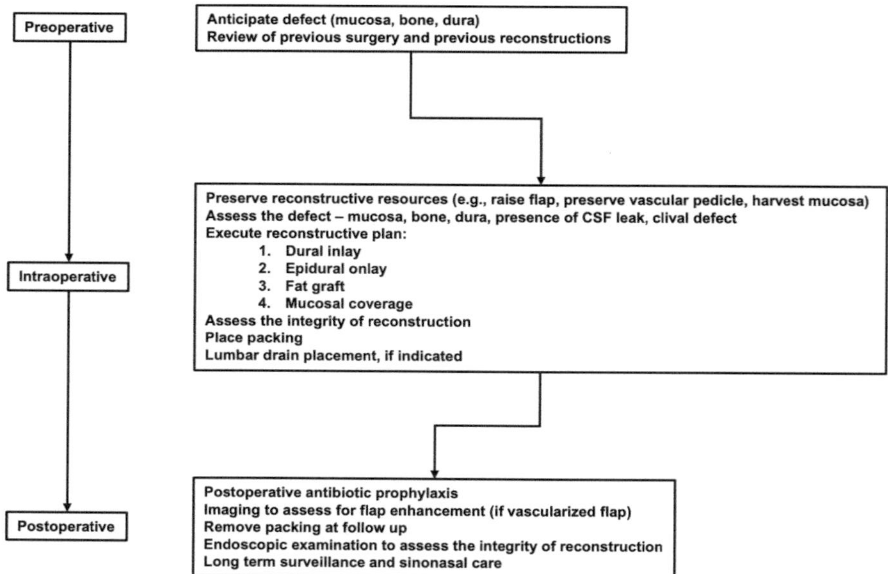

Fig. 23.3 Overview of the steps of reconstruction

Free Mucosal Grafts

Free mucosal grafts are often harvested from the middle turbinate (which is frequently removed during endoscopic skull base surgery) or the nasal floor. Previous studies have demonstrated the relative equivalency in preventing post-operative CSF leaks between free mucosal grafts and vascularized reconstruction when there is either no intraoperative or a low-flow intraoperative CSF leak [2]. By contrast, Soudry et al. found in a systematic review that high-flow intraoperative CSF leaks were better managed with vascularized tissue reconstruction in lieu of free mucosal grafts—4% post-operative CSF leak rate with vascularized reconstruction vs. 18% post-operative CSF leak rate with free mucosal graft reconstruction [4]. Moreover, Soudry et al. reported a 60% success rate with free mucosal graft reconstruction for clival defects compared to a 75–100% success rate with vascularized tissue reconstruction. Based on the best available evidence, vascularized reconstruction is critical following surgery of the posterior cranial fossa and craniocervical junction that involves dissection of the prepontine cistern or results in a high-flow CSF leak, while a free mucosal graft may be an option if the surgery does not result in an intraoperative CSF leak.

Local Pedicled Flaps: Nasoseptal Flap, Lateral Nasal Wall Flap, and Rhinopharyngeal Flap

The nasoseptal flap is a local flap of septal mucosa and perichondrium/periosteum that is pedicled posteriorly by the posterior septal branch of the sphenopalatine artery. The flap was popularized by Hadad et al. in 2006 and has since become the workhorse flap for endonasal skull base reconstruction [5]. Modifications that can be performed include an extension to include the nasal floor and inferior meatal mucosa for clival defects as well as the ability to raise rescue flaps for craniocervical defects. Its premier position as the workhorse reconstructive flap is based on a robust vascular supply, ability for rapid flap elevation, minimal donor site morbidity, ease of access within the surgical field, and total available surface area. Within the context of clival and craniocervical junction reconstruction, the arc of rotation relative to the vascular pedicle may limit the coverage that it can provide. In this situation, mobilization of the vascular pedicle to the internal maxillary artery in the pterygopalatine fossa has been described to maximize the reach of the flap [6]. Care must be taken not to injure the pedicle during transclival surgery as the course of the posterior septal branch is at the same level as the mid-clivus in an axial plane. Careful preoperative planning of the anticipated defect is essential, and supplementation with other grafts or flaps across the reconstructive ladder may be required to address particularly low or extensive defects of the clivus and/or craniocervical junction. An endoscopic view of a multilayer reconstruction of a clival defect with fascia lata, abdominal fat, and an extended nasoseptal flap is presented in Fig. 23.4.

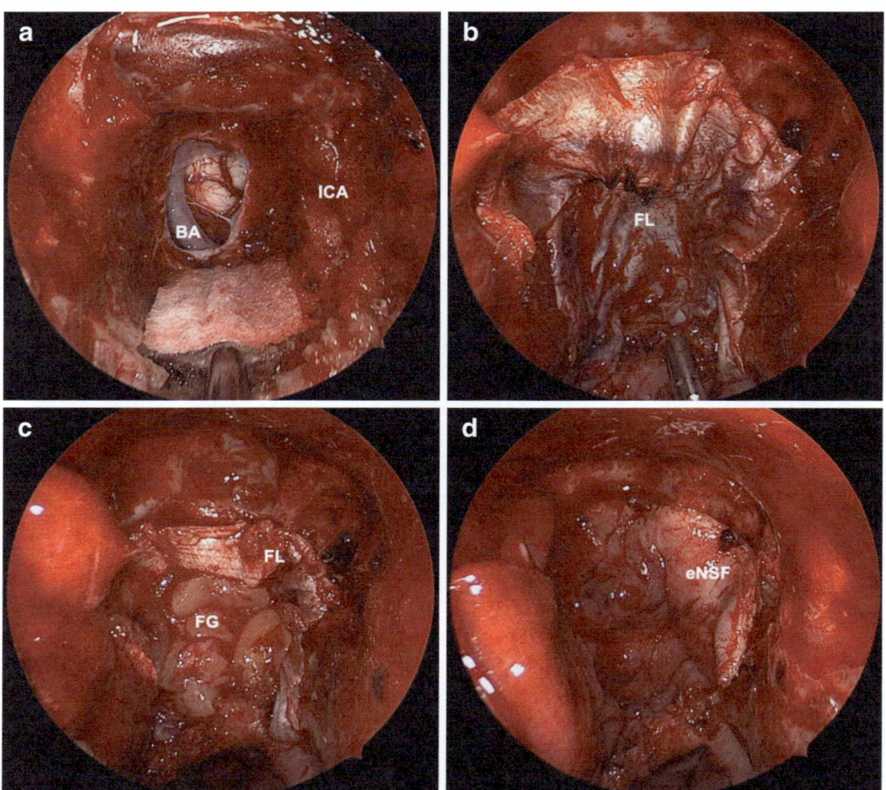

Fig. 23.4 Multilayer reconstruction of a clival defect. (**a**) A clival defect with exposure of the posterior cranial fossa contents, including the basilar artery. Half-inch cottonoid included for scale. (**b**) A fascia lata graft has been placed over the defect after placement of a collagen matrix inlay (not shown). (**c**) Placement of a free abdominal fat graft to reduce the clival defect. (**d**) Placement and positioning of the extended nasoseptal flap to complete the multilayer reconstruction. *ICA* internal carotid artery, *BA* basilar artery, *FL* fascia lata, *FG* fat graft, *eNSF* extended nasoseptal flap

As previously noted, vascularized flaps, with the nasoseptal flap being the most commonly analyzed, are superior to free mucosal grafts for clival reconstruction with regard to post-operative CSF leak rates. Fraser et al. performed a retrospective review of 615 patients who underwent skull base reconstruction and found that posterior fossa tumors had the highest rates of post-operative CSF leaks (32.6%, compared to 9.9% of sellar/suprasellar defects). This group also found that vascularized flap utilization was associated with lower rates of post-operative CSF leaks compared to free grafts: 13.5% vs. 27.8% [7]. Direct comparisons of mucosal grafts and vascularized flaps in reconstruction of posterior fossa defects were not included, but the authors determined that posterior cranial fossa defects should be considered to be an indication for reconstruction with a vascularized flap rather than a free graft.

The mucosa of the lateral nasal wall and inferior turbinate has also been employed in skull base reconstruction. In 2007, Fortes et al. described a mucoperiosteal inferior turbinate flap pedicled posteriorly on the artery to the inferior turbinate for the reconstruction of three clival defects [8]. Previous studies had demonstrated that a similar flap pedicled anteriorly could offer approximately 5 cm^2 of surface area for reconstruction [9], but the authors noted that flap size could be augmented by raising bilateral flaps or extending the incisions to include the nasal floor and middle meatus. All patients in the original report recovered without post-operative complications or CSF leak. Lavigne et al. performed an anatomic cadaveric study characterizing the vascular pedicle of the lateral nasal wall flap and found that the deep branch of the artery of the inferior turbinate was the dominant supply to the flap, rather than the superficial branch [10]. The authors also described the clinical outcomes of 24 lateral nasal wall flaps used when a nasoseptal flap was unavailable, there was a post-operative CSF leak from nasoseptal flap necrosis, or there was a post-operative leak due to insufficient flap tissue. They noted an overall success rate of 75%—while an anatomic subsite-specific analysis was not included, a majority of the flaps (18/24) were used in clival and craniocervical junction reconstruction. The authors note the particular suitability of this flap for posterior fossa reconstruction given the pedicle location and orientation. Anteriorly pedicled lateral nasal wall flaps have also been well described but based on the pedicle location are not suitable for reconstruction of clival or craniocervical junction defects.

The soft tissue of the nasopharynx and upper oropharynx can either be removed or elevated as an inferiorly pedicled flap to access the lower clivus or craniocervical junction, referred to as a rhinopharyngeal flap. The mucosa of the nasopharynx is incised with a needle-tip electrocautery in an inverted-U with the sphenoid floor forming the superior boundary and the fossae of Rosenmüller and salpingopharyngeus muscles forming the lateral boundaries. The position of the parapharyngeal carotid arteries should be assessed preoperatively on imaging and intraoperatively with Doppler ultrasound to avoid inadvertent injury with flap elevation. During reconstruction, the soft tissue of the rhinopharyngeal flap is typically positioned over the edges of the fascia lata used as an extradural onlay graft, thus limiting a direct avenue of egress of CSF into the lumen of the oropharynx and nasopharynx. If another vascularized flap is being employed for reconstruction (e.g., a nasoseptal flap), care is taken to minimize mucosal overlap so that the mucoperichondrium and mucoperiosteum of both flaps are in contact with the deeper layers of the multilayer reconstruction. The endoscopic views of an odontoidectomy defect, elevation of the rhinopharyngeal flap, and final flap placement and stabilization with tissue glue are presented in Fig. 23.5.

Champagne et al. performed a retrospective case-control study evaluating the lower clival and craniocervical junction reconstruction with and without a rhinopharyngeal flap [11]. Sixty patients underwent surgery of the clivus or craniocervical junction of which 30 had a rhinopharyngeal flap and 30 patients did not have a rhinopharyngeal flap. There was no significant difference in the rates of CSF leaks between the flap and no-flap group; however, there was a significantly higher rate of nasoseptal flap necrosis (no-flap 20% vs. flap 3%) and surgical site infection

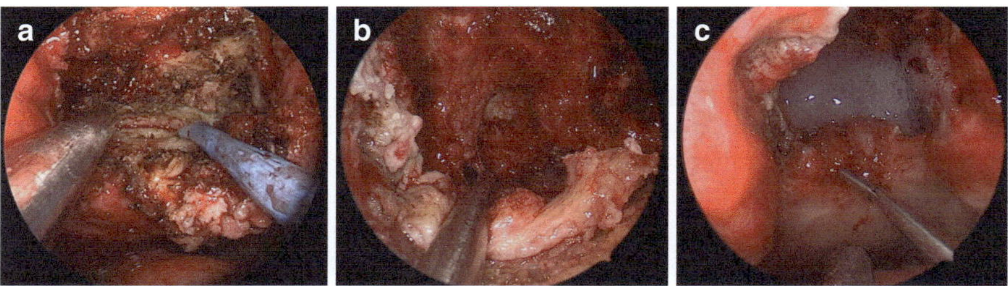

Fig. 23.5 Craniocervical junction defect and rhinopharyngeal flap. (**a**) Elevation of the rhinopharyngeal flap—the flap is elevated using electrocautery in a superior to inferior direction. (**b**) A craniocervical junction defect after removal of the odontoid process. (**c**) After the craniocervical junction work is done, the rhinopharyngeal flap is reflected superiorly and can be stabilized in this position using a fibrin tissue glue

(no-flap 27% vs. flap 3%) in the group reconstructed without a rhinopharyngeal flap between post-operative CSF leaks. All rhinopharyngeal flaps were found to be well vascularized as shown by contrast enhancement on post-operative gadolinium-enhanced MRI. Though the exact, causal relationship between the nasoseptal flap, rhinopharyngeal flap, flap necrosis, and infection remains unclear, the flap does appear to improve the integrity of low-clival and craniocervical junction reconstruction when available. It may serve as a soft tissue "floor" akin to the sphenoid sinus floor in supporting the inferior aspect of the reconstruction and serve as a barrier to prevent contamination from the oropharynx.

Vascularized Regional Flaps: Pericranial Flap, Temporoparietal Fascia Flap, and Palatal Flap

Many other reconstructive flaps have been described in the literature; however, no other flap has been studied as extensively as the nasoseptal flap, and there are no head-to-head studies comparing outcomes across reconstructive outcomes. As such, in reviewing other reconstructive flaps, comparisons are made based on logistical as well as technical advantages and disadvantages rather than evidence-based, functional performance. However, all of these regional flaps do benefit from a robust vascular supply and are thus considered to be functionally superior to free mucosal grafts when reconstructing complex cranial base defects with high-flow CSF leaks. This assumption is supported by evidence provided by Patel et al. who reported only 1 CSF leak across 34 cases reconstructed with secondary flaps (i.e., non-nasoseptal flap reconstructions); this rate was found to be equivalent to the success rate achieved with nasoseptal flap reconstruction [12].

The pericranial flap is a subgaleal flap of scalp pericranium pedicled on the supratrochlear and supraorbital arteries. The flap has a long history of use in open craniofacial and anterior skull base reconstruction. Theoretically the flap can extend from the vascular pedicle to the occiput, providing a very large, vascularized graft. Moreover, its robust vascular supply allows the flap to survive on one vascular pedicle. The pericranial flap initially suffered with the transition to endoscopic endonasal surgery as there was not a reliable, minimally invasive/endoscopic harvest technique. However, in more recent years, endoscopic harvest and tunneling techniques have been described; in these reports, large flaps of pericranium were used to reconstruct the entirety of the anterior skull base from frontal sinus to the planum sphenoidale [13]. After endoscopic-assisted harvest, the flap is transposed intranasally via a tunnel drilled through the nasion. Follow-up studies provided a radiologic methodology to estimate the size of pericranium needed to reach particular defects, including clival and posterior cranial fossa defects [14]. To identify risk factors for persistent CSF leak, Torres-Bayona et al. performed a case-control study of 7 patients with persistent post-operative CSF leaks (requiring more than 1 repair) matched to 25 patients who underwent similar surgeries but did not develop persistent CSF leaks [15]. All patients, both case and control, underwent transclival/posterior cranial fossa surgery and had high-flow intraoperative CSF leaks during the index surgery. There was a significantly higher proportion of obese patients in the persistent leak group than the matched controls. Furthermore, the authors reported that five of the seven patients with persistent leak were ultimately salvaged with a pericranial flap. The pericranial flap is particularly useful when the septal mucosa is not a viable flap either due to previous procedures or septal involvement with a malignancy, if a clival defect is confluent with a large anterior cranial base defect, or in the setting of a persistent CSF leak in an obese patient.

The temporoparietal fascia flap is pedicled on the anterior branch of the superficial temporal artery (one of the terminal branches of the external carotid artery) and utilizes the temporoparietal fascia of the temporal region for reconstruction (the inferior continuation of the galea aponeurotica of the scalp and the superior continuation of the superficial musculoaponeurotic system of the face). Although previously described in the head and neck and plastic surgery literature for the reconstruction of the scalp, auricle, orbit, and oral cavity defects, in 2007 Fortes et al. described a novel methodology for transposing the flap endonasally via a trans-infratemporal fossa/pterygopalatine fossa approach [16] that was well illustrated in a surgical video published by London et al. in 2020 [17]. The lateral positioning of the vascular pedicle makes this flap geometrically well suited to reconstruction of clival and craniocervical junction with defects extensive enough to involve the foramen magnum [16, 18]. Relative to the endoscopically harvested pericranial flap or nasoseptal flap, the temporoparietal fascia flap does require an external, hemicoronal (and sometimes bicoronal) incision. The authors recommend using the flap in scenarios where the nasoseptal flap is not available for reconstruction and further recommend using the flap, if available, on the ipsilateral side of the defect. Particular pitfalls to be aware of with the temporoparietal fascia flap are a history of superficial temporal artery biopsy or scalp radiation which may compromise the vascular pedicle.

Palatal mucoperiosteal flaps have also been used in clival and posterior cranial fossa reconstruction. Oliver et al. described a method to transpose a hemi- or complete palatal mucoperiosteal flap via the greater palatine canal pedicled on the descending palatine vessels endonasally for skull base reconstruction [19]. The authors noted a potential flap surface area of up to 18.5 cm^2 that allowed easy coverage of clival defects and craniocervical junction defects to the level of the foramen magnum. Patel et al. reported two clinical cases of the palatal transposition flap used for clival reconstruction and noted no post-operative complications [12].

Microvascular Free Tissue Transfer

Microvascular reconstruction has been described in reconstruction of skull base defects but is generally considered to be a last-resort option in extensive defects and/or if no viable locoregional pedicle flap options exist. A variety of donor sites have been described including radial forearm free flaps [20, 21], anterolateral thigh free flaps [22], and the fibula free flap [23]. Technically, the vascular pedicle of these flaps is oftentimes tunneled through the maxillary sinus and a lateral maxillotomy for anastomosis with the recipient vessels of the neck, oftentimes the facial vessels [24], though other techniques have been described where the pedicle is externalized via a burr-hole craniotomy [25]. The plethora of local, pedicled flaps has mitigated the need for regular microvascular free tissue transfer, but they remain an important component of the reconstructive ladder.

Perioperative Management

Packing

Numerous options exist for nasal packing in endoscopic skull base surgery. The role of packing is to bolster the skull base reconstruction in the acute phases of healing but may provide the added benefit of hemostasis and maintenance of nasal patency. Both absorbable options (NasoPore, Gelfoam, Surgicel) and nonabsorbable options (Merocel, strip gauze packing) exist. The choice and combination of agents to use in packing are best left to surgeon experience given the lack of evidence for or against particular agents. Within the context of clival and craniocervical junction defects, packing has to be very carefully placed to bolster the reconstruction of a potentially high-flow CSF leak but without overpacking and exerting pressure on the delicate structures of the brainstem and posterior cranial fossa. For reconstructions involving high-flow CSF leaks, the authors use Merocel (Medtronic Inc., Minneapolis, MN, USA) to buttress the reconstruction; conversely, NasoPore (Stryker, Kalamazoo, Michigan, USA) is used for packing in extradural reconstructions without CSF leaks.

Antibiotics

Data assessing the use of perioperative antibiotics in endoscopic skull base surgery is particularly heterogenous. Agents, duration, and indications with respect to CSF leak and nasal packing as well as pathology-specific usage vary widely across studies and from institution to institution [2]. Rosen et al. performed a systematic review of perioperative prophylactic antibiotics in endoscopic skull base surgery and was unable to perform a meta-analysis due to the heterogeneity of the included reports [26]. Milanese et al. found significantly higher rates of meningitis in patients with post-operative CSF leaks (OR 20.8; 95% CI 5.6–76.6) and surgery for malignancy (OR 8.3; 95% CI 1.2–36.8). Higher-quality studies assessing the risk factors for post-operative infection and the role of prophylactic antibiotics are necessary to address these unanswered questions [27]. Based on this, an evidence-based statement on the use perioperative use of prophylactic antibiotics is not possible; it is the authors' practice, though, to provide IV ceftriaxone for 48 h post-operatively, thereafter, switching to 5 days of cefuroxime for the duration of nasal packing.

Lumbar Drain

Perioperative lumbar can be used to augment multilayered closures and vascularized tissue coverage in posterior fossa defects and minimize post-operative CSF leaks. Placement of a lumbar drain creates a low-resistance avenue of egress for CSF thus potentially reducing the pressure on the skull base reconstruction. Wang et al. performed a meta-analysis of 7 studies with 1131 cases of endoscopic skull base surgery—the average odds ratio or post-operative leak for patients with a lumbar drain compared to those without was 1.14 (95% CI 0.7954–1.6496) suggesting an equivocal effect [2]. Of note, the studies that were used for the meta-analysis often did not provide pathology- or subsite-specific leak rates with and without lumbar drain placement. Zwagerman et al. performed a prospective randomized-controlled clinical trial of lumbar drain placement in patients who developed an intraoperative high-flow CSF leak [1]. Eighty-five patients were randomized to receive a lumbar drain, and 85 patients were randomized to no drain. The trial was ended early due to a clear benefit of lumbar drain placement on interim analysis—CSF leak rate in patients without a lumbar drain was 21.2% compared to 8.2% in the experimental group. Fifty patients in the study had posterior fossa pathology—among these patients, the leak rate for those with a drain was 12.5% compared to 30.8% without a drain. Based on these data, the authors advocate for lumbar drain placement in transclival or craniocervical junction surgery that results in a high-flow CSF leak or a large dural defect (>1 cm^2). Surgery that does not result in an intraoperative CSF leak or a dural defect does not require lumbar drain placement.

Conclusions

Endoscopic reconstruction of clival and craniocervical junction defects poses unique challenges to the skull base surgery team. The clival recess, the proximity of the prepontine cistern and potential for high-flow CSF leaks, the proximity of key neurovascular structures, the orientation of clival and craniocervical defects, and the types of the pathologies seen in these regions all require careful consideration during the reconstructive process. For defects in this area that result in a CSF leak, vascularized, multilayered closure provides superior results; the use of abdominal fat grafts also helps reduce the rates of pontine herniation for clival reconstruction. Additionally, fat can fill the clival recess, flatten the defect, and decrease the coverage area of vascularized mucosal flap. When possible, nasopharyngeal mucosa should be preserved to create a rhinopharyngeal flap for closure of nasopharyngeal and craniocervical junction defects. Finally, while the nasoseptal flap is a versatile flap that is a key component of clival, craniocervical, and posterior fossa reconstruction, the cranial base team must be prepared to utilize secondary vascular flaps in the salvage setting or when the nasoseptal flap is not available.

References

1. Zwagerman NT, Wang EW, Shin SS, Chang Y-F, Fernandez-Miranda JC, Snyderman CH, et al. Does lumbar drainage reduce postoperative cerebrospinal fluid leak after endoscopic endonasal skull base surgery? A prospective, randomized controlled trial. J Neurosurg. 2018:1–7.
2. Wang EW, Zanation AM, Gardner PA, Schwartz TH, Eloy JA, Adappa ND, et al. ICAR: endoscopic skull-base surgery. Int Forum Allergy Rhinol. 2019;9(S3):S145–365.
3. Koutourousiou M, Filho FVG, Costacou T, Fernandez-Miranda JC, Wang EW, Snyderman CH, et al. Pontine encephalocele and abnormalities of the posterior fossa following transclival endoscopic endonasal surgery. J Neurosurg. 2014;121(2):359–66.
4. Soudry E, Turner JH, Nayak JV, Hwang PH. Endoscopic reconstruction of surgically created skull base defects: a systematic review. Otolaryngol Head Neck Surg. 2014;150(5):730–8.
5. Hadad G, Bassagasteguy L, Carrau RL, Mataza JC, Kassam A, Snyderman CH, et al. A novel reconstructive technique after endoscopic expanded endonasal approaches: vascular pedicle nasoseptal flap. Laryngoscope. 2006;116(10):1882–6.
6. Pinheiro-Neto CD, Peris-Celda M, Kenning T. Extrapolating the limits of the nasoseptal flap with pedicle dissection to the internal maxillary artery. Oper Neurosurg. 2019;16(1):37–44.
7. Fraser S, Gardner PA, Koutourousiou M, Kubik M, Fernandez-Miranda JC, Snyderman CH, et al. Risk factors associated with postoperative cerebrospinal fluid leak after endoscopic endonasal skull base surgery. J Neurosurg. 2018;128(4):1066–71.
8. Fortes FSG, Carrau RL, Snyderman CH, Prevedello D, Vescan A, Mintz A, et al. The posterior pedicle inferior turbinate flap: a new vascularized flap for skull base reconstruction. Laryngoscope. 2007;117(8):1329–32.
9. Murakami CS, Kriet JD, Ierokomos AP. Nasal reconstruction using the inferior turbinate mucosal flap. Arch Facial Plast Surg. 1999;1(2):97–100.
10. Lavigne P, Vega MB, Ahmed OH, Gardner PA, Snyderman CH, Wang EW. Lateral nasal wall flap for endoscopic reconstruction of the skull base: anatomical study and clinical series. Int Forum Allergy Rhinol. 2020;10(5):673–8.

11. Champagne P-O, Zenonos GA, Wang EW, Snyderman CH, Gardner PA. The rhinopharyngeal flap for reconstruction of lower clival and craniovertebral junction defects. J Neurosurg. 2021;12:1–9.
12. Patel MR, Taylor RJ, Hackman TG, Germanwala AV, Sasaki-Adams D, Ewend MG, et al. Beyond the nasoseptal flap: outcomes and pearls with secondary flaps in endoscopic endonasal skull base reconstruction. Laryngoscope. 2014;124(4):846–52.
13. Zanation AM, Snyderman CH, Carrau RL, Kassam AB, Gardner PA, Prevedello DM. Minimally invasive endoscopic pericranial flap: a new method for endonasal skull base reconstruction. Laryngoscope. 2009;119(1):13–8.
14. Patel MR, Shah RN, Snyderman CH, Carrau RL, Germanwala AV, Kassam AB, et al. Pericranial flap for endoscopic anterior skull-base reconstruction: clinical outcomes and radioanatomic analysis of preoperative planning. Neurosurgery. 2010;66(3):506–12; discussion 512.
15. Bayona-Torres S, Velasquez N, Nakassa A, Eguiluz-Melendez A, Hernandez V, et al.. Risk factors and reconstruction techniques for persistent cerebrospinal fluid leak in patients undergoing endoscopic endonasal approach to the posterior fossa. J Neurol Surg B Skull Base. 2021 Feb 24 [cited 2021 June 8]. https://www.thieme-connect.com/products/ejournals/abstract/10.1055/s-0041-1729904.
16. Fortes FSG, Carrau RL, Snyderman CH, Kassam A, Prevedello D, Vescan A, et al. Transpterygoid transposition of a temporoparietal fascia flap: a new method for skull base reconstruction after endoscopic expanded endonasal approaches. Laryngoscope. 2007;117(6):970–6.
17. London NR, Mohyeldin A, Silveira-Bertazzo G, Prevedello DM, Carrau RL. Video demonstration of a tunneled temporoparietal fascia flap: how I do it. Laryngoscope. 2021;131(4):E1088–93.
18. Reconstruction of the cranial base following endonasal skull base surgery: regional tissue flaps. Oper Tech Otolaryngol Head Neck Surg 2010;21(1):83–90.
19. Oliver CL, Hackman TG, Carrau RL, Snyderman CH, Kassam AB, Prevedello DM, et al. Palatal flap modifications allow pedicled reconstruction of the skull base. Laryngoscope. 2008;118(12):2102–6.
20. Hackman TG. Endoscopic adipofascial radial forearm flap reconstruction of a clival defect. Plast Reconstr Surg Glob Open. 2016;4(11):e1109.
21. Mady LJ, Kaffenberger TM, Baddour K, Melder K, Godse NR, Gardner P, et al.. Anatomic considerations of microvascular free tissue transfer in endoscopic endonasal skull base surgery. J Neurol Surg B Skull Base. 2021 Feb 22 [cited 2021 May 3]. http://www.thieme-connect.de/DOI/DOI?10.1055/s-0041-1722935.
22. Bell EB, Cohen ER, Sargi Z, Leibowitz J. Free tissue reconstruction of the anterior skull base: a review. World J Otorhinolaryngol Head Neck Surg. 2020;6(2):132–6.
23. Heredero S, Solivera J, García B, Dean A. Osteomyocutaneous peroneal artery perforator flap for reconstruction of the skull base. Br J Oral Maxillofac Surg. 2016;54(1):99–101.
24. Moy JD, Gardner PA, Sridharan S, Wang EW. Radial forearm free tissue transfer to clival defect. J Neurol Surg B Skull Base. 2019;80(Suppl 4):S380–1.
25. Minchew HM, Karadaghy OA, Camarata PJ, Chamoun RB, Beahm DD, Przylecki WH, et al. Outcomes and utility of intracranial free tissue transfer. Ann Otol Rhinol Laryngol. 2022;131:94.
26. Rosen SAB, Getz AE, Kingdom T, Youssef AS, Ramakrishnan VR. Systematic review of the effectiveness of perioperative prophylactic antibiotics for skull base surgeries. Am J Rhinol Allergy. 2016;30(2):e10–6.
27. Milanese L, Zoli M, Sollini G, Martone C, Zenesini C, Sturiale C, et al. Antibiotic prophylaxis in endoscopic endonasal pituitary and skull base surgery. World Neurosurg. 2017;106:912–8.

Part V
Lateral Skull Base Reconstruction

Chapter 24
Management of Cerebrospinal Fluid Leaks During Otologic Surgery

Matthew A. Shew, David Lee, and James Lin

Introduction

Cerebrospinal fluid (CSF) leaks are rare and sometimes unavoidable in otologic and lateral skull base surgery. While there are multiple etiologies for CSF leaks, they all originate from an abnormal communication between the subarachnoid space and the air-containing spaces of the temporal bone. CSF leaks clinically present from three primary anatomic barriers: the tympanic membrane (CSF otorrhea), the eustachian tube (CSF rhinorrhea), and/or violated skin (incisional or traumatic). Ultimately, CSF fluid will percolate through the aerated temporal bone in the middle ear and present through any of these communication pathways. It is imperative to understand that CSF leaks can occur in any otologic surgery from a routine stapes operation to large complex lateral skull base operations. CSF leaks in otologic surgery can be classified as congenital and acquired, with acquired CSF leaks being far more common. There is no consensus on the exact incidence of acquired temporal bone CSF fistula. However acquired CSF leaks have been estimated to be present in about 17% of temporal bone fractures [1], 1% of all revision chronic ear surgeries [2], and 10–20% following vestibular schwannoma surgery [3]. Congenital CSF leaks, while less common, may also present from different congenital cochlear or peri-labyrinthine anomalies. Although some CSF leaks remain indolent for many years, unrepaired fistulas may lead to highly morbid complications like meningitis

M. A. Shew (✉) · D. Lee
Department of Otolaryngology Head and Neck Surgery, Washington University School of Medicine, St. Louis, MO, USA
e-mail: mshew@wustl.edu

J. Lin
Department of Otolaryngology Head and Neck Surgery, University of Kansas School of Medicine, Kansas City, KS, USA
e-mail: jlin2@kumc.edu

or brain abscess. Thorough preoperative planning, anticipation, prompt recognition, a comprehensive understanding of temporal bone anatomy, and an arsenal of techniques for the management of CSF fistulas are critical for a surgeon to best take care of patients within an otology and neurotology practice.

Preoperative Considerations

Role of Imaging and Avoidance

The simplest method for managing CSF leaks is early preoperative recognition and avoidance. Judicious use of imaging, either computed tomography (CT) scan or magnetic resonance imaging (MRI) of the temporal bones, is often performed prior to otologic surgery for surgical planning. CT is often best to delineate the bony anatomy and identify temporal bone air cell tracks that may provide routes for CSF leaks. MRI can help provide additional information on meningoceles as well as identify T2 hyperintense fluid within the temporal bone or middle ear. MRI can also be helpful in identifying alternative signs for patients that are at increased risk for CSF fistula, such as patients with an empty sella or compressed optic nerve suggestive of uncontrolled intracranial hypertension [4].

In cochlear implantation, at least one if not both modalities is often chosen to aid in the detection of a patent cochlear duct, cochlear malformation, cochlear patency, and the presence of a cochlear nerve. The latter is only demonstrable with high-resolution MRI. These imaging modalities for the early recognition of potential CSF fistulas are particularly prudent in patients with any type of suspected congenital hearing loss. Because of risk of radiation exposure, the CT scan may be potentially omitted in the pediatric population [5], in cases of postlingually deafened adults when cochlear nerve deficiency is not suspected, and in symmetric hearing losses with normal examination [6]. When one or both of these imaging modalities are obtained preoperatively, the cochlea must be carefully evaluated for malformations that may predispose to CSF leak upon fenestration prior to electrode array insertion. With early recognition and careful planning, the surgeon may take steps as delineated below to deal with the leak intraoperatively and, equally as important, counsel the patient or caregiver preoperatively and postoperatively the potential for postoperative CSF rhinorrhea or wound collection/leak.

In patients with conductive hearing loss and possible otosclerosis, the role of imaging is less defined prior to exploring the middle ear and performing ossicular chain reconstruction or stapedectomy. Some clinicians advocate for preoperative imaging, but many will argue there is no role for routine imaging provided that the hearing loss is clearly acquired without history of head trauma or chronic ear disease and that the audiogram demonstrates absent acoustic reflexes on the ear in question. The feared complication following stapedotomy or stapedectomy is a CSF gusher [7]. Occasionally, a dilated IAC or vestibule on CT may suggest possible

CSF gusher [8]. However, studies have shown that preoperative CT fails to accurately predict perilymph gusher following stapes footplate fenestration [7, 9]. Therefore CT should be not be heavily relied upon for preoperative diagnosis of CSF gusher. In patients with chronic inflammatory ear disease, this author performs preoperative CT scanning in patients with evidence of cholesteatoma, revision mastoid surgery, or suspicion for CSF leak preoperatively. Imaging is usually deferred in individuals with dry or clearly infectious draining perforations, regardless of size and location.

Perioperative Discussion

Given the potential risk of CSF leak and its intracranial sequelae, it should be discussed with all patients undergoing mastoidectomy for chronic ear disease, skull base procedure, or cochlear implantation. This should be emphasized in revision surgeries as scarring, residual or recidivistic disease, and effaced landmarks all pose additional challenges to the surgeon, placing the patient at a greater risk of complications. When attempting a surgery with imaging findings of inner ear malformation, encephalocele, or dural exposure, those findings should be discussed preoperatively with the patient as it prepares him or her for postoperative precautions should a CSF leak occur. Additionally, if a CSF leak is encountered in surgery and repaired, the location and method of repair should be documented in the operative report and discussed with the patient. The better the patient understands what was performed may play a role in weighing the benefit versus risk of any future procedures on the ear. Secondly, individuals who may be at a higher risk of developing meningitis should strongly be encouraged to receive pneumococcal vaccination prior to surgery.

Operative Repair of Congenital and Acquired CSF Leak

General Considerations

When managing a CSF leak during an otologic procedure, one must consider the patient's comorbidities, hearing status of both ears, location and size/rate of the leak, and infectious state of the ear undergoing surgery (Figs. 24.1 and 24.2). Location plays an import role when considering options to repair a CSF leak and the surrounding anatomy and potential sequelae. For example, a CSF leak surrounding the inner ear cannot undergo vigorous packing in a patient with normal acoustic hearing without significant risk. Similarly, a CSF leak repair surrounding the epitympanum and ossicles may result in significant dampening of the ossicular chain and result in a large conductive hearing loss. On the other hand, in a CSF

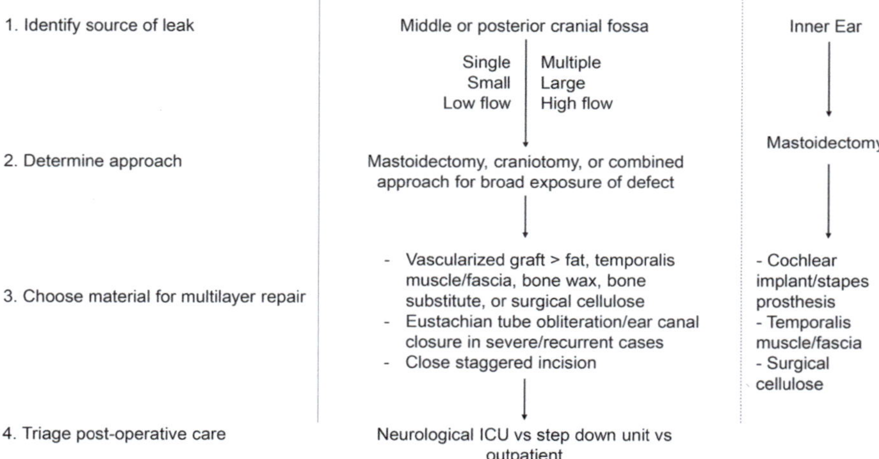

Fig. 24.1 Flow chart of CSF leak repair guiding principles

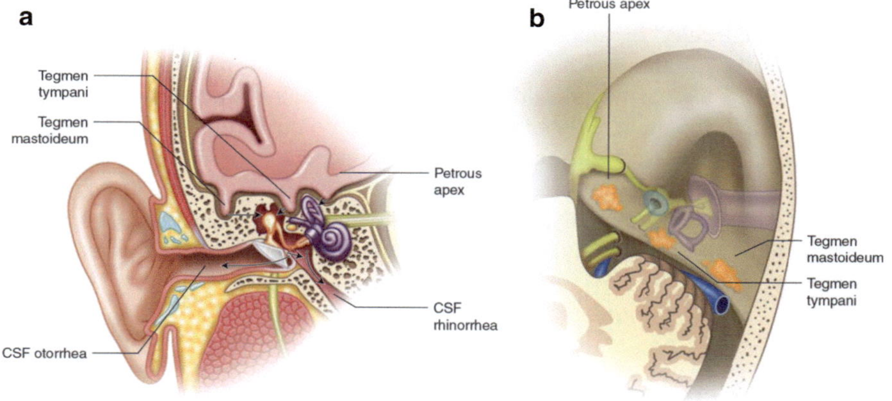

Fig. 24.2 Common locations of CSF leaks, routes of egress, and common approaches. Coronal (**a**) and axial (**b**) illustrations of skull base defects from the mastoid tegmen to the petrous apex. These are typically repaired through either a transmastoid approach for small defects, and middle cranial fossa or combined approaches for large defects. CSF percolates through the aerated temporal bone, eventually draining through the eustachian tube or into the ear canal in the presence of a tympanic membrane perforation

leak within the mastoid, packing may be more vigorous with less risk to the acoustic auditory apparatus. In leaks that occur from the inner ear, the more severe the existing hearing loss, the more aggressive one may be in packing the leak and other potential routes of CSF egress. The more tenuous the repair of the leak, the more consideration should be made to CSF diversion postoperatively. Secondly, the infectious state of the inner ear intraoperatively plays a significant role in management. In patients with obvious and substantial infections, surgeons should strongly consider not only a longer and directed antibiotic therapy but also the use of vascularized tissue for the repair. However, vascularized tissue may not always be available to conform to the dural or bony defect, in which case autologous free tissue should also be considered as an alternative option. Finally, allograft or synthetic material should be used as the last resort in an inflamed mastoid or middle ear.

Avoidance and Detection of Intraoperative CSF Leaks

The dura can be exposed in any procedure that involves a mastoidectomy. Limited dura exposure alone can be common and, given its robust support, often does not require treatment. However, direct dural injury resulting in CSF leak is a complication that is infrequent but should be promptly recognized and treated accordingly. The use of the drill is intuitively the most common cause of iatrogenic CSF leak. Other inciting factors include overuse of cautery, sharp instrumentation, or curettes. Cutting burs are more dangerous than their diamond bur counterparts, and although somewhat counterintuitive, smaller burs are more dangerous than larger burs because of their smaller contact surface. During chronic ear surgery mastoidectomy, dural injury and CSF leak can occur along the middle fossa plate and less commonly along the posterior fossa dura. One must also be cognizant of iatrogenic fistula during performance of a canalplasty in a very contracted ear with a low-lying tegmen above the ear canal. Similarly, extremely obese patients with uncontrolled intracranial hypertension can be at risk of brain herniation and obliteration of the mastoid cavity. This places them at risk of dural injury when elevating the mucoperiosteal flap to expose the underlying mastoid bone for any type of otologic procedure (Fig. 24.1). Patients are at risk for CSF leak during endolymphatic sac surgery because exposure of the endolymphatic sac necessiates exposure of the posterior fossa. Patient who undergo endolymphatic shunt require an incision in the posterior fossa dura fold, utlimately putting them at an even higher risk for a CSF leak.

Although the technique of mastoidectomy is too elementary for this chapter, key principles and techniques to any otologic drilling should be emphasized. It behooves the surgeon to drill from lateral to medial using a wide exposure, parallel to key structures, and one layer at a time. This emphasizes the early identification of key anatomical structures including the tegmen superiorly, external auditory canal anteriorly, and sigmoid sinus posteriorly. These principles are even more critical when operating on a chronic and/or retracted ear to help avoid trauma to the temporal lobe or posterior fossa. Particularly in a chronically inflamed mastoid, there is bleeding that interferes with good visualization of the tegmen; switching to a diamond bur will aid in drying up bleeding sources, presumably by packing bone dust into the offending vascular channels along the tegmen. Furthermore, larger diamond burs are less traumatic to underlying dura should the tegmen be violated. At some point after the mastoidectomy and all drilling is complete, this author visually inspects the middle and posterior fossa bony plates to make sure they are intact. Palpation with a blunt instrument will aid in differentiating an inflamed air cell from exposed dura. Simply exposed dura will usually not develop into a problem, but if there is a leak or the dura is at all compromised, then encephalocele, meningoencephalocele, or CSF leak is at risk of developing in the future [10, 11]. Secondly, some leaks may not be obvious, particularly in the setting of inflamed mucosa; therefore, careful inspection at the conclusion of any otologic procedure is prudent. This may include a Valsalva by the anesthesiologist to increase intrathoracic pressure, decrease intracranial venous outflow, and increase intracranial pressure to elicit leaking if present. Typically, CSF leaks that occur along the tegmen typically have the benefit of temporal lobe expansion intracranially, which aids in blocking the route of CSF egress into the mastoidectomy cavity after repair. On the other hand, the cerebellum is unlikely to expand in such fashion to aid in posterior fossa defects. It is important to identify if dura exposure or disruption occurs during mastoidectomy as persistent CSF leak may lead to meningitis or the development of encephalocele may lead to pain, seizures, or even cosmetic deformity [11] (picture of postoperative encephalocele).

Management of Intraoperative CSF Leak

Soft Tissue Work

Managing a mastoidectomy CSF leak starts with thoughtful perioperative planning. The first step in any otologic surgery that is either in preparation to repair a CSF leak or precautionary for the potential sequelae of an iatrogenic CSF leak includes methodical skin and soft tissue incisions. The steps of making a postauricular incision are relatively straightforward, but one must adhere to good routine soft tissue technique. Staggering the incision through layers and creating a large anteriorly based musculoperiosteal flap not only aids in obliterating a potential canal wall down defect, but it also provides a potential soft tissue flap to plug low posterior fossa CSF leaks that may occur during surgery. If not used for mastoid obliteration or CSF leak plugging, the careful approximation of staggered layers decreases the likelihood of CSF egress through the wound. One should be mindful to minimize cautery-induced shrinkage of the soft tissue flaps when opening an ear as well. In primary cases of chronic ear surgery, temporalis fascia should be readily available for harvest and would be harvested in advance for tympanic membrane defects. In revision cases where temporalis fascia may not be readily available from prior use, scar tissue can be harvested between the cutaneous and mucoperiosteal layers. A second option for a reconstructive graft is periosteum, which can be readily harvested immediately below the temporalis muscle.

Repair of Small Defects

A small bony and dural defect may simply be patched with a free temporalis muscle plug that is placed in such fashion to "dumbbell" on the inside and just outside the dura (Fig. 24.3). This method works well for both middle and posterior fossa dura defects. This technique may be used alone for the small defect or performed

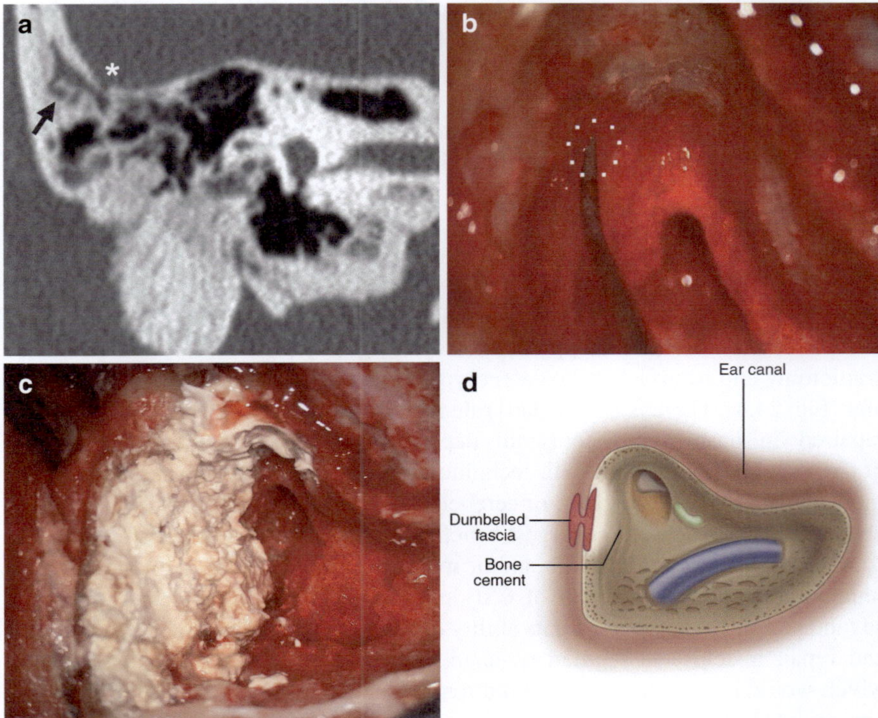

Fig. 24.3 Coronal view of a temporal bone CT (**a**) demonstrating a lateral 1 mm mastoid tegmen dehiscence (*) with CSF accumulating in the mastoid air cells (arrow). Given the defect's pinpoint size and lateral position, a transmastoid approach was taken. The defect and compromised dura are outlined at the tip of the instrument (**b**). The defect was repaired in multiple layers, including "dumbelled" temporalis fascia plugging the defect and overlaying bone substitute (**c**). It is important to "dumbell" the fascia into the dehiscence to create a water-tight seal (**d**; representative illustration)

concomitantly with resurfacing techniques for larger defects or in the setting of poor-quality or exposed dura surfaces. A second technique for repair of small defects includes a small inlay technique. If a dural tear and leak are identified, many will advocate for removing surrounding 5 mm of bone not only to aid in inspection of the brain and dura but also to facilitate an inlay repair [12]. With exposed normal dura, often resurfacing techniques can be accomplished either through the bony defect or around the bony defect and rely on a layer of soft tissue, which may be free or pedicled. Typically, the authors prefer an inlay technique, where soft tissue or cartilage is placed between the bony defect and dura. This method does require elevating dura intracranially circumferentially around the edges of the bony defect using angled blunt instruments; however, it often ensures a more secured repair. Sometimes careful bipolar cautery of a pinpoint leak leads to its cessation; however, the compromised dura benefits from resurfacing of the exposed area through the defect intracranially. Furthermore, careful use of bipolar can aid in contracting the dura to facilitate an easier repair. This technique of addressing the pathology directly is often advocated by many surgeons for transmastoid CSF leak repair and applies many of the same principles [13–15]. In addition to fascia or other soft tissue, some surgeons will advocate for the use of autologous bone, cartilage, and many different forms of tissue sealant.

Repair of Large or Multiple Defects

A second and more robust approach to repairing CSF leaks is through a separate craniotomy and resurfacing the defect typically from a top-down approach or from afar (Fig. 24.4). There is no standard rule regarding the size of defect that should be repaired via separate craniotomy; this depends on the experience and comfort level of the surgeon. By its nature, this technique requires more soft tissue dissection and more aggressive dura, cerebral, or cerebellar retraction but enables a more comprehensive repair. However, the largest benefit of this approach is that it allows visualization and resurfacing of large and/or multiple cranial defects. Although using a separate craniotomy for repair of CSF leaks remains a topic of debate, the main advantages of this approach are its ability to address multiple cranial defects at once and repair a dehiscent tegmen tympani without sacrificing the ossicular heads, which would have otherwise required removal to access the defect with a mastoid approach [16, 17]. Using a separate craniotomy is typically reserved for CSF leaks arising from the tegmen and middle fossa. Repair of posterior fossa CSF leaks theoretically may be performed through this approach; however, it requires exposure and significant compression of the sigmoid sinus, potentially occluding its blood flow and leading to thrombosis and is not recommended.

If a surgeon encounters an unexpected temporal CSF leak during a mastoidectomy and considers a temporal craniotomy to repair the defect, the patient's age,

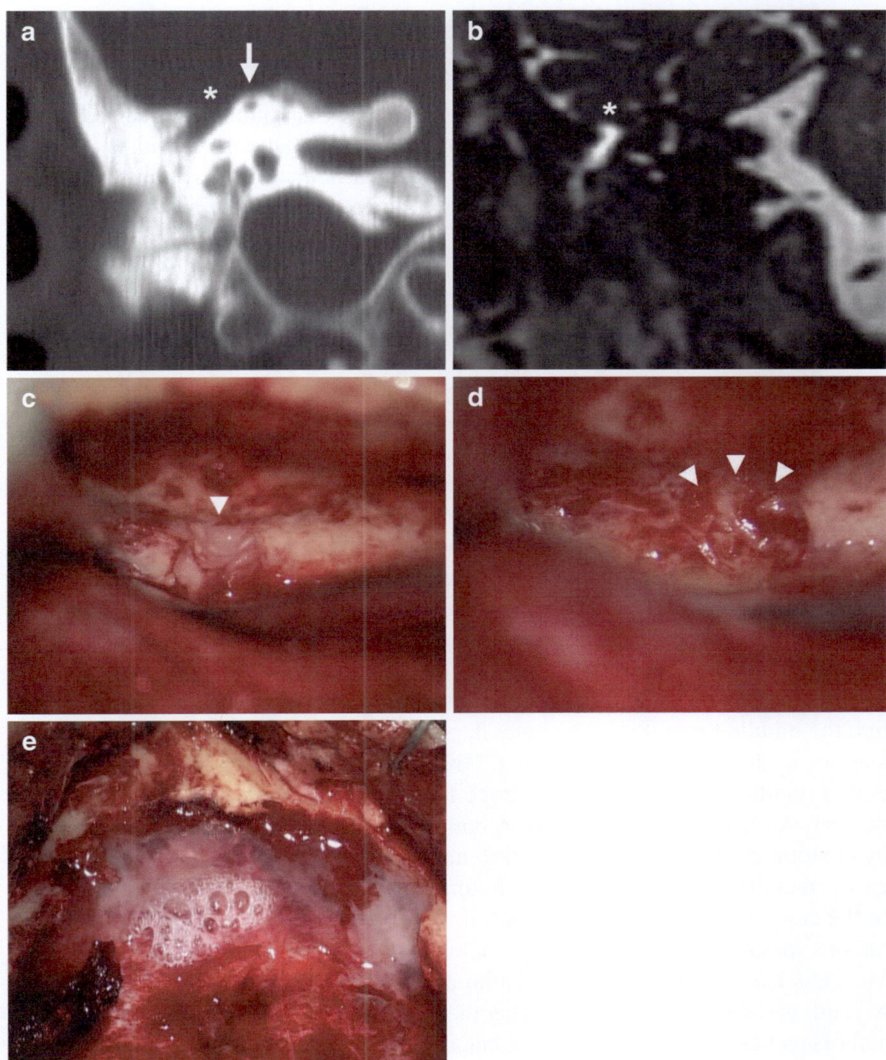

Fig. 24.4 Coronal views of a temporal bone CT (**a**) and T2 MRI (**b**) demonstrating a 10 mm mastoid tegmen dehiscence (*) lateral to the superior semicircular canal (arrow). A middle cranial fossa approach was performed because of the size and location of the defect. A transmastoid approach for repair was limited by a sclerotic mastoid and anteriorly positioned sigmoid sinus (not shown). Arrowheads indicate a T2 hyperintense encephalocele protruding through the tegmen defect before electrocautery (**c**) and after removal with handheld instruments (**d**). There was no involvement of the ossicular chain. The defect was repaired in multiple layers, including temporalis fascia, bone graft from the craniotomy flap, surgical cellulose, and fibrin sealant (**e**)

comorbidities, quality of the dura, and side of the temporal lobe requiring retraction should be considered before proceeding with a separate craniotomy. In general, older patients tend to have weaker and more adherent dura as well as worse tolerance of temporal lobe retraction. Creating a separate craniotomy risks further injury to the dura and temporal lobe that may compound patient morbidity. In most patients, the left temporal lobe is dominant for articulation of speech; prolonged retraction or trauma to the left temporal lobe increases the potential of postoperative aphasia.

Middle Fossa Craniotomy for Repair of Tegmen Defects

The standard middle fossa craniotomy for tumor removal is often larger in size (typically no smaller than 5 cm), allowing wide dural elevation to access medial and anterior based pathology along the petrous apex. Fortunately, defects in the tympanic and mastoid tegmen are usually lateral and posterior, enabling for a smaller craniotomy for access to the affected middle fossa floor [18, 19]. When using this approach, soft tissue incisions between the skin and temporalis muscle should once again be staggered, and they can often be connected and extended off the mastoid periosteum incisions. The temporalis muscle should be incised posteriorly as to pedicle it anterior and inferior, preserving its superficial and deep temporal artery vascular blood supply. Cautery along the undersurface of the temporalis should be kept to a minimum to optimize its viability in case it is chosen as a pedicled flap to line the middle fossa floor. The bone flap should typically sit 1/3 posterior and 2/3 anterior to the visible tegmen defect. Given that these defects are easier to access with a middle fossa approach, the bone flap height and width can be limited, particularly for lateral tegmen defects. A bone flap is created using the otologic drill or by creation of bur holes and a craniotome. Under microscopy, the temporal lobe is elevated to expose at least a 1.5 cm circumference around the bony and dural defect. In the case of spontaneous CSF leaks, it is best to maximize exposure of the entire middle fossa floor. This exposure includes from the superior petrosal sinus to Meckel's cave anteriorly and as medial as possible being (at least one centimeter beyond the arcuate eminence). The method of repair varies between different authors and even within institutions, but a multilayered approach is often favored in reconstruction of spontaneous leaks (Fig. 24.4) [17, 20, 21]. Repair may be extradural or intradural, with increased risk of temporal lobe trauma in the latter. The extradural repairs demonstrate high rates of success and are often preferred [22]. Materials described in multilayer repairs include cartilage, fascia, temporoparietal fascia, pedicled temporalis muscle, bone flap, dural substitute, bone pate, and hydroxyapatite cement. At our institutions, we favor the use of a multilayered approach with fascia, dural substitute, and bone flap with a high success rate for spontaneous middle fossa temporal bone encephaloceles with or without cerebrospinal fluid leaks. All exposed temporal lobe is relined with dural substitute and extended over the exposed lateral temporal lobe dura. If the dura is of poor quality, then dural substitute is used to cover the entire area under the bone flap with edges tucked underneath the craniotomy. The bone flap is subsequently replaced and secured with miniplates and screws with or without use of injectable bone substitute.

Repair of Mastoid Defects

Mastoid CSF leaks can be repaired either through the mastoid (transmastoid) or through a separate craniotomy for tegmen defects. Mastoid CSF leak repairs can often be reinforced through the mastoid side by obliterating the mastoid itself. If the leak is arising from the posterior fossa, they can often be repaired through mastoid obliteration as the mastoid posterior fossa sites are typically distant from the hearing apparatus. Typical materials for mastoid obliteration include autologous fat, collected bone pate, and/or injectable bony substitute. Using autologous fat is an attractive option for plugging the mastoid because it is easy to harvest, molds and plugs into temporal bone air cells, and results in a scarring type of mechanism in its repair. Cranioplasty mesh can be used to place the fat under pressure to prevent CSF percolating through the defect and the fat. However, it is critical that one takes hearing status into consideration, particularly if there is concern that the autologous fat graft may herniate on to the ossicles and potentially cause a conductive hearing loss. In such cases, one may use a cranioplasty mesh to bolster the graft and hold it in place to prevent untoward migration on to middle ear structures. Other strategies to help mitigate fat herniation include placing Gelfilm (for fat) or Gelfoam (bone pate or bony substitute) along the mastoid antrum over the ossicles to prevent herniation onto the ossicles. Furthermore, it is important to consider the infectious state of the temporal bone, as adding an autologous fat graft into an infected field can lead to persistent infection down the line. In a very well pneumatized mastoid, obliterating exposed air cells with bone wax is a reasonable consideration.

In most cases, the material used for CSF leak repair is a matter of preference, and the more important considerations are determining the extent of the defect(s) and achieving a multilayered repair. However, as aforementioned, chronically inflamed and infected mastoids are unique because their pro-inflammatory environments require more durable and robust materials used in repairs. Utilizing avascular autologous or allogeneic material in these situations may lead to irreversible contamination of the graft material, potentially threatening the integrity of the repair and exacerbating the inciting insult. Therefore, vascularized tissue is preferred for reconstruction in chronically inflamed and infected mastoids because their blood supply offers substantially more support than their avascular or synthetic counterparts. However, vascularized tissue is not always available. In such circumstances, it is important for surgeons to weigh the benefits and risks of implanting autologous or allogeneic material in an infected mastoid cavity after copious antibiotic irrigation versus none at all. It is the authors' opinion that it is more important to maximize control of the leak with an autologous graft during the surgery and maintain systemic antibiotics in the postoperative period.

The Canal Wall Down Mastoid Cavity

A CSF leak in a canal wall down cavity is a challenging and unique situation. The mastoid cavity is intentionally created for the purpose of communication with the outside to minimize trapped keratinizing squamous epithelium. The safest and most conservative measure to repair a CSF leak in a canal wall down cavity is to close off the ear canal, obliterate the mastoid cavity and middle ear, and plug the eustachian tube (see section "Eustachian Tube Obliteration and Ear Canal Closure"). However, the drawback to this technique is the consequences to hearing. When obliterating a cavity, one must make every effort to remove keratinizing squamous epithelium as failure to do so will lead to trapped cholesteatoma in a closed space and is a serious risk that should be discussed with patients undergoing this procedure. With this risk, Oghalai describes a layered procedure to repair tegmen defects without necessitating ear canal closure using a bone graft, pedicled temporalis flap, and fascial dural repair [23]. Oghalai and colleagues use a pedicled temporalis flap and tuck it through a middle fossa craniotomy so that it sits between the bony defect and the dura. Variations of this technique may be used to repair smaller defects in a mastoid cavity along the tegmen. A temporalis muscle flap or Palva flap may also be used to repair CSF leaks by plugging the leak from the mastoid side and resurfacing the exposed dura with the vascular flap. Given the decreased ability to pack the leak site with vigor, a lumbar drain may also be placed postoperatively for 3–5 days to take pressure off the repair site.

Eustachian Tube Obliteration and Ear Canal Closure

The most conservative and longstanding method to repair a temporal bone CSF leak is through closure of the ear canal and obliteration of the eustachian tube. This approach is typically performed in patients with poor hearing and/or the leak persists after several attempts to control it through various other methods. The advantage of this procedure is that it obviates the need to perform a craniotomy for control of the leak. Secondly, one can directly visualize and pack the mastoid cavity and eustachian tube thoroughly. The disadvantage of this approach, however, is that by closing off the ear and obliterating the cavity, the end result is a maximal conductive hearing loss. The second disadvantage of this approach is the potential and risk of iatrogenic cholesteatoma further down the line.

A postauricular incision is typically performed in staggered layers. An anteriorly based Palva flap is elevated to expose the posterior ear canal. Attention is first turned to closing off the ear canal. This can be done in a variety of techniques, but the preferred method of the authors is the modified Rambo meatoplasty [24, 25]. Briefly, in the canal an incision is made along the anterior aspect of the ear canal skin to raise an anteriorly based tragal skin flap followed by removal of the underlying tragal cartilage. The tragal skin flap is laid along the concha bowl to approximate the closure, and the posterior concha bowl skin is marked out and excised or alternatively lateralized to form a second layer of closure supporting the skin closure. The remainder of the circumferential ear canal skin is elevated from a lateral to medial direction along the previous incision sites, where it can be later removed along with the tympanic membrane. The tragal skin flap is then sutured to the free edge of the conchal bowl skin using an interrupted vertical mattress to ensure full eversion and minimize the risk of any iatrogenic cholesteatoma.

Next, the ear canal is entered from the postauricular incision, and the remainder of the medial ear canal skin is removed. If there is a functional inner ear, the tympanic membrane is lifted posteriorly, the incudostapedial joint is sharply cut, and the incus is removed. The medial ear canal skin and tympanic membrane may be removed en bloc or piecemeal. Using various size diamond burs, a wide canalplasty is performed along every surface of the bony ear canal, with emphasis on the anterior and medial bony annulus, just lateral to the eustachian tube opening. A wide and complete canaloplasty helps ensure all keratinizing epithelium is removed from the bony ear canal. Once complete, it is important to carefully inspect all routes of CSF egress within the middle ear and eustachian tube and meticulously pack them. Routes for CSF egress include, but are not limited to, the mastoid antrum, facial recess posteriorly, and/or hypotympanic air cells. Packing and/or plugging can be accomplished with bone wax, fat, bone substitute, or other material to ensure a watertight seal. A wide canalplasty and removal of the posterior ear canal will allow a near direct view down the lumen of the eustachian tube. The eustachian tube obliteration is usually performed with two or more materials, including soft tissue, muscle, surgical cellulose, the incus, bone wax, or other bone substitute. When packing the eustachian tube, one must be cognizant of any type of pulsations that may indicate a dehiscent carotid, as vigorous packing may lead to potential catastrophic cerebrovascular event.

When closing off the ear in a canal wall down cavity, removal of the skin within the cavity can be difficult and poses a higher risk of iatrogenic cholesteatoma. It is the authors' experience that this is best accomplished when removing the skin en bloc and maximizing the use of diamond burs to polish off any skin-lined bony surfaces. Following complete skin removal, eustachian tube obliteration, and ear canal closure, one can turn their attention to the CSF leak pathology using the above-described methods. The advantage of the ear canal closure prior to repairing a CSF leak is that the mastoid and middle ear can be packed and further reinforce the repair. This can be accomplished with either a free fat graft for a relatively clean cavity or pedicled flap if it is infected or inflamed. Furthermore, a cranioplasty plate may also aid in securing the tissue of a mastoid obliteration more firmly into place. The postauricular incision is then closed in multiple layers in a watertight fashion.

Cerebrospinal Fluid Leaks from the Inner Ear

CSF leak from the inner ear classically originates from the round window or oval window, typically during stapes procedures or cochlear implantation. As discussed above, preoperative imaging can sometimes help anticipate potential CSF leaks, but they are not always 100% sensitive. Therefore, surgeons should be adequately trained and prepared to deal with inner ear CSF leaks should they occur. Preoperative imaging can typically help identify potential CSF leaks upon opening up the inner ear by identifying congenital abnormalities, inner ear abnormalities, and/or other aberrant connections between the subarachnoid and perilymphatic spaces [7–9, 26, 27]. Typical CT findings that may indicate an aberrant connection between the subarachnoid space and perilymph include a dilated IAC, enlarged vestibular aqueduct, and/or a large cochlear aqueduct.

When a potential CSF gusher or CSF leak is anticipated, certain steps preoperatively, intraoperatively, and postoperatively are critical. Preoperatively, it is vital that the surgeon carefully counsels the patient on potential sensorineural hearing loss (with a stapes gusher), postoperative CSF leak, meningitis, and possible need for a lumbar drain. Intraoperatively, it is important that the surgeon is adequately prepared to deal with the CSF leak prior to opening the inner ear. This includes a wide exposure to maximize the view of the anatomy, easy access to the eustachian tube for potential packing, and contingency plans to harvest temporalis muscle or other material to seal off the inner ear opening.

If a CSF leak is encountered upon opening up the inner ear, it is important to raise the head of the bed. When a CSF leak is encountered during cochlear implantation, the electrode is inserted. Then, muscle or fascia is used to pack circumferentially around the electrode array using a small pick, allowing some tissue to "dumbbell" across the cochleostomy for a watertight seal. Systematic and careful packing around the electrode is important for repairing the CSF leak without displacing the electrode, and one should not hesitate to restart packing should a small leak persist. Others have advocated for cutting a piece of muscle or fascia ring around the electrode prior to insertion, which can then carefully be advanced to seal off the leak following insertion [28]. Further consideration can be given to additional tissue sealant with muscle or fascia or surgical cellulose around the packing site. In certain CI CSF leak cases, further consideration can be given to packing the eustachian tube. A Valsalva to 20–40 cmH$_2$O pressure will help reassure the surgeon that the packing around the electrode array or stapes prosthesis is solid.

CSF leaks that occur during stapedectomy are rare and occur less than 1% of the time and may be a result of a fundal defect or large cochlear aqueduct with the former leading to more profuse CSF leakage or a "gusher" [26, 29]. Regardless of whether the operator performs stapedotomy, partial stapedectomy, or total stapedectomy, if a CSF gusher is suspected, then surgeons should start with a small fenestra that can be easily packed with fascia or perichondrium. A "gusher" is detectable once fenestration occurs, and a profuse leak may be packed, with or without a prosthetic placed [29]. The head should be elevated, and excess fluid should be carefully suctioned out because the defect is difficult to pack while actively leaking. It is critical to avoid over-suctioning fluid because this may increase the risk of flow trauma and larger sensorineural hearing loss. Secondly, it is critical to avoid over-suctioning CSF prior to elevating the head of the bed, as this may lead to an air embolus within the inner ear in a CSF-depleted patient. Similar to a cochlear implant gusher, packing is best accomplished with either circumferential packing around the new stapes prosthesis and/or laying fascia over the opening [29]. In both cases, the prosthesis is often helpful in securing the packing over the oval window. A Valsalva is helpful to determine success of the closure after the patient is laid flat once again. Despite a relatively higher incidence of sensorineural hearing loss when a gusher is encountered, hearing loss is not a foregone conclusion, and natural anatomy should be left as intact as possible. It follows that eustachian tube packing, ear canal closure, and further removal of ossicles should not be attempted at the time of initial surgery, but reserved for failure of initial CSF leak repair.

Middle Ear CSF Leaks

The middle ear can also be a rare site for CSF leaks to occur. CSF egress in such circumstances arise from either air cell dehiscence connecting different CSF spaces to the middle ear or congenital bony defects like Hyrtl's fissure or the fallopian canal [30, 31]. When the etiology of CSF egress is arising from the tegmen tympani, repair can be approached in two techniques. First, it can be repaired using a traditional middle fossa craniotomy, which often maximizes the visualization of the defect from a top-down approach. A second option can be performed through a transmastoid approach; however, this often necessitates removal of the ossicular head (incus ± malleus head) to maximize the view and quality of repair. The surgeon must be cognizant of the ear's hearing status. In these cases, the leak cannot be packed vigorously because of the acoustic apparatus, and selective, gentle packing into the defects can be performed to avoid trauma to the inner ear, facial nerve, and the middle ear vibratory components. CSF diversion should also be considered to take pressure off the repair.

Postoperative Considerations

Postoperatively, the patient should, at a minimum, be placed on CSF leak precautions. These include head-of-bed elevation, stool softeners, open-mouth sneezing, and sometimes bed rest. In cases with a high flow or if the integrity of the repair is at all questionable, then one may also consider serial lumbar punctures or placing a lumbar drain for 3–5 days to divert CSF. CSF leaks in the canal wall down mastoid cavity have decreased ability to pack the leak site with vigor, so a lumbar drain requires particular consideration in these rare cases. For cases involving a craniotomy, most patients should be observed in the neurologic ICU to monitor for acute neurologic changes related to surgery (stroke, hemorrhage, cerebral edema, and hydrocephalus). A standard course would include neurological checks every hour for the first 24 h, followed by every 2–4 h until the patient is well enough for transfer out of the ICU. In the setting of infection, postoperative systemic antibiotics are critical, especially if grafting material was placed to repair the CSF leak. Lastly, patients should be educated on postoperative signs of CSF leak and meningitis, including clear otorrhea, salty or metallic taste, high fever, symptoms of meningitis, and changes in mentation. Patients should follow up with the operating surgeon at 1 week, 1 month, and every 6 months as needed thereafter.

References

1. Brodie HA, Thompson TC. Management of complications from 820 temporal bone fractures. Am J Otol. 1997;18(2):188–97.
2. Wootten CT, Kaylie DM, Warren FM, Jackson CG. Management of brain herniation and cerebrospinal fluid leak in revision chronic ear surgery. Laryngoscope. 2005;115(7):1256–61. https://doi.org/10.1097/01.Mlg.0000165455.20118.E3.
3. Selesnick SH, Liu JC, Jen A, Newman J. The incidence of cerebrospinal fluid leak after vestibular schwannoma surgery. Otol Neurotol. 2004;25(3):387–93. https://doi.org/10.1097/00129492-200405000-00030.
4. Chen BS, Meyer BI, Saindane AM, Bruce BB, Newman NJ, Biousse V. Prevalence of Incidentally detected signs of intracranial hypertension on magnetic resonance imaging and their association with papilledema. JAMA Neurol. 2021;78(6):718–25. https://doi.org/10.1001/jamaneurol.2021.0710.
5. Ehrmann-Müller D, Shehata-Dieler W, Kaulitz S, et al. Cochlear implantation in children without preoperative computed tomography diagnostics. Analysis of procedure and rate of complications. Int J Pediatr Otorhinolaryngol. 2020;138:110266. https://doi.org/10.1016/j.ijporl.2020.110266.
6. Brown CS, Choi KJ, Kaylie DM. Preoperative imaging findings and cost in adults with postlingual deafness prior to cochlear implant. Ann Otol Rhinol Laryngol. 2018;127(4):270–4. https://doi.org/10.1177/0003489418759114.
7. Glasscock ME III. The Stapes Gusher. Arch Otolaryngol. 1973;98(2):82–91. https://doi.org/10.1001/archotol.1973.00780020088004.
8. Jackler RK, Hwang PH. Enlargement of the cochlear aqueduct: fact or fiction? Otolaryngol Head Neck Surg. 1993;109(1):14–25. https://doi.org/10.1177/019459989310900104.
9. Krouchi L, Callonnec F, Bouchetemblé P, Tollard E, Dehesdin D, Marie J-P. Preoperative computed tomography scan may fail to predict perilymphatic gusher. Ann Otol Rhinol Laryngol. 2013;122(6):374–7. https://doi.org/10.1177/000348941312200605.
10. Neely JG, Kuhn JR. Diagnosis and treatment of iatrogenic cerebrospinal fluid leak and brain herniation during or following mastoidectomy. Laryngoscope. 1985;95(11):1299–300. https://doi.org/10.1288/00005537-198511000-00001.
11. Moore GF, Nissen AJ, Yonkers AJ. Potential complications of unrecognized cerebrospinal fluid leaks secondary to mastoid surgery. Am J Otol. 1984;5(4):317–23.
12. Paparella MM. Mastoidectomy and tympanoplasty. Otolaryngology. 1991:1405–39.
13. Kim L, Wisely CE, Dodson EE. Transmastoid approach to spontaneous temporal bone cerebrospinal fluid leaks: hearing improvement and success of repair. Otolaryngol Head Neck Surg. 2014;150(3):472–8. https://doi.org/10.1177/0194599813518173.
14. Perez E, Carlton D, Alfarano M, Smouha E. Transmastoid repair of spontaneous cerebrospinal fluid leaks. J Neurol Surg B Skull Base. 2018;79(5):451–7. https://doi.org/10.1055/s-0037-1617439.
15. Karkas A, Khneisser E. Trans-mastoid approach for cerebrospinal fluid leak repair. Curr Opin Otolaryngol Head Neck Surg. 2019;27(5):334–8. https://doi.org/10.1097/moo.0000000000000565.

16. Lobo BC, Baumanis MM, Nelson RF. Surgical repair of spontaneous cerebrospinal fluid (CSF) leaks: A systematic review. Laryngoscope Investig Otolaryngol. 2017;2(5):215–24. https://doi.org/10.1002/lio2.75.

17. Tolisano AM, Kutz JW Jr. Middle fossa approach for spontaneous cerebrospinal fluid fistula and encephaloceles. Curr Opin Otolaryngol Head Neck Surg. 2019;27(5):356–60. https://doi.org/10.1097/moo.0000000000000560.

18. Kuhweide R, Casselman JW. Spontaneous cerebrospinal fluid otorrhea from a tegmen defect: transmastoid repair with minicraniotomy. Ann Otol Rhinol Laryngol. 1999;108(7 Pt 1):653–8. https://doi.org/10.1177/000348949910800706.

19. Walia A, Lander D, Durakovic N, Shew M, Wick CC, Herzog J. Outcomes after mini-craniotomy middle fossa approach combined with mastoidectomy for lateral skull base defects. Am J Otolaryngol. 2021;42(1):102794. https://doi.org/10.1016/j.amjoto.2020.102794.

20. Cheng E, Grande D, Leonetti J. Management of spontaneous temporal bone cerebrospinal fluid leak: a 30-year experience. Am J Otolaryngol. 2019;40(1):97–100. https://doi.org/10.1016/j.amjoto.2018.09.018.

21. Kutz JW Jr, Husain IA, Isaacson B, Roland PS. Management of spontaneous cerebrospinal fluid otorrhea. Laryngoscope. 2008;118(12):2195–9. https://doi.org/10.1097/MLG.0b013e318182f833.

22. Kutz JW Jr, Tolisano AM. Diagnosis and management of spontaneous cerebrospinal fluid fistula and encephaloceles. Curr Opin Otolaryngol Head Neck Surg. 2019;27(5):369–75. https://doi.org/10.1097/moo.0000000000000568.

23. McMurphy AB, Oghalai JS. Repair of iatrogenic temporal lobe encephalocele after canal wall down mastoidectomy in the presence of active cholesteatoma. Otol Neurotol. 2005;26(4):587–94. https://doi.org/10.1097/01.mao.0000178119.46290.e1.

24. Rambo JH. Primary closure of the radical mastoidectomy wound: a technique to eliminate post-operative care. Laryngoscope. 1958;68(7):1216–27. https://doi.org/10.1002/lary.5540680707.

25. Meyerhoff WL, Pollock KJ, Roland PS, Mickey B. Modified Rambo meatoplasty in trans-labyrinthine tumor removal. Otolaryngol Head Neck Surg. 1991;104(1):100–2. https://doi.org/10.1177/019459989110400118.

26. Quesada JL, Cammaroto G, Bonanno L, Galletti F, Quesada P. Cerebrospinal fluid leak during stapes surgery: gushing leaks and oozing leaks, two different phenomena. Ear Nose Throat J. 2017;96(8):302–10. https://doi.org/10.1177/014556131709600817.

27. Eftekharian A, Amizadeh M. Cerebrospinal fluid gusher in cochlear implantation. Cochlear Implants Int. 2014;15(3):179–84. https://doi.org/10.1179/1754762814y.0000000069.

28. Tolisano AM, Wick CC, Kutz JW Jr. A novel surgical technique for the management of cerebrospinal fluid gusher encountered during cochlear implantation. Otol Neurotol. 2020;41(9):e1177. https://doi.org/10.1097/mao.0000000000002828.

29. Alicandri-Ciufelli M, Molinari G, Rosa MS, Monzani D, Presutti L. Gusher in stapes surgery: a systematic review. Eur Arch Otorhinolaryngol. 2019;276(9):2363–76. https://doi.org/10.1007/s00405-019-05538-x.

30. Lovin BD, Appelbaum EN, Makoshi L, Whitehead WE, Sweeney AD. Spontaneous congenital perilabyrinthine cerebrospinal fluid fistulas. Ann Otol Rhinol Laryngol. 2021;130(12):1360–8. https://doi.org/10.1177/00034894211007242.

31. Dey JK, Van Gompel JJ, Lane JI, Carlson ML. Fallopian canal meningocele with spontaneous cerebrospinal fluid otorrhea: case report and systematic review of the literature. World Neurosurg. 2019;122:e285–90. https://doi.org/10.1016/j.wneu.2018.10.021.

Chapter 25
General Repair Principles Following Posterior Cranial Base Surgery

Mehdi Abouzari, Karen Tawk, Dae Bo Shim, Harrison W. Lin, and Hamid R. Djalilian

Introduction

Since the 1960s, collaborations between neurotologists and neurosurgeons have led to less invasive techniques, improved results, and reduced complications in skull base surgery. The ultimate goal of posterior skull base surgery for tumors is safe tumor extirpation with minimal complications. The three conventional approaches—middle fossa, retrosigmoid, and translabyrinthine for vestibular schwannoma resection—have cerebrospinal fluid (CSF) leakage as one of the most common and reducible complications. CSF leakage is due to a communication between the intradural space, containing the CSF, with the middle ear, the mastoid, and/or the Eustachian tube. CSF leaks usually present with rhinorrhea, otorrhea, subcutaneous collection, and incisional leak [1]. CSF rhinorrhea results from a leak of the CSF from the dural incision, into the tympanomastoid space, and through the Eustachian tube to the nasopharynx [2]. Rarely, CSF leakage can present as a chronic dry cough, which occurs as CSF drains into the hypopharynx resulting in irritation and a cough reflex. The otorrhea is explained by either a perforation of the tympanic membrane or a laceration in the external auditory canal skin [3]. Therefore, meticulous repair following skull base surgery is crucial to diminish surgical complications.

M. Abouzari · K. Tawk · D. B. Shim
Department of Otolaryngology-Head and Neck Surgery, University of California, Irvine, CA, USA
e-mail: mabouzar@hs.uci.edu

H. W. Lin · H. R. Djalilian (✉)
Department of Otorhinolaryngology, Hanyang University College of Medicine, Goyang, South Korea
e-mail: harriswl@hs.uci.edu; hdjalili@hs.uci.edu

© The Author(s), under exclusive license to Springer Nature Switzerland AG 2023
E. C. Kuan et al. (eds.), *Skull Base Reconstruction*,
https://doi.org/10.1007/978-3-031-27937-9_25

355

CSF leak prevention is an issue that the surgeon needs to consider in all steps of the surgery. Preoperative assessment of the temporal bone anatomy and air cell tracts is critical in knowing where air cells may be encountered and which cells need to be sealed at the end of surgery. Starting with the incision, we avoid excessive monopolar cautery to reduce tissue destruction and to optimize rapid healing. Meticulous preservation of the dura in some approaches (e.g., retrosigmoid) by keeping the dura moist and flipped under the dural incision prevents desiccation and shrinkage/destruction by the drill. The critical areas to address at closure are mastoid air cells, petrous apex air cells, openings into the middle ear, air cells around the internal auditory canal, lacerations of the canal skin, dural closure, incisional closure, and dressing. Lumbar drain will be discussed in a separate chapter. Generally, a single layer of closure is never deemed sufficient to prevent CSF leakage, and the general principle of "belts and suspenders," i.e., using multiple methods for tamponading the CSF, is critical. In general, if CSF leaks into the mastoid but does not communicate with the middle ear or if CSF leaks through the dural closure but does not get into the air cells or come out of the wound, the leak has no way to "flow" out and thus will be self-controlled. A non-flowing leak may not require treatment.

Closure After Middle Cranial Fossa Approach

Once the tumor is removed from the internal auditory canal (IAC) or the middle fossa floor (e.g., facial nerve tumor or epidermoid) and hemostasis is achieved, air cells surrounding the IAC and other petrous apex cells need to be meticulously closed using bone wax. This is best accomplished using bone wax that is pressed into the cell using small cottonoids or cotton balls. The second layer of closure is accomplished with pieces of the temporalis muscle or fascia lata which are placed over the air cells, thus allowing the released temporal lobe to expand and to hold the packing in place. We routinely use a layer of fibrin glue to hold the fascia in place. While the fibrin glue cannot be relied upon to hold a CSF leak, it allows the fascia graft to heal in place without movement. Alternatively, a fat graft may be placed in the IAC which can seal the air cells secondarily after bone wax placement. If there is a middle ear opening, that area is plugged with an on-lay or dumbbell fascia graft. Mastoid air cells, if open, are waxed as well and covered with fascia. Finally, attention should be paid to the edges of the craniotomy as zygomatic root air cells or a very well pneumatized temporal bone will have air cells at the edges which can allow CSF leak to reach the middle ear and thus the nose. After controlling all sources of CSF leak and flow, the bone flap is replaced and attached to the edges of the craniotomy. Dural tacking sutures are placed to prevent epidural blood collection. The wound is closed in three layers (temporalis, subcutaneous, and cutaneous) in a watertight fashion. We prefer using Prolene sutures for skin edges rather than staples for better sealing. The blue color of the suture is easier to distinguish from hair when it has to be removed. Thereafter, a compression bandage is applied for 48

h. Given the limited air cell opening of the middle fossa approach, it is associated with a lower incidence of postoperative CSF fistulas relative to other approaches [4–6].

Closure After Retrosigmoid or Lateral Suboccipital Approach

Once the tumor is completely removed, the surgical field is thoroughly rinsed, and hemostasis is achieved. The surgeon carefully checks the bone of the IAC and the edge of the craniotomy for air cells and seals them with tissue or bone wax to fill the gaps and prevent CSF from penetrating the mastoid and middle ear. To ensure that all the cells are filled, a 30-degree rigid endoscope is usually used to inspect the drilled surfaces of the IAC that may be out of microscopic line of sight. This step is critical to close all air cells and reduce rates of CSF leakage. Then, a layer of fascia or a portion of muscle or fat graft is inserted into the IAC to further prevent postoperative CSF leakage. The dura flaps that were kept moist to facilitate subsequent closure are closed in a watertight fashion with a 4-0 silk suture in several layers. In case a watertight seal cannot be achieved, a pericranial graft or dural substitute (e.g., DuraGen) is usually used to fill the remaining gap or as an only graft with fibrin glue sealant. Then, the bone flap is replaced, and absorbable sutures are used to close the muscular layer. Finally, the skin is closed with running sutures, and a pressure dressing is applied for 5 days [4, 5, 7].

Closure After Translabyrinthine Approach

During the translabyrinthine approach, the surgeon enters the middle ear through the mastoid, which might create a potential pathway for CSF leakage. Accordingly, the Eustachian tube should be identified and entirely filled with obstructive materials, such as fascia. Some surgeons use muscle or Surgicel, but we avoid muscle due to its atrophy and non-patient biomaterials to obtain better healing and sealing of the Eustachian tube. We will sometimes use the incus (after separation of the incudostapedial joint) to wedge the fascia strips that were placed into the Eustachian tube for better control. The middle ear can also be filled with abdominal fat grafts though we prefer fascia which can be directly placed into the Eustachian tube in a strip-by-strip format and pushed in with an annulus elevator. Facial recess should be minimally opened, and if open, all air cells should be closed with bone wax. A large fascia graft is used to cover the entire mastoid-middle ear connection. The flaps of the dura are re-approximated, and a large piece of temporalis fascia is used to cover the dura and the facial nerve as it passes in the IAC. The mastoid is filled with strips of abdominal fat graft, and fibrin glue can be used additionally. Some surgeons use hydroxyapatite to seal the mastoid or to counterpressure the fat graft. We prefer not to use bone cement for closure of the translabyrinthine approach as cement can break down with tissue fluids and CSF, and a rapid approach to the skull base in the rare case of a postoperative hemorrhage is not possible. Ideally, the mastoid periosteum should be closed with 3-0 Vicryl watertight sutures. If due to tissue contraction, we will use a thin titanium mesh that can be compressed after securing with screws to hold the fat graft in place and provide better seal. This also prevents the sinking in of the skin and soft tissues. The skin is closed with continuous 4-0 nylon sutures. Every effort is made to ensure a watertight seal to prevent postoperative CSF leakage. A compression bandage is applied for 5 days, and the patient is admitted to the intensive care unit for overnight monitoring [4–6, 8].

Outcomes for Reconstruction of Posterior Skull Base Defects

Middle Cranial Fossa Approach

The middle cranial fossa (MCF) approach is usually used for the resection of small-to medium-sized vestibular schwannomas, as well as lateral skull base lesions. It offers the possibility of both hearing and facial nerve function preservation [9–11]. Similarly to all skull base surgeries, CSF leakage is the most common complication following MCF approach, with a rate of up to 10% [10]. Subsequently, various closure techniques have been developed in an attempt to prevent CSF leakage. In Table 25.1, we have summarized the various studies on the topic.

Retrosigmoid or Lateral Suboccipital Approach

The retrosigmoid approach is one of the most commonly used approaches to access the cerebellopontine angle (CPA) as it provides a broad view—from the tentorium cerebelli to the foramen magnum [14]. It is usually preferred by many surgeons as it is a relatively safe approach, it can be used for tumors of all sizes, and hearing can be preserved (as the otic capsule is not violated during this approach) [1, 15]. Nevertheless, CSF leakage remains a common complication (with an incidence of 2–30% [12]) associated with an increased risk of intracerebral infection and prolonged hospital stay [16]. CSF leak commonly occurs through the perilabyrinthine air cells, the mastoidal air cells, and the apical air cells [17]. An unusual leak through an intracochlear air cell tract was described in the literature [18].

Several studies identified the risk factors associated with CSF leakage [19–24]. Firstly, young patients were at a higher risk of CSF leak when compared to older patients (>65 years) [19–21], as with age the production of CSF decreases as well as intracranial pressure [25, 26]. A high body mass index (BMI) was also reported as a risk factor, as obesity increases intracranial pressure and is associated with decreased dural cicatrization [19, 22, 23]. Furthermore, when compared to other tumor resections (meningioma, facial schwannoma, trigeminal schwannoma, etc.),

Table 25.1 Prophylactic techniques in middle cranial fossa approach and postoperative cerebrospinal fluid (CSF) leakage incidences

Study	Patients (*n*)	Reconstructive technique	CSF leakage (%)	Comments
Becker et al. (2003) [12]	100 patients	Air cells of the IAC were filled with bone wax; IAC defects were closed with temporalis muscle or abdominal adipose tissue	10	CSF leak rates were similar between the retrosigmoid, translabyrinthine, and middle fossa approaches; it was also comparable to other studies conducted during the last decade
Fishman et al. (2004) [13]	24 patients	Abdominal fat was used to obliterate open-air cells; air cells of the floor of the middle fossa were sealed with fascia; dural defects were repaired with fat and sutures	12	Plugging air cells with abdominal fat has significantly decreased CSF leakage
Khan et al. (2014) [8]	8 patients	Titanium mesh plate, autologous temporalis fascia graft, and synthetic fibrin sealant were used for reconstruction	12.5	Titanium mesh plate could be used as an alternative to bone grafts in reconstruction of the middle cranial fossa skull base
Scheich et al. (2016) [14]	148 patients	Temporalis muscle graft and fibrin glue were used to close the IAC; wax and fibrin sealant patch were used to seal temporal bone cells	13	Pneumatization of the temporal bone is associated with a higher rate of CSF leakage
Lipschitz et al. (2019) [10]	161 patients	The dura was sutured in a watertight fashion; bone wax was used to obliterate open-air cells; temporalis muscle was placed in the IAC; MCF was covered with temporalis fascia, fibrin sealant, and Duraform dural graft	3	MCF can be used for vestibular schwannoma resection, with hearing preservation and low-rate CSF leakage

vestibular schwannoma resection was reported to be associated with a higher risk of CSF leak as it requires drilling of the petrous bone of the IAC [24].

Following a retrosigmoid approach, several techniques for repairing the dura mater have been proposed to reduce the rate of CSF leak (Table 25.2). In addition, Hoffman reported a significantly decreased incidence of CSF leaks when the IAC was not drilled (0% versus 16% when drilled) [44]. However, since drilling is an inevitable step for complete tumor resection, it is crucial to seal open-air cells of the posterior wall of the IAC and retrosigmoid air cells [16, 44]. An interesting finding was that the incidence of CSF leak was <1% following a series of steps suggested by Date et al. The most important step was the careful suturing of the dura and the use of fibrin glue to perform the cranioplasty [45]. In another series of patients, no CSF leak was reported in patients with Palacos cranioplasty.

Table 25.2 Studies of the retrosigmoid approach and various closure techniques and likelihood of CSF leakage

Study	Patients (*n*)	Reconstructive technique	CSF leakage (%)	Comments
Gal and Bartels (1999) [28]	35 patients	Bone wax was used to seal perisigmoid air cells and to cover the defect in the porus acusticus	2.9	Bone wax is an effective, safe, and time-efficient way to prevent CSF from entering the residual air cell system
Yamakami et al. (2004) [42]	50 patients	Resection of the posterior wall of the internal auditory meatus was minimized and was then reconstructed to avoid CSF leakage; after watertight dural closure, cranioplasty was performed using an autobone or artificial bone	4	The evaluation of the temporal bone pneumatization, the reconstruction of the IAC, the watertight dural closure, and the absence of an epidural or subcutaneous drain prevented CSF leakage
Cueva and Mastrodimos (2005) [30]	160 patients	Bone wax was used to seal the IAC and air cells; dura mater was closed with 4-0 woven nylon suture; a patch of blood-impregnated microfibrillar collagen hemostat is used to fill the craniectomy defect	0	The technique described was useful to achieve the lowest rate of CSF leakage
Galer et al. (2006) [31]	31 patients	Hydroxyapatite-titanium mesh was used for cranioplasty, and closed suction drainage was used postoperatively	3.2	The use of closed suction drainage reduces CSF leak rate
Baird et al. (2007) [32]	280 patients	130 patients underwent surgery for reconstruction of the posterior wall of the drilled porus acusticus with hydroxyapatite cement (HAC); 150 patients underwent the same surgical approach but without the HAC reconstruction	10% in HAC group and 18.7% in control group	Statistically significant difference in rate of CSF rhinorrhea was reported; no statistically significant difference in the incisional leak rate between the two groups
Ludemann et al. (2008) [33]	420 patients	In 283 patients, muscle was used to seal opened air cells at the IAC and mastoid bone; in 137 patients, fat tissue was used for this purpose	5.7% after muscle use and 2.2% after application of fat tissue	Sealing air cells with fat tissue was superior to muscle for the prevention of CSF leakage

Table 25.2 (continued)

Study	Patients (*n*)	Reconstructive technique	CSF leakage (%)	Comments
Bayazit et al. (2009) [34]	412 patients	Repair of retrosigmoid dura was achieved by watertight closure; the mastoid air cells and open-air cells in the petrous bone were filled with bone wax; tight mastoid dressing was used for 3 days	7.7	Vestibular schwannoma resection was associated with a higher incident of CSF leakage, probably due to the drilling of the internal acoustic meatus; in this case, endoscopes might be useful
Stieglitz et al. (2010) [35]	519 patients	In addition to fibrin glue, muscle tissue and subcutaneous fat were used to seal air cells at the drilled IAC; open mastoid air cells were sealed with fat tissue and glue; dura mater was closed and sealed with glue; bony defect was closed with Palacos	4.2	The perilabyrinthine air cells (extend into the posterior wall of the IAC), the mastoidal air cells (posteromedial to the sigmoid sinus), and the apical air cells (superior to the IAC) should be sealed to avoid CSF fistulas
Samii et al. (2010) [36]	50 patients	Opened air cells around the IAC and mastoid are occluded by pieces of muscle sealed with fibrin glue; bone wax is only applied for hemostasis; Gelfoam is placed on the dura mater, and craniectomy is reconstructed with methyl methacrylate	6	Large and giant vestibular schwannomas were associated with a higher incident of CSF leakage although there was no significant difference

(continued)

Table 25.2 (continued)

Study	Patients (*n*)	Reconstructive technique	CSF leakage (%)	Comments
Arlt et al. (2011) [17]	81 patients	In 41 cases, the dura was closed using the sandwich technique and non-autologous materials (TissueFleece, Spongostan, TachoSil); in 40 cases, the dura was closed in a monolayer fashion with epidural TachoSil; in 5 cases, Palacos was used during the cranioplasty. In the 76 other cases, the bone flaps were fixed using miniplates; drilled posterior wall of the meatus acusticus internus and opened mastoid cells were obliterated using an autologous muscle patch from the neck musculature that was fixed with fibrin glue	8.6	By comparing the two techniques: 7.3% CSF leakage with the sandwich technique and 10% with the monolayer technique with no statistically significant difference between the two groups; there was no association between the mean operation time and rate of CSF leakage; no CSF leakage when Palacos was used during cranioplasty (however the number of patients allows no conclusion)
Chovanec et al. (2012) [37]	89 patients	Microsurgical tumor resection (MS) and endoscopy-assisted microsurgical tumor resection (EA-MS); in both groups, open-air cells were plugged with muscle and fibrin glue	MS: 20 EA-MA: 8	The use of endoscopy helped identify the pathways for CSF leakage when compared to the microscope
Heman-Ackah et al. (2012) [38]	197 patients	An anterior retraction of the dura and sigmoid sinus was created, thus allowing a maximum visualization of the CPA; air cells were sealed with bone wax; fat was used to seal the drill-out defect	6.6	The modified retrosigmoid approach provides a better access to seal air cells (extracranial, mastoid, and retrofacial)

Table 25.2 (continued)

Study	Patients (*n*)	Reconstructive technique	CSF leakage (%)	Comments
Fredrickson and Sekula (2013) [39]	79 patients	Calcium phosphate cement was used for cranioplasty	0	Calcium phosphate cement provides a watertight, nonporous barrier for the CSF; in a previous study, the authors used titanium mesh cranioplasty which constitutes a porous barrier, and the rate of CSF leak was reported to be 2%
Ling et al. (2014) [3]	58 patients	Dura was closed using a watertight fashion, and a dural allograft patch was used when needed; bone wax was used to seal mastoid air cells; if needed, IAC air cells were sealed with wax and small autologous fat graft; fat graft was then placed over the sutures and the waxed off mastoid cells; finally, a cranioplasty is performed with a Medpor Titan implant that was secured to the bone edges with titanium screws	0	After performing the described technique, the use of additional tissue dural sealants or postoperative lumbar drainage did not appear to be necessary to prevent postoperative CSF leakage
Foster et al. (2016) [40]	672 patients	336 patients underwent calcium phosphate cement (CPC) cranioplasty, and 336 underwent polyethylene mesh cranioplasty	0% in cement group and 6% in mesh group	CPC could be used as an alternative to titanium as it reduces the risk of CSF leakage
Azad et al. (2016) [41]	24 patients	IAC defect and air cells were sealed with bone wax; then, autologous fat graft from the abdomen was used; this was then reinforced with Surgicel and fibrin glue; the dural opening was closed with watertight sutures and reinforced with muscle or fat graft; mastoid pressure dressing	0	The use of fat graft is a viable long-term barrier to prevent CSF leakage following vestibular schwannoma resection, due to its ability to revascularized

(continued)

Table 25.2 (continued)

Study	Patients (n)	Reconstructive technique	CSF leakage (%)	Comments
Luryi et al. (2017) [43]	19 patients	Hydroxyapatite cement was used for cranioplasty	0	Hydroxyapatite could be considered as an alternative to traditional retrosigmoid craniotomy repair methods
Venable et al. (2018) [46]	86 patients	Bone wax or paste was used to seal mastoid air cells; dura was kept moist to avoid desiccation; dura was closed with 4-0 Nurolon sutures; DuraSeal tissue glue was added on top of the sutures; Gelfoam was then place in the epidural space, and titanium mesh was used to reconstruct the bone defect	0	Primary dural closure should be a goal in retrosigmoid approaches to avoid CSF leaks
Hwa et al. (2021) [47]	196 patients	IAC reconstruction: bone wax and muscle plug; Norian hydroxyapatite bone cement; Cranios hydroxyapatite bone cement	15.6 % with no bone cement, 6.3% with Norian cement, and 1% with Cranios cement	CSF leak is significantly reduced when Cranios hydroxyapatite was used for reconstruction; tumor size or age did not affect CSF leak rate

However, the insufficient number of cases allowed no conclusion [16]. Three series described the retrosigmoid approach without the use of graft (allo- or auto-). In these studies, the incidence of the CSF leak varied between 0% and 4% [27, 28, 42]. Finally, in the last two decades, the use of hydroxyapatite bone cement for the reconstruction of retrosigmoid craniectomy became widespread. However, it could be associated with the formation of seroma and subsequently life-threatening infection [46].

Translabyrinthine Approach

Patients with a lack of serviceable hearing are suitable for the translabyrinthine approach. It allows the preservation of the other cranial nerves and the early identification of the facial nerve and does not require cerebellar retraction. Several single-treatment arm studies investigating complications from treating vestibular schwannomas via the translabyrinthine approach have been published [22, 47–51]. CSF leakage has been one of the most common postoperative complications that resulted in meningitis, increased rate of re-operation, and prolonged hospital stay

Table 25.3 Studies of the translabyrinthine approach and various closure techniques and corresponding CSF leakage chance

Study	Patients (n)	Reconstructive technique	CSF leakage (%)	Comments
Wu et al. (1999) [54]	277 patients	1st group, fascia fat was used to obliterate the operative cavity; 2nd group, fascia-fat-flap technique was used; 3rd group, fat-flap technique	1st group, 28.2%; 2nd group, 21.7%; and 3rd group, 7.4%	Filling the operative cavity with fat directly, without fascia, significantly reduced the rate of CSF leakage
Fayad et al. (2007) [55]	389 patients	After translabyrinthine tumor removal, patients underwent titanium mesh cranioplasty	3.3	CSF leaks seem to be reduced after titanium mesh cranioplasty
Merkus et al. (2010) [56]	1803 patients	After the incus is disarticulated, the attic and middle ear are plugged with dry periosteum; bone wax is used to plug open cells; the operative site is obliterated with long strips of abdominal fat with part of the strips protruding into the CPA; dural edges are not sutured; the fasciomusculoperiosteal flaps are sutured in a watertight fashion	0.8	The technique used in this series reduced CSF leak to an absolute minimum
Manjila et al. (2013) [57]	42 patients	Patients underwent a multilayered closure using titanium mesh—hydroxyapatite cement cranioplasty with dural substitute and fat grafts; temporalis muscle and Eustachian tube obliteration were not used	0	The described technique was successful in preventing postoperative CSF leakage
Hunter et al. (2015) [58]	53 patients	Bone defects were closed with a dural substitute, layered fat graft, and a resorbable mesh plate secured with screws	1.9	The use of fat graft with mesh reduced the rate of CSF leakage
Zhu et al. (2016) [59]	382 patients	332 patients underwent classic enlarged translabyrinthine approach (ETLA), 28 patients underwent ETLA with blind sac technique and middle ear eradication, and 22 patients underwent vestibular schwannoma resection via transotic approach	4.8% via classic ETLA, 0% via ETLA with blind sac technique, and 0% via transotic approach	CSF leakage can be reduced in large vestibular schwannoma resection using the blind sac technique

(continued)

Table 25.3 (continued)

Study	Patients (n)	Reconstructive technique	CSF leakage (%)	Comments
Volsky et al. (2017) [66]	369 patients	Patients underwent hydroxyapatite cement cranioplasty with or without fat graft	1.9	The use of HAC with fat is superior to fat alone following translabyrinthine approach
Russel et al. (2017) [60]	275 patients	Eustachian tube was obliterated with multilayer of temporalis muscle and biological glue; bone pate, biological glue, and wax were used to obliterate cells of the middle ear, the infralabyrinthine, and apical mastoid; abdominal fat and biological glue were used to obliterate the operative cavity; the musculoperiosteal flap and the cutaneous incision were sutured close	12	Young patients, male sex, long duration of surgery, and high BMI were associated with a higher rate of CSF leakage; the most important way to prevent CSF leakage was to obliterate the petromastoid cavity
Luryi et al. (2020) [61]	52 patients	Hydroxyapatite cement was used for cranioplasty without any fat graft or any other material	3.8	Hydroxyapatite cement is an acceptable alternative to fat grafting
Totten et al. (2021) [62]	77 patients	21 patients underwent multilayer repair using small intestinal submucosal xenografts, and 56 patients underwent multilayer reconstruction using fascia autograft	4.8% in xenograft group and 16% autograft group	Xenografts are robust alternative for closure, thus reducing CSF leakage
Selleck et al. (2021) [63]	132 patients	Mesh cranioplasty versus watertight periosteal closure	12.8% in titanium mesh closure group and 0% via periosteal closure	Periosteal approach statistically reduced CSF leakage when compared to titanium mesh closure technique

Table 25.3 (continued)

Study	Patients (n)	Reconstructive technique	CSF leakage (%)	Comments
Cooper et al. (2021) [53]	23 patients	Air cells are sealed with soft tissue packing, hydroxyapatite cement, and bone cement; facial grafts are pressed and draped over the IAC and the aditus ad antrum; primary closure of the dural flaps is achieved when possible; the remaining defect is plugged with fascia or fat in a dumbbell fashion; cranioplasty with titanium mesh if desired; wound closure in a watertight fashion; tight mastoid dressing is finally applied	4.3	It is crucial to identify and obstruct all potential cell tracts to avoid CSF leakage
Christopher et al. (2021) [64]	204 patients	In 102 patients, facial recess approach was used during translabyrinthine surgery for schwannoma, and 102 patients underwent translabyrinthine surgery without facial recess approach	3.9% in group who underwent facial recess approach and 4.9% in control group	CSF leak was not affected whether or not facial recess approach was used to pack the Eustachian tube
Martinez-Perez et al. (2022) [65]	69 patients	34 patients underwent cranioplasty with hydroxyapatite cement and fat, and 35 patients underwent fat-only cranioplasty	2.9% in HAC + fat group and 8.6% in fat-only group	The use of hydroxyapatite for cranial reconstruction after translabyrinthine approaches showed superiority in preventing percutaneous postoperative CSF leaks

[52]. Subsequently, since the development of the translabyrinthine approach in 1960 [53], surgeons have been working to develop new reconstruction and closure techniques to minimize the risk of CSF leaks (Table 25.3) [52].

Conclusion

A collaboration between neurotologists and neurosurgeons and meticulous attention to detail in every step of the operation including pre-op assessment, intraoperative closure, and immediate post-op care can help reduce the likelihood of CSF leakage. Every source of leak—incision, canal skin laceration, tympanic membrane perforation, mastoid air cells, middle ear cavity/opening, petrous apex cells, and especially the IAC air cells—needs to be addressed to reduce the likelihood of CSF leak. Multiple layers of closure for each area should be considered to keep a CSF leak to a minimum.

References

1. Charalampakis S, Koutsimpelas D, Gouveris H, Mann W. Post-operative complications after removal of sporadic vestibular schwannoma via retrosigmoid-suboccipital approach: current diagnosis and management. Eur Arch Otorhinolaryngol. 2011;268:653–60.
2. Yang H, Sun S, Zheng X, Ding F, Bie Y. Effect of subdural muscle packing in repairing dura mater after retrosigmoid craniotomy. J Int Med Res. 2020;48:299.
3. Ling PY, Mendelson ZS, Reddy RK, Jyung RW, Liu JK. Reconstruction after retrosigmoid approaches using autologous fat graft-assisted Medpor Titan cranioplasty: assessment of postoperative cerebrospinal fluid leaks and headaches in 60 cases. Acta Neurochir. 2014;156:1879–88.
4. Glasscock ME, Shambaugh GE. Surgery of the ear. Philadelphia: W.B. Saunders; 1990.
5. Donald PJ. Surgery of the skull base. Basel: Karger; 1994. p. 624.
6. Régis J, Roche P-H. Modern management of acoustic neuroma: 41 tables. Basel: Karger; 2008.
7. Hildmann H, Sudhoff H, Bernal-Sprekelsen M. Middle ear surgery. Cham: Springer; 2006.
8. Khan A, Lapin A, Eisenman DJ. Use of titanium mesh for middle cranial fossa skull base reconstruction. J Neurol Surg B Skull Base. 2014;75:104–9.
9. Chamoun R, MacDonald J, Shelton C, Couldwell WT. Surgical approaches for resection of vestibular schwannomas: translabyrinthine, retrosigmoid, and middle fossa approaches. Neurosurg Focus. 2012;33:E9.
10. Lipschitz N, et al. Cerebrospinal fluid leak rate after vestibular schwannoma surgery via middle cranial fossa approach. J Neurol Surg B Skull Base. 2019;80:437–40.
11. Angeli S. Middle fossa approach: indications, technique, and results. Otolaryngol Clin N Am. 2012;45:417–38.
12. Becker SS, Jackler RK, Pitts LH. Cerebrospinal fluid leak after acoustic neuroma surgery: a comparison of the translabyrinthine, middle fossa, and retrosigmoid approaches. Otol Neurotol. 2003;24:107–12.
13. Fishman AJ, Marrinan MS, Golfinos JG, Cohen NL, Roland JT. Prevention and management of cerebrospinal fluid leak following vestibular schwannoma surgery. Laryngoscope. 2004;114:501–5.
14. Scheich M, Ginzkey C, Ehrmann-Müller D, Shehata-Dieler W, Hagen R. Management of CSF leakage after microsurgery for vestibular schwannoma via the middle cranial fossa approach. Eur Arch Otorhinolaryngol. 2016;273:2975–81.
15. Rajput MSA, et al. Preservation of hearing and facial nerve function with the microsurgical excision of large vestibular schwannomas: experience with the retrosigmoid approach. Cureus. 2018;10:e3684.
16. Kolagi S, Herur A, Ugale M, Manjula R, Mutalik A. Suboccipital retrosigmoid surgical approach for internal auditory canal—a morphometric anatomical study on dry human temporal bones. Indian J Otolaryngol Head Neck Surg. 2010;62:372–5.
17. Arlt F, et al. Cerebrospinal fluid leak after microsurgical surgery in vestibular schwannomas via retrosigmoidal craniotomy. Neurol Res. 2011;33:947–52.
18. Spiegel R, et al. Ginkgo biloba extract EGb 761 alleviates neurosensory symptoms in patients with dementia: a meta-analysis of treatment effects on tinnitus and dizziness in randomized, placebo-controlled trials. CIA. 2018;13:1121–7.
19. Ondik MP, Benson AG, Djalilian H. An unusual site of a CSF Leak following resection of a retrosigmoid acoustic neuroma. Ear Nose Throat J. 2006;85:164–7.

20. Sathaporntheera P, Saetia K. Risk factors associated with CSF leakage and complications after retrosigmoid surgery. Interdiscip Neurosurg. 2020;22:100865.
21. Kehler U, et al. CSF leaks after cranial surgery — a prospective multicenter analysis. Innov Neurosurg. 2013;1:49–53.
22. Alattar AA, et al. Risk factors for readmission with cerebrospinal fluid leakage within 30 days of vestibular schwannoma surgery. Neurosurgery. 2018;82:630–7.
23. Copeland WR, Mallory GW, Neff BA, Driscoll CLW, Link MJ. Are there modifiable risk factors to prevent a cerebrospinal fluid leak following vestibular schwannoma surgery? J Neurosurg. 2015;122:312–6.
24. O'Connell BP, Rizk HG, Stevens SM, Nguyen SA, Meyer TA. The relation between obesity and hospital length of stay after elective lateral skull base surgery: an analysis of the American College of Surgeons national surgical quality improvement program. ORL J Otorhinolaryngol Relat Spec. 2015;77:294–301.
25. Montano N, et al. Factors associated with cerebrospinal fluid leak after a retrosigmoid approach for cerebellopontine angle surgery. Surg Neurol Int. 2021;12:258.
26. Fleischman D, et al. Cerebrospinal fluid pressure decreases with older age. PLoS One. 2012;7:e52664.
27. Date I, Asari S, Ohmoto T. Tips for preventing cerebrospinal fluid rhinorrhea after acoustic neurinoma surgery. Skull Base Surg. 1998;8:181–3.
28. Gal TJ, Bartels LJ. Use of bone wax in the prevention of cerebrospinal fluid fistula in acoustic neuroma surgery. Laryngoscope. 1999;109:167–9.
29. Benson AG, Djalilian HR. Complications of hydroxyapatite bone cement reconstruction of retrosigmoid craniotomy: two cases. Ear Nose Throat J. 2009;88:1–4.
30. Cueva RA, Mastrodimos B. Approach design and closure techniques to minimize cerebrospinal fluid leak after cerebellopontine angle tumor surgery. Otol Neurotol. 2005;26:1176–81.
31. Galer C, Bowdino B, Leibrock L, Moore GF. Complication rate of retrosigmoid craniotomy with and without closed-suction wound drainage. Skull Base. 2006;16:A090.
32. Baird CJ, et al. Reduction of cerebrospinal fluid rhinorrhea after vestibular schwannoma surgery by reconstruction of the drilled porus acusticus with hydroxyapatite bone cement. J Neurosurg. 2007;107:347–51.
33. Lüdemann WO, Stieglitz LH, Gerganov V, Samii A, Samii M. Fat implant is superior to muscle implant in vestibular schwannoma surgery for the prevention of cerebrospinal fluid fistulae. Neurosurgery. 2008;63:38–42; discussion 42-43.
34. Bayazit YA, Celenk F, Duzlu M, Goksu N. Management of cerebrospinal fluid leak following retrosigmoid posterior cranial fossa surgery. ORL. 2009;71:329–33.
35. Stieglitz LH, et al. Petrous bone pneumatization is a risk factor for cerebrospinal fluid fistula following vestibular schwannoma surgery. Neurosurgery. 2010;67:509–15.
36. Samii M, Gerganov VM, Samii A. Functional outcome after complete surgical removal of giant vestibular schwannomas. J Neurosurg. 2010;112:860–7.
37. Chovanec M, et al. Impact of video-endoscopy on the results of retrosigmoid-transmeatal microsurgery of vestibular schwannoma: prospective study. Eur Arch Otorhinolaryngol. 2013;270:1277–84.
38. Heman-Ackah SE, Cosetti MK, Gupta S, Golfinos JG, Roland JT Jr. Retrosigmoid approach to cerebellopontine angle tumor resection: surgical modifications. Laryngoscope. 2012;122:2519–23.
39. Frederickson AM, Sekula RF. The utility of calcium phosphate cement in cranioplasty following retromastoid craniectomy for cranial neuralgias. Br J Neurosurg. 2013;27:808–11.
40. Foster KA, Shin SS, Prabhu B, Fredrickson A, Sekula RF. Calcium phosphate cement cranioplasty decreases the rate of cerebrospinal fluid leak and wound infection compared with titanium mesh cranioplasty: retrospective study of 672 patients. World Neurosurg. 2016;95:414–8.
41. Azad T, Mendelson ZS, Wong A, Jyung RW, Liu JK. Fat graft-assisted internal auditory canal closure after retrosigmoid transmeatal resection of acoustic neuroma: technique for prevention of cerebrospinal fluid leakage. J Clin Neurosci. 2016;24:124–7.

42. Yamakami I, Uchino Y, Kobayashi E, Yamaura A, Oka N. Removal of large acoustic neurinomas (vestibular schwannomas) by the retrosigmoid approach with no mortality and minimal morbidity. J Neurol Neurosurg Psychiatry. 2004;75:453–8.
43. Luryi AL, Bulsara KR, Michaelides EM. Hydroxyapatite bone cement for suboccipital retrosigmoid cranioplasty: a single institution case series. Am J Otolaryngol. 2017;38:390–3.
44. Pedersen SH, Lilja-Cyron A, Andresen M, Juhler M. The relationship between intracranial pressure and age-chasing age-related reference values. World Neurosurg. 2018;110:e119–23.
45. Hoffman RA. Cerebrospinal fluid leak following acoustic neuroma removal. Laryngoscope. 1994;104:40–58.
46. Venable GT, Roberts ML, Lee RP, Michael LM. Primary dural closure for retrosigmoid approaches. J Neurol Surg B Skull Base. 2018;79:330–4.
47. Hwa TP, et al. Impact of reconstruction with hydroxyapatite bone cement on CSF leak rate in retrosigmoid approach to vestibular schwannoma resection: a review of 196 cases. Otol Neurotol. 2021;42:918–22.
48. Ölander C, Gudjonsson O, Kinnefors A, Laurell G, Edfeldt L. Complications in translabyrinthine surgery of vestibular schwannoma. Acta Otolaryngol. 2018;138:639–45.
49. Ben Ammar M, Piccirillo E, Topsakal V, Taibah A, Sanna M. Surgical results and technical refinements in translabyrinthine excision of vestibular schwannomas: the Gruppo Otologico experience. Neurosurgery. 2012;70:1481–91; discussion 1491.
50. Sanna M, Taibah A, Russo A, Falcioni M, Agarwal M. Perioperative complications in acoustic neuroma (vestibular schwannoma) surgery. Otol Neurotol. 2004;25:379–86.
51. Brackmann DE, Cullen RD, Fisher LM. Facial nerve function after translabyrinthine vestibular schwannoma surgery. Otolaryngol Head Neck Surg. 2007;136:773–7.
52. Springborg JB, et al. Outcome after translabyrinthine surgery for vestibular schwannomas: report on 1244 patients. J Neurol Surg B Skull Base. 2012;73:168–74.
53. Cooper MW, Ward BK, Sharon J, Francis HW. Reducing the risk of cerebrospinal fluid rhinorrhea following translabyrinthine surgery of the posterior fossa. World J Otorhinolaryngol Head Neck Surg. 2021;7:82–7.
54. Wu H, Kalamarides M, Garem HE, Rey A, Sterkers O. Comparison of different wound closure techniques in translabyrinthine acoustic neuroma surgery. Skull Base Surg. 1999;9:239–42.
55. Fayad JN, Schwartz MS, Slattery WH, Brackmann DE. Prevention and treatment of cerebrospinal fluid leak after translabyrinthine acoustic tumor removal. Otol Neurotol. 2007;28:387–90.
56. Merkus P, Taibah A, Sequino G, Sanna M. Less than 1% cerebrospinal fluid leakage in 1,803 translabyrinthine vestibular schwannoma surgery cases. Otol Neurotol. 2010;31:276–83.
57. Manjila S, Weidenbecher M, Semaan MT, Megerian CA, Bambakidis NC. Prevention of postoperative cerebrospinal fluid leaks with multilayered reconstruction using titanium mesh-hydroxyapatite cement cranioplasty after translabyrinthine resection of acoustic neuroma. J Neurosurg. 2013;119:113–20.
58. Hunter JB, et al. Prevention of postoperative cerebrospinal fluid leaks after translabyrinthine tumor resection with resorbable mesh cranioplasty. Otol Neurotol. 2015;36:1537–42.
59. Zhu ZJ, Zhu WD, Chen HS, Wang ZY, Wu H. Decision making in dissection range of temporal bone: refinements to enlarged translabyrinthine approach. Eur Arch Otorhinolaryngol. 2016;273:1115–21.
60. Russel A, Hoffmann CP, Nguyen DT, Beurton R, Parietti-Winkler C. Can the risks of cerebrospinal fluid leak after vestibular schwannoma surgery be predicted? Otol Neurotol. 2017;38:248–52.
61. Luryi AL, Schutt CA, Michaelides E, Kveton JF. Hydroxyapatite cement cranioplasty for translabyrinthine surgery: a single institution experience. Laryngoscope. 2020;130:206–11.
62. Totten DJ, et al. Comparison of small intestinal submucosal graft and autologous tissue in prevention of CSF leak after posterior fossa craniotomy. J Neurol Surg B Skull Base. 2021;82:695–9.

63. Selleck AM, Hodge SE, Brown KD. Cerebrospinal fluid leak following translabyrinthine vestibular schwannoma surgery-is mesh cranioplasty necessary for prevention? Otol Neurotol. 2021;42:e593–7.
64. Christopher L, Slattery W, Lekovic GP, Mehta GU, Miller M. Matched cohort analysis of the effect of the facial recess approach on cerebrospinal fluid leak after translabyrinthine surgery for schwannoma. Otol Neurotol. 2021;42:1394–8.
65. Martinez-Perez R, et al. Hydroxyapatite cement cranioplasty for reconstruction of translabyrinthine approach: aesthetic results, long-term satisfaction, quality of life, and complications. Acta Neurochir. 2022;164:669–77.
66. Volsky PG, et al. Hydroxyapatite cement cranioplasty following translabyrinthine approach: long-term study of 369 cases. Laryngoscope. 2017;127:2120–5.

Chapter 26
Reconstruction of the Middle Cranial Fossa Floor

Judith S. Kempfle and Aaron K. Remenschneider

Introduction

Congenital and acquired lateral skull base defects can involve isolated or combined defects of the tegmen mastoideum, the tegmen tympani, and the petrous apex. Defects may result in herniating meningoencephaloceles with or without cerebrospinal fluid (CSF) leakage into the mastoid air cells and/or the middle ear [1–4]. Mounting evidence points toward a direct connection between encephaloceles, CSF leaks and increased body mass index (BMI), which is concerning given the rise in BMI at the US population level [5, 6]. Obesity and elevated intracranial pressure have been directly linked to skull base thinning and resultant skull base defects with encephaloceles and CSF leaks [7]. Other etiologies of skull base defects include tegmen mastoideum defects, which are often caused by erosion related to cholesteatoma or iatrogenic injuries during mastoidectomy. These defects generally represent smaller, more posterior and lateral dehiscences of the middle cranial fossa floor. Defects of the tegmen tympani involve dehiscences of the anterior and medial aspects of the middle cranial fossa floor, are more often congenital in nature and larger or multiple, and can affect the ossicular chain and the geniculate ganglion. Patients may present with a range of symptoms from mild ear blockage and conductive hearing loss to CSF otorrhea and otogenic meningitis. Regardless of

J. S. Kempfle
Department of Otolaryngology, University Medical Center, Tübingen, Germany
e-mail: judith.kempfle@umassmemorial.org

A. K. Remenschneider (✉)
Department of Otolaryngology, UMass Memorial Medical Center, Worcester, MA, USA

UMass Chan Medical School, Worcester, MA, USA
e-mail: Aaron.Remenschneider@umassmemorial.org

location, the primary goal of surgical management of lateral skull base defects is to guard against devastating intracranial complications from progressive disease as well as to address symptoms affecting patient quality of life.

Tegmen defects are most commonly repaired via one of three approaches: a transmastoid approach, a middle fossa craniotomy (MFC), or a combined transmastoid–middle fossa approach [8]. The transmastoid approach circumvents a craniotomy and allows for exposure and repair of smaller posterior and lateral tegmen mastoideum defects. Larger or multiple defects that extend more medially and involve or expose the ossicular chain are preferably treated with a MFC approach, which provides better visualization of the entire lateral skull base all the way to the level of the petrous apex [9, 10]. Combined approaches are often used in cases of eroding middle ear and mastoid cholesteatoma and large meningoencephalocele [11, 12].

Various materials have been utilized for lateral skull base repair. Single layer or multilayer repair involving autologous materials (e.g., fascia, calvarial bone graft, cartilage, bone pate, or vascularized flaps) and allogenic materials (e.g., bone cement, bone wax, polyethylene scaffold, or synthetic dura) are overall safe and effective in recreating a watertight boundary and reconstructing the lateral skull base [8, 13, 14]. This chapter covers methods and materials used in reconstruction of the middle cranial fossa floor.

Surgical Techniques

Middle Fossa Craniotomy for Repair of Spontaneous Tegmen Defects With or Without Meningoencephalocele and CSF Leak

We commonly use this approach for most of our lateral skull base repairs, including dehiscences of the tegmen mastoideum, the tegmen tympani, and for treatment of superior canal dehiscence syndrome. This intracranial, extradural technique provides a stable dural closure in cases of dural defects with CSF leaks and allows excellent visualization for extradural reduction and resection of meningoencephaloceles, as well as repair of bony dehiscence. Exposure of the entire tegmen mastoideum and tegmen tympani without disruption of the ossicular chain is a major advantage of this approach. The disadvantages of this approach compared to a transmastoid approach however include a slightly higher risk of temporal lobe injury, seizure, subdural or epidural hematoma, and a required hospital stay [8].

Preoperatively, we recommend obtaining a thin-cut CT scan of the temporal bone and, in cases of suspected meningoencephalocele with or without CSF leak, an MRI. This will allow for identification of single or multiple meningoencephaloceles, concurrent superior canal dehiscence (SCD), dehiscent facial nerve at the geniculate ganglion, and surgical landmarks necessary for safe craniotomy technique.

Classically, a C-shaped or "horseshoe" incision has been created, curving from slightly anteriorly to the tragus and about 3–4 cm superiorly to the auricle at the level of the external auditory canal. This creates a prominent incision that at times may lie outside of the hairline [15]. In contrary to previous publications [10, 15], we favor a smaller, 4–5 cm long, S-shaped incision centered over the external auditory canal that can be easily hidden in the hairline (Fig. 26.1a, a′). We recommend marking the incision on the awake, upright sitting patient in the preoperative area, to best predict the location of the defect and to compose the incision line accordingly (Fig. 26.1a).

After induction of general anesthesia, the patient is then positioned supine, and the head is rotated to the contralateral side. Facial nerve monitoring is advisable, given the close relationship of many tegmen defects to the geniculate ganglion. The location of the facial nerve should also be appreciated on preoperative imaging. A Mayfield headholder for head fixation has been successfully employed and described by many others [10, 15] but is not necessary in our experience. A small donut, tape, and a shoulder roll are generally sufficient to limit head movement. A foley catheter is placed at the start of the procedure to permit diuresis and decrease cerebrospinal fluid pressure, which will assist in decreasing temporal lobe retraction.

Minimal hair removal is necessary with this modified incision (Fig. 26.1a′), and the patient is then prepped and draped in normal sterile fashion. An S-shaped curvilinear incision is then made along the previously marked line, from behind the hairline, and above the auricle down over the supra-auricular fold and into the postauricular crease. By keeping the incision posterior to the hairline, the frontal branch of the facial nerve is protected. The incision is carried down through the subcutaneous soft tissues to the level of the temporalis fascia. This plane is elevated anteriorly and posteriorly, and a small retractor can be placed to reflect the ear forward. Next, a fascia graft should be harvested from the temporalis fascia. An anteriorly based temporalis flap is then incised and reflected anteriorly to expose the squamous portion of the temporal bone (Fig. 26.1b).

To create the craniotomy, an otologic drill with #4 cutting drill bit and #3 diamond bur is sufficient. Under the surgical microscope, a typical bone flap of approximately 3 × 2 cm is then outlined, which should be centered along the long axis directly above the external auditory canal, with its inferior border positioned roughly along the floor of the middle fossa, corresponding to the root of the zygoma (Fig. 26.1c). Larger bone flaps may be necessary for anterior or more medially located middle fossa floor defects. The margins of the craniotomy are carried down to the level of the dura, taking care to keep the dura intact. The bone flap is then elevated by careful dissection from the underlying dura using a Woodson or Freer elevator (Fig. 26.1d). If air cells are encountered over the zygoma or mastoid during the craniotomy, these should be sealed with bone wax to prevent CSF leaks (Fig. 26.1e). Additional bone from the inferior border of the craniotomy obstructing the direct view of the anterior skull base floor should be removed. At this point, the surgeon should reposition himself/herself at the top of the head, as this position provides a superior en face view of the middle fossa floor.

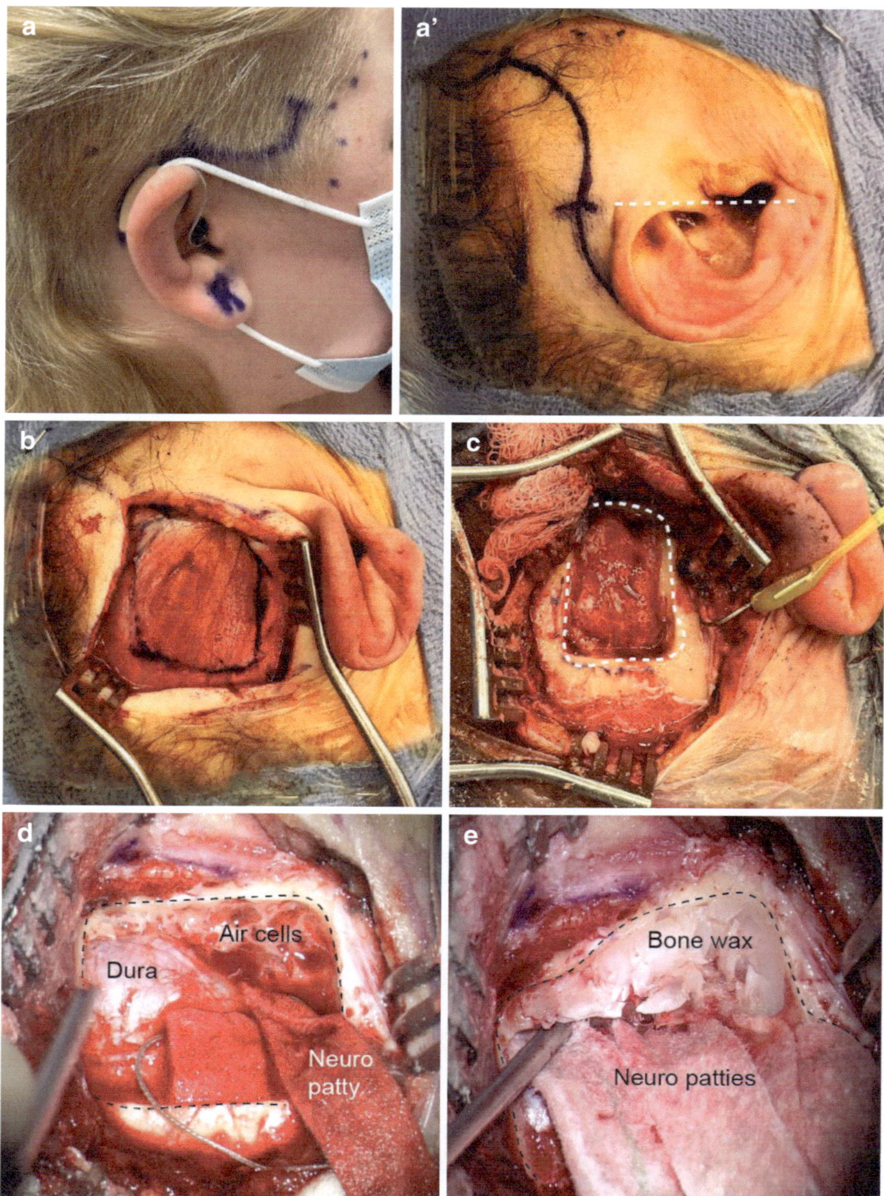

Fig. 26.1 Middle fossa craniotomy for tegmen repair. (**a**) Incision is planned behind the hair line of the awake, upright, sitting patient. (**a′**) Incision should be centered over the external auditory canal (dashed line). (**b**) Fascia graft is harvested, and an anteriorly based temporalis flap is created (blue marker). (**c**) Craniotomy is performed, and bone flap is removed (dashed white line). (**d**) Brain and dura are carefully elevated to expose the skull base. (**e**) Exposed air cells are sealed with bone wax

The dura is then carefully elevated with a Freer elevator from the middle fossa floor, starting from posteriorly to anteriorly under constant suction irrigation (Fig. 26.2a). This trajectory protects the greater superficial petrosal nerve and inadvertent damage to a dehiscent geniculate ganglion [10]. Once the posterior petrous ridge is identified, dissection proceeds anteriorly and medially to identify additional landmarks such as the arcuate eminence and geniculate ganglion as well as any bony defects over the tegmen tympani and/or mastoideum (Fig. 26.2a, b). If the geniculate ganglion is dehiscent, a nerve stimulator probe may be employed to confirm the location and function of the nerve (and monitor) prior to reconstruction.

At this point, the nature of the defect should then be further characterized and documented. Several important questions must be asked to verify CT/MRI findings with the intraoperative exam.

1. Is there concurrent mastoid or middle ear disease that needs to be addressed via mastoidectomy?
2. Is there significant encephalocele penetrating into the mastoid or the tympanic cavity?
3. Is CSF encountered from the defect?
4. If there is a tegmen tympani defect present, are the ossicular heads exposed, and how does the defect relate to a (potentially dehiscent) facial nerve in that area?

These intraoperative findings will ultimately guide decision-making for reconstruction. Mastoid and middle ear disease should be known prior to the procedure, but if unanticipated findings are encountered, then a mastoidectomy and middle ear exploration should be performed. If a large encephalocele/temporal herniation is present, the stalk is identified and cauterized before it is resected at its base. In case of a broad base, the encephalocele can be coagulated to produce tissue shrinkage followed by amputation. Typically, this can be safely done, as the herniated encephalocele generally represents nonfunctional brain tissue. The resected portion of the brain is then sent for pathology to confirm the initial diagnosis. Disease present in the mastoid may be removed through the middle fossa floor defect prior to reconstruction. Dural defects may occur following amputation of herniated tissue or because of thin or dehiscent dura and addressing the resultant CSF leak will typically require a multilayered approach. Finally, tegmen tympani defects must be cautiously approached given their proximity to the facial nerve and the potential to iatrogenically introduce ossicular trauma.

We favor multilayer repair of the dura and lateral skull base, using a combination of non-autologous collagen matrix for dural onlay, a split calvarial bone graft for bony reconstruction, and autologous soft tissue (temporalis fascia) against the skull base defect to obtain a tight seal (Fig 26.2c). For bony reconstruction, the previously harvested bone flap is split using a sagittal saw in order to generate a bone chip that will provide the main solid reconstruction of middle fossa floor (Fig. 26.2d). Although rarely observed, if there is a concern of contact between the bone graft and the ossicular heads, it can be positioned with the concave side over the ossicles to minimize contact [15]. Next, a piece of synthetic dura is placed over the dura in an onlay fashion (Fig. 26.2e). The previously harvested fascia is then wrapped

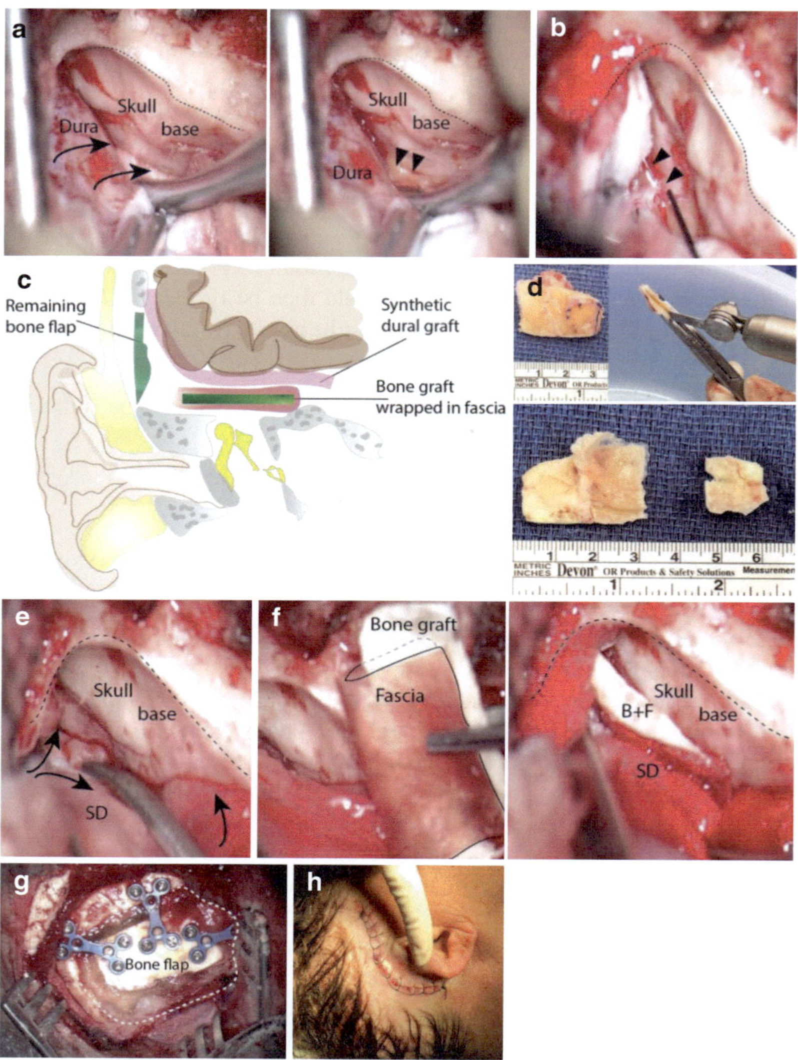

Fig. 26.2 Intracranial, extradural repair of tegmen defect. (**a**) Dura is carefully elevated from the skull base posteriorly to anteriorly under constant suction irrigation (arrows), until the petrous ridge and the arcuate eminence are visualized (arrowheads). (**b**) The tegmen defect is identified and characterized, meningocele (arrowheads) or meningoencephaloceles are reduced. (**c**) Schematic of the skull base repair via multilayer reconstruction. (**d**) The calvarial bone flap is split using a sagittal saw, and the resulting bone chip is saved to be used as rigid reinforcement of the skull base. (**e**) A dural replacement graft/synthetic dura (SD) is placed over the brain to protect native dura and repair dural defects in onlay fashion. (**f**) A bone-fascia "taco" is created (**b+f**), which is then slid between the dural graft and the bony skull base defect. The open side of the reconstruction is facing laterally. (**g**) The lateral cranial defect is reconstructed with the remaining bone flap and fixed with titanium plates. (**h**) Watertight multilayer closure of soft tissue and skin

around the bone graft to create a soft surface on each side, and the bone chip is placed superior to the bony defect and inferior to the dural replacement graft, ensuring that the open side of the bone "taco" is facing laterally (Fig. 26.2c, f). In cases of a dehiscent geniculate ganglion, great care should be taken during this maneuver to avoid pushing the bone chip too far medially to impinge on the nerve. Fibrin glue is then used throughout the reconstruction and lateral to the temporal lobe dura to complete the repair. In cases where bone cement is used to repair a defect, absorbable materials (e.g., gelatin sponge) or autologous fascia can be used over the exposed ossicles to prevent fixation and associated conductive hearing loss [8, 14]. In cases of simple dural defects, a patch with dural replacement matrix (bovine pericardium, alloderm, collagen substitute, or temporalis fascia) may be performed in an onlay technique. Alternatively, a primary dural closure can be attempted with 4.0 Nurolon suture (Johnson & Johnson, New Brunswick, NJ) [10]. If an additional superior canal dehiscence is unexpectedly identified intraoperatively, the defect can be plugged at the same time using bone wax as described below, or with bone wax and bone cement [8]. In cases of small middle fossa floor defects, a bone graft is not necessarily required. Inlay grafts of synthetic dura and extradural temporalis fascia have also demonstrated high success rates [15].

The calvarial bone flap is then replaced and secured using at least three titanium mini plates and 4 mm titanium self-tapping self-drilling screws. The anterior inferior corner of the craniotomy should be protected with the bone flap (Fig. 26.2g). Alternatively, resorbable plates and screws can be used to cover the defect. In cases where the calvarial bone is thin or is used in its entirety for reconstruction of the tegmental floor, a titanium mesh cranioplasty provides a viable alternative [16]. The use of an alloplastic graft has been shown to shorten the overall mean operating time compared to autologous grafts [10]. Absorbable hemostatic agents are excellent choices for hemostasis and to cover and seal any remaining bony defects around the cranioplasty. To obtain a watertight closure, the temporalis muscle flap is then replaced and reapproximated, and the skin is closed in multiple layers (Fig. 26.2h). To avoid postoperative hematomas or CSF hygromas, a mastoid pressure dressing should be applied over the incision and left in place for at least 5 days.

Middle Fossa Craniotomy for Superior Canal Dehiscence Repair

A comparable intracranial, extradural approach as described above is employed for superior canal dehiscence (SCD) repair (Fig. 26.3). In select cases, for example, revisions or where the defect is located adjacent to the superior petrosal sinus, or located medially along a downsloping tegmen, a transmastoid canal plugging may be more favorable [17]. In this chapter, we focus on the middle fossa approach.

Preoperative evaluation and intraoperative positioning and incision are identical to the approach described above. Once the dura is elevated from the middle fossa

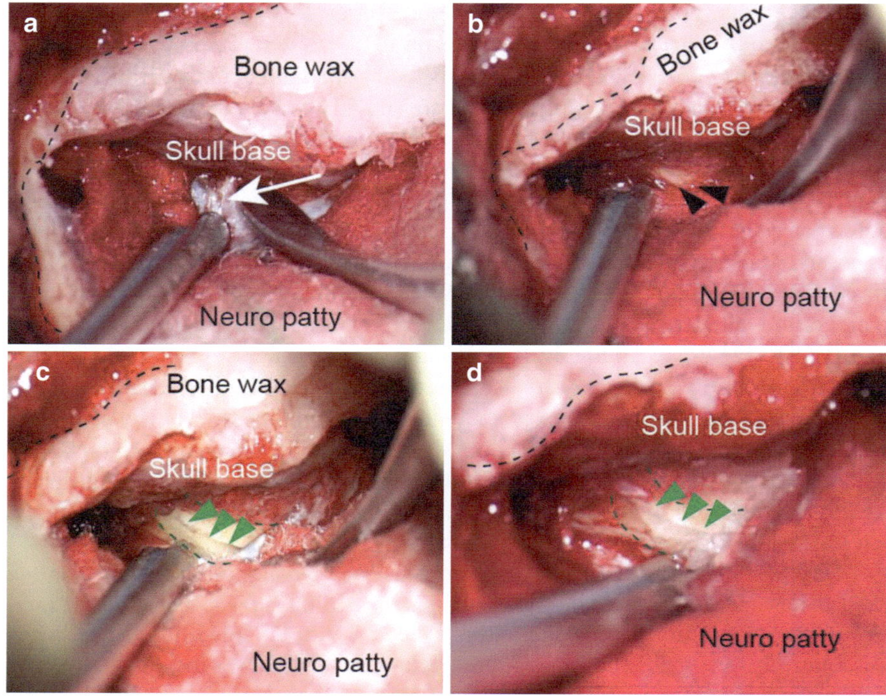

Fig. 26.3 Middle fossa repair of SCD. (**a**) Dura is elevated off the skull base under constant suction irrigation. (**b**) Petrous ridge and arcuate eminence are exposed (arrowheads). (**c**) Bony defect (green arrowheads) of the superior semicircular canal (green dashed line) is identified. (**d**) Defect is plugged with prewarmed bone wax (green arrowheads)

floor (Fig. 26.3a), the petrous ridge is identified to guide the dissection toward the arcuate eminence (Fig. 26.3b). Preoperative CT imaging can aid in identifying the defects of the superior semicircular canal intraoperatively and any relationship to additional tegmen defects or a dehiscent geniculate ganglion. Distance measurements from the inner table to the arcuate eminence in the coronal plane can provide helpful guidance in cases where the defect is not readily visualized.

Once the bony dehiscence is identified (Fig. 26.3c), several prewarmed spheres of bone wax are carefully pressed into the defect to occlude both the ampulated end and the crus cummune it in its entirety [18]. A Neuro patty and a Freer elevator can be employed to apply additional pressure [19]. The area over the defect is then irrigated with warm saline to "test" the durability of the reconstruction (Fig. 26.3d). The repair can be reinforced with a bone "taco" of temporalis fascia, split calvarial bone graft, and synthetic dura as described above, as well as bone cement, cartilage, or fascia, but is ultimately not required if an adequate bone wax seal can be obtained and no other middle fossa floor defects are identified [8, 20].

Transmastoid Repair of Posterior and Lateral Tegmen Defects

A transmastoid approach to tegmental defect repair avoids a craniotomy and allows for resection of concurrent mastoid and middle ear disease [8]. This approach has been thoroughly described in the literature for repair of small tegmen mastoideum defects or for disease originating in the mastoid with minimal penetration of the middle cranial fossa [12, 21–24]. In experienced hands, the transmastoid approach can also be successfully used to repair tegmen tympani defects but usually requires disarticulation of the ossicular chain, often with removal of the incus and the malleus head for adequate exposure to the epitympanum. Repair of larger defects may be compromised and destabilized by continued intracranial pressure, which may lead to recurrence of meningoencephalocele and/or CSF leak [13].

In terms of surgical technique, the patient is positioned supine with the head turned to the contralateral side. After induction of general anesthesia, a conventional C-shaped postauricular incision is carried through the soft tissues to expose the root of zygoma and spine of Henle of the external auditory canal, and a standard mastoidectomy is performed. In cases of a lateral tegmen mastoideum defect, the mastoidectomy can be carried to the level of the antrum. The tegmen and the sigmoid sinus are bluelined, and bone over the tegmen is further removed to reveal the site of the bony defect with the meningoencephalocele or meningeal herniation with CSF leak (Fig. 26.4). Granulation tissue and reactive bone may be present around the defect, and diamond burs are recommended to avoid additional injury to surrounding structures. In cases of brain or meningeal herniation, the stalk can be resected at its base using bipolar electrocautery in a similar fashion as described above.

Next, the tegmen mastoideum defect is prepared for extradural, intracranial reconstruction of the bony defect via transmastoid graft placement: through the tegmental defect, the dura is carefully elevated from the middle cranial fossa floor,

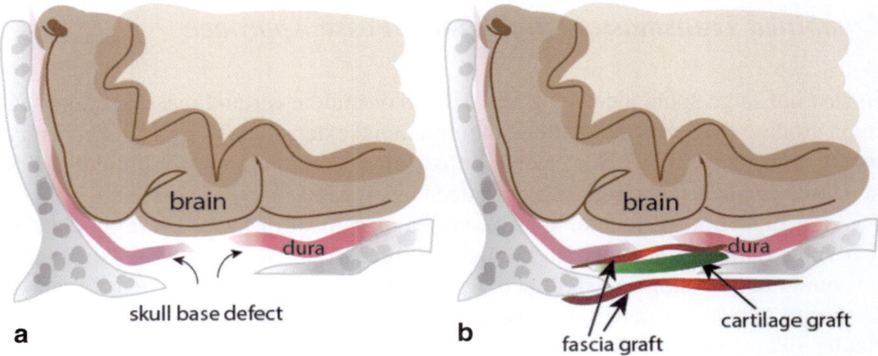

Fig. 26.4 Schematic of transmastoid repair of lateral skull base defect. (**a**) Elevation of dura to create an intracranial, extradural pocket from below. (**b**) Fascia graft is placed below the dural defect, and key-hole cartilage graft is slid intracranially, below the fascia graft. A second fascia graft is placed extracranially to cover the mastoid tegmen defect

roughly reaching a circumferential extradural pocket 1–2 mm circumferential to the bony defect (Fig. 26.4a). For reconstruction of the tegmen mastoideum, a cartilage graft (e.g., conchal cartilage) and temporalis fascia are harvested. The cartilage is sized into a piece slightly larger than the defect. Next, a piece of fascia (or alternatively a dural replacement graft) is placed intracranially for protection of the dura, followed by the cartilage graft. Sizing the graft generously with extension beyond the bony defect will stabilize the cartilage intracranially, in addition to the weight added from the temporal lobe. Using the previously described multilayer technique, a second piece of fascia is placed underneath, covering the tegmen defect from the mastoid cavity (Fig. 26.4b). Additional treatment with fibrin glue or obliteration of the mastoid cavity with adipose tissue can be beneficial to secure the reconstruction. Care must be taken not to inadvertently immobilize the ossicular chain during the repair.

In cases of tegmen tympani involvement or multiple small defects of the tegmen mastoideum and tegmen tympani, the mastoidectomy is extended by a posterior tympanotomy in order to expose the epi- and mesotympanum and to reach the defect. This generally entails disarticulation and removal of the incus and malleus head. The bony tegmental defect is then reconstructed in a similar manner, using a sandwich technique, consisting of fascia or dural onlay graft followed by cartilage and reinforced by a temporalis fascia onlay. If feasible, reconstruction of the ossicular chain can be performed in the same surgery via the posterior tympanotomy, using the previously removed incus as an interposition graft, or with a partial ossicular replacement prosthesis (PORP).

After layered closure of the postauricular incision, similar to a standard postauricular closure, a mastoid pressure dressing should be applied. Transmastoid repair of a tegmen defect may be performed as an outpatient surgery, and patients doing well can often be discharged home the same day [13].

Combined Transmastoid and Middle Fossa Approach

In cases of large spontaneous tegmen defects or middle ear and mastoid cholesteatoma eroding the tegmental bone with intracranial extension or a resulting encephalocele with or without CSF leakage, repair via a combined mastoid/middle fossa approach can achieve a high success rate [12, 24, 25].

After induction of general anesthesia and placement of facial nerve monitoring leads, the patient is prepped and draped in the normal sterile fashion. A standard postauricular incision is combined with our minimal supra-auricular C-shaped C-shaped incision as detailed above. As such, the incision is created in the postauricular sulcus and extended in curvilinear fashion above the auricle but behind the hairline over the supra-auricular fold. A large temporalis fascia graft should be harvested for skull base repair, and an inferiorly based periosteal flap can be created at this point to obliterate the mastoid defect later in the case. A canal wall-up or, if necessary, a canal-wall down mastoidectomy is performed next to remove disease from the mastoid cavity in case of cholesteatoma and to expose any defects of the lateral tegmen mastoideum. Careful dissection is needed in areas of tegmen erosion to not violate the dura. Involvement and dehiscence of the tegmen tympani will likely require removal of the incus and malleolar head [12].

During mastoidectomy, the tympanic and mastoid portion of the facial nerve are identified and can help during the craniotomy to identify the geniculate ganglion, which may be dehiscent in cases of extensive cholesteatoma. Next, the craniotomy is performed as described above. After the dura is elevated from the middle fossa floor, the petrous ridge is identified, and defects in the tegmen can be visualized from above and below. At this point, an encephalocele can be easily reduced and resected, or cholesteatoma extending intracranially can be thoroughly assessed and safely mobilized and delivered through the mastoid cavity. Dural defects can be repaired in onlay fashion using synthetic dura before attention is turned to repair of the bony defects. The middle cranial fossa floor is reconstructed in multilayer fashion with dural onlay, split calvarial bone, and autologous tissue from above, and a cranioplasty using autologous or allogenic materials is performed. Depending on nature of the mastoid defect, the cavity can be obliterated with a combination of cartilage, bone pate, an inferiorly based periosteal flap, temporalis fasci, or non-autologous tissuesa. A mastoid pressure dressing covering the postauricular and temporal defect should be placed postoperatively. Consideration should be given for a postoperative lumbar drain in combined approaches if large dural defects and high flow CSF leaks are encountered and repaired. Persistent postoperative CSF otorrhea may compromise the middle ear and mastoid reconstruction, or even lead to meningitis.

Modified Approaches

Endoscopic Assisted Middle Fossa Craniotomy Approach

In cases of unfavorable skull base topography where visualization of bony dehiscences and defects under the microscope can be impaired, rigid endoscopes have been successfully used to detect "hidden" defects [19]. Endoscopes of a 0 and 30° angle with diameter between 2.7 and 4.0 mm, and a length between 11 and 18 cm, are sufficient to explore the middle cranial fossa and can provide a high magnification view even of small tegmental dehiscences or bluelined superior canal defects [19]. In addition, endoscopic approaches may theoretically reduce the extent of temporal lobe retraction as visualization of the defect will not require direct line of sight.

Keyhole Middle Fossa Approach

A small retrospective case series investigated the success rate of a minimally invasive keyhole middle fossa craniotomy [16]. This approach exposes the middle cranial fossa base through a limited 1 × 2 cm craniectomy, thereby reducing the retraction of the temporal lobe, need for a lumbar drain, and length of hospital stay. In order to additionally reduce the operating time, multilayer reconstruction was performed only with allogenic material, consisting of synthetic dural collagen graft and fetal bovine collagen dural substitute for dural repair, as well as a titanium mesh for the skull base. In cases of large tegmen defects, a porous polyethylene implant was added for additional support between the titanium mesh and the bony dehiscence. This resulted in an average reported operating time of 77 min [16]. A keyhole middle fossa approach can also be combined with endoscope-assisted visualization of a tegmental defect [26]. Success rates of tegmental repair procedures using this approach are not yet known.

3D Printed Implants for Lateral Skull Base Repair

The search for a durable, rapid, and patient-specific reconstruction of the middle cranial fossa in order to minimize associated risk of extended temporal lobe retraction and anesthesia has prompted the development of 3D-printed rigid biocompatible implants [4, 27]. CT imaging of the temporal bone from cadavers as well as three index patients was processed using a 3D modeling and segmentation program to create a 3D model of their temporal bones. These were then 3D printed with a commercial grade FDM printer using polylactic acid (PLA) or acrylonitrile butadiene styrene (ABS) to visualize defects within the tegmen [4]. Tegmental plates matching the unique characteristics of a patients' skull base defect were then 3D printed in Poly-Ether-Ketone-Ketone (PEKK), a semicrystalline thermoplastic material, and successfully used for intraoperative tegmen repair with a dural replacement graft in three patients who underwent MFC. While placement of the personalized implant significantly reduced operative time, it was limited somewhat by overestimation of defects in the 3D printed models [27].

Materials

Small defects of the middle cranial fossa can be repaired by soft materials alone; however, there are limitations in regard to durability and support of the defect repair. In the past, autologous and allogenic materials such as temporalis muscle flaps, temporalis fascia, and dural substitutes have been described [2, 4–7]. More commonly, for increased support of large defects and defects involving the tegmen tympani with exposed ossicular heads, these materials are now combined with a rigid graft, such as cartilage, calvarial bone graft, hydroxyapatite bone cement, porous polyethylene implants, or titanium mesh [14, 27–29].

Rigid reconstruction is less pliable and conforms less to the irregular bone of the lateral skull base, in addition to carrying a higher risk of injury to surrounding structures such as the temporal lobe or a dehiscent geniculate ganglion. Therefore, a

Table 26.1 Reconstructive materials

Material	Approach	References
Autologous		
Temporalis fascia, in multilayer	TM, MFC, CA, SCD	[8, 13, 24, 29, 30]
Cartilage	TM	[13, 29]
Bone pate	CA, TM, MFC	[30, 31]
Bone particulate	TM	[32]
Calvarial bone graft	MFC, CA, SCD	[8, 15, 29, 33]
Muscle flap	MFC, CA	[1, 25]
Alloplastic		
Bone wax	MFC, SCD	[1, 18, 20, 34]
Synthetic dural replacement graft	MFC, CA, TM	[1, 8, 14, 15, 30]
Hydroxyapatite bone cement	MFC, TM, CA	[8, 14]
Titanium mesh	MFC	[16, 24]
Porous polyethylene implant	MFC	[16]
Semicrystalline thermoplastic	MFC	[4, 27]

MFC, middle fossa craniotomy; *TM,* transmastoid approach; *CA,* combined approach; *SCD,* superior canal dehiscence repair

"taco technique" is frequently used, which supports rigid constructs with soft materials on either side. This also improves a watertight 'onlay' seal of the skull base. Allogenic materials may be chosen in order to reduce operating time and temporal lobe retraction with potential trauma to the temporal lobe [9]. They do however carry an increased risk of postoperative infection [8], as well as breakdown with disease recurrence [24]. Table 26.1 lists various materials for repair of lateral temporal bone defects as they relate to the surgical approaches.

Perioperative Considerations

Thoughtful pre- and postoperative management of patients with middle cranial fossa defects is essential to enable the successful repair of the defect as well as ensure the patient progresses through the perioperative period safely. We strongly recommend infectious and seizure prophylaxis during MFC, and we and others commonly use a CSF penetrating prophylactic antibiotic and monotherapy with an anticonvulsant such as Levetiracetam. Dexamethasone, osmotic diuretics (e.g., mannitol), loop diuretics (e.g., Lasix), and induced hypocapnia via hyperventilation are effective in reducing intracranial pressure and promoting temporal lobe relaxation during surgery [10]. For 24 h postoperatively, patients are closely monitored in a surgical intensive care unit or step-down bed, while assessment for changes in neurological status is performed. Antibiotic and anticonvulsant therapy can be stopped at 24 h, and many patients can be discharged home on postoperative day 1 or 2 if doing well. Postoperative restrictions include CSF leak precautions such as avoidance of straining or voluntary elevation in ICP. In general, placement of a lumbar drain preoperatively to reduce intracranial pressure is not necessary in our practice. It is controversially discussed in the literature, as it carries a potential risk of tension pneumocephalus, subdural or subarachnoid hemorrhage, local site infection, and meningitis [10, 15, 35]. Postoperative lumbar drain may be necessary if persistent CSF otorrhea or rhinorrhea is encountered following reconstruction of the middle cranial fossa floor. A short period of CSF flow diversion may be helpful to ensure the new repair adequately seals prior to being challenged with normal or elevated intracranial CSF pressure.

Conclusion

Reconstruction of the middle cranial fossa floor can be done safely and successfully using either a middle fossa craniotomy or transmastoid approach. Ultimately, the success of the utilized approach depends upon the surgeon's comfort with the technique, the location, and extent of the disease and appropriate patient management during the perioperative period.

References

1. Savva A, Taylor MJ, Beatty CW. Management of cerebrospinal fluid leaks involving the temporal bone: report on 92 patients. Laryngoscope. 2003;113(1):50–6.
2. Brown NE, Grundfast KM, Jabre A, Megerian CA, O'Malley BW Jr, Rosenberg SI. Diagnosis and management of spontaneous cerebrospinal fluid-middle ear effusion and otorrhea. Laryngoscope. 2004;114(5):800–5.
3. Sanna M, Fois P, Russo A, Falcioni M. Management of meningoencephalic herniation of the temporal bone: personal experience and literature review. Laryngoscope. 2009;119(8):1579–85.
4. Ahmed S, VanKoevering KK, Kline S, Green GE, Arts HA. Middle cranial fossa approach to repair tegmen defects assisted by three-dimensionally printed temporal bone models. Laryngoscope. 2017;127(10):2347–51.
5. Stucken EZ, Selesnick SH, Brown KD. The role of obesity in spontaneous temporal bone encephaloceles and CSF leak. Otol Neurotol. 2012;33(8):1412–7.
6. Kutz JW Jr, Tolisano AM. Diagnosis and management of spontaneous cerebrospinal fluid fistula and encephaloceles. Curr Opin Otolaryngol Head Neck Surg. 2019;27(5):369–75.
7. Rabbani CC, Saltagi MZ, Nelson RF. The role of obesity, sleep apnea, and elevated intracranial pressure in spontaneous cerebrospinal fluid leaks. Curr Opin Otolaryngol Head Neck Surg. 2019;27(5):349–55.
8. Kutz JW Jr, Johnson AK, Wick CC. Surgical management of spontaneous cerebrospinal fistulas and encephaloceles of the temporal bone. Laryngoscope. 2018;128(9):2170–7.
9. Gonen L, Handzel O, Shimony N, Fliss DM, Margalit N. Surgical management of spontaneous cerebrospinal fluid leakage through temporal bone defects–case series and review of the literature. Neurosurg Rev. 2016;39(1):141–50; discussion 50.
10. Hoang S, Ortiz Torres MJ, Rivera AL, Litofsky NS. Middle cranial fossa approach to repair tegmen defects with autologous or alloplastic graft. World Neurosurg. 2018;118:e10–7.
11. Falcioni M, Aristegui M, Landolfi M, Saleh E, Taibah AK, Russo A, et al. Meningoencephalic herniation into the middle ear. Acta Otorhinolaryngol Ital. 1995;15(4):305–11.

12. Marchioni D, Bonali M, Alicandri-Ciufelli M, Rubini A, Pavesi G, Presutti L. Combined approach for tegmen defects repair in patients with cerebrospinal fluid otorrhea or herniations: our experience. J Neurol Surg B Skull Base. 2014;75(4):279–87.
13. Semaan MT, Gilpin DA, Hsu DP, Wasman JK, Megerian CA. Transmastoid extradural-intracranial approach for repair of transtemporal meningoencephalocele: a review of 31 consecutive cases. Laryngoscope. 2011;121(8):1765–72.
14. Alwani MM, Saltagi MZ, MacPhail ME, Nelson RF. Middle cranial fossa repair of temporal bone spontaneous CSF leaks with hydroxyapatite bone cement. Laryngoscope. 2021;131(3):624–32.
15. Kenning TJ, Willcox TO, Artz GJ, Schiffmacher P, Farrell CJ, Evans JJ. Surgical management of temporal meningoencephaloceles, cerebrospinal fluid leaks, and intracranial hypertension: treatment paradigm and outcomes. Neurosurg Focus. 2012;32(6):E6.
16. Wong AK, Shinners M, Wong RH. Minimally invasive repair of tegmen defects through keyhole middle fossa approach to reduce hospitalization. World Neurosurg. 2020;133:e683–e9.
17. McCall AA, McKenna MJ, Merchant SN, Curtin HD, Lee DJ. Superior canal dehiscence syndrome associated with the superior petrosal sinus in pediatric and adult patients. Otol Neurotol. 2011;32(8):1312–9.
18. Mikulec AA, Poe DS, McKenna MJ. Operative management of superior semicircular canal dehiscence. Laryngoscope. 2005;115(3):501–7.
19. Cheng YS, Kozin ED, Lee DJ. Endoscopic-assisted repair of superior canal dehiscence. Otolaryngol Clin N Am. 2016;49(5):1189–204.
20. Chemtob RA, Noij KS, Qureshi AA, Klokker M, Nakajima HH, Lee DJ. Superior canal dehiscence surgery outcomes following failed round window surgery. Otol Neurotol. 2019;40(4):535–42.
21. Rao AK, Merenda DM, Wetmore SJ. Diagnosis and management of spontaneous cerebrospinal fluid otorrhea. Otol Neurotol. 2005;26(6):1171–5.
22. Oliaei S, Mahboubi H, Djalilian HR. Transmastoid approach to temporal bone cerebrospinal fluid leaks. Am J Otolaryngol. 2012;33(5):556–61.
23. Perez E, Carlton D, Alfarano M, Smouha E. Transmastoid repair of spontaneous cerebrospinal fluid leaks. J Neurol Surg B Skull Base. 2018;79(5):451–7.
24. Carlson ML, Copeland WR, Driscoll CL, Link MJ, Haynes DS, Thompson RC, et al. Temporal bone encephalocele and cerebrospinal fluid fistula repair utilizing the middle cranial fossa or combined mastoid-middle cranial fossa approach. J Neurosurg. 2013;119(5):1314–22.
25. Tabuchi K, Yamamoto T, Akutsu H, Suzuki K, Hara A. Combined transmastoid/middle fossa approach for intracranial extension of middle ear cholesteatoma. Neurol Med Chir. 2012;52(10):736–40.
26. Roehm PC, Tint D, Chan N, Brewster R, Sukul V, Erkmen K. Endoscope-assisted repair of CSF otorrhea and temporal lobe encephaloceles via keyhole craniotomy. J Neurosurg. 2018;128(6):1880–4.
27. VanKoevering KK, Gao RW, Ahmed S, Green GE, Arts HA. A 3D-printed lateral skull base implant for repair of tegmen defects: a case series. Otol Neurotol. 2020;41(8):1108–15.
28. Lobo BC, Baumanis MM, Nelson RF. Surgical repair of spontaneous cerebrospinal fluid (CSF) leaks: a systematic review. Laryngosc Investig Otolaryngol. 2017;2(5):215–24.
29. Cheng E, Grande D, Leonetti J. Management of spontaneous temporal bone cerebrospinal fluid leak: a 30-year experience. Am J Otolaryngol. 2019;40(1):97–100.
30. Sergi B, Passali GC, Picciotti PM, De Corso E, Paludetti G. Transmastoid approach to repair meningoencephalic herniation in the middle ear. Acta Otorhinolaryngol Ital. 2013;33(2):97–101.
31. Dutt SN, Mirza S, Irving RM. Middle cranial fossa approach for the repair of spontaneous cerebrospinal fluid otorrhoea using autologous bone pate. Clin Otolaryngol Allied Sci. 2001;26(2):117–23.
32. Greene AK, Poe DS. Repair of tegmen defect using cranial particulate bone graft. Am J Otolaryngol. 2015;36(2):292–5.

33. Leonetti JP, Marzo S, Anderson D, Origitano T, Vukas DD. Spontaneous transtemporal CSF leakage: a study of 51 cases. Ear Nose Throat J. 2005;84(11):700, 2-4, 6.
34. Cheng YS, Kozin ED, Remenschneider AK, Nakajima HH, Lee DJ. Characteristics of wax occlusion in the surgical repair of superior canal dehiscence in human temporal bone specimens. Otol Neurotol. 2016;37(1):83–8.
35. Governale LS, Fein N, Logsdon J, Black PM. Techniques and complications of external lumbar drainage for normal pressure hydrocephalus. Neurosurgery. 2008;63(4):379–84; discussion 84.

Chapter 27
Reconstruction of Large Temporal Bone Defects

Michael H. Berger, Kelsey Roman, and Yarah M. Haidar

Introduction

The complex anatomy of the lateral skull base presents unique challenges for the reconstructive surgeon. Defects within this region are often a consequence of tumor resection but may also be related to trauma, infection, congenital lesions, or necrosis secondary to irradiation [1]. Tumors may be either benign or malignant, with squamous cell and basal cell carcinomas among the more common malignancies [2]. Benign lesions include paragangliomas, meningiomas, schwannomas, cholesteatomas, and granulomas [3].

Although many lesions of the lateral skull base are small and uncomplicated, larger tumors may place critical anatomical structures at risk. They may involve the cranial cavity, the middle ear, or the parotid gland and overlying facial nerve plexus. Depending on the size and location of the tumor, surgical management may require temporal bone resection, ablation of the external auditory canal or middle ear, partial or total parotidectomy, and facial nerve sacrifice. The loss of these structures coupled with resulting large volume defects leaves patients with devastating functional and aesthetic deficits that are challenging to resolve.

Because these complex lesions are rare, algorithms for surgical management are limited. However, reconstruction of the lateral skull base has several important goals. First, extracranial and intracranial spaces must be separated to prevent cerebrospinal fluid leakage [2]. With advancements in tissue transfer techniques, vascularized tissue has become the gold standard to achieve a watertight dural seal [2, 4, 5]. It can also be used to eliminate dead space within the surgical defect to optimize tissue contour and promote wound healing. In cases of partial or total auriculectomy, auricle reconstruction and positioning also becomes a concern [6]. Facial

M. H. Berger · K. Roman · Y. M. Haidar (✉)
University of California Irvine Medical Center, Irvine, CA, USA
e-mail: michael.berger2@mountsinai.org; haidary@hs.uci.edu

E. C. Kuan et al. (eds.), *Skull Base Reconstruction*,
https://doi.org/10.1007/978-3-031-27937-9_27

389

nerve reanimation may be indicated for patients with facial paralysis secondary to resection or other injury. The surgeon may also face challenges posed by patient-specific factors like prior skull base surgery or planned radiation therapy [7].

This chapter discusses reconstruction of lateral skull base defects with an emphasis on vascularized tissue and facial nerve reanimation. We review the relevant regional anatomy, discuss reconstructive goals and complications, and present current standards for local, regional, and free tissue transfer.

Anatomy of Lateral Skull Base

In 1993, Irish et al. proposed three anatomical regions of the skull base according to common tumor growth patterns and surgical approaches for resection [8]. Region I is located in the anterior cranial fossa and includes the area from the clivus to the foramen magnum. Region II involves the middle cranial fossa, the infratemporal fossa, and the pterygopalatine fossa. Region III, which mainly consists of the temporal bone, includes the posterior cranial fossa and part of the middle cranial fossa. Here, we focus on the anatomy of regions II and II, which comprise the lateral skull base.

Region II begins at the posterior orbital wall, extends to the petrous part of the temporal bone within the middle cranial fossa, and communicates with the infratemporal and pterygopalatine fossae [8]. The internal carotid artery passes through region II via the carotid canal. Other key structures include the maxillary (V2) and mandibular (V3) branches of the trigeminal nerve. V3 exits the skull base through the foramen spinosum to enter the infratemporal fossa, which lies deep and inferior to the zygomatic arch and deep to the ramus of the mandible. The chorda tympani of the facial nerve (CN VII), otic ganglion, and maxillary artery are also located here. The maxillary artery passes from the infratemporal fossa into the pterygopalatine fossa deep to the apex of the orbit, where it is joined by V2 as it exits the cranium via the foramen rotundum. Region II tumors originating in the infratemporal or pterygopalatine fossa may invade the middle cranial fossa through one of these cranial foramina [8].

Skull base region III encompasses the posterior region of the middle cranial fossa and the posterior cranial fossa [8]. Major structures include the internal jugular vein, the glossopharyngeal nerve (CN IX), the vagus nerve (CN X), and spinal accessory (CN XI), which pass through the jugular foramen. Medial to the jugular foramen is the hypoglossal canal, which conveys CN XII. The facial nerve (CN VII) and vestibulocochlear nerve (VIII) pass laterally through the internal acoustic meatus. Region III tumors that originate within or around the temporal bone may extend into the middle or posterior cranial fossae [8].

The tortuous anatomy of the facial nerve (CN VII) is an important consideration in surgery of the lateral skull base. The facial nerve passes from the internal acoustic meatus into the facial canal and proceeds a short distance within the temporal bone before turning abruptly to course along the medial wall of the tympanic cavity.

Inside the facial canal, it gives off the greater petrosal nerve, the nerve to the stapedius, and the chorda tympani. It then exits the cranial cavity via the stylomastoid foramen, gives off the posterior auricular nerve, and enters the parotid gland. After it pierces the gland, the facial nerve typically bifurcates into two trunks, which further divide into the five major branches of the parotid plexus: the temporal, zygomatic, buccal, marginal, and cervical branches. However, there is significant anatomical variation in branching patterns [9]. These nerves course through the tissue of the parotid gland superficial to the retromandibular vein and external carotid artery and ultimately terminate on muscles of facial expression. Surgical management of parotid gland tumors typically requires complete or partial resection of the gland. In addition, advanced parotid tumors may necessitate sacrifice of the facial nerve [9].

The lateral skull base is also associated with the middle ear, which is implicated in many pathologies requiring surgical management. The tympanic cavity of the middle ear is an irregularly shaped six-walled space located within the petrous portion of the temporal bone below the middle cranial fossa. It contains three auditory ossicles, which communicate with the tympanic membrane laterally and the oval window medially to transmit sound into the inner ear. The tympanic cavity is separated from the middle cranial fossa superiorly by a thin layer of bone called the tegmen tympani. Damage to this region can lead to dura injury and CSF leakage [10].

Important Considerations for Reconstruction

The intricate anatomy of the lateral skull base presents reconstructive challenges. Surgical management of pathologies in this region may involve partial or total parotidectomy with or without facial nerve sacrifice, external auditory canal resection, and partial or total resection of the temporal bone. Dural exposure is often necessary but risks cerebrospinal (CSF) fluid leakage. An effective reconstructive approach will eliminate communication between intracranial and extracranial spaces and optimize tissue coverage within the defect to preserve function and cosmesis. Technical considerations include CSF leak prevention, elimination of dead space with vascularized tissue transfer, and auricle reconstruction.

Malignancies limited to the cartilaginous or bony ear canal are generally treated with lateral temporal bone resection, selective neck dissection, and parotidectomy, with the resulting defects often amenable to primary closure of the ear canal and filling the temporal bone defect with abdominal fat. However, it is important to note that fat grafts will atrophy with time and when postoperative radiotherapy is required, so overpacking of the defect is generally necessary [11].

Auricle reconstruction is an important consideration following partial or total auriculectomy and in cases where the external ear has been surgically displaced to access underlying structures. Advanced cases requiring total or subtotal temporal bone resection may necessitate sacrifice of the external auditory canal and pinna with prosthetic reconstruction, particularly in patients with risk factors for tissue necrosis like prior or planned radiation therapy [12]. When possible, preserving all or part of the auricle results in better cosmetic and functional outcomes. Canaloplasty, meatoplasty, and stenting of the external auditory canal can help prevent complications like canal stenosis and otitis externa [1]. Necrosis of the auricular tissue is less likely to occur when its collateral blood supply is well preserved [1, 6].

In cases of subtotal auriculectomy, auricle repositioning can be challenging due to underlying bony and soft tissue defects. Tissue transferred during reconstruction tends to droop over time postoperatively, pulling the auricle downward such that the two ears become vertically asymmetrical [8]. Optimal long-term positioning of the external ear depends on careful preoperative and intraoperative planning. If all or part of the temporal bone remains after resection, the dermis of the transferred tissue should be rigidly sutured to the underlying bone to prevent displacement of the auricle over time [6].

Reconstruction becomes more complicated, and CSF leak is encountered and is associated with higher patient morbidity and greater hospital expense [5]. The surgeon must establish a watertight dural seal by creating a tissue barrier between the exposed dura and the external environment. Free abdominal fat or skin grafts may be used to seal small defects but often are inadequate in large defects. Vascularized tissue transfer has become the reconstructive method of choice for preventing CSF leak complications associated with larger defects [2, 5, 7].

Vascularized tissue is also used to eliminate dead space within the surgical defect, which reduces postoperative complications and improves tissue contour to maximize the aesthetic outcome. Reconstructive options are diverse and include local tissue flaps, regional flaps, and free flaps. Flap selection depends on the size and location of the skull base defect. Donor site morbidity and total operating time are additional considerations.

Reconstructive Methods

Local Tissue Flaps

Local tissue is harvested from regions directly abutting the defect and remains connected to the local blood supply. Because the flap is advanced directly into the defect, it has the advantage of low morbidity and requires less operating time to complete [1]. However, local tissue is often only suitable for filling smaller defects because it usually provides less bulk than regional or free flaps. In cases of smaller defects, local tissue reconstructive options include pericranial flaps [13–15], galeal, or galeal-myofascial flaps [16], though these flaps are not traditionally used for lateral skull base defects given difficulty of reach [2]. Cervicofacial advancement flaps may be used as well but are limited in patients with history of prior irradiation to the neck or heavy smokers; additionally, they lack sufficient bulk to fill large defects effectively [17].

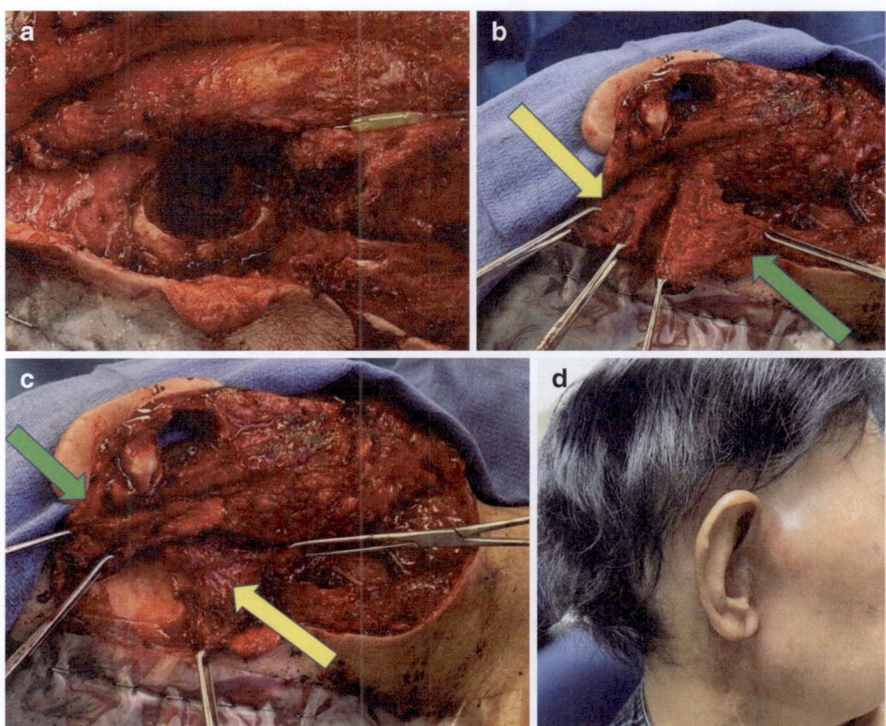

Fig. 27.1 Panel (**a**) represents the surgical defect after a lateral temporal bone resection. Panel (**b**) demonstrates the temporalis flap (yellow arrow) and the temporoparietal fascia flap (green arrow) raised. In panel (**c**), the temporalis flap (yellow arrow) is used to fill the lateral temporal bone defect, and the temporoparietal fascia flap (green arrow) is used to reduce temporal hollowing. Panel (**d**) shows the reconstruction 6 months postoperatively

For small lateral skull base defects, temporalis muscle flaps are a good option given its relative proximity to the expected defect (Fig. 27.1) [1]. The temporalis muscle flap vascular supply is derived from the anterior and posterior branches of the deep temporal artery, with additional blood supply from the middle temporal artery, which is itself a branch of the superficial temporal artery [12]. When harvested, the temporalis muscle flap can provide a length of 12–16 cm, a thickness of 0.5–1.0 cm, and a surface of 4 × 5 cm [18]. Morbidity associated with the temporalis muscle flap includes temporal hollowing and alopecia, though techniques to reduce postoperative temporal hollowing have been described, including preservation of the anterior portion of the muscle, preservation of the temporal fat pad, and postoperative fat transfer to the temporal fat pad [19]. While the temporalis muscle flap is a myofascial flap, a split thickness skin graft can be placed over the muscular fascia when a cutaneous defect is present.

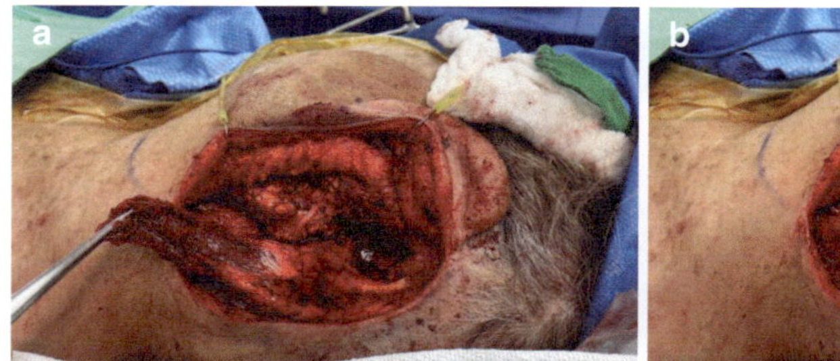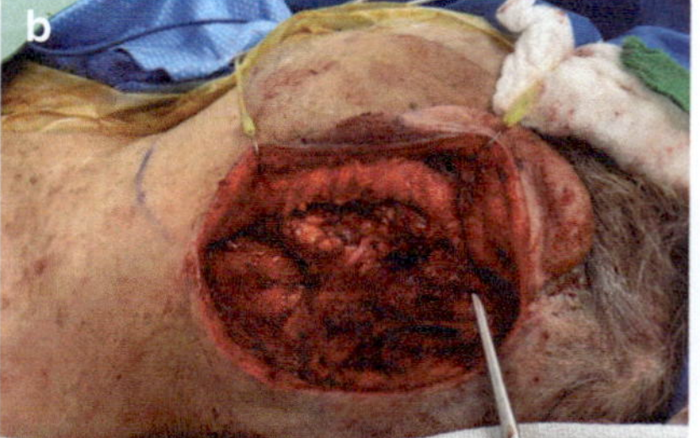

Fig. 27.2 Panel (**a**) demonstrates the sternocleidomastoid flap raised. The sternocleidomastoid flap is then used to reconstruct the lateral temporal bone defect in panel (**b**)

Similar to the temporalis muscle flap, the temporoparietal fascia flap (TPFF) may also be used in skull base reconstruction. The vascular supply is from the superficial and middle temporal arteries, in addition to the occipital and posterior auricular arteries [20]. Important risks of flap harvest include injury to the frontal branch of the facial nerve as well as alopecia [3]. The temporoparietal fascia flap is thin but still can be used to control CSF leaks in skull base surgery, particularly when combined with autologous fat grafting, as discussed by Patel et al. [21] Notably, the temporoparietal flap may be inadequate in size for large postresection defects. Similarly, in large resections or in patients with prior radiation, the vascular supply to the flap may be compromised. Fig. 27.1 demonstrates the use of both temporalis and the TPFF for reconstruction. The temporalis flap is used to reconstruct a lateral temporal bone defect, and the TPFF is used to reduce temporal hollowing.

Another option for filling small defects of the lateral skull base is the sternocleidomastoid muscle flap (Fig. 27.2) [22]. The blood supply of the sternocleidomastoid muscle is from the transverse cervical artery, occipital artery, and superior thyroid artery. The flap is pedicled superiorly as the blood supply enters high in the neck [23]. The drawback of the sternocleidomastoid muscle flap is that the blood supply to the muscle may be impacted by a concurrent neck dissection. Similarly, in patients with malignant appearing cervical lymph nodes, there is a theoretical risk of introducing tissue that may seed tumor into the temporal bone defect [23].

Regional Flaps

Regional pedicled myocutaneous or fasciocutaneous flaps may be employed to fill defects requiring a larger tissue volume or in cases where the local blood supply has been compromised by surgery or prior irradiation. They are harvested from the general vicinity of the defect, remain attached by a pedicle to their original blood supply, and are rotated into the recipient site. Donor tissue from more distant regions may be tunneled under the skin or subcutaneous tissue to reach the defect. Regional flaps are generally a good match for skin color and type at the recipient site, which is important from a cosmetic standpoint [1].

The lower trapezius island flap may be harvested as a myocutaneous versus a muscle only flap [24]. It was initially described as being based off the transverse cervical artery [25], but later anatomical studies noted that the dominant pedicle can also be from the dorsal scapular artery [26]. Therefore, the transverse cervical artery and the dorsal scapular artery may both need to be preserved during harvest [24]. Additionally, to reduce shoulder mobility, efforts should be made to preserve the upper trapezius fibers during harvest [11, 26]. The flap can be harvested in the lateral decubitus position, but the pedicle is at risk in cases of a level 4 neck dissection due to potential risk of damaging the transverse cervical artery pedicle [1].

The supraclavicular flap and the pectoralis major flap both are appropriate pedicled flap options that can be harvested without re-positioning the patient. The supraclavicular flap is a fasciocutaneous flap based off the supraclavicular vessels branching from the thyrocervical trunk. The advantages of the flap are excellent skin color and texture match, ability to reach lateral skull base, and decreased operative time compared to free flaps [27]. Additionally, given that it is based off the transverse cervical artery, there is a risk of pedicle injury with level 4 neck dissections [1]. Emerick et al. reported 16 patients with parotid and/or lateral skull base defects that were reconstructed with supraclavicular flaps, with no complete flap loss and only one case of partial flap dehiscence. The average flap harvested in the aforementioned case series was 7×10 cm, allowing for limited donor site defect with primary site closure [28]. However, with defects larger than 10–15 cm in width, the supraclavicular flap angiosome may be inadequate in addition to the challenge of primary closure with such a large skin paddle [29]. In these larger defects, the supraclavicular flap may be inappropriate. An additional limitation of the supraclavicular flap is the lack of a muscle component, which may be necessary with large defects particularly in those that would be at high risk for CSF leaks as vascularized muscle is excellent in its ability to seal off skull base defects [30].

The pectoralis major flap can be raised as a myofascial or a myocutaneous flap, similar to the latissimus dorsi flap. It is based off the pectoral branch of the thoracoacromial artery. It is a frequently used flap in head and neck reconstruction as it is reliable and relatively easy to harvest. In lateral temporal reconstruction, it has traditionally been thought of as best utilized in defects inferior to the external auditory canal due to concerns that the flap length would be insufficient for more cranial defects and would have higher propensity for venous congestion [17]. Another concern with the pectoralis flap in lateral skull base reconstruction is the significant bulk of the flap would cause poor contour match and lead to excess tension, thus increasing risk of flap dehiscence [29]. However, Resto et al. reported a case of eight lateral skull base defects superior to the temporal line reconstructed with pectoralis muscle flaps, and no cases of dehiscence or infection were noted [31]. Several modifications were suggested in their harvest of the pectoralis flap to mitigate the commonly reported risks, such as extending the skin paddle over the entire length of the incision, dividing the motor nerves to the muscle (lateral and medial pectoral nerves), and incorporating superior rectus fascia, which can be used to close the dural defect or suspend the flap to minimize tension [31].

The submental flap was first described in 1990 and is based off the submental artery and vein and can be harvested with a generous cuff of muscle that may include the bilateral anterior bellies of the digastric muscle and the bilateral mylohyoid muscles [32]. It additionally has a favorable arc of rotation, making it an ideal candidate for lateral skull base reconstruction (Fig. 27.3), particularly given its muscular component that can be used to fill larger defects. A series of 31 patients with lateral temporal bone defects was presented by Howard et al., with 16 of these patients having a submental flap to reconstruct. The remaining patients were either reconstructed with pedicled latissimus dorsi flaps or anterolateral thigh free flaps. In the series, there was 100% survival of the submental flaps. Additionally, the submental flaps had a shorter operative time and hospital stay compared to free flaps and were less likely to require debulking procedures compared to latissimus dorsi and anterolateral thigh flaps [30]. Notably, the submental flap may not be available in all cases, as the vascular pedicle can be damaged in patients who have received prior or concurrent level 1A or 1B neck dissections, prior reconstructive procedures, or prior radiation [29].

The latissimus dorsi flap can be raised as a myocutaneous versus a muscle only flap and is based off the thoracodorsal artery and vein. It has the largest surface area and greatest arc of rotation of all pedicled flaps, so it has utility in coverage of large cephalad defects, such as a temporal bone defect [30, 33]. This flap can be raised as a pedicled or as a free flap. One drawback to the pedicled latissimus flap is the need to place the patient in the lateral decubitus position as well as risk of kinking the pedicle while rotating the flap cephalad. Additionally, as is the case with pedicled flaps, there is a risk of partial flap necrosis, with the most likely location of necrosis at the flap tip, which would most likely correspond with the location of the defect being covered [34]. However, techniques have been described to increase the reach

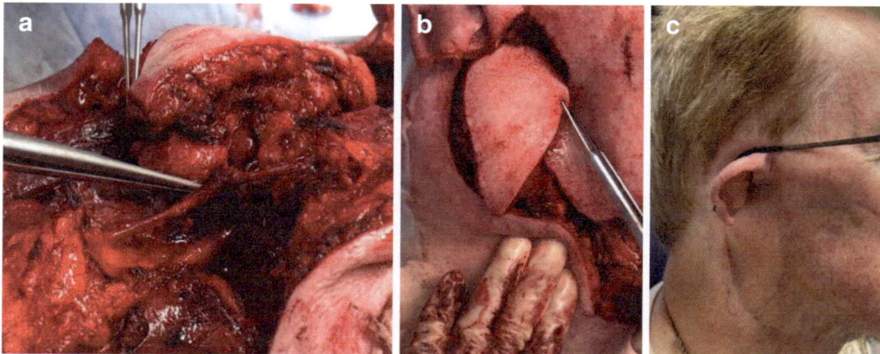

Fig. 27.3 Panel (**a**) shows the submental vessels isolated for submental flap. Panel (**b**) demonstrates the submental flap rotated for closure of right temporal bone defect. Panel (**c**) shows the same patient 2 years postoperatively

of a pedicled latissimus flap, including an otter-tail skin paddle design allowing inclusion of more perforators, preservation of circumflex scapular branches from the subscapular artery, and keeping the latissimus tendon attached until pedicle dissection is completed to prevent inadvertent traction injury to the pedicle [33]. The latissimus dorsi flap may also be raised as a free tissue transfer as well, which mitigates the risk associated with attempts at reaching the pedicled flap across a long distance.

For very large surgical defects, local and regional flaps may fail to provide sufficient tissue bulk to obliterate dead space and restore tissue contour. Regional transfer may also may not be an option when local tissues have been compromised by radiotherapy or if the arc of rotation for regional flaps is limited to close the respective defects [19, 35]. In these cases, reconstruction with free tissue transfers—or free flaps—is preferred [35, 36].

Free Flaps

A free flap is a section of tissue taken from a donor site remote from the recipient site. The donor tissue must contain intact vasculature that can be anastomosed with vessels at the recipient site. Common free flap donor sites for lateral skull base reconstruction include the radial forearm, anterolateral thigh, and rectus abdominis muscle, though many other sites may be considered [1]. No longer dependent on local tissues, the surgeon has more reconstructive freedom when working with free tissue. The flap can be tailored to fit the unique parameters of the skull base defect. However, free flaps are associated with greater donor site morbidity, longer operating times and hospital stays, and higher failure rates than other types of tissue transfer [37].

The radial forearm free flap (RFFF) is commonly used in head and neck reconstruction, given its reliability, large vessels, and favorable vessel geometry. It is a fasciocutaneous flap based off of the radial artery. Given the thin, pliable nature of the RFFF, it has been proposed that its primary use in lateral skull base reconstruction should be for small defects as its soft tissue component would be inadequate for larger defects [38]. However, in a series of 17 patients with lateral skull base defects requiring free tissue transfer, radial forearms were used with a "double layer" technique modification, in which a large fat pad is incorporated surrounding the proximal pedicle in addition to the skin paddle. In this way, the authors obtained a bulkier flap than typical and used the fat component to fill the lateral skull base defect [39]. The authors noted excellent outcomes that were favorable when compared to other commonly used free flaps for lateral skull base defects. An additional benefit of the RFFF is the ability to harvest the median antebrachial cutaneous nerve or the palmaris longus, which may be used if immediate facial reanimation is to be attempted [1].

The rectus abdominis flap has been one of the workhorses for lateral skull base reconstruction given the ability to harvest a skin and muscle to obliterate postsurgical defects [29]. It is supplied by the inferior epigastric artery and is harvested with the patient in the supine position, allowing for a two-team approach. The pedicle length is roughly 8–10 cm but with an extended intramuscular dissection, up to a 19 cm pedicle length may be achieved [40]. Other advantages of the flap include that the donor site can be closed primarily, and an additional devascularized fat graft can be harvested from the same incision if further bulk is necessary to fill the lateral temporal bone defect. However, there are well-described morbidities associated with the rectus flap, including abdominal hernias, bulges, and weakness [41]. Prior studies have promoted the use of the rectus abdominis flap [34, 42]; however, other authors have found higher morbidity and high rate of revision of flaps with rectus flaps compared to other free flaps, particularly the anterolateral thigh flap [38].

The anterolateral thigh (ALT) free flap may be raised as a fasciocutaneous or a myocutaneous perforator flap, depending on the extent of the defect. The muscle component of the flap when utilized is the vastus lateralis. The blood supply is derived from the descending branch of the lateral femoral circumflex artery. It allows for a similar size skin paddle compared to the rectus flap, but proponents of the ALT feel it better matches the contour lateral skull base defects [2, 38]. Additional advantages include the ability to simultaneously harvest tensor fascia lata grafts, nerve grafts, and vein grafts from the same incision [43]. The ALT is also be harvested in the supine position, allowing for a two-team approach, and has low donor site morbidity allowing for early ambulation [44]. The ALT also is unique in its ability to be thinned down to a thickness of about 0.5 cm [45], allowing the flap to be adjusted to better match the contour of the defect. Given the aforementioned features of the ALT, it has gained favor at multiple institutions as a primary means of reconstruction for moderate to large-sized lateral skull base defects [7, 19, 38, 46]. Figs. 27.4 and 27.5 demonstrate the use of the ALT for reconstruction in lateral temporal bone defects.

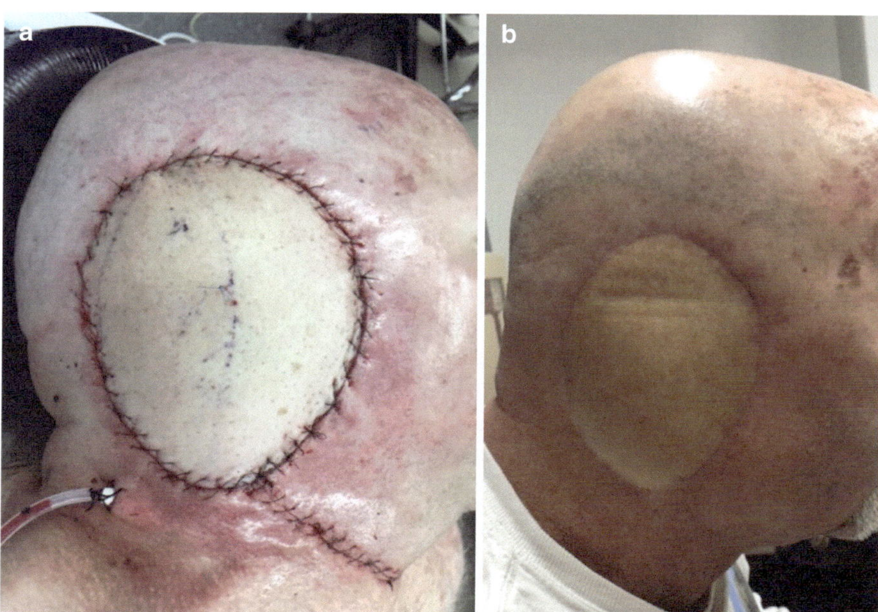

Fig. 27.4 Panel (**a**)—anterolateral thigh flap after inset intraoperatively. Panel (**b**)—the same patient 2 years postoperatively

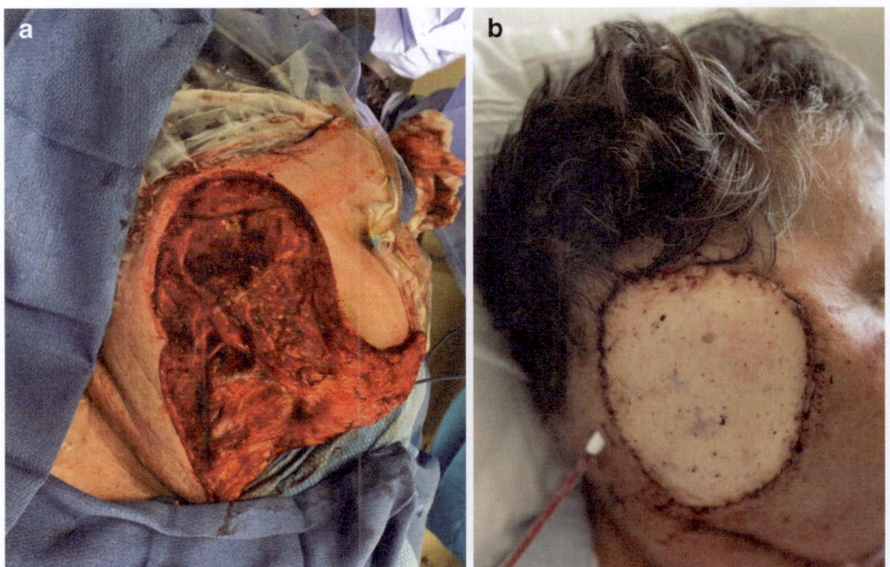

Fig. 27.5 Panel (**a**) represents a large lateral temporal bone defect intraoperatively. The defect was closed with an anterolateral thigh free flap, with the reconstruction shown in Panel (**b**) at postoperative day 1

Approach to Reconstruction

It is difficult to determine a precise algorithm that can be employed consistently across all lateral skull base defects, particularly given that multiple reconstructive methods may be suitable. Rosenthal et al. introduced a classification system for lateral skull base defects. Class I defects consisted of preauricular defects with skin loss and preservation of the external auditory canal, with or without a mastoidectomy. In Class I defects, the authors proposed local tissue advancement versus RFFF for reconstruction. Class II defects involved lateral temporal bone resection with middle ear obliteration but with preservation of most of the auricle. In these defects, the authors proposed using ALT versus RFFF for reconstruction. Finally, Class III defects included lateral temporal bone resections, total auriculectomy with middle ear obliteration and with or without a parotidectomy. For these larger defects, the authors proposed use of ALT versus rectus abdominis for reconstruction [38].

While such a classification system is helpful in categorizing lateral skull base defects, it primarily favors free tissue transfer in reconstruction. Richmon et al. proposed an algorithm categorized based on the size of temporal bone defect and involvement of skin and auricle. In small temporal bone defects with intact skin and auricle, free fat graft alone or TPFF is recommended. In large temporal bone defects with intact skin and auricle, the temporalis flap, TPFF, and possible fat graft are recommended. If there is skin loss but the external auditory canal is preserved, the

RFFF, supraclavicular flap, and temporalis flap with or without a skin graft are recommended. If there is a lateral temporal bone resection and partial auriculectomy, the RFFF, ALT, supraclavicular flap, and temporalis with or without skin graft and recommended. Finally in lateral temporal bone resections with total auriculectomy and parotidectomy, the recommended reconstructive methods include the RFFF, ALT, rectus abdominis, or latissimus flaps [1].

Hanasono et al. similarly suggested that in small defects near the ear and mastoid region, a temporalis flap can be used, with resultant decreased surgical times and decreased hospital stays when compared to free flap patients. However, they further note that in patients with prior radiation or patients with prior surgery in region or patients with large defects, free flap reconstruction should be favored, with preference for the ALT [19]. In contrast, other centers have advocated for the use of regional pedicled flaps, including the submental and supraclavicular flap in particular cases as opposed to free tissue transfer [28, 30].

Patel et al. also proposed an algorithm for lateral skull base defects [22]. In their approach, patients without anticipated postoperative radiation, preservation of the auricle, and lack of CSF leak (or a CSF leak without a large dural defect), a nonvascularized fat graft, versus temporalis flap, versus primary closure with or without a skin graft would be sufficient for reconstruction. However, any patient with a CSF leak with a large dural defect should have reconstruction with a free or pedicled flap. They further discuss that defects well above the zygomatic arch should have free flap reconstruction as opposed to pedicled flap reconstruction, given the anticipated challenge of poor reach in the pedicled flap group.

There is no widely accepted consensus for reconstruction of lateral skull base defects, as demonstrated by the variability in the literature in terms of approaches. However, when weighing the options for possible reconstructions, consideration should be made for patient comorbidities, prior or anticipated radiation, prior surgery, volume of defect, presence of CSF leak, patient goals, and surgeon comfort with particular methods.

References

1. Richmon JD, Yarlagadda BB, Wax MK, Patel U, Diaz J, Lin DT. Locoregional and free flap reconstruction of the lateral skull base. Head Neck. 2014;37:1387–91.
2. Thurnher D, Novak CB, Neligan PC, Gullane PJ. Reconstruction of lateral skull base defects after tumor ablation. Skull Base. 2007;17(1):79–88. https://doi.org/10.1055/s-2006-959338.
3. Patel R, Buchmann LO, Hunt J. The use of the temporoparietal fascial flap in preventing CSF leak after lateral skull base surgery. J Neurol Surg. 2013;74(5):311–6. https://doi.org/10.1055/s-0033-1349059.
4. Bertelsen C, Simsolo E, Maceri D, Sinha U, Kokot N. Outcomes of reconstruction after temporal bone resection for malignancy. J Cranio-Maxillofac Surg. 2018;46(10):1856–61. https://doi.org/10.1016/j.jcms.2018.08.002.
5. Kaylie DM, O'Malley M, Aulino JM, Jackson CG. Neurotologic surgery for glomus tumors. Otolaryngol Clin N Am. 2007;40(3):625–49. https://doi.org/10.1016/j.otc.2007.03.009.

6. Tanaka K, Yano T, Homma T, et al. A new method for selecting auricle positions in skull base reconstruction for temporal bone cancer. Laryngoscope. 2018;128(11):2605–10. https://doi.org/10.1002/lary.27170.
7. O'Connell DA, Teng MS, Mendez E, Futran ND. Microvascular free tissue transfer in the reconstruction of scalp and lateral temporal bone defects. J Craniofac Surg. 2011;22(3):801–4. https://doi.org/10.1097/SCS.0b013e31820f3730.
8. Irish JC, Gullane PJ, Gentili F, et al. Tumors of the skull base: outcome and survival analysis of 77 cases. Head Neck. 1994;16(1):3–10. https://doi.org/10.1002/hed.2880160103.
9. Gandolfi MM, Slattery W. Parotid gland tumors and the facial nerve. Otolaryngol Clin N Am. 2016;49(2):425–34. https://doi.org/10.1016/j.otc.2015.12.001.
10. Luers JC, Hüttenbrink KB. Surgical anatomy and pathology of the middle ear. J Anat. 2016;228(2):338–53. https://doi.org/10.1111/joa.12389.
11. Marzo SJ, Leonetti JP, Petruzzelli GJ, Vandevender D. Closure of complex lateral skull base defects. Otol Neurotol. 2005;26(3):522–4. https://doi.org/10.1097/01.mao.0000169771.38915.ad.
12. Eldaly A, Magdy EA, Nour YA, Gaafar AH. Temporalis myofascial flap for primary cranial base reconstruction after tumor resection. Skull Base. 2008;18(4):253–64. https://doi.org/10.1055/s-2007-1016958.
13. Argenta LC, Friedman RJ, Dingman RO, Duus EC. The versatility of pericranial flaps. Plast Reconstr Surg. 1985;76(5):695–702.
14. Smith JE, Ducic Y. The versatile extended pericranial flap for closure of skull base defects. Otolaryngol Head Neck Surg. 2004;130(6):704–11. https://doi.org/10.1016/j.otohns.2004.01.004.
15. Safavi-Abbasi S, Komune N, Archer JB, et al. Surgical anatomy and utility of pedicled vascularized tissue flaps for multilayered repair of skull base defects. J Neurosurg. 2016;125(2):419–30. https://doi.org/10.3171/2015.5.JNS15529.
16. Jackson IT, Adham MN, Marsh WR. Use of the galeal frontalis myofascial flap in craniofacial surgery. Plast Reconstr Surg. 1986;77(6):905–10.
17. Gal TJ, Kerschner JE, Futran ND, et al. Reconstruction after temporal bone resection. Laryngoscope. 1998;108(4):476–81. https://doi.org/10.1017/S0022215100096420.
18. Smith JE, Ducic Y, Adelson RT. Temporalis muscle flap for reconstruction of skull base defects. Head Neck. 2010;32:199–203.
19. Hanasono MM, Silva AK, Yu P, Skoracki RJ, Sturgis EM, Gidley PW. Comprehensive management of temporal bone defects after oncologic resection. Laryngoscope. 2012;122(12):2663–9. https://doi.org/10.1002/lary.23528.
20. Stow NW, Gordon DH, Eisenberg R. Technique of temporoparietal fascia flap in ear and lateral skull base surgery. Otol Neurotol. 2010;31(5):964–7.
21. Patel UA, Moore BA, Wax M, et al. Impact of pharyngeal closure technique on fistula after salvage laryngectomy. JAMA Otolaryngol Head Neck Surg. 2013;139(11):1156–62. https://doi.org/10.1001/jamaoto.2013.2761.
22. Patel NS, Modest MC, Brobst TD, et al. Surgical management of lateral skull base defects. Laryngoscope. 2016;126(8):1911–7. https://doi.org/10.1002/lary.25717.
23. McCraw JB, Magee WP, Kalwaic H. Uses of the Trapezius and sternomastoid myocutaneous flaps in head and neck reconstruction. Plast Reconstr Surg. 1979;63(1):49–57. https://doi.org/10.1097/00006534-197901000-00009.
24. Zenga J, Sharon JD, Santiago P, et al. Lower trapezius flap for reconstruction of posterior scalp and neck defects after complex occipital-cervical surgeries. J Neurol Surg. 2015;76(5):397–408. https://doi.org/10.1055/s-0034-1544123.
25. Baek S-M, Biller HF, Krespi YP, Lawson W. The lower trapezius island myocutaneous flap. Ann Plast Surg. 1980;5(2):108–14.
26. Netterville JL, Wood DE. The lower trapezius flap: vascular anatomy and surgical technique. Arch Otolaryngol Neck Surg. 1991;117(1):73–6. https://doi.org/10.1001/archotol.1991.01870130079020.

27. Chiu ES, Liu PH, Friedlander PL. Supraclavicular artery island flap for head and neck oncologic reconstruction: indications, complications, and outcomes. Plast Reconstr Surg. 2009;124(1):115–23. https://doi.org/10.1097/PRS.0b013e3181aa0e5d.

28. Emerick KS, Herr MW, Lin DT, Santos F, Deschler DG. Supraclavicular artery island flap for reconstruction of complex parotidectomy, lateral skull base, and total auriculectomy defects. JAMA Otolaryngol Head Neck Surg. 2014;140(9):861–6. https://doi.org/10.1001/jamaoto.2014.1394.

29. Arnaoutakis D, Kadakia S, Abraham M, Lee T, Ducic Y. Locoregional and microvascular free tissue reconstruction of the lateral skull base. Semin Plast Surg. 2017;31(4):197–202. https://doi.org/10.1055/s-0037-1606556.

30. Howard BE, Nagel TH, Barrs DM, Donald CB, Hayden RE. Reconstruction of lateral skull base defects: a comparison of the submental flap to free and regional flaps. Otolaryngol Head Neck Surg. 2016;154(6):1014–8. https://doi.org/10.1177/0194599816634296.

31. Resto VA, McKenna MJ, Deschler DG. Pectoralis major flap in composite lateral skull base defect reconstruction. Arch Otolaryngol Head Neck Surg. 2007;133(5):490–4. https://doi.org/10.1001/archotol.133.5.490.

32. Martin D, Baudet J, Mondie JM, Peri G. The submental island skin flap. A surgical protocol. Prospects of use. Ann Chir Plast Esthet. 1990;35(6):480–4.

33. Hayden RE, Kirby SD, Deschler DG. Technical modifications of the latissimus dorsi pedicled flap to increase versatility and viability. Laryngoscope. 2000;110(3):352–7. https://doi.org/10.1097/00005537-200003000-00004.

34. Disa JJ, Rodriguez VM, Cordeiro PG. Reconstruction of lateral skull base oncological defects: the role of free tissue transfer. Ann Plast Surg. 1998;41(6):633–9.

35. Heth JA, Funk GF, Karnell LH, et al. Free tissue transfer and local flap complications in anterior and anterolateral skull base surgery. Head Neck. 2002;24(10):901–12. https://doi.org/10.1002/hed.10147.

36. Wax MK, Burkey BB, Bascom D, Rosenthal EL. The role of free tissue transfer in the reconstruction of massive neglected skin cancers of the head and neck. Arch Facial Plast Surg. 2003;5(6):479–82. https://doi.org/10.1001/archfaci.5.6.479.

37. Frederick JW, Sweeny L, Carroll WR, Peters GE, Rosenthal EL. Outcomes in head and neck reconstruction by surgical site and donor site. Laryngoscope. 2013;123(7):1612–7. https://doi.org/10.1002/lary.23775.

38. Rosenthal EL, King T, McGrew BM, Carroll W, Magnuson JS, Wax MK. Evolution of a paradigm for free tissue transfer reconstruction of lateral temporal bone defects. Head Neck. 2008;30:589–94.

39. Lin AC, Lin DT. Reconstruction of lateral skull base defects with radial forearm free flaps: the double-layer technique. J Neurol Surg. 2015;76(4):257–61. https://doi.org/10.1055/s-0035-1548551.

40. Cordeiro PG, Santamaria E. The extended, pedicled rectus abdominis free tissue transfer for head and neck reconstruction. Ann Plast Surg. 1997;39(1):53–9.

41. Vyas RM, Dickinson BP, Fastekjian JH, Watson JP, DaLio AL, Crisera CA. Risk factors for abdominal donor-site morbidity in free flap breast reconstruction. Plast Reconstr Surg. 2008;121(5):1519–26. https://doi.org/10.1097/PRS.0b013e31816b1458.

42. Teknos TN, Smith JC, Day TA, Netterville JL, Burkey BB. Microvascular free tissue transfer in reconstructing skull base defects: lessons learned. Laryngoscope. 2002;112(10):1871–6. https://doi.org/10.1097/00005537-200210000-00032.

43. Hanasono MM, Sacks JM, Goel N, Ayad M, Skoracki RJ. The anterolateral thigh free flap for skull base reconstruction. Otolaryngol Head Neck Surg. 2009;140(6):855–60. https://doi.org/10.1016/j.otohns.2009.02.025.

44. Hanasono MM, Skoracki RJ, Yu P. A prospective study of donor-site morbidity after anterolateral thigh fasciocutaneous and myocutaneous free flap harvest in 220 patients. Plast Reconstr Surg. 2010;125(1):209–14. https://doi.org/10.1097/PRS.0b013e3181c495ed.

45. Yang WG, Chiang YC, Wei FC, Feng GM, Chen K. Thin anterolateral thigh perforator flap using a modified perforator microdissection technique and its clinical application for foot resurfacing. Plast Reconstr Surg. 2006;117(3):1004–8. https://doi.org/10.1097/01. prs.0000200615.77678.f1.
46. Trojanowski P, Szymański M, Trojanowska A, Andrzejczak A, Szczepanek D, Klatka J. Anterolateral thigh free flap in reconstruction of lateral skull base defects after oncological resection. Eur Arch Oto-Rhino-Laryngol. 2019;276(12):3487–94. https://doi.org/10.1007/ s00405-019-05627-x.

Part VI
Postoperative Care

Chapter 28
Postoperative Management Following Skull Base Reconstruction

Peter Papagiannopoulos, Pete S. Batra, and Bobby A. Tajudeen

Introduction

Anterior skull base cerebrospinal fluid (CSF) leaks may be congenital, iatrogenic, traumatic, or spontaneous, related to benign intracranial hypertension. Repair of these lesions is of clinical imperative for prevention of complications including pneumocephalus, meningitis, or intracranial abscess [1]. Historically, these defects were repaired by neurosurgeons through a transcranial approach for adequate visualization, which requires a large degree of brain retraction for access to the skull base [1, 2]. However, in the last 20 years, there has been significant advancement in the endoscopic endonasal approach (EEA) to the skull base. While the endoscopic approach was initially used for endoscopic sinus surgery (ESS), indications quickly expanded to include endoscopic repair of encephaloceles as well as resection of sinonasal tumors, pituitary lesions, and, more recently, completely intracranial lesions such as meningiomas and craniopharyngiomas [3–7]. Technical and technological advancements have even allowed for application of the EEA techniques to anterior skull base surgery and CSF leak repair in pediatric patients as young as 23 months [3] (Figs. 28.1 and 28.2).

These endoscopic advancements are largely due to increased anatomic understanding, newly developed sinonasal instrumentation, and improved image-guidance systems. Additionally, advancements in successful skull base reconstruction include

P. Papagiannopoulos · P. S. Batra · B. A. Tajudeen (✉)
Department of Otolaryngology—Head and Neck Surgery, Section of Rhinology and Skull Base Surgery, Rush University Medical Center, Chicago, IL, USA
e-mail: Peter_Papagiannopoulos@rush.edu; Pete_Batra@rush.edu;
Bobby_tajudeen@rush.edu

E. C. Kuan et al. (eds.), *Skull Base Reconstruction*,
https://doi.org/10.1007/978-3-031-27937-9_28

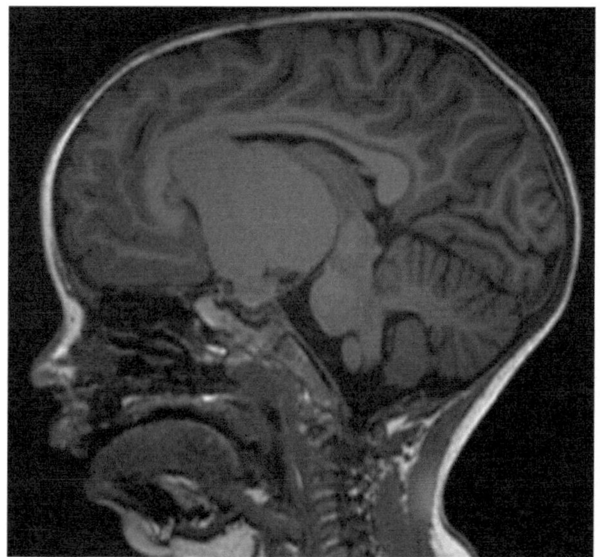

Fig. 28.1 23 month old female with craniopharyngioma extending into the suprasellar cistern. T1, contrast enhanced MRI, sagittal view

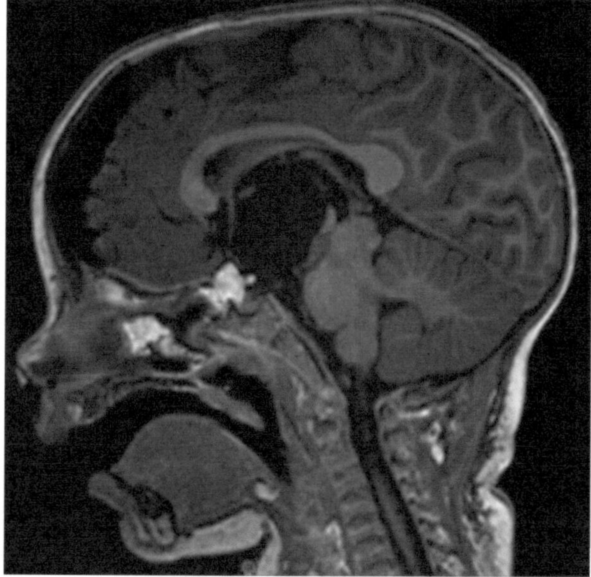

Fig. 28.2 Post-operative MRI, T1, contrast enhanced. 3 months after EEA with gross total resection, CSF leak reconstructed with fat, fascia lata underlay and NSF overlay with fibrin glue sealant. Note NSF enhancement with contrast

the development of novel synthetic grafting materials and vascularized pedicled flaps [8], which have been covered in detail elsewhere in this text. Critical to successful reconstruction is effective postoperative management, which will be the focus of this chapter.

Skull Base Reconstruction Intranasal Bolstering

Sealant Layer

Once the final layer of closure of the skull base defect has been positioned (nasoseptal flap, free mucosal graft, etc.), it is critical to stabilize the graft in the desired position to promote healing and to ensure a good seal against the skull base so as to avoid the risk of graft migration. Tissue sealants are frequently used as a final step of the reconstruction [5, 9]. There are several commercially available tissue sealants that have been evaluated with in vitro and in vivo models [10].

Within the broader category of tissue sealants, there are both fibrin-based and non-fibrin sealants. Fibrin-based sealants Beriplast (CSL-Behring, Tokyo, Japan) and Tisseel (Baxter Inc., Mississauga, ON, Canada) stimulate the final phase of the coagulation cascade while non-fibrin sealants Bioglue (Cryolife Inc., Kennesaw, GA) and Duraseal (Integra LifeSciences Corporation, Plainsboro, NJ) function as a tissue glue. For both types of sealants, studies show improved graft adherence and overall increased ability to withstand burst pressure compared to the control arm [10–12] and, therefore, are widely used as part of a multilayer closure of skull base reconstructions (Fig. 28.3).

Despite the ability of sealants to increase the ability to withstand pressure, the evidence to support their use in skull base reconstruction is limited to small, single-institution, retrospective studies [10–12] limiting broad recommendations regarding tissue sealants. Despite this lack of evidence, they are commonly used as part of a robust multilayered reconstruction.

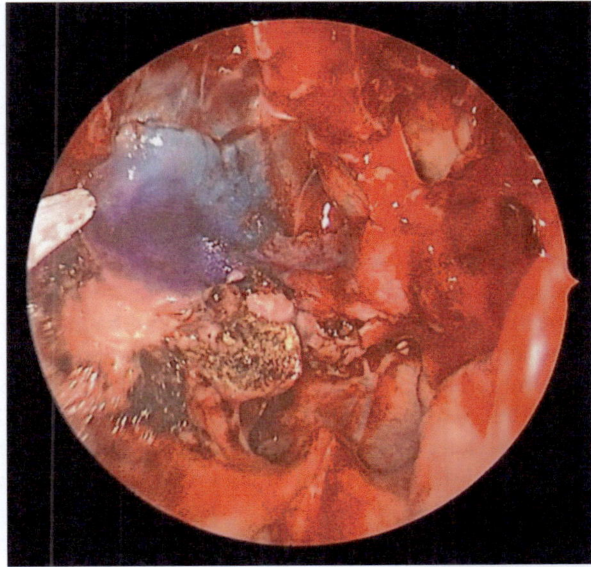

Fig. 28.3 Tissue sealant being used the stabilize a nasoseptal flap being used to reconstruct a right sphenoid defect

Nasal Packing

Nasal packing is often used to line the nasal and sinus cavities at the conclusion of endoscopic skull base surgery. There are several theorized benefits for nasal packing: first, to promote hemostasis; second, to provide a barrier to avoid pneumocephalus should positive pressure ventilation be emergently required; and third, and most importantly, to act as a bolster to decrease the risk of graft migration and to provide physical support of the reconstruction. This allows time for epithelization of the defect and for fortification against rapid changes of intracranial pressure in the immediate postoperative due to straining or vomiting [13].

There are both absorbable and nonabsorbable options for nasal packing. Absorbable options include Surgicel, Nasopore (Stryker, Kalamazoo, MI), Gelfoam (Pfizer Inc., New York, NY), and Merogel (Medtronic, Minneapolis, MN). Nonabsorbable packing products include Telfa (Kendall Company, Walpole, MA) Merocel sponges (Medtronic, Minneapolis, MN), Xeroform strip gauze, and finally Foley catheter balloon for buttressing of the skull base. Nonabsorbable packing requires removal and antibiotic prophylaxis.

The decision and the type of packing used is based on surgeon preference. Although there are theoretical benefits and deterrents for use of packing, the scientific literature investigating this issue is not adequate to make any definitive conclusions [10].

Postoperative Imaging

The need for immediate postoperative imaging (within 24–72 h) to identify complications or residual disease is often ordered on a patient-specific basis [10]. CT brain without contrast can help identify pneumocephalus or intracranial hemorrhage. MRI scans with and without contrast are used to assess for residual disease although this may be limited due to postop inflammation and packing materials.

Recent studies have tried to assess whether imaging can help detect postoperative CSF leak, which remains the most common complication following endoscopic skull base surgery. A recent meta-analysis showed a fairly low postoperative leak rate of 2% in endoscopic trans-sphenoidal surgery for pituitary lesions [14] but a postoperative leak rate as high as 22% and 25% for chordomas and meningiomas, respectively [15]. While high volume skull base centers tend to have much lower postoperative CSF leak rates [4, 16] for these extended skull base approaches, CSF leak still remains the most common postoperative complication.

Studies assessing the ability of imaging to detect CSF leak have largely been expert opinion papers [10] and while contrast-enhanced MRI can determine whether a nasoseptal flap is perfused, it does not necessarily correlate with a decreased rate of postoperative CSF leak [17].

As a result, identifying CSF leaks continues to be largely a clinical diagnosis.

Skull Base Precautions

The research available assessing postoperative skull base precautions is largely expert opinion, and each skull base center tends to have its own regimen, making it difficult to formulate definitive recommendations. At our institution, if a CSF leak was repaired, the patient's head of bed is kept elevated at 30°, and systolic blood pressure is regulated to be less than 140 mmHg, if possible, for the first 48 h post-surgically. The patient is typically monitored on surgical floor unless the patient requires ICU level care typically for lumbar drain management or for ICU level care after removal of an intracranial tumor.

Skull base reconstruction typically includes a period of bedrest, 48 hours postoperatively. Additionally, the use of antiemetics and cautious advancement of diet to avoid emesis is critical. Further, it is important the patient is given instructions to avoid Valsalva maneuvers, nose blowing, bending at the waist, or lifting anything heavier than 20 pounds. Stool softeners are also very commonly used in the postoperative period, if needed. Typically, these precautions are extended for a duration of 6 weeks.

Antibiotics

Judicious use of antibiotics is an important consideration given the inherently contaminated nature of the paranasal sinuses and potential intracranial infectious sequela from surgery. The presence of a normal sinonasal microbes and, in patients with sinusitis, pathogenic bacteria portends a theoretical risk of postoperative intracranial infection with these procedures [10]. However, despite this, the risk of postoperative meningitis is low [18], and antibiotic use has several risks, including adverse effects, allergic reaction, disruption of the normal gastrointestinal flora, and development of drug-resistant organisms [18].

Further, the literature for perioperative antibiotics in endoscopic skull base surgery is limited by being largely retrospective in nature, not having consistent pathology, and not having consistent antibiotic regimens between studies [19–21]. As a result, this does not allow for definitive conclusions regarding the safety and impact of antibiotics on postoperative infectious complications [10].

The studies available do suggest a low rate of meningitis with short-term perioperative antibiotics and as a result should be considered postoperatively [19–21]. A higher rate of infectious complications has been found in patients with postoperative CSF leak and those undergoing surgery for malignancy, and therefore, there may be a larger role of antibiotics in these settings. Further, for those surgeons choosing to use nonabsorbable packing material, antibiotics should be considered until removal of the packing.

At our institution, we give ceftriaxone intraoperatively and then for 48 h postoperatively before transitioning to Augmentin until nonabsorbable packing is removed, typically for 10–14 days.

Lumbar Drain

In most cases of skull base surgery, routine placement of lumbar drain in the postoperative period is not needed given the preponderance of potential harm over benefit [10]. Potential negative effects of lumbar drain include potential for post-spinal headaches, which may require blood patch, meningitis, pneumocephalus, retained catheter fragment, and complications of intracranial hypotension. However, lumbar drain usage can be considered for administration of intrathecal fluorescein and to confirm water-tight closure. Further, it may be of utility in high-risk cases, such as difficult anatomic sites (i.e., lateral pterygoid recess of sphenoid, clivus), high-flow cerebrospinal fluid leaks, or patients with extremely high BMIs and should be determined on a case-by-case basis [10].

Debridement

The schedule for follow-up nasal debridement after endoscopic skull base surgery is lacking [22]. At our institution, debridement is critical to ensure proper healing and to evaluate for complications such as infection and CSF leak. Patients are seen for their first debridement approximately 7 days after surgery. During the initial debridement, nasal crusting is carefully removed from the anterior portion of the nasal cavity to help facilitate breathing. Packing directly overlying the reconstruction is also gently removed. After this first visit, saline irrigations can be initiated to facilitate additional removal of nasal crusting. At the second postoperative visit, typically 4–6 weeks after surgery, the patient undergoes a more complete debridement with continued caution at the site of reconstruction.

The patient should continue saline irrigations at least twice daily. We recommend following the patient endoscopically until the health of their nasal cavity (minimal or no crusting, non-edematous well-healed mucosa, no CSF leak) is clearly established. Once the sinonasal cavity is well-healed, future follow-up visits are guided by the surveillance required for the disease process being managed.

References

1. Komotar RJ, et al. Endoscopic endonasal versus open repair of anterior skull base CSF leak, meningocele, and encephalocele: a systematic review of outcomes. J Neurol Surg A Cent Eur Neurosurg. 2013;74(4):239–50.

2. Lindstrom DR, et al. Management of cerebrospinal fluid rhinorrhea: the Medical College of Wisconsin experience. Laryngoscope. 2004;114(6):969–74.
3. Khalili S, Palmer JN, Adappa ND. The expanded endonasal approach for the treatment of intracranial skull base disease in the pediatric population. Curr Opin Otolaryngol Head Neck Surg. 2015;23(1):65–70.
4. Zanation AM, et al. Nasoseptal flap reconstruction of high flow intraoperative cerebral spinal fluid leaks during endoscopic skull base surgery. Am J Rhinol Allergy. 2009;23(5):518–21.
5. Conger A, et al. Evolution of the graded repair of CSF leaks and skull base defects in endonasal endoscopic tumor surgery: trends in repair failure and meningitis rates in 509 patients. J Neurosurg. 2018;130(3):861–75.
6. Karnezis TT, et al. Factors impacting cerebrospinal fluid leak rates in endoscopic sellar surgery. Int Forum Allergy Rhinol. 2016;6(11):1117–25.
7. Rawal RB, et al. Endoscopic resection of sinonasal malignancy: a systematic review and meta-analysis. Otolaryngol Head Neck Surg. 2016;155(3):376–86.
8. Lam K, et al. Use of autologous fat grafts for the endoscopic reconstruction of skull base defects: indications, outcomes, and complications. Am J Rhinol Allergy. 2018;32(4):310–7.
9. Campbell RG, et al. Cerebrospinal fluid rhinorrhea secondary to idiopathic intracranial hypertension: long-term outcomes of endoscopic repairs. Am J Rhinol Allergy. 2016;30(4):294–300.
10. Wang EW, et al. ICAR: endoscopic skull-base surgery. Int Forum Allergy Rhinol. 2019;9(S3):S145–365.
11. Fandiño M, et al. Determining the best graft-sealant combination for skull base repair using a soft tissue in vitro porcine model. Int Forum Allergy Rhinol. 2013;3(3):212–6.
12. Oshino S, Saitoh Y, Yoshimine T. Withstand pressure of a simple fibrin glue sealant: experimental study of mimicked sellar reconstruction in extended transsphenoidal surgery. World Neurosurg. 2010;73(6):701–4.
13. Hannan CJ, Kelleher E, Javadpour M. Methods of skull base repair following endoscopic endonasal tumor resection: a review. Front Oncol. 2020;10:1614.
14. Thomas R, Chacko AG. Principles in skull base reconstruction following expanded endoscopic approaches. J Neurol Surg B Skull Base. 2016;77(4):358–63.
15. Borg A, Kirkman MA, Choi D. Endoscopic endonasal anterior skull base surgery: a systematic review of complications during the past 65 years. World Neurosurg. 2016;95:383–91.
16. Patel MR, et al. Beyond the nasoseptal flap: outcomes and pearls with secondary flaps in endoscopic endonasal skull base reconstruction. Laryngoscope. 2014;124(4):846–52.
17. Adappa ND, et al. Radiographic enhancement of the nasoseptal flap does not predict postoperative cerebrospinal fluid leaks in endoscopic skull base reconstruction. Laryngoscope. 2012;122(6):1226–34.
18. Lai LT, et al. The risk of meningitis following expanded endoscopic endonasal skull base surgery: a systematic review. J Neurol Surg B Skull Base. 2014;75(1):18–26.
19. Milanese L, et al. Antibiotic prophylaxis in endoscopic endonasal pituitary and skull base surgery. World Neurosurg. 2017;106:912–8.
20. Brown SM, et al. Role of perioperative antibiotics in endoscopic skull base surgery. Laryngoscope. 2007;117(9):1528–32.
21. Orlando R, et al. Retrospective analysis of a new antibiotic chemoprophylaxis regimen in 170 patients undergoing endoscopic endonasal transsphenoidal surgery. Surg Neurol. 2007;68(2):145–8; discussion 148.
22. Tien DA, et al. Comprehensive postoperative management after endoscopic skull base surgery. Otolaryngol Clin N Am. 2016;49(1):253–63.

Chapter 29
Management of the Postoperative Leak

Duncan C. Watley, Nyall R. London, and Nicholas R. Rowan

Introduction

Successful closure of skull base defects during endoscopic tumor resection is of paramount importance. By effectively closing the pathway between the microbiologically colonized nasal cavity from the sterile subarachnoid space, significant morbidity and mortality can be avoided. Evidence exists showing increased duration of primary hospitalization, need for prolonged mechanical ventilation, postoperative readmission, reoperation, meningitis, pneumocephalus, and development of deep venous thrombosis in the setting of postoperative CSF leaks [1]. Historically, the incidence of meningitis following microscopic transsphenoidal and open craniotomy surgery is 0.7–3.1% and 0.9–2.5%. The incidence of meningitis following endoscopic skull base surgery in a large review performed by the Pittsburgh group in 2011 showed an overall rate of 1.8% [2]. Risk factors identified in this review included a history of previous surgery, presence of ventriculoperitoneal shunt or external ventricular drain, higher complexity intradural surgeries, and male sex. Notably, 72% of the patients that ultimately developed meningitis had concomitant postoperative CSF fistula. Rates of meningitis may be as high as 13% in patients with postoperative CSF leak, compared with 0.1% in patients who undergo uncomplicated endoscopic skull base surgery [3].

Though postoperative CSF leaks cannot be completely avoided, the incidence of postoperative CSF leak has significantly declined as surgeon familiarity with multilayered and vascularized reconstruction techniques has improved [4, 5]. Several recent studies have shown overall postoperative CSF leak rate to approximate <5%

D. C. Watley · N. R. London · N. R. Rowan (✉)
Department of Otolaryngology, Johns Hopkins University School of Medicine, Baltimore, MD, USA
e-mail: nlondon2@jhmi.edu; nrowan1@jhmi.edu

E. C. Kuan et al. (eds.), *Skull Base Reconstruction*, https://doi.org/10.1007/978-3-031-27937-9_29

[1, 5–7], but this rate varies considerably with certain patient and tumor characteristics. The successful skull base surgical team carefully evaluates perioperative risk factors prior to taking their patient to the operating room for complex reconstruction. Risk factors predisposing the patient to postoperative CSF leak vary widely but can be roughly divided into patient and surgical characteristics.

This chapter aims to review factors associated with the formation of a postoperative CSF leak, diagnostic considerations, and management strategies.

Patient Characteristics

Obesity

Obesity is a well-understood risk factor for both the development of spontaneous and postoperative CSF leak. The exact etiology of increased risk of postoperative CSF leaks is unknown; however, it is well known that BMI has a positive direct linear relationship with intracranial opening pressure [8]. Some authors have suggested a theoretical pathophysiologic pathway in which obesity ultimately leads to decreased CSF drainage into the sagittal sinus, resulting in increased intracranial CSF pressure [9]. Multiple groups have identified obesity as an independent risk factor for postoperative CSF leak [10–15]. A large retrospective evaluation of the Pittsburgh experience demonstrated a significant difference in leak rate when overweight individuals (BMI > 25) were compared to individuals with healthy weight (BMI < 25) (18.8% CSF leak rate in overweight vs. 11.6% in healthy weight) [10].

OSA

Obstructive sleep apnea (OSA) is an increasingly prevalent disease worldwide that provides a distinct challenge to the skull base surgeon on multiple levels. First, common symptoms of OSA such as headache, daytime sleepiness, and brain fog are shared presenting indicators of neurologic complication following skull base surgery. Additionally, patients with OSA, especially untreated, have increased intracranial pressure, thus theoretically increasing their risk of failed reconstruction [16, 17].

Repeated escalation of intra-abdominal and intra-thoracic pressure during sleep are hallmark for obstructive sleep apnea. Due to decreased CSF outflow and thus increased intracranial pressure during these events, it is suspected that OSA can increase the risk of graft failure. A group of healthy individuals with normal ICP were artificially able to increase their ICP to a mean of 32.3 cmH_2O when performing a voluntary Valsalva maneuver [18]. This result is well above the normal range and is further evidence that apneic events followed by straining in the OSA population may put increased tension on the reconstruction.

Additionally, the treatment of OSA may be associated with increased risk in the immediate postoperative period. Application of positive pressure devices such as CPAP increase intranasal pressure at approximately 85% of applied CPAP pressure [19]. Positive pressure has the potential for disruption of the reconstruction site or tension pneumocephalus. Tension pneumocephalus, although extremely rare, has associated significant morbidity and increased risk of mortality. Work by Castle-Kirszbaum et al. reported two incidences in which positive pressure was applied to immediate postoperative ESBS patients, both resulting in prolonged admission and reoperation [20]. Chitguppi et al. showed in a cadaver study that sellar multilayered reconstructions with a naso-septal flap were able to tolerate CPAP with pressures up to 20 cmH$_2$O [21], but this finding has yet to be confirmed in vivo [21]. Resumption of postoperative positive pressure therapy varies by surgical team with the majority falling between 2 and 6 weeks postoperatively [22].

Radiation Exposure

Ionizing radiation is associated with poor wound healing due to tissue cellular depletion, stromal cell dysfunction, aberrant collagen deposition, and microvascular damage [23]. Intuitively, prior radiation therapy may predispose patients for failed reconstruction. This finding was confirmed in two large multicenter trials. Exposure to ionizing radiation yielded a statistically significant increased odds (2.67) for postoperative CSF leak [1] as well as a higher than typical rate (28.6%) [11]. Although both studies compiled data from multiple high-volume centers, each had small patient cohorts with prior irradiation. With the advent of modern radiotherapy techniques, continued investigation will be needed to understand the associated risk for postoperative reconstruction failures.

Revision Surgery

Multiple studies in the skull base reconstructive literature have examined revision surgery as a potential risk factor for CSF fistula. The vast majority have shown comparable rates of postoperative leak in primary and revision surgery [14, 24–26]. Zhou et al. showed in a large series of pituitary patients, an increased rate of intra-operative CSF leak during revision (30% revision vs. 16.4% index), but it was not statistically significant on multivariate analysis [6]. Additionally, no difference was seen on postoperative leak rates. Ultimately, the aggregate grade of evidence derived by international skull base guidelines on the topic was grade C in favor of no increased risk [27].

Surgical Characteristics

Surgical Subsite

Many authors have characterized rates of postoperative CSF leaks by anatomical subsites, as well as the associated pathologies and respective surgical defects. In the following section, these subsites will be explored and will be divided into sellar, parasellar/suprasellar, anterior cranial fossa (ACF), and posterior cranial fossa (PCF) tumors.

Sella Turcica

Much of the overall surgical subsite literature involves patients with pituitary neoplasms due to the relative frequency in which these lesions are seen in comparison to pathologies of other locations. Sellar defects have a known range of postoperative CSF leak rates from 0% to 13.5% [27], but many of the studies involved in this calculation include patients without intraoperative CSF leak, thus artificially lowering their rate of postoperative leak. Fraser et al. specifically excluded patients without intraoperative leak in their combined review of sellar and parasellar pathologies, showing an aggregate leak rate of 10% [10]. The total aggregate leak rate for pituitary lesions totaled by the international skull base guidelines demonstrated a fistula rate of 4.8% [27].

Parasellar/Suprasellar

Surgery beyond the sella is generally associated with greater risk of postoperative CSF leak rates. Parasellar defects, including the tuberculum, suprasellar space, and cavernous sinus, may represent additional risk. Examining the literature on the subject is challenging as many authors have combined populations of sellar tumors, with parasellar, and suprasellar. Two recent systematic reviews showed postoperative CSF leak rates of 15.3% [28] and 21% [29] for endoscopic resection of tuberculum meningioma. A recent international consensus statement aggregated all reported parasellar tumors with an overall 9.0% postoperative leak rate [27].

Anterior and Posterior Cranial Fossa

Tumors of the anterior and posterior cranial fossa are typically associated with larger surgical defects, and pathologies that often extend intradurrally. The most common tumors of the ACF include olfactory groove meningioma and esthesioneuroblastoma, both of which are largely asymptomatic until large in size. In the PCF, the tightly adherent dura to the posterior wall of the clivus and proximity to the pre-pontine cistern often lead to high-flow CSF leaks during tumor resection. Zwagerman et al. showed an average dural defect of 7.2 cm in ACF and 3.8 cm in PCF tumor resections, which was significantly larger than any other subsite [26] (Figs. 29.1, 29.2, and 29.3). High flow intraoperative CSF leak patients with ACF and PCF tumors were at greater risk of postoperative leak compared with parasellar tumors (parasellar 7%, ACF 20%, PCF 22%) [26]. This difference resolved with use of postoperative LD use (parasellar 4.7%, ACF 11%, PCF 13%). Increased risk of postoperative failure was also reported in two other large systematic reviews

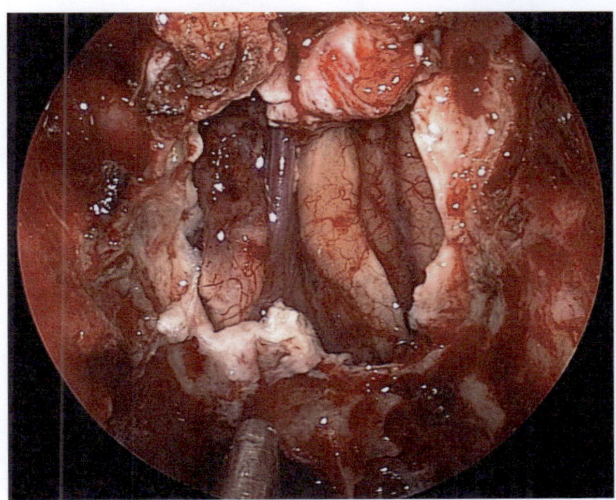

Fig. 29.1 Large anterior cranial fossa defect utilizing a transcribriform approach

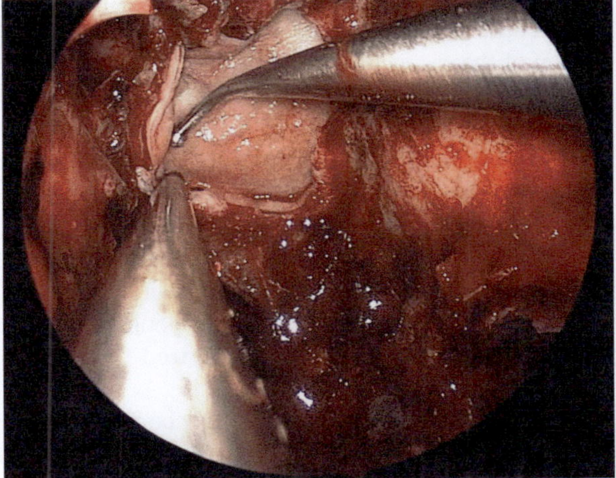

Fig. 29.2 Collagen matrix dural inlay used as the first layer of a multi-layered reconstruction

Fig. 29.3 Right sided nasoseptal pedicled flap used as the final step of multi-layered reconstruction

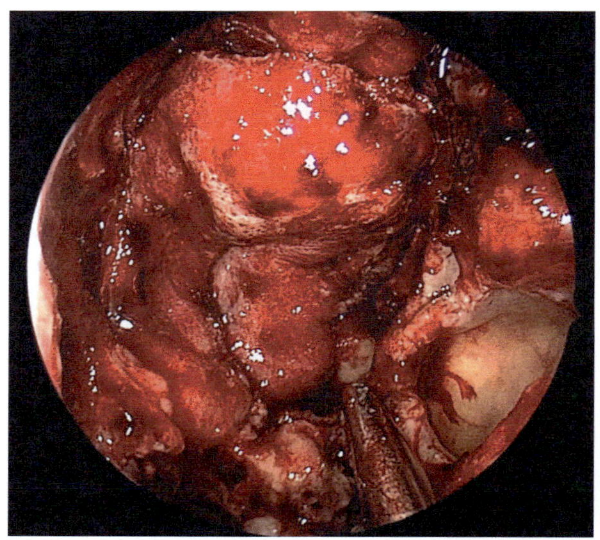

showing a 16.5% [3] and 20% [30] CSF fistula rate in PCF tumor resections. The international consensus statement aggregate failure rate was 13% for ACF and 19.1% for PCF tumors [27].

Technical Errors

Multiple technical errors can be made during endoscopic skull base surgery that may contribute to failed reconstruction. First, properly positioning graft materials is of utmost importance. Dural underlays with synthetic or autogenic materials are commonly used as a part of multilayered closure. Placing these grafts is challenging as the entire rim of the graft must be under the edges of the dural defect. A small portion of the reconstructive graft that is not completely within the dura can easily allow egress of CSF. The grafts then must be firmly apposed to the bony defect and supported by packing materials. Inadequate support of the multilayered closure is a common source of immediate postoperative CSF leak.

Prior to reconstruction, the recipient site must be prepared by removing sinonasal mucosa near the bony defect. Retained mucosa can be the source of immediate or delayed reconstruction failure due to poor opposition of reconstructive layers to the bone and evolving mucocele formation. Additionally, meticulous hemostasis should be achieved to decrease risk of pooling between layered reconstructive elements. Blood retained under vascularized flaps can lead to flap migration in the postoperative period.

Finally, some grafting materials may be inadvertently porous as a result of failure during production, in the case of artificial materials, or during harvest, in the case of autologous tissue. For instance, traumatic elevation of a nasoseptal flap off of a deviated nasal septum may result in an inadvertent tear or perforation of the vascularized flap. Nonetheless, several authors have demonstrated that although perhaps increasing risk of postoperative CSF leak, these vascularized flaps remain a reliable option for reconstruction [31].

Identification and Localization of Postoperative CSF Leak

Early identification of postoperative CSF leaks is of paramount importance to the skull base surgeon due to the evolving risk of intracranial complications including infection and pneumocephalus. Conservative, nonsurgical management of iatrogenic or traumatic CSF leaks has an established meningitis rate of 10%–37% in the literature [32–35]. The risk of meningitis increases the longer the fistula persists with one report showing 1.3% risk added per day for the first 2 weeks [33]. This finding is in line with a robust retrospective cohort that reported meningitis in 13% of patients with a postoperative CSF leak [2]. Accurate identification and localization of the postoperative leak is of utmost importance in the prompt management of the complication. Commonly used techniques to confirm the presence of CSF in the postoperative patient include physical exam with or without accompanying provocation maneuvers, nasal endoscopy, high resolution CT, and laboratory evaluation including β2-transferrin.

Physical Exam

Physical exam findings when attempting to identify a postoperative CSF leak range from diagnostic, such as in the case of a high-volume leak with persistent continuous clear anterior or posterior nasal drainage that worsens with provocation, to subtle. Bedside endoscopy can be extremely useful in visualizing the location of the leak or shifted reconstructive elements in the postoperative patient. It additionally can be further improved by having the patient perform a Valsalva maneuver while visualizing the reconstruction. Placing the patient in a Trendelenburg position is also useful due to associated increase in intracranial pressure. Physical exam and full visualization of the reconstruction may be limited by nasal packing in the postoperative patient. Endoscopy in the operating room with removal of packing is appropriate for patients with high clinical suspicion for CSF leak.

Additionally, the historical "halo sign" is a physical exam test used for many years to identify CSF admixed with blood. When the two fluids are dripped onto a white medium, they will separate forming a rim of clear fluid surrounding a central patch of red blood. The accuracy and reproducibility of this test has been called into question by many texts as many clear fluids mixed with blood will separate with the same halo effect. Dula et al. showed blood mixed with CSF, normal saline, tap water, and typical nasal rhinorrhea all produced halo signs on white filter paper [36]. Due to the high potential for misdiagnosis, the use of the halo sign for CsF leak confirmation should be avoided [37].

Laboratory Investigation

Two immunologic laboratory assays can be performed on collected nasal drainage suspected to be cerebrospinal fluid. These laboratory examinations rely on protein compositional differences between CSF and other bodily secretions.

β-Trace Protein

First, β-trace protein, a secretory protein involved in transportation of small lipophilic substances within the CSF, is often utilized as a biomarker for CSF. β-Trace protein is found both in CSF and serum but at vastly different concentrations [38]. Exceptional cases in which the biomarker is unreliable include end-stage renal disease and bacterial meningitis [39]. It has a tested sensitivity of 91–100% and specificity of 93–99% [40, 41]. Although extremely useful, this laboratory exam is only performed in Europe.

β2-Transferrin

β2-Transferrin is the second biomarker used and is exclusively performed in the United States. It is a brain-specific form of transferrin involved in the transportation and utilization of iron. It has been identified in CSF, perilymph, and aqueous humor and is notably absent from serum in normal healthy adults [42]. Exceptional cases in which the protein may be found in serum are patients with chronic alcohol-related cirrhosis and inborn errors of glycoprotein metabolism [43, 44]. Analysis for the presence of the biomarker is possible with as little as 0.17 mL of collected fluid [45]. Skull base procedures with known intraoperative CSF leaks have the potential to increase the rate of false-positive results as the protein may be found in the patient's rhinorrhea for some time [46]. In-house testing for this protein can lead to rapid identification of CSF leak, but many hospitals use outside laboratories, which may take several days to result. β2-Transferrin has a tested sensitivity of 93–99% and specificity of 95–97% [41, 47].

Imaging

High-Resolution Computed Tomography

High-resolution computed tomography (HRCT) is typically the first imaging choice selected during the workup for postoperative CSF leak. It provides high resolution of sinonasal anatomy and excellent reproduction of bony architecture. Not only is HRCT readily available in most hospital settings, it is typically much less costly ($504) when compared to both radionuclide cisternography ($2800), magnetic resonance cisternography ($1800), and CT cisternography ($1800) [48]. Radiologic signs worrisome for CSF leak when seen on HRCT include expanding pneumocephalus, obvious bony defects without corresponding graft coverage, and enhancement surrounding reconstructive layers on contrasted images.

The reported sensitivity and specificity vary significantly depending on the study, but a recent metanalysis showed sensitivity from 44% to 100% and specificity from 45% to 100% with the majority of articles in the upper range [37]. Some authors recommend routine postoperative HRCT for early detection of postoperative complications including pneumocephalus, CSF leak, and intracranial bleeding [49, 50]. Nadimi et al. showed in their retrospective review that routine postoperative imaging was generally not helpful and of the patients that did ultimately develop surgical complications all exhibited clinical symptoms such as persistent rhinorrhea, nausea, vomiting, headache, or altered mental status [51].

Magnetic Resonance Imaging

Magnetic resonance imaging is a commonly utilized imaging modality to delineate similar soft tissue densities, nervous structures, and dura. MRI has been used extensively in the postoperative period to assess for complications of surgery as well as extent of tumor resection. It additionally can also be employed for the primary diagnosis of CSF leak with a reported sensitivity ranging from 11.8 to 100% but with the majority of studies showing >80% [52]. Recent advances including 3D sequences have shown performance benefit when compared to HRCT and traditional MRI [53, 54].

Magnetic Resonance Cisternography

Magnetic resonance cisternography (MRC) is a noninvasive imaging modality frequently used to identify postoperative CSF leaks. CSF fistula would appear either as a high signal intensity extending from the subarachnoid space into the adjacent paranasal sinuses, or herniation of brain parenchyma through a bony defect. However, in the postoperative patient, nonspecific mucosal inflammation surrounding the operative repair may mimic the appearance of a CSF leak and lead to a false-positive diagnosis [55, 56].

MRC can be further enhanced with intrathecally injected gadolinium. This imaging modality improves contrast between CSF and surrounding structures on T1 and fat-suppressed magnetic resonance imaging. Theoretical risks associated with intrathecal injection of contrast material include behavior change, seizure, allergic reaction, intracerebral hemorrhage, and altered mental status. However, multiple studies have shown that these are rare reactions, and the most common complication is self-limited headache [57–59]. MRC without intrathecal gadolinium has a studied sensitivity of 56%–94% and specificity of 57%–100% [37]. MRC with intrathecal gadolinium has a sensitivity ranging from 61% to 100% and specificity from 66% to 80% [37].

Computed Tomography Cisternography

Computed tomography cisternography (CTC) combines HRCT with intrathecally injected water-soluble nonionic contrast to better differentiate CSF from surrounding neurologic structures. It can be used like MRC for diagnosis and anatomic localization of CSF fistula. Evidence exists that it is a less reliable evaluative tool when compared to MRC (MRC sensitivity 72%, specificity 93%) (CTC sensitivity 33%, specificity 67%) [56]. Like MRC, there are similar theoretical risks associated with intrathecal contrast injection; additionally, rare reports of cerebral edema have been published [60]. CTC remains an option for evaluation of CSF fistula, but due to poor performance when compared to other exams and the invasive nature of intrathecal contrast injection, it is generally not recommended for routine diagnosis and localization [37].

Radionuclide Cisternography

Radionuclide cisternography (RNC) is a confirmational exam in which a radioisotope is intrathecally injected through a lumbar puncture. Dry cottonoid pledgets are then placed into the patient's nasal cavities and are left in place for several hours in an effort to collect the radioisotope as it drains intranasally through a CSF fistula. The exam is unable to pinpoint the exact location of fistula as the radioisotope may leave the subarachnoid space in one position and contact the pledget in another, especially when the pledgets are in a dependent position. Additionally, due to this same concept, RNC is also unable to differentiate anterior skull base CSF leaks from lateral, as CSF may drain through the eustachian tube and contact the pledgets in the nasopharynx [37]. RNC has an established sensitivity of 76–100% and specificity of 100% [48, 61, 62], but due to its invasive nature, relatively high cost [48], and poor performance when compared to laboratory confirmational studies, it is not a recommended exam [37]. Though nasal endoscopy, laboratory evaluation of rhinorrhea, and imaging are the preferred modalities, RNC can be considered in complex cases when a potential leak cannot be located. This is generally not used in the immediate postoperative period and has increased utility in patients with spontaneous CSF rhinorrhea of unknown origin.

Intrathecal and Topical Fluorescein

Fluorescein is an organic dye that can be used both intrathecally and topically for localization of CSF fistula. The dye has a distinct green-orange color when mixed with CSF, which sharply contrasts the normal sinonasal mucosa allowing easy endoscopic localization (Fig. 29.4). It can also be used with endoscopic blue light filters further contrasting the color into a bright green shade. The dye has been implicated in dose-dependent adverse effects including cranial nerve deficits, seizure, lower extremity weakness, and even death [63, 64]. The standard intrathecal dose is 0.1–2 mL of 5% fluorescein diluted in CSF [65]. The authors' preference is 0.1 mL of 10% fluorescein diluted in 10 mL of CSF. This dose is orders of power lower than doses known to cause systemic adverse events (500–1250 mg) [63]. Intrathecal fluorescein has a studied success rate of 46–100% in the localization of CSF leaks [37, 66, 67].

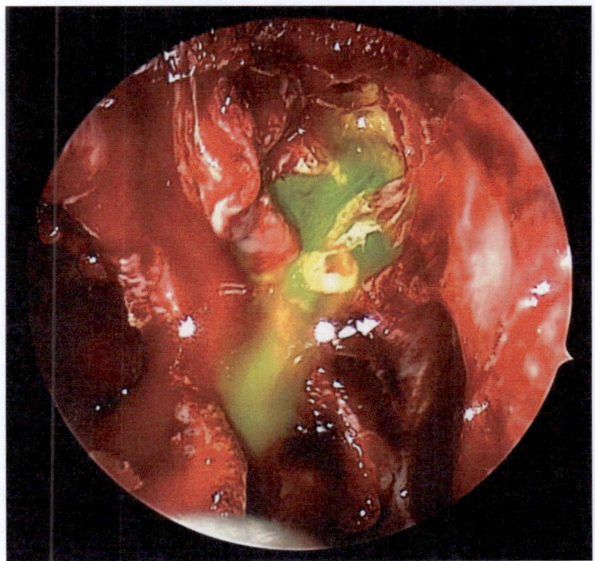

Fig. 29.4 Characteristic green hue of intrathecal fluorescein mixed with CSF

Topical fluorescein is a technique that avoids the potential adverse reactions associated with intrathecal injection. Five percent fluorescein is applied to cottonoid pledgets and inserted in the middle meatus, roof of the cribriform plate, and sphenoethmoidal recess and left to rest for a few moments. Then when removed, the sinonasal cavity is inspected for color change from orange-brown to green, which signifies mixing of the dye with CSF. Topical fluorescein has a reported accuracy of 100%, but few studies have reported thus far in the literature, and the authors suspect that while specific, this test may not have 100% sensitivity [68–70]. No major complications associated with the topical use of fluorescein have been reported [68].

Conservative Measures/Surgical Adjuncts

After identification of a postoperative CSF leak, the skull base surgeon must decide between conservative management and surgical reoperation. It is the authors viewpoint that postoperative leaks, especially during the index hospitalization, typically represent a technical error or shifting of the reconstructive materials and would be best suited for prompt reoperation and interrogation of the reconstruction site. This viewpoint, however, is not shared by all, with some surgeons reporting successful closure of leaks with lumbar drainage and bedrest alone [30].

Lumbar Drain

Lumbar drains are potentially helpful adjuncts to the reconstruction of skull base defects. The insertion of a drain into the lumbar subarachnoid cistern allows egress for cerebrospinal fluid at a set rate per hour. This egress decreases intracranial CSF pressure, thereby decreasing pressure on the newly reconstructed skull base defect. The use of lumbar drains during the postoperative period has changed significantly over time; however, there is little consensus in the literature on the optimal use of this adjunct. The recently published international consensus document evaluated and summarized the known literature on lumbar drain use in sellar-based defects and concluded that very little evidence suggests significant benefit in CSF fistula rate [27]. Despite this, many centers routinely employ lumbar drains especially in high-risk patient groups, or during treatment of a postoperative CSF leak. Zwagerman et al. performed one of the only randomized controlled trials to delineate the benefits of drainage in high risk patients, which included patients with skull base defects >1 cm, extensive arachnoid dissection, or dissection into a ventricle [26]. This inclusion criteria specifically selected for patients with "high-flow" intraoperative leaks. The trial was stopped early after revealing significant benefit of the adjunct (lumbar drain: 8.2% postoperative leak, control: 21.2%) for combined tumor subsites. The difference was even more pronounced in high-risk subsites such as the ACF (LD 11.1%, control 35.3%) and PCF (LD 12.5%, control 30.8%) [26].

Complications associated with lumbar drainage include headache, meningitis, pneumocephalus, radiculopathy, intracranial hemorrhage, and decreased patient mobility in the postoperative period. Postoperative CT scans are often employed prior to drainage as lumbar drainage can exacerbate intracranial bleeding and pneumocephalus. Many large series have identified these complications as rare, with the most common being headache [26].

Medical Adjuncts

Acetazolamide is a carbonic anhydrase inhibitor whose action in the proximal tubule of the kidney causes increased excretion of sodium, bicarbonate, and chloride leading to diuresis. This diuresis decreases intracranial pressure, blood pressure, and intraocular pressure.

Acetazolamide is an option during the perioperative period in patients with suspected increased intracranial pressure. Its use is well established in patients with spontaneous CSF leaks due to intracranial hypertension, but its utility has not been well studied outside of this population [71].

Chaaban et al. showed an approximate decrease of 10 mmH_2O with a single 500 mg dose of acetazolamide in a population of spontaneous CSF leak patients [72]. It is suspected that it also may be a useful adjunct in patients with elevated BMI, as they are at higher risk of intracranial hypertension [8, 73]. The use of this medication is typically recommended as an adjunct rather than primary treatment of both postoperative and spontaneous CSF leak.

A wide variety of adverse effects are possible with acetazolamide including malaise, nausea, diarrhea, metabolic acidosis, kidney stones, and taste disturbance. Additionally, specific patient groups should not use this medication including patients with sulfonamide allergy, chronic kidney disease, patients on long term salicylates, anti-folates, amphetamines, lithium, and pregnant women.

Surgical Treatment of Postoperative CSF Leak

Surgical reexploration remains the mainstay of postoperative CSF leak management. The timing of reoperation and techniques practiced vary widely with no clear optimal surgical protocols. Much of these nuanced decisions incorporate patient and surgical factors, as well as the findings at the time of reoperation. As described above, the majority of CSF fistulas during the index hospitalization, or less than 1 week following surgery, are the result of technical mistake or shifting of reconstructive materials. Both instances are often managed with revision of reconstruction. A wide variety of options for smaller defects exist, including the use of free mucosal grafts, fat grafts to bolster the reconstruction, fascial or alloplastic grafts with high levels of success [30, 35, 74]. Use of a vascularized pedicled flaps also associated with improved closure rates and even more pronounced in patients with high-flow leaks. Multiple reviews have shown greater than 50% reduction in the rate of postoperative CSF fistula when vascularized flaps are utilized in this population [30, 75, 76]. In the setting of flap necrosis, an alternate vascularized reconstruction may be required.

Proper orientation and support of reconstructive materials is also of the utmost importance. Often during the index surgery, the reconstruction is watertight, but upon reoperation, the bolstering materials that were meant to support the dural inlay have moved. This can result from insufficient packing, or too rapid of dissolution in the case of absorbable materials.

A recent, large retrospective series highlights the importance of timing on the treatment paradigm for postoperative leaks. In a cohort of 1017 patients, 17 cases (2%) presented with a delayed CSF leak, which was defined as more than 2 weeks following index surgery [77]. This cohort had a variety of identifiable reasons for failure including nasoseptal flap dehiscence, partial or complete flap necrosis, inappropriate folding of the pedicled flap, or an inciting event such as a robust sneeze or vomiting episode. All patients were managed with reoperation, and based on the size of the defect and the viability of the previously placed nasoseptal flap, a variety of reconstructions were performed. The majority of patients presented between 1 and 2 weeks from surgery and were treated with either a large bolstering abdominal fat graft, or a collagen matrix inlay and fat graft. In patients were the nasoseptal flap was folded or severely mispositioned, it was completely freed and reoriented to a better position. In the instance of complete or partial pedicled flap necrosis, a new local flap was utilized. Two patients in this series presented in a delayed fashion from their index surgery with a CSF leak in the setting of adjuvant radiation therapy. Radiation therapy is the direct cause of osteoradionecrosis of the skull base, and both patients ultimately required free flap coverage of their defects due to poor blood supply to the area and concern for continued poor healing. Lee et al. also reported a small population of delayed CSF leaks thought to be at least partially related to radiation exposure [78]. These patients presented at a median of 137 months following the completion of their treatment, and all were successfully repaired with a pedicled flap.

The pediatric patient population provides different sources for reconstruction failure and different nuances for management of postoperative CSF leaks. One management consideration for young children should be a preoperative assessment of general temperament and ability to adhere to decreased activity and other postoperative conservative measures. If the child is suspected to be unable to avoid Valsalva maneuvers, postoperative sedation for several days could be employed [79, 80]. Additionally, children can present with congenital bony deficiencies and large encephaloceles. These may require more rigid reconstruction such as a split calvaria graft.

Ultimately, the surgical techniques employed for repair of postoperative CSF leaks vary widely between surgeons and are largely guided by experience. Additional research is required in this area to further delineate the optimal paradigm for management.

Conclusion/Summary

Successful reconstruction of skull base defects is of paramount importance to reduce the risk of postoperative meningitis. Despite significant effort by endoscopic skull base teams, CSF leaks do occur, and there should be consistent suspicion for this complication in the postoperative period. High-risk patients including those with obesity, obstructive sleep apnea, surgical defects outside the sella turcica, and those with high-flow intraoperative leaks should warrant increased wariness and attention. When a postoperative CSF leak is suspected, thorough physical exam and nasal endoscopy at bedside, or in the operating room, can rapidly diagnose the complication. HRCT and MRI are often useful in the diagnosis and surgical planning of CSF fistula. The treatment of postoperative leaks varies widely between teams, but revision reconstruction remains the mainstay of treatment, though there is a role for adjunctive measures such as lumbar drainage especially in the setting of high-flow intraoperative leaks and high-risk patients.

References

1. Shahangian A, Soler ZM, Baker A, Wise SK, Rereddy SK, Patel ZM, et al. Successful repair of intraoperative cerebrospinal fluid leaks improves outcomes in endoscopic skull base surgery. Int Forum Allergy Rhinol. 2017;7:80–6.
2. Kono Y, Prevedello DM, Snyderman CH, Gardner PA, Kassam AB, Carrau RL, et al. One thousand endoscopic skull base surgical procedures demystifying the infection potential: incidence and description of postoperative meningitis and brain abscesses. Infect Control Hosp Epidemiol. 2011;32:77–83.
3. Lai LT, Trooboff S, Morgan MK, Harvey RJ. The risk of meningitis following expanded endoscopic endonasal skull base surgery: a systematic review. J Neurol Surg B Skull Base. 2014;75:18–26.
4. Cavallo LM, Frank G, Cappabianca P, Solari D, Mazzatenta D, Villa A, et al. The endoscopic endonasal approach for the management of craniopharyngiomas: a series of 103 patients: clinical article. J Neurosurg. 2014;121:100–13.
5. Paluzzi A, Paluzzi A, Fernandez-Miranda JC, Fernandez-Miranda JC, Tonya Stefko S, Tonya Stefko S, et al. Endoscopic endonasal approach for pituitary adenomas: a series of 555 patients. Pituitary. 2014;17:307–19.
6. Zhou Q, Yang Z, Wang X, Wang Z, Zhao C, Zhang S, et al. Risk factors and management of intraoperative cerebrospinal fluid leaks in endoscopic treatment of pituitary adenoma: analysis of 492 patients. World Neurosurg. 2017;101:390–5.
7. Han Z-L, He D-S, Mao Z-G, Wang H-J. Cerebrospinal fluid rhinorrhea following transsphenoidal pituitary macroadenoma surgery: experience from 592 patients. Clin Neurol Neurosurg. 2008;110:570–9.
8. Berdahl JP, Fleischman D, Zaydlarova J, Stinnett S, Allingham RR, Fautsch MP. Body mass index has a linear relationship with cerebrospinal fluid pressure. Invest Ophthalmol Vis Sci. 2012;53:1422–7.
9. Fleischman GM, Ambrose EC, Rawal RB, Huang BY, Ebert CS, Rodriguez KD, et al. Obstructive sleep apnea in patients undergoing endoscopic surgical repair of cerebrospinal fluid rhinorrhea. Laryngoscope. 2014;124:2645–50.

10. Fraser S, Gardner PA, Koutourousiou M, Kubik M, Fernandez-Miranda JC, Snyderman CH, et al. Risk factors associated with postoperative cerebrospinal fluid leak after endoscopic endonasal skull base surgery. J Neurosurg. 2018;128:1066–71.
11. Karnezis TT, Baker AB, Soler ZM, Wise SK, Rereddy SK, Patel ZM, et al. Factors impacting cerebrospinal fluid leak rates in endoscopic sellar surgery. Int Forum Allergy Rhinol. 2016;6:1117–25.
12. Boling CC, Karnezis TT, Baker AB, Lawrence LA, Soler ZM, Vandergrift WA, et al. Multi-institutional study of risk factors for perioperative morbidity following transnasal endoscopic pituitary adenoma surgery. Int Forum Allergy Rhinol. 2016;6:101–7.
13. Dlouhy BJ, Madhavan K, Clinger JD, Reddy A, Dawson JD, O'Brien EK, et al. Elevated body mass index and risk of postoperative CSF leak following transsphenoidal surgery: clinical article. J Neurosurg. 2012;116:1311–7.
14. Ivan ME, Bryan Iorgulescu J, El-Sayed I, McDermott MW, Parsa AT, Pletcher SD, et al. Risk factors for postoperative cerebrospinal fluid leak and meningitis after expanded endoscopic endonasal surgery. J Clin Neurosci. 2014;22:48–54.
15. Cohen S, Schwartz T, Anand V. Lumbar drains decrease the risk of post-operative cerebrospinal fluid (CSF) leak following extended endonasal endoscopic surgery for suprasellar meningiomas in patients with high BMI. J Neurol Surg B Skull Base. 2016;77:P020.
16. Sugita Y, Iijima S, Teshima Y, Shimizu T, Nishimura N, Tsutsumi T, et al. Marked episodic elevation of cerebrospinal fluid pressure during nocturnal sleep in patients with sleep apnea hypersomnia syndrome. Electroencephalogr Clin Neurophysiol. 1985;60:214–9.
17. Jennum P, Børgesen SE. Intracranial pressure and obstructive sleep apnea. Chest. 1989;95:279–83.
18. Neville L, Egan RA. Frequency and amplitude of elevation of cerebrospinal fluid resting pressure by the valsalva maneuver. Can J Ophthalmol. 2005;40:775–7.
19. Reilly EK, Huntley CT, Boon MS, Epps G, Vimawala S, Chitguppi C, et al. Qualitative assessment of the effect of continuous positive airway pressure on the nasal cavity. Am J Rhinol Allergy. 2020;34:487–93.
20. Castle-Kirszbaum M, Wang YY, King J, Uren B, Kim M, Danks RA, et al. Tension pneumocephalus from positive pressure ventilation following endoscopic skull base surgery: case series and an institutional protocol for the management of postoperative respiratory distress. World Neurosurg. 2020;141:357–62.
21. Chitguppi C, Rimmer RA, Garcia HG, Koszewski IJ, Fastenberg JH, Nyquist GG, et al. Evaluation of cranial base repair techniques utilizing a novel cadaveric CPAP model. Int Forum Allergy Rhinol. 2019;9:795–803.
22. Gravbrot N, Jahnke H, White WL, Little AS. Resumption of positive-pressure ventilation devices for obstructive sleep apnea following transsphenoidal surgery: an institutional experience of a surgical cohort. J Neurol Surg Part B Skull Base. 2020;81:237–43.
23. Jacobson LK, Johnson MB, Dedhia RD, Niknam-Bienia S, Wong AK. Impaired wound healing after radiation therapy: a systematic review of pathogenesis and treatment. JPRAS Open. 2017;13:92–105.
24. Przybylowski CJ, Dallapiazza RF, Williams BJ, Pomeraniec IJ, Xu Z, Payne SC, et al. Primary versus revision transsphenoidal resection for nonfunctioning pituitary macroadenomas: matched cohort study. J Neurosurg. 2017;126:889–96.
25. Gruss CL, Al Komser M, Aghi MK, Pletcher SD, Goldberg AN, McDermott M, et al. Risk factors for cerebrospinal leak after endoscopic skull base reconstruction with nasoseptal flap. Otolaryngol Head Neck Surg. 2014;151:516–21.
26. Zwagerman NT, Wang EW, Shin SS, Chang Y-F, Fernandez-Miranda JC, Snyderman CH, et al. Does lumbar drainage reduce postoperative cerebrospinal fluid leak after endoscopic endonasal skull base surgery? A prospective, randomized controlled trial. J Neurosurg. 2018;131:1–1178.
27. Wang EW, Zanation AM, Gardner PA, Schwartz TH, Eloy JA, Adappa ND, et al. ICAR: endoscopic skull-base surgery. Int forum allergy Rhinol. 2019;9:S145–365.

28. Turel MK, Tsermoulas G, Reddy D, Andrade-Barazarte H, Zadeh G, Gentili F. Endonasal endoscopic transsphenoidal excision of tuberculum sellae meningiomas: a systematic review. J Neurosurg Sci. 2016;60:463–75.
29. Clark AJ, Jahangiri A, Garcia RM, George JR, Sughrue ME, McDermott MW, et al. Endoscopic surgery for tuberculum sellae meningiomas: a systematic review and meta-analysis. Neurosurg Rev. 2013;36:349–59.
30. Soudry E, Turner JH, Nayak JV, Hwang PH. Endoscopic reconstruction of surgically created skull base defects: a systematic review. Otolaryngol Head Neck Surg. 2014;150:730–8.
31. Huntley C, Iloreta AMC, Nyquist GG, Otten M, Garcia H, Farrell C, et al. Perforation of a nasoseptal flap does not increase the rate of postoperative cerebrospinal fluid leak. Int Forum Allergy Rhinol. 2015;5:353–5.
32. Eftekhar B, Ghodsi M, Nejat F, Ketabchi E, Esmaeeli B. Prophylactic administration of ceftriaxone for the prevention of meningitis after traumatic pneumocephalus: results of a clinical trial. J Neurosurg. 2004;101:757–61.
33. Eljamel MS, Foy PM. Acute traumatic CSF fistulae: the risk of intracranial infection. Br J Neurosurg. 1990;4:381–5.
34. Bernal-Sprekelsen M, Alobid I, Mullol J, Trobat F, Tomás-Barberán M. Closure of cerebrospinal fluid leaks prevents ascending bacterial meningitis. Rhinology. 2006;43:277–81.
35. Hegazy HM, Carrau RL, Snyderman CH, Kassam A, Zweig J. Transnasal endoscopic repair of cerebrospinal fluid rhinorrhea: a meta-analysis. Laryngoscope. 2000;110:1166–72.
36. Dula DJ, Fales W. The 'ring sign': is it a reliable indicator for cerebral spinal fluid? Ann Emerg Med. 1993;22:718–20.
37. Oakley GM, Alt JA, Schlosser RJ, Harvey RJ, Orlandi RR. Diagnosis of cerebrospinal fluid rhinorrhea: an evidence-based review with recommendations. Int Forum Allergy Rhinol. 2016;6:8–16.
38. Felgenhauer K, Schädlich HJ, Nekic M. β trace-protein as marker for cerebrospinal fluid fistula. Klin Wochenschr. 1987;65:764–8.
39. Meco C, Oberascher G, Arrer E, Moser G, Albegger K. β-trace protein test: new guidelines for the reliable diagnosis of cerebrospinal fluid fistula. Otolaryngol Head Neck Surg. 2003;129:508–17.
40. Bachmann G, Michel O. Clinical experience with beta-trace protein as a marker for cerebrospinal fluid. Ann Otol Rhinol Laryngol. 2000;109:1099–102.
41. Arrer E, Meco C, Oberascher G, Piotrowski W, Albegger K, Patsch W. β-trace protein as a marker for cerebrospinal fluid rhinorrhea. Clin Chem. 2002;48:939–41.
42. Nandapalan V, Watson ID, Swift AC. Beta-2-transferrin and cerebrospinal fluid rhinorrhoea. Clin Otolaryngol Allied Sci. 1996;21:259–64.
43. Sloman AJ, Kelly RH. Transferrin allelic variants may cause false positives in the detection of cerebrospinal fluid fistulae. Clin Chem. 1993;39:1444–5.
44. Stibler H. Carbohydrate-deficient transferrin in serum: a new marker of potentially harmful alcohol consumption reviewed. Clin Chem. 1991;37:2029–37.
45. Papadea C, Schlosser RJ. Rapid method for β2-transferrin in cerebrospinal fluid leakage using an automated immunofixation electrophoresis system. Clin Chem. 2005;51:464–70.
46. Bleier BS, Debnath I, O'Connell BP, Vandergrift WA, Palmer JN, Schlosser RJ. Preliminary study on the stability of beta-2 transferrin in extracorporeal cerebrospinal fluid. Otolaryngol Head Neck Surg. 2011;144:101–3.
47. Skedros DG, Cass SP, Hirsch BE, Kelly RH. Beta-2 transferrin assay in clinical management of cerebral spinal fluid and perilymphatic fluid leaks. J Otolaryngol. 1993;22:341–4.
48. Zapalac JS, Marple BF, Schwade ND. Skull base cerebrospinal fluid fistulas: a comprehensive diagnostic algorithm. Otolaryngol Head Neck Surg. 2002;126:669–76.
49. Ransom ER, Chiu AG. Prevention and management of complications in intracranial endoscopic skull base surgery. Otolaryngol Clin North Am. 2010;43:875–95.
50. Wagenmann M, Schipper J. The transnasal approach to the skull base. From sinus surgery to skull base surgery. GMS Curr Top Otorhinolaryngol Head Neck Surg. 2011;10:Doc08.

51. Nadimi S, Caballero N, Carpenter P, Sowa L, Cunningham R, Welch KC. Immediate postoperative imaging after uncomplicated endoscopic approach to the anterior skull base: is it necessary? Int Forum Allergy Rhinol. 2014;4:1024–9.
52. Eljazzar R, Loewenstern J, Dai JB, Shrivastava RK, Iloreta AM. Detection of cerebrospinal fluid leaks: is there a radiologic standard of care? A systematic review. World Neurosurg. 2019;127:307–15.
53. Xie T, Sun W, Zhang X, Liu T, Ding H, Hu F, et al. The value of 3D-FIESTA MRI in detecting non-iatrogenic cerebrospinal fluid rhinorrhoea: correlations with endoscopic endonasal surgery. Acta Neurochir. 2016;158:2333–9.
54. Zhang Y, Wang F, Chen X, Zhang Z, Meng X, Yu X, et al. Cerebrospinal fluid rhinorrhea: evaluation with 3D-SPACE sequence and management with navigation-assisted endonasal endoscopic surgery. Br J Neurosurg. 2016;30:643–8.
55. Hegarty SE, Millar JS. MRI in the localization of CSF fistulae: is it of any value? Clin Radiol. 1997;52:768–70.
56. Goel G, Ravishankar S, Jayakumar PN, Vasudev MK, Shivshankar JJ, Rose D, et al. Intrathecal gadolinium-enhanced magnetic resonance cisternography in cerebrospinal fluid rhinorrhea: road ahead? J Neurotrauma. 2007;24:1570–5.
57. Aydin K, Guven K, Sencer S, Jinkins JR, Minareci O. MRI cisternography with gadolinium-containing contrast medium: its role, advantages and limitations in the investigation of rhinorrhoea. Neuroradiology. 2004;46:75–80.
58. Aydin K, Terzibasioglu E, Sencer S, Sencer A, Suoglu Y, Karasu A, et al. Localization of cerebrospinal fluid leaks by gadolinium-enhanced magnetic resonance cisternography: a 5-year single-center experience. Neurosurgery. 2008;62:584–9.
59. Nacar Dogan S, Kizilkilic O, Kocak B, Isler C, Islak C, Kocer N. Intrathecal gadolinium-enhanced MR cisternography in patients with otorhinorrhea: 10-year experience of a tertiary referral center. Neuroradiology. 2018;60:471–7.
60. Kelley BC, Roh S, Johnson PL, Arnold PM. Malignant cerebral edema following CT myelogram using Isovue-M 300 intrathecal nonionic water-soluble contrast: a case report. Radiol Res Pract. 2011;2011:212516.
61. Stone JA, Castillo M, Neelon B, Mukherji SK. Evaluation of CSF leaks: high-resolution CT compared with contrast-enhanced CT and radionuclide cisternography. AJNR Am J Neuroradiol. 1999;20:706–12.
62. Flynn BM, Butler SP, Quinn RJ, McLaughlin AF, Bautovich GJ, Morris JG. Radionuclide cisternography in the diagnosis and management of cerebrospinal fluid leaks: the test of choice. Med J Aust. 1987;146:82–4.
63. Moseley JI, Carton CA, Stern WE. Spectrum of complications in the use of intrathecal fluorescein. J Neurosurg. 1978;48:765–7.
64. Keerl R, Weber RK, Draf W, Wienke A, Schaefer SD. Use of sodium fluorescein solution for detection of cerebrospinal fluid fistulas: an analysis of 420 administrations and reported complications in Europe and the United States. Laryngoscope. 2004;114:266–72.
65. Antunes P, Perdigão M. The use of intrathecal fluorescein in cerebrospinal fluid leak repair: management from an anesthesiologist's point-of-view. Acta Anaesthesiol Scand. 2016;60:1323–7.
66. Demarco RC, Tamashiro E, Valera FCP, Anselmo-Lima WT. Use of a hypodense sodium fluorescein solution for the endoscopic repair of rhinogenic cerebrospinal fluid fistulae. Am J Rhinol. 2007;21:184–6.
67. Javadi SAH, Samimi H, Naderi F, Shirani M. The use of low-dose intrathecal fluorescein in endoscopic repair of cerebrospinal fluid rhinorrhea. Arch Iran Med. 2013;16:264–6.
68. Saafan ME, Ragab SM, Albirmawy OA. Topical intranasal fluorescein: the missing partner in algorithms of cerebrospinal fluid fistula detection. Laryngoscope. 2006;116:1158–61.
69. Hai-sheng L, Ye-tao C, Dong W, Hui L, Yunpeng W, Shi-jie W, et al. The use of topical intranasal fluorescein in endoscopic endonasal repair of cerebrospinal fluid rhinorrhea. Surg Neurol. 2009;72:341–5.

70. Jones ME, Reino T, Gnoy A, Guillory S, Wackym P, Lawson W. Identification of intranasal cerebrospinal fluid leaks by topical application with fluorescein dye. Am J Rhinol. 2000;14:93–6.
71. Campbell RG, Farquhar D, Zhao N, Chiu AG, Adappa ND, Palmer JN. Cerebrospinal fluid rhinorrhea secondary to idiopathic intracranial hypertension: long-term outcomes of endoscopic repairs. Am J Rhinol Allergy. 2016;30:294–300.
72. Chaaban MR, Illing E, Riley KO, Woodworth BA. Acetazolamide for high intracranial pressure cerebrospinal fluid leaks. Int Forum Allergy Rhinol. 2013;3:718–21.
73. Daniels AB, Liu GT, Volpe NJ, Galetta SL, Moster ML, Newman NJ, et al. Profiles of obesity, weight gain, and quality of life in idiopathic intracranial hypertension (pseudotumor cerebri). Am J Ophthalmol. 2007;143:635–641.e1.
74. Harvey RJ, Parmar P, Sacks R, Zanation AM. Endoscopic skull base reconstruction of large dural defects: a systematic review of published evidence. Laryngoscope. 2012;122:452–9.
75. McCoul ED, Anand VK, Singh A, Nyquist GG, Schaberg MR, Schwartz TH. Long-term effectiveness of a reconstructive protocol using the nasoseptal flap after endoscopic skull base surgery. World Neurosurg. 2014;81:136–43.
76. Dehdashti AR, Stofko D, Okun J, Obourn C, Kennedy T. Endoscopic endonasal reconstruction of skull base: repair protocol. J Neurol Surg Part B Skull Base. 2016;77:271–8.
77. London NR, Mohyeldin A, Montaser AS, Tanjararak K, Prevedello DM, Otto BA, et al. Contributing factors for delayed postoperative cerebrospinal fluid leaks and suggested treatment algorithm. Int Forum Allergy Rhinol. 2020;10:779–84.
78. Lee JJ, Kim HY, Dhong H-J, Chung S-K, Kong D-S, Nam D-H, et al. Delayed cerebrospinal fluid leakage after treatment of skull base tumors: case series of 9 patients. World Neurosurg. 2019;132:e591–8.
79. London NR, Rangel GG, Onwuka A, Carrau RL, Prevedello DM, Leonard JA, et al. Reconstruction of pediatric skull base defects: a retrospective analysis emphasizing the very young. Int J Pediatr Otorhinolaryngol. 2020;133:109962.
80. Rawlins KW, Governale LS, Leonard JR, Elmaraghy CA, Walz PC. Recurrent cerebrospinal leak after endonasal cranial base surgery in a 4-year-old male: challenges for postoperative management. Ear Nose Throat J. 2019;100:472S.

Chapter 30
Other Complications Following Skull Base Reconstruction

Amarbir S. Gill and Gretchen M. Oakley

Introduction

The ability to perform highly complex procedures such as skull base tumor resections using minimally invasive endoscopic approaches has been a tremendous advance in the field. These approaches are associated with shorter operation times, less morbidity, and shorter hospital stays [1, 2]. However, although overall morbidity is lower with endoscopic skull base surgical approaches, the standard complications associated with any intracranial surgery can still occur, including cerebrospinal fluid leaks, orbital and vascular injury, and permanent neurologic disability. In addition, sinonasal morbidity is unique to the endonasal endoscopic approach. Thus, it is critical for the surgeon to familiarize him/herself with the potential complications and their management to optimize preparedness, mitigate harm, and manage sequelae when they do occur.

Tension Pneumocephalus

Tension pneumocephalus can be defined as intracranial air resulting from a ball valve phenomenon, where air is able to enter the postoperative intracranial cavity but cannot exit [3]. This can occur when pressure within the nasal cavity exceeds that of the intracranial cavity in the setting of inadequate skull base repair; air is then able to enter the postoperative cavity but cannot escape due to coaptation of the repair barrier [4]. The air continues to build up and compress the intracranial contents, resulting in mental status changes. Alternative suggested mechanisms include

A. S. Gill · G. M. Oakley (✉)
Department of Otolaryngology-Head and Neck Surgery, University of Utah,
Salt Lake City, UT, USA
e-mail: amarbir.gill@hsc.utah.edu; gretchen.oakley@hsc.utah.edu

© The Author(s), under exclusive license to Springer Nature
Switzerland AG 2023
E. C. Kuan et al. (eds.), *Skull Base Reconstruction*,
https://doi.org/10.1007/978-3-031-27937-9_30

the potential intracranial negative pressure created from CSF continuing to leak out versus intracranial infection with anaerobic, or gas forming, bacteria [3–6]. Recently, Castle-Kirzbaum et al. reported two cases of tension pneumocephalus in the setting of positive pressure ventilation (PPV) that was performed post-procedure for hypoxia resuscitation [4]. If ignored, progressive tension pneumocephalus can result in permanent neurologic deficits, brain herniation, and even death.

Presentation and Diagnosis

The typical presentation of tension pneumocephalus can include a postoperative headache, seizures, and rhinorrhea in the setting of a sudden change in mental status. It can be difficult to distinguish a normal amount of non-tension pneumocephalus, which is self-limiting and can be present after any neurosurgical procedure, from the surgical emergency of tension pneumocephalus, and a high degree of suspicion is needed [3]. One tool that can be helpful in making the diagnosis is a computed tomography (CT) scan. Classically, in the setting of tension pneumocephalus, a Mt. Fuji sign is observed, where the frontal poles are peaked and both surrounded and, to a lesser degree, divided by the presence of intracranial air with mass effect (Fig. 30.1) [3]. Moreover, tension pneumocephalus typically presents with

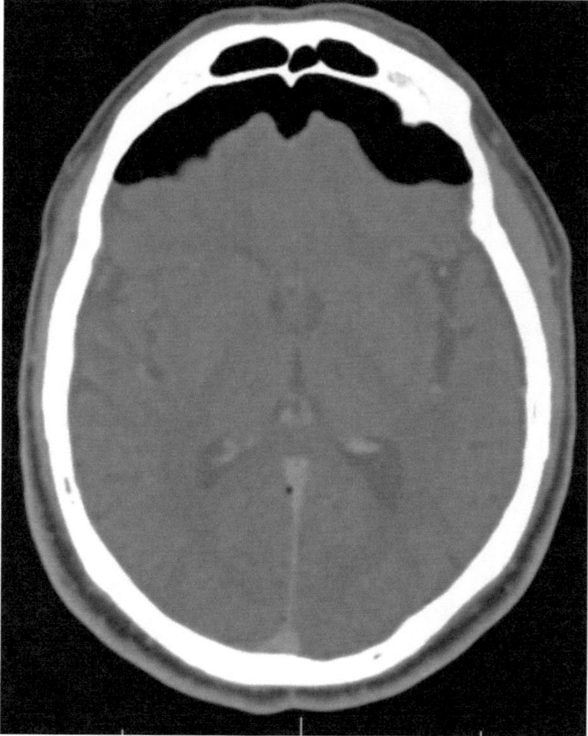

Fig. 30.1 Axial CT scan on postoperative day 1 demonstrating a Mt. Fuji sign (peaked frontal lobes surrounded and divided by intracranial air) in a patient who underwent endoscopic resection of sinonasal adenocarcinoma

progressive neurologic decline that can result in hemodynamic changes and instability, including eventual cardiac arrest [4]. In a recent literature review of tension pneumocephalus after skull base surgery, Biju et al. found only 11 reported cases, noting complete recovery among all but one patient and suggested this is to be a rare complication in the setting of endoscopic skull base surgery (ESBS) [3].

Management

Treatment includes evacuation of the air in an expedited fashion followed by definitive repair of the defect that is allowing the air to enter and build up, using a multi-layered approach [3]. While awaiting evacuation of air and repair, conservative measures, such as elevation of the head of bed, bed rest, and 100% inspired oxygen, may be initiated [3]. Castle-Kirzbaum et al. argue for avoidance of PPV in the postoperative setting; if first-line measures fail, such as oxygenation with a non-rebreather, then authors suggest initiation of intubation over PPV [4].

Orbital Complications

There is limited data available regarding orbital complications after ESBS. In a single institution review of 58 cases over a 6-year period, Naunheim et al. noted that only two patients (3.4%) experienced a temporary decrease in vision after surgery [7]. One patient (1.7%) noted new onset diplopia after surgery, which resolved within 150 days; one patient (1.7%) noted new onset epiphora, which did not resolve within the study follow-up period [7].

Yano et al. examined ESBS outcomes and complications in the setting of giant pituitary adenomas causing preoperative visual deficits [8]. The authors noted that 23/25 (92%) cases of preoperative visual impairment improved after surgery and one case of sixth nerve palsy resolved. No orbital complications were noted in their case series of 34.

Wang et al. performed a similar retrospective review at their institution focusing on an extended endonasal transsphenoidal approach to tuberculum sellae meningiomas [9]. The authors noted that of the 12 patients with confirmed preoperative visual deficits, 11 improved after surgery; in fact, 5 out of 12 patients had complete normalization of their vision. No patients experienced worsening of their vision after surgery.

The most comprehensive review of orbital complications after ESBS was performed by Borg et al. [10]. The authors examined 82 studies and 7460 cases over the last 65 years. They noted an overall complication rate of 17.1%, with an orbital complication rate of only 0.8%. Interestingly, when broken down by tumor type, esthesioneuroblastoma resections were associated with the greatest number of orbital complications at 6%, followed by clival lesions at 4%.

Ultimately, the literature provides limited information about the prevalence of orbital complications after ESBS. The overall rate of orbital complications appears to be minimal, ranging between 0.8% and 1.7% [7, 10]. However, evidence is hindered by poor study design, small sample sizes, and significant heterogeneity. Additional prospective studies with standardization of tumor types and definition of orbital complications are needed.

Intracranial Bleeding

Although the prevalence of intraoperative arterial injury is very low, the consequences can be dire and ultimately result in permanent neurologic deficits and/or death. Consequently, despite the lack of robust evidence (i.e., no randomized controlled trials, primarily case series and expert opinions), it is of the utmost importance that the surgeon be able to recognize these injuries and understand how to manage them based on the available literature.

Carotid Injury

Injury to the internal carotid artery (ICA) during ESBS is the most published about arterial injury and for good reason, given its potential to result in devastating sequelae. Based on the recent International Consensus Statement on Allergy and Rhinology for Endoscopic Skull-Base Surgery (ICAR: ESBS), the prevalence of ICA injury during ESBS ranges from 0.016 to 1%; the mortality associated with this injury is approximated at 10% [11]. The injury typically presents with a sudden gush of blood when working to expose and dissect tumor at the cranial base [11]. The injury occurs most commonly on the left side with a ratio of 1.3:1 [12]. It has been theorized this may be secondary to most surgeons being right-handed [12]. The most commonly injured site is the parasellar carotid [11]. Although not statistically significant, increased risk of injury has been demonstrated in the setting of the transclival/transpterygoid approach (4/534 cases) compared to the transsellar approach (3/1004 cases) [13]. Similarly, when broken down by tumor type, the greatest number of injuries occurred with chondroid tumors [13]. The risk is also increased in the setting of growth hormone-secreting pituitary adenomas and complex anatomy of the sphenoid sinus [14]. Additional risk factors for ICA injury include history of prior surgery, radiation, chemotherapy, and use of bromocriptine for pituitary tumors [11].

Initial management of an ICA injury in the endonasal endoscopic approach typically consists of recognizing the injury and packing the nasal cavity to achieve hemostasis. This allows time for the surgical team to discuss more definitive ICA preserving options, such as bipolar cautery, aneurysm clip placement, or muscle patch. Wang et al. demonstrated that regardless of which of these options (temporary packing or permanent control) was utilized, most patients subsequently underwent angiography to determine extent of injury and/or quality of repair [11]. The most commonly reported sequela from ICA injury in this setting was pseudoaneurysm of the carotid artery, although complete carotid occlusion/stenosis, dissection, active extravasation, thromboembolic events, and carotid cavernous fistulas were also observed [11]. Endovascular options for repair included endoluminal reconstruction/stenting, embolization of the pseudoaneurysm, or unilateral carotid sacrifice; the latter option was associated with a 21.7% risk of permanent neurologic deficits (Fig. 30.2) [11]. Most studies discussing carotid complications in the setting of ESBS recommend postoperative surveillance imaging to ensure no delayed sequelae of repair and/or injury develop [11]. However, there is no consensus on the type of imaging modality that should be used and no recommendation on the timing of imaging. Several studies have recommended close follow-up during the first month, as delayed ICA pathology has been identified during this period despite an initial negative angiogram [11]. Different studies have suggested an initial angiogram at 1-week post-repair, followed by additional imaging around 4–6 weeks, 3 months, 6 months, and possibly again at 12 months [11, 13, 15].

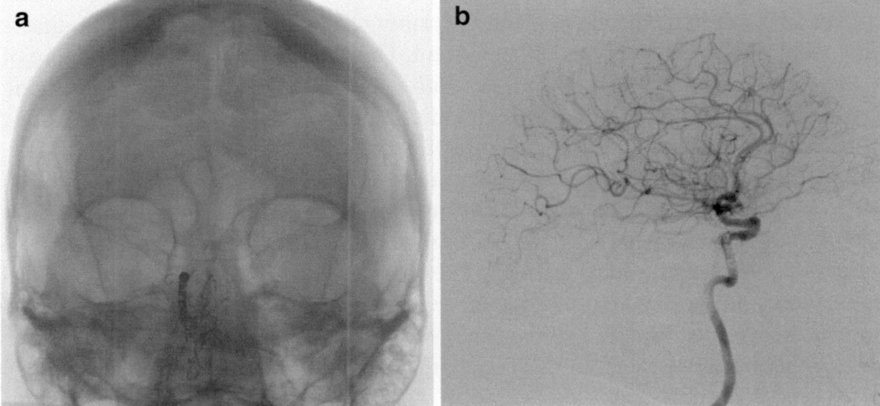

Fig. 30.2 Cerebral angiogram images of a patient who suffered a right internal carotid injury at the distal cavernous segment, proximal to the ophthalmic artery, at the time of endoscopic revision pituitary tumor resection. She was packed and taken immediately to the Neurosurgical Interventional Radiology suite where right ICA endovascular occlusion was performed with use of a pipeline stent (**a**). Angiogram images following this occlusion demonstrated perfusion through the anterior communicating artery to the right side of the brain (**b**)

Other Arterial and Vascular Injury

Postoperative subdural hematoma (SDH) after ESBS is a rare entity and has been reported only in a minority of case reports [16–20]. There is evidence to support that excess drainage of CSF can result in SDH [21, 22]. Theorized pathophysiology of the SDH in most of the previously mentioned cases of ESBS is predicated on a negative pressure related to significant CSF drainage, often in the setting of ongoing postoperative CSF rhinorrhea, resulting in a subdural collection [20]. Dallan et al. explain that high-flow CSF leaks can cause significant negative pressure and thus place tension on the bridging veins of the subarachnoid space, predisposing them to rupture and subsequent SDH formation [20]. For this reason, the authors recommend postoperative imaging within the first 24–48 h after ESBS. Additionally, postoperative intracranial hemorrhage can occur from partial resection of intracranial tumors such as pituitary adenomas, resulting in apoplexy that can further be complicated by vasospasm, or from unidentified arterial injury during surgery [23].

Babgi et al. reported a case of intradural arterial injury (anterior communicating artery) during ESBS for a planum sphenoidale meningioma and performed a literature review of other similar injuries related to endoscopic skull base surgeries [24]. The authors noted that these are rare occurrences with only 11 other reported cases described in the literature; in their review, additional injuries were noted to the anterior cerebral artery, posterior cerebral artery, ophthalmic artery, frontopolar artery, basilar artery, and posterior communicating artery [25–31]. The authors noted that these are typically avulsion injuries of perforator vessels in the setting of significant manipulation and/or tumor dissection [24]. Not uncommonly, the injury to the parent vessel is not immediately evident, but rather results in a pseudoaneurysm that is later localized on angiography or angiogram. The authors note the critical nature of the angiogram in the setting of intraoperative, intradural arterial injury, observing that many of the described cases required complete sacrifice of the parent artery, usually in the setting of adequate collateral circulation.

In general, the management of non-carotid arterial injuries is based mostly on surgeon-specific anecdote without evidence-based guidelines. Nevertheless, it is useful to understand what options the surgeon has at his or her disposal to manage intraoperative bleeding during ESBS. The muscle patch has been touted as a reliable, vessel-preserving option to manage major arterial bleeding; a randomized controlled trial (RCT) with varying types of artificially created carotid injuries in a sheep model demonstrated 100% efficacy in hemostasis with the muscle patch [32]. A retrospective analysis of nine cases of ICA injury treated with muscle patch similarly noted complete success in achieving hemostasis with only one instance of pseudoaneurysm [11]. In a separate animal model RCT comparing muscle patch, floseal, surgicel, chitosan gel, and U-clip, the authors noted that both the clip and patch demonstrated complete hemostasis with less overall blood loss during the encounter [33]. Although human RCTs are lacking, case series have demonstrated that additional effective hemostatic agents in the setting of venous bleeding during intracranial ESBS include fibrin and gelatin-thrombin matrix flowable agents, as well as warm saline irrigation, although the latter may take some time to take effect [11].

Ultimately, the quality of the evidence surrounding major arterial vessel injury and its management is limited to case series and expert opinions, as well as animal model studies. Although the occurrence of these complications is low, the associated consequences, including neurologic morbidity and potential mortality, can be disastrous. Thus, it is of paramount importance that the surgeon review and understand anatomic variations, practice meticulous technique and preparedness, and familiarize him/herself with available strategies and techniques to manage such injuries if they were to occur.

Sinonasal Morbidity Following ESBS

Although ESBS is considered minimally invasive, executing a safe and effective procedure of this type necessitates wide surgical access. This means that structures en route to the skull base are often altered, compromised, or resected to create a surgical field amenable to easy visualization, endoscopic instrument mobility, and frequent bi-nostril, two-surgeon technique. Depending on the surgical approach, common steps can include septectomy, inferior, middle, or superior turbinate resection, sinus surgery, and harvest of various sizes of nasal mucosa for planned skull base reconstruction. There is a tradeoff in the surgical insult to these sinonasal structures for the benefit of accessing ventral skull base pathology, which can result in patients experiencing significant nasal crusting, scarring, septal perforation, nasal structural compromise, sinonasal mucosal dysfunction, and sinusitis (Fig. 30.3). These can be further compounded by adjuvant therapies, such as radiation and chemotherapy.

Postoperative Sinonasal Quality of Life

In a systematic review of sinonasal morbidity following ESBS, the most commonly reported sinonasal symptoms experienced by patients were nasal crusting (50.8%), nasal discharge (40.4%), nasal obstruction (40.1%), and smell dysfunction (26.7%) [34]. These symptoms were worst in the immediate postoperative period but resolved within 3–4 months postoperatively, although some studies demonstrated this could take up to 6–12 months [35, 36]. Patients' postoperative sinonasal symptoms did not appear to be worse beyond the 3 month mark between endoscopic versus microscopic approaches [37], or based on whether or not a nasoseptal flap was utilized [38, 39]. Factors that did predispose to worse postoperative sinonasal symptoms included surgical extent secondary to increased complexity, anterior cranial fossa surgery versus central surgery, and overall patient health status [40–42]. Although long-term nasal crusting does not appear to be worse following use of a

Fig. 30.3 Coronal CT scan of a patient who is status post a combined open and endoscopic resection and adjuvant chemoradiation for a rare and highly aggressive sinonasal teratocarcinosarcoma. Post-treatment, he had ongoing mucosal dysfunction and nasal crusting requiring regular postoperative visits for management

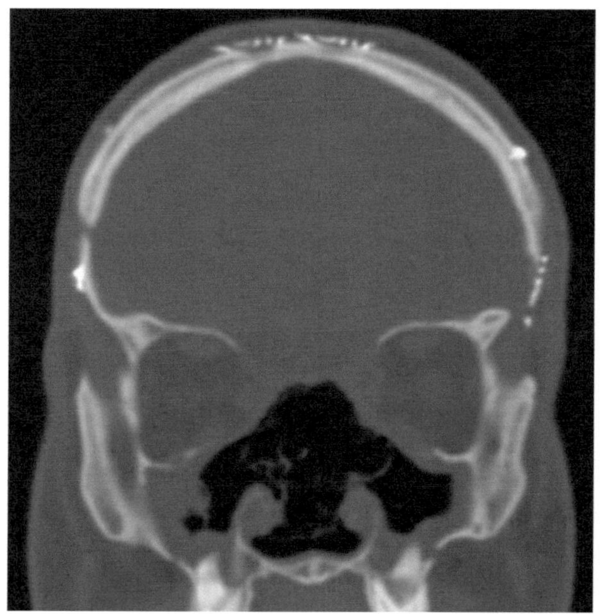

nasoseptal flap for reconstruction, the exposure of the septal cartilage and bone from harvest of the nasoseptal flap can be associated with significant crusting in the immediate postoperative period lasting a mean duration of 126 days [43]. This symptom, along with associated nasal obstruction, can be managed effectively with postoperative debridement, saline irrigations, and mitigation techniques such as placement of silastic sheeting to cover the donor site for 3–4 weeks while healing by secondary intention takes place (Fig. 30.4). Additional prevention options that have been described by some surgeons include use of a "rescue flap" instead of a nasoseptal flap when possible to minimize cartilage exposure and donor site morbidity [44, 45], as well as secondary coverage of the exposed cartilage with a reverse flap or a free mucosa grafts [46–48] in an effort to speed up remucosalization.

Nasal Structural Changes

Nasal structural changes appear to be uncommon complications of ESBS. Excluding the creation of a posterior septectomy, an intentional step in many skull base surgical approaches to provide necessary surgical access, unintended postoperative septal perforation is reported in more recent studies with larger patient series to occur in less than 1% of cases and is associated with use of a nasoseptal flap [49, 50]. A large series of post-ESBS nasal complications also reported nasal dorsal collapse to occur in 5.8% of patients, presumably secondary to septal devascularization [50]. In a series of 41 patients following ESBS, internal nasal valve collapse occurred in

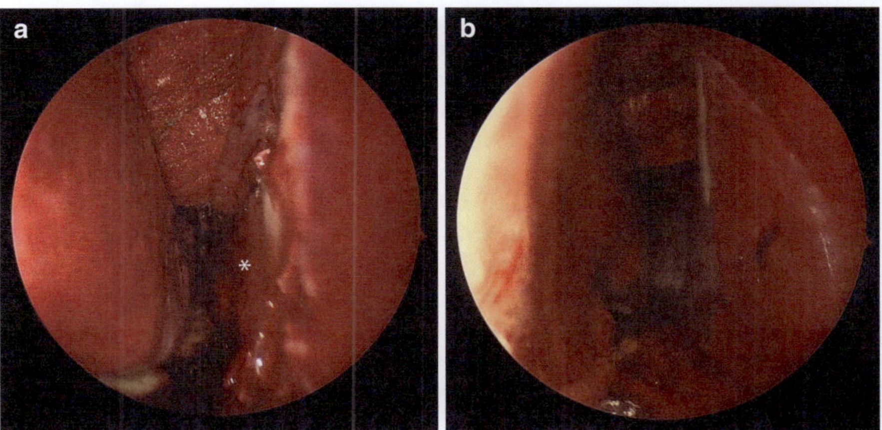

Fig. 30.4 Intraoperative images of a patient who underwent endoscopic resection of esthesioneuroblastoma with nasoseptal flap reconstruction. She had harvest of a right nasoseptal flap, with subsequent exposure of the septal cartilage (asterisk) (**a**). This donor site was then covered with a 0.51 mm silastic sheet secured to the septum with prolene suture (**b**). It was left in place for 4 weeks, allowing for complete remucosalization of the donor site with minimal crusting

14.6% of patients, while synechiae formation was present in 19.5% [51]. Careful intraoperative technique by the surgical team, utilization of dressings like silastic sheeting where appropriate, and regular postoperative debridement may help mitigate these nasal complications. Overall, a good understanding of these potential complications is important, since they can lead to prolonged patient quality of life impairment or even the need for a future nasal reconstructive surgery.

Sinusitis

The disturbance of otherwise healthy sinus anatomy and sinonasal mucosa as a necessary component of ESBS raises concern for the development of sinusitis as a common sequela. However, there is little evidence to demonstrate the development of ongoing sinusitis following ESBS beyond the immediate postoperative period. Although sinonasal symptoms typically occur for a few months following ESBS, these symptoms typically resolve thereafter; true chronic rhinosinusitis involves both subjective and objective diagnostic criteria for more than 12 weeks. In a review of 51 patients following transnasal transsphenoidal surgery, Deconde et al. reported an increase in anterior ethmoid mucosal thickening seen on 3 and 6 month postoperative CT imaging on the side of the surgical corridor compared to the control side [52]. This finding was associated with middle turbinate resection, maxillary antrostomy, and harvest of nasoseptal flap, with a lower incidence of this finding when native anatomy was preserved. In a similar size series by Langdon et al., patients had both Lund-Mackay scores and sinonasal symptoms evaluated before and after

ESBS. The authors demonstrated worse Lund-Mackay scores at 12 months postoperatively compared to baseline, especially in patients requiring nasoseptal flap reconstruction. However, sinonasal symptoms did not correlate with this change, having returned to baseline by 12 months postoperatively [53].

In a systematic review of post-ESBS sinonasal morbidity, mucocele formation was reported in 8% of cases across all age groups and up to 25% of pediatric cases. The latter observation is likely related to the delayed maturation of frontal sinuses in children, resulting in an already narrow frontal recess made even narrower and more prone to obstruction by an adjacent nasoseptal flap [34]. In addition to mucocele formation secondary to sinus stenosis, poor attention to the principles of sinonasal mucociliary clearance can lead to an increased rate of mucus recirculation if natural sinus ostia are not incorporated into surgical ostia. Although this should be standard practice in any functional endoscopic sinus surgery, adherence to this principle may be overshadowed by the skull base pathology and overall complex surgical plan, leading to symptomatic and ongoing post-nasal drip in these patients. Similarly, mucosal stripping beyond what is necessary for skull base access should be avoided due to the risk of mucociliary dysfunction development at these sites. The fact that rhinoogists are the most common surgeons performing these joint ESBS approaches with neurosurgeons helps minimize these risks, since their understanding of these principles is entrenched in their training.

Conclusion

The advent of endoscopic surgical approaches and reconstruction for skull base pathology has been a significant advance in the field. Although relatively infrequent, neurologic, vascular, orbital, and sinonasal complications do occur. The skull base surgeon must be aware and fully capable of managing these complications to optimize patient safety and surgical outcomes.

References

1. Goffart Y, Jorissen M, Daele J, et al. Minimally invasive endoscopic management of malignant sinonasal tumours. Acta Otorhinolaryngol Belg. 2000;54(2):221–32.
2. Kim BJ, Kim DW, Kim SW, et al. Endoscopic versus traditional craniofacial resection for patients with sinonasal tumors involving the anterior skull base. Clin Exp Otorhinolaryngol. 2008;1(3):148–53.
3. Biju RD, Wu J, Hussain Z. Tension pneumocephalus after skull base surgery. A case report and review of literature. J Clin Neurosci. 2020;75:218–20.
4. Castle-Kirszbaum M, Wang YY, King J, et al. Tension pneumocephalus from positive pressure ventilation following endoscopic skull base surgery: case series and an institutional protocol for the management of postoperative respiratory distress. World Neurosurg. 2020;141:357–62.

5. Kerr EE, Prevedello DM, Jamshidi A, Ditzel Filho LF, Otto BA, Carrau RL. Immediate complications associated with high-flow cerebrospinal fluid egress during endoscopic endonasal skull base surgery. Neurosurg Focus. 2014;37(4):E3.

6. Yin C, Chen BY. Tension pneumocephalus from skull base surgery: a case report and review of the literature. Surg Neurol Int. 2018;9:128.

7. Naunheim MR, Sedaghat AR, Lin DT, et al. Immediate and delayed complications following endoscopic skull base surgery. J Neurol Surg B Skull Base. 2015;76(5):390–6.

8. Yano S, Hide T, Shinojima N. Efficacy and complications of endoscopic skull base surgery for giant pituitary adenomas. World Neurosurg. 2017;99:533–42.

9. Wang Q, Lu XJ, Ji WY, et al. Visual outcome after extended endoscopic endonasal transsphenoidal surgery for tuberculum sellae meningiomas. World Neurosurg. 2010;73(6):694–700.

10. Borg A, Kirkman MA, Choi D. Endoscopic endonasal anterior skull base surgery: a systematic review of complications during the past 65 years. World Neurosurg. 2016;95:383–91.

11. Wang EW, Zanation AM, Gardner PA, et al. ICAR: endoscopic skull-base surgery. Int Forum Allergy Rhinol. 2019;9(S3):S145–365.

12. Chin OY, Ghosh R, Fang CH, Baredes S, Liu JK, Eloy JA. Internal carotid artery injury in endoscopic endonasal surgery: a systematic review. Laryngoscope. 2016;126(3):582–90.

13. Gardner PA, Tormenti MJ, Pant H, Fernandez-Miranda JC, Snyderman CH, Horowitz MB. Carotid artery injury during endoscopic endonasal skull base surgery: incidence and outcomes. Neurosurgery. 2013;73(2 Suppl Operative):ons261–9; discussion ons269-270.

14. Zada G, Cavallo LM, Esposito F, et al. Transsphenoidal surgery in patients with acromegaly: operative strategies for overcoming technically challenging anatomical variations. Neurosurg Focus. 2010;29(4):E8.

15. Padhye V, Valentine R, Wormald PJ. Management of carotid artery injury in endonasal surgery. Int Arch Otorhinolaryngol. 2014;18(Suppl 2):S173–8.

16. Menon G, Bahuleyan B, Nair S. Acute subdural hematoma after transsphenoidal surgery. J Clin Neurosci. 2009;16(1):160–2.

17. Tanaka Y, Kobayashi S, Hongo K, Tada T, Kakizawa Y. Chronic subdural hematoma after transsphenoidal surgery. J Clin Neurosci. 2002;9(3):323–5.

18. Fukuhara N, Nishioka H, Yamada S. Acute subdural hematoma immediately after extended transsphenoidal surgery for craniopharyngioma. Turk Neurosurg. 2017;27(2):309–11.

19. Eloqayli HCJ, Vik A. Acute spontaneous subdural hematoma after transsphenoidal surgery. Acta Neurochir. 2006;148:587–90.

20. Dallan I, Lenzi R, Muscatello L, Bignami M, Battaglia P, Castelnuovo P. Subdural haematoma after endoscopic skull base surgery: case report and lesson learned. Clin Neurol Neurosurg. 2011;113(6):496–8.

21. Gaucher DJ Jr, Perez JA Jr. Subdural hematoma following lumbar puncture. Arch Intern Med. 2002;162(16):1904–5.

22. Mizuno J, Mummaneni PV, Rodts GE, Barrow DL. Recurrent subdural hematoma caused by cerebrospinal fluid leakage. Case report. J Neurosurg Spine. 2006;4(2):183–5.

23. Vaz-Guimaraes F, Su SY, Fernandez-Miranda JC, Wang EW, Snyderman CH, Gardner PA. Hemostasis in endoscopic endonasal skull base surgery. J Neurol Surg B Skull Base. 2015;76(4):296–302.

24. Babgi M, Alsaleh S, Babgi Y, Baeesa S, Ajlan A. Intracranial intradural vascular injury during endoscopic endonasal transsphenoidal surgery: a case report and literature review. J Neurol Surg Rep. 2020;81(3):e52–8.

25. Romero A, Lal Gangadharan J, Bander ED, Gobin YP, Anand VK, Schwartz TH. Managing arterial injury in endoscopic skull base surgery: case series and review of the literature. Oper Neurosurg (Hagerstown). 2017;13(1):138–49.

26. Ciceri EF, Regna-Gladin C, Erbetta A, et al. Iatrogenic intracranial pseudoaneurysms: neuroradiological and therapeutic considerations, including endovascular options. Neurol Sci. 2006;27(5):317–22.

27. Kassam AB, Prevedello DM, Carrau RL, et al. Endoscopic endonasal skull base surgery: analysis of complications in the authors' initial 800 patients. J Neurosurg. 2011;114(6):1544–68.

28. Cinar C, Bozkaya H, Parildar M, Oran I. Endovascular management of vascular injury during transsphenoidal surgery. Interv Neuroradiol. 2013;19(1):102–9.
29. Rodriguez-Hernandez A, Huang C, Lawton MT. Superior cerebellar artery-posterior cerebral artery bypass: in situ bypass for posterior cerebral artery revascularization. J Neurosurg. 2013;118(5):1053–7.
30. Lee CH, Chen SM, Lui TN. Posterior cerebral artery pseudoaneurysm, a rare complication of pituitary tumor transsphenoidal surgery: case report and literature review. World Neurosurg. 2015;84(5):1493.e1491–3.
31. Morinaga Y, Nii K, Sakamoto K, Inoue R, Mitsutake T, Hanada H. Stent-assisted coil embolization for a ruptured posterior communicating artery pseudoaneurysm after endoscopic transsphenoidal surgery for pituitary adenoma. World Neurosurg. 2019;123:301–5.
32. Padhye V, Valentine R, Paramasivan S, et al. Early and late complications of endoscopic hemostatic techniques following different carotid artery injury characteristics. Int Forum Allergy Rhinol. 2014;4(8):651–7.
33. Valentine R, Boase S, Jervis-Bardy J, Dones Cabral JD, Robinson S, Wormald PJ. The efficacy of hemostatic techniques in the sheep model of carotid artery injury. Int Forum Allergy Rhinol. 2011;1(2):118–22.
34. Awad AJ, Mohyeldin A, El-Sayed IH, Aghi MK. Sinonasal morbidity following endoscopic endonasal skull base surgery. Clin Neurol Neurosurg. 2015;130:162–7.
35. Balaker AE, Bergsneider M, Martin NA, Wang MB. Evolution of sinonasal symptoms following endoscopic anterior skull base surgery. Skull Base. 2010;20(4):245–51.
36. Davies BM, Tirr E, Wang YY, Gnanalingham KK. Transient exacerbation of nasal symptoms following endoscopic transsphenoidal surgery for pituitary tumors: a prospective study. J Neurol Surg B Skull Base. 2017;78(3):266–72.
37. Little AS, Kelly DF, Milligan J, et al. Comparison of sinonasal quality of life and health status in patients undergoing microscopic and endoscopic transsphenoidal surgery for pituitary lesions: a prospective cohort study. J Neurosurg. 2015;123(3):799–807.
38. Harvey RJ, Malek J, Winder M, et al. Sinonasal morbidity following tumour resection with and without nasoseptal flap reconstruction. Rhinology. 2015;53(2):122–8.
39. McCoul ED, Patel AS, Bedrosian JC, Anand VK, Schwartz TH. Intranasal cross-sectional area and quality of life changes following endoscopic transsphenoidal skull base surgery. Int Forum Allergy Rhinol. 2015;5(12):1124–8.
40. de Almeida JR, Snyderman CH, Gardner PA, Carrau RL, Vescan AD. Nasal morbidity following endoscopic skull base surgery: a prospective cohort study. Head Neck. 2011;33(4):547–51.
41. de Almeida JR, Witterick IJ, Gullane PJ, et al. Physical morbidity by surgical approach and tumor location in skull base surgery. Head Neck. 2013;35(4):493–9.
42. Little AS, Kelly D, Milligan J, et al. Predictors of sinonasal quality of life and nasal morbidity after fully endoscopic transsphenoidal surgery. J Neurosurg. 2015;122(6):1458–65.
43. Pant H, Bhatki AM, Snyderman CH, et al. Quality of life following endonasal skull base surgery. Skull Base. 2010;20(1):35–40.
44. Rawal RB, Kimple AJ, Dugar DR, Zanation AM. Minimizing morbidity in endoscopic pituitary surgery: outcomes of the novel nasoseptal rescue flap technique. Otolaryngol Head Neck Surg. 2012;147(3):434–7.
45. Rivera-Serrano CM, Snyderman CH, Gardner P, et al. Nasoseptal "rescue" flap: a novel modification of the nasoseptal flap technique for pituitary surgery. Laryngoscope. 2011;121(5):990–3.
46. Caicedo-Granados E, Carrau R, Snyderman CH, et al. Reverse rotation flap for reconstruction of donor site after vascular pedicled nasoseptal flap in skull base surgery. Laryngoscope. 2010;120(8):1550–2.
47. Kasemsiri P, Carrau RL, Otto BA, et al. Reconstruction of the pedicled nasoseptal flap donor site with a contralateral reverse rotation flap: technical modifications and outcomes. Laryngoscope. 2013;123(11):2601–4.

48. Yoo F, Kuan EC, Bergsneider M, Wang MB. Free mucosal graft reconstruction of the septum after nasoseptal flap harvest: a novel technique using a posterior septal free mucosal graft. J Neurol Surg B Skull Base. 2017;78(2):201–6.
49. Cheng Y, Xue F, Wang TY, et al. Analyses and treatments of postoperative nasal complications after endonasal transsphenoidal resection of pituitary neoplasms. Medicine (Baltimore). 2017;96(15):e6614.
50. Rowan NR, Wang EW, Gardner PA, Fernandez-Miranda JC, Snyderman CH. Nasal deformities following nasoseptal flap reconstruction of skull base defects. J Neurol Surg B Skull Base. 2016;77(1):14–8.
51. Dolci RLL, Miyake MM, Tateno DA, et al. Postoperative otorhinolaryngologic complications in transnasal endoscopic surgery to access the skull base. Braz J Otorhinolaryngol. 2017;83(3):349–55.
52. Deconde AS, Vira D, Thompson CF, Wang MB, Bergsneider M, Suh JD. Radiologic assessment of the paranasal sinuses after endoscopic skull base surgery. J Neurol Surg B Skull Base. 2013;74(6):351–7.
53. Langdon C, Ensenat J, Rioja E, et al. Long-term radiological findings after endonasal endoscopic approach to the skull base. Am J Otolaryngol. 2016;37(2):103–7.

Chapter 31
Outcomes of Anterior Skull Base Reconstruction

Jacob G. Eide, Tapan D. Patel, Nithin D. Adappa, and James N. Palmer

Introduction

Since the advent of endoscopic endonasal approach (EEA) for intradural pathology, EEA has allowed the skull base surgeon to access the entire ventral skull base, including the anterior, middle, and posterior cranial fossae [1]. Reconstruction of defects created during these approaches presents a unique challenge. Multiple factors need to be considered when reconstructing the skull base defect, including the size of the defect, availability of grafts and vascular flaps, technical difficulty, effects of postoperative radiation, and morbidity to the patient. In general, smaller defects may be repaired with avascular grafts, while larger defects with higher flow CSF leaks may require vascularized flaps for reliable reconstruction [2].

Goals of anterior skull base reconstruction, whether open or endoscopic, remain the same: a multilayered watertight closure of the skull base defect in order to prevent a postoperative cerebrospinal fluid (CSF) leak and prevent the possibility of future pneumocephalus or ascending infection from the nasal cavity [3]. As skull base defects are rarely exactly alike, a reconstructive plan must always be tailored to the individual patient. In certain clinical scenarios, a commonly used reconstructive method may not be available and may warrant one that is less often used. Therefore, it is important for the reconstructive surgeon to be comfortable with

J. G. Eide · T. D. Patel · N. D. Adappa
Department of Otorhinolaryngology, University of Pennsylvania, Philadelphia, PA, USA
e-mail: jeide1@hfhs.org; tapan.patel@pennmedicine.upenn.edu;
Nithin.adappa@pennmedicine.upenn.edu

J. N. Palmer (✉)
Division of Rhinology and Skull Base Surgery, Department of Otorhinolaryngology, University of Pennsylvania, Philadelphia, PA, USA

Division of Rhinology and Skull Base Surgery, Hospital of the University of Pennsylvania, Philadelphia, PA, USA
e-mail: james.palmer@pennmedicine.upenn.edu

© The Author(s), under exclusive license to Springer Nature Switzerland AG 2023
E. C. Kuan et al. (eds.), *Skull Base Reconstruction*,
https://doi.org/10.1007/978-3-031-27937-9_31

variety of different surgical techniques. Here, we review the reconstructive options for reconstruction of the anterior skull base and their outcomes published in the literature.

Avascular Grafts

A variety of materials are available for reconstruction of the anterior skull base defects that are smaller than 1 cm. Avascular grafts including autologous grafts, acellular human dermis grafts, and engineering collagen grafts are available. Autologous grafts include fat, fascia, bone, cartilage, and free mucosal grafts harvested from the patient. A multitude of options are available, but the most common include intranasal free mucosal grafts, septal cartilage, fat from abdomen or leg, temporalis fascia or fascia lata, and free bone grafts. While they have fallen somewhat out of favor since the advent of vascularized nasoseptal flaps, free grafts remain a useful adjunct for large defects or primary reconstruction in recurrent defects of the skull base without other reconstructive options.

Middle turbinate grafts are the most commonly used intranasal graft, and most free grafts are fully integrated into the mucosa in 8 weeks [4]. Free grafts have limited donor site morbidity and are often quick to harvest; however, it has been reported that free grafts have an approximately 20% decrease in size and should be harvested larger than the skull base defect [5]. While outcome data is limited, endoscopic repair of CSF leak with free mucosal graft has been reported to be 94.4% by Lanza et al. in retrospective review [6]. Larger meta-analyses and reviews would suggest a slightly lower initial success rate of 90–91% with an overall success rate of 97–98% after revision endoscopic repair [7, 8]. However, it should be noted that in large (>2 cm) skull base defects, free grafts have had leak rates as high as 20–30% [9]. Complications related to free graft harvest include crusting, nasal septal perforation, and, if an extranasal site is used for harvest, hematoma, infection, and scarring. Fortunately, all of the aforementioned complications remain uncommon [10]. Meningitis following repair was reported in 2.5% of patients, significantly lower than the rate of meningitis in patients with active CSF leak without treatment [7].

Vascularized Intranasal Flaps

Initially described by Hadad et al., the nasoseptal flap (NSF) remains the mainstay of endoscopic skull base reconstruction and was reported in the initial retrospective review of 50 patients to have a 95% initial success rate [11]. The ease of harvest, reliability, and ability to tailor the flap to the skull base defect have made the NSF ubiquitous in skull base reconstruction. Anatomic studies suggest that the NSF has sufficient mobility and length to cover the entirety of the anterior skull base [12]. While good outcomes with avascular grafts have been reported, the success rate falls to 50–70% in high flow CSF leaks, which are encountered if dissection is required into arachnoid cistern or ventricle [2]. Success rates have been reported variably, with one retrospective review noting a 4% overall CSF leak rate, with a 6.7% rate if a high flow intraoperative CSF leak was encountered [2]. A systematic review of CSF leak rate outcomes would suggest a somewhat higher leak rate with a 15.6% leak rate for free grafts and a 6.7% leak rate for vascularized flap closure [13].

Morbidity apart from CSF leak remains low with septal perforation (1.3%), mucocele formation (0.7%), and prolonged skull base crusting (5.3%), especially following radiation therapy, being reported [14]. Importantly, as NSFs are used more commonly, surgeons have had to increasingly manage previous reconstruction to access the skull base for recurrent or persistent lesions. Initial data suggests that previous NSF repair can be carefully removed from the skull base and re-used after lesion resection without devascularization of the flap [15]. The rate of necrosis of has also been investigated. In a review of 601 patients who underwent NSF by Chabot et al., 49 patients (8.2%) returned to the OR for CSF leak or suspicion of meningitis [16]. Of these patients, eight patients (1.3% overall) had necrotic NSFs with two patients (0.3% overall) who were noted to have an epidural empyema with a viable NSF. They also noted that non-enhancement of the flap on contrasted MRI, fat graft, and previous surgery was associated with cases of NSF necrosis [16].

While NSFs are by far the most common vascularized intranasal flaps performed, in multiply recurrent lesions or sinonasal malignancies involving the septum, they may not be available. Vascularized flaps based off the inferior and middle turbinate as well as nasal side wall have all been successfully used. Initial results are promising, but it should be noted that these flaps are often used in salvage situations where the NSF is not available or challenging cases where more coverage is needed [17, 18]. For instance, in a review of their experience with lateral nasal wall flaps, Lavigne et al. found that they had an initial success rate of 75%, significantly lower than reported for NSF [19]. However, these flaps were performed in cases where the NSF was previously used for surgical repair (41.7%), patients had CSF leak after NSF partial loss (41.7%), or CSF leak due to insufficient NSF coverage (16.6%) [19]. Clearly, these patients represent a more challenging reconstruction. Middle turbinate flap outcomes have been reported in only small series with initial results showing successful middle turbinate flap use in ten patients undergoing transsphenoidal surgery with one other study showing one of the two middle turbinate flaps undergoing necrosis after repair [18, 20].

Locoregional Flaps

A variety of locoregional flaps have been used for the skull base with the pericranial flap being the most commonly used. Typically, a pericranial flap is harvested via a coronal incision although a modified endoscopic harvest technique has been described [21]. The flap offers a large amount of pliable tissue that can be used to reconstruct defects in the posterior table of the frontal sinus or ethmoid roof. Similarly, temporoparietal fascia tunneled flaps have also been utilized as well as submental locoregional flaps. Number of reported cases for both of these flaps remains low, but initial data suggests they are reasonable alternatives [22–24].

Local flaps have been estimated to fail in 0–10% of cases (including both partial and total flap failure) with CSF leak rates reported from 0–14% and pneumocephalus in 0–7% of cases in a recent systematic review [25]. Another smaller retrospective review showed a similar success rate of 87.5% with 11.1% rate of CSF leak and meningitis [26]. Interestingly, when compared, local and free flaps had a similar, relatively high rate of major complications (35% and 31%, respectively); however, this data is based on a small cohort primarily before the endoscopic era, so it is unclear if this conclusion remains true with newer techniques [27].

Free Tissue Transfer

Currently, the role of free tissue transfer in anterior skull base reconstruction has remained limited primarily due to the reliability of other reconstruction options as well as the increased operative time and need for additional surgical training. However, in large open craniofacial resections, multiply recurrent tumors, and patients who have persistent reconstruction failure due to radiation therapy, microvascular free flap reconstruction remains an important tool in skull base reconstruction. Choice of free flap reconstruction is outside the scope of this chapter, but radial forearm and anterolateral thigh free flaps are commonly used, although fibula, scapula, latissimus dorsi, and rectus abdominis flaps have all been described [28].

In a recent systematic review of 22 studies including retrospective data on 1628 patients undergoing free flap reconstruction, reported outcomes were heterogeneous. Of note, some authors reported combined free and local flap reconstruction, and there is sparse data in regard to outcomes by free flap type. However, the authors estimate a flap complication rate of 0–14%, a partial flap failure rate of 4.1%, and a 7.7% total flap failure rate [25]. The rate of postoperative CSF leak ranged from 1.6–13.5%, and postoperative pneumocephalus was reported between 1.6% and 7.1%. Finally, the operative mortality of free flap reconstruction ranged from 0 to 7%, highlighting the complexity and challenge of repairing large or recalcitrant skull base defects [25]. Donor site morbidity was not reported in these studies but is also a consideration when performing free tissue transfer.

Quality of Life Outcomes

As surgeons have become more facile at reliably reconstructing the skull base, there has naturally been increased attention on long-term quality of life metrics and efforts to reduce morbidity. One retrospective study suggested that SNOT-22

(Sinonasal Outcome Test) scores improved or stayed the same in 63% of patients and worsened in the remaining 37% in long-term follow-up (>3 years) [29]. Interestingly, a recent systematic review of adult patients undergoing skull base surgery suggested that patients with impaired sinonasal function prior to skull base surgery were improved immediately after surgery and in long-term follow-up. Patients with low preoperative SNOT-22 scores did not worsen over the same time period, suggesting that endoscopic skull base surgery does not worsen sinonasal function [30]. Of note, while commonly used in the skull base literature, SNOT-22 has only been validated for chronic rhinosinusitis, so it may not be a valid metric for this patient population [31]. There have been efforts to make a skull base surgery-specific quality of life tool, but reporting remains variable [32].

Preservation of olfaction can be challenging in skull base malignancies given the need to disrupt olfactory tissue for exposure or need to resect the olfactory cleft if involved with tumor. Furthermore, there is frequent need for postoperative radiation therapy, which further diminishes sense of smell. Interestingly, there is conflicting data on the impact of skull base surgery on the disruption of olfaction [33]. The most robust study to date was completed by Kim and colleagues in 2014 in which 226 patients underwent preoperative and 6 month olfactory testing with the Visual Analog Scale, Connecticut Chemosensory Clinical Research Center Test, and Cross-Cultural Smell Identification Test. They found significant decreases in olfaction in patients over 30 years of age and in those who had bilateral nasoseptal flaps (NSF) or unilateral NSF with contralateral rescue flap [34].

Other data attempting to determine the impact of skull base surgery on olfaction is more contradictory. Rotenberg et al. were the first to describe postoperative symptomatic hyposmia, as measured by the University of Pennsylvania Smell Identification Test (UPSIT) [35]. Meanwhile, prospective data by Bedrosian et al. found transient decreases in smell and taste 6 weeks postoperatively but normalization of both sense to preoperative levels at 12-month follow-up as measured by the Anterior Skull Base Questionnaire [36]. Hart et al. found similar transient decreases in olfaction after pituitary surgery that later normalized, and Sowerby et al. found no difference in olfaction [37, 38]. Yet another study showed improved or stable smell in 88% of patients undergoing pituitary surgery with worsening olfaction in the remaining 12% [39]. Li and colleagues looked specifically at surgical manipulation of the superior turbinate given its density of olfactory fibers. They compared partial resection versus preservation of the turbinate with lateralization, and although the 6-month postoperative threshold test was diminished in the resection group, overall olfaction measured by smell identification ("Sniffin Sticks") test was the same [40].

Given the conflicting data, it is difficult to make broad generalizations on olfactory outcomes after skull base reconstruction. The heterogeneity of approaches, variations in surgical technique, lack of standardization in olfactory testing methods, and relatively small number of patients make it difficult to establish firm rates of olfactory loss of surgery. However, given the state of data, further study is warranted, and patients should be counseled that loss of smell is possible when undergoing skull base resection and reconstruction.

Conclusion

Skull base reconstruction has improved over the last two decades, and there are more options for repair than ever before. In general, outcomes remain excellent for reconstruction with appropriate technique, and attention has turned to improving post-treatment quality of life. The main impediment to the current state of the research is a lack of standardization in reporting making it difficult to compare data.

References

1. Snyderman CH, Pant H, Carrau RL, Prevedello D, Gardner P, Kassam AB. What are the limits of endoscopic sinus surgery?: the expanded endonasal approach to the skull base. Keio J Med. 2009;58(3):152–60.
2. Patel MR, Stadler ME, Snyderman CH, et al. How to choose? Endoscopic skull base reconstructive options and limitations. Skull Base. 2010;20(6):397–404. https://doi.org/10.1055/s-0030-1253573.
3. Wang EW, Zanation AM, Gardner PA, et al. ICAR: endoscopic skull-base surgery. Int Forum Allergy Rhinol. 2019;9(S3):S145–s365. https://doi.org/10.1002/alr.22326.
4. Reyes C, Mason E, Solares CA. Panorama of reconstruction of skull base defects: from traditional open to endonasal endoscopic approaches, from free grafts to microvascular flaps. Int Arch Otorhinolaryngol. 2014;18(Suppl 2):S179–86. https://doi.org/10.1055/s-0034-1395268.
5. Hosemann W, Goede U, Sauer M. Wound healing of mucosal autografts for frontal cerebrospinal fluid leaks–clinical and experimental investigations. Rhinology. 1999;37(3):108–12.
6. Lanza DC, O'Brien DA, Kennedy DW. Endoscopic repair of cerebrospinal fluid fistulae and encephaloceles. Laryngoscope. 1996;106(9):1119–25. https://doi.org/10.1097/00005537-199609000-00015.
7. Banks CA, Palmer JN, Chiu AG, O'Malley BW Jr, Woodworth BA, Kennedy DW. Endoscopic closure of CSF rhinorrhea: 193 cases over 21 years. Otolaryngol Head Neck Surg. 2009;140(6):826–33. https://doi.org/10.1016/j.otohns.2008.12.060.
8. Hegazy HM, Carrau RL, Snyderman CH, Kassam A, Zweig J. Transnasal endoscopic repair of cerebrospinal fluid rhinorrhea: a meta-analysis. Laryngoscope. 2000;110(7):1166–72. https://doi.org/10.1097/00005537-200007000-00019.
9. Liu JK, Schmidt RF, Choudhry OJ, Shukla PA, Eloy JA. Surgical nuances for nasoseptal flap reconstruction of cranial base defects with high-flow cerebrospinal fluid leaks after endoscopic skull base surgery. Neurosurg Focus. 2012;32(6):E7. https://doi.org/10.3171/2012.5.Focus1255.
10. Dadgostar A, Okpaleke C, Al-Asousi F, Javer A. The application of a free nasal floor mucoperiosteal graft in endoscopic sinus surgery. Am J Rhinol Allergy. 2017;31(3):196–9. https://doi.org/10.2500/ajra.2017.31.4430.
11. Hadad G, Bassagasteguy L, Carrau RL, et al. A novel reconstructive technique after endoscopic expanded endonasal approaches: vascular pedicle nasoseptal flap. Laryngoscope. 2006;116(10):1882–6. https://doi.org/10.1097/01.mlg.0000234933.37779.e4.
12. Pinheiro-Neto CD, Ramos HF, Peris-Celda M, et al. Study of the nasoseptal flap for endoscopic anterior cranial base reconstruction. Laryngoscope. 2011;121(12):2514–20. https://doi.org/10.1002/lary.22353.
13. Harvey RJ, Parmar P, Sacks R, Zanation AM. Endoscopic skull base reconstruction of large dural defects: a systematic review of published evidence. Laryngoscope. 2012;122(2):452–9. https://doi.org/10.1002/lary.22475.

14. Thorp BD, Sreenath SB, Ebert CS, Zanation AM. Endoscopic skull base reconstruction: a review and clinical case series of 152 vascularized flaps used for surgical skull base defects in the setting of intraoperative cerebrospinal fluid leak. Neurosurg Focus. 2014;37(4):E4. https://doi.org/10.3171/2014.7.Focus14350.

15. Zanation AM, Carrau RL, Snyderman CH, et al. Nasoseptal flap takedown and reuse in revision endoscopic skull base reconstruction. Laryngoscope. 2011;121(1):42–6. https://doi.org/10.1002/lary.21162.

16. Chabot JD, Patel CR, Hughes MA, et al. Nasoseptal flap necrosis: a rare complication of endoscopic endonasal surgery. J Neurosurg. 2018;128(5):1463–72. https://doi.org/10.3171/2017.2.Jns161582.

17. Choby GW, Pinheiro-Neto CD, de Almeida JR, et al. Extended inferior turbinate flap for endoscopic reconstruction of skull base defects. J Neurol Surg B Skull Base. 2014;75(4):225–30. https://doi.org/10.1055/s-0033-1358791.

18. Patel MR, Taylor RJ, Hackman TG, et al. Beyond the nasoseptal flap: outcomes and pearls with secondary flaps in endoscopic endonasal skull base reconstruction. Laryngoscope. 2014;124(4):846–52. https://doi.org/10.1002/lary.24319.

19. Lavigne P, Vega MB, Ahmed OH, Gardner PA, Snyderman CH, Wang EW. Lateral nasal wall flap for endoscopic reconstruction of the skull base: anatomical study and clinical series. Int Forum Allergy Rhinol. 2020;10(5):673–8. https://doi.org/10.1002/alr.22534.

20. Simal Julián JA, Miranda Lloret P, Cárdenas Ruiz-Valdepeñas E, Barges Coll J, Beltrán Giner A, Botella AC. Middle turbinate vascularized flap for skull base reconstruction after an expanded endonasal approach. Acta Neurochir. 2011;153(9):1827–32. https://doi.org/10.1007/s00701-011-1064-8.

21. Zanation AM, Snyderman CH, Carrau RL, Kassam AB, Gardner PA, Prevedello DM. Minimally invasive endoscopic pericranial flap: a new method for endonasal skull base reconstruction. Laryngoscope. 2009;119(1):13–8. https://doi.org/10.1002/lary.20022.

22. Chang BA, Ryan Hall S, Howard BE, et al. Submental flap for reconstruction of anterior skull base, orbital, and high facial defects. Am J Otolaryngol. 2019;40(2):218–23. https://doi.org/10.1016/j.amjoto.2018.11.008.

23. Ferrari M, Vural A, Schreiber A, et al. Side-door temporoparietal fascia flap: a novel strategy for anterior skull base reconstruction. World Neurosurg. 2019;126:e360–70. https://doi.org/10.1016/j.wneu.2019.02.056.

24. Fortes FS, Carrau RL, Snyderman CH, et al. Transpterygoid transposition of a temporoparietal fascia flap: a new method for skull base reconstruction after endoscopic expanded endonasal approaches. Laryngoscope. 2007;117(6):970–6. https://doi.org/10.1097/MLG.0b013e3180471482.

25. Lim X, Rajagopal R, Silva P, Jeyaretna DS, Mykula R, Potter M. A systematic review on outcomes of anterior skull base reconstruction. J Plast Reconstr Aesthet Surg. 2020;73(11):1940–50. https://doi.org/10.1016/j.bjps.2020.05.044.

26. Jalisi S, O'Gara B, Toshkezi G, Chin L. Local vascularized flap reconstruction of the skull base-clinical outcomes and analysis. World Neurosurg. 2015;83(1):87–92. https://doi.org/10.1016/j.wneu.2012.11.073.

27. Califano J, Cordeiro PG, Disa JJ, et al. Anterior cranial base reconstruction using free tissue transfer: changing trends. Head Neck. 2003;25(2):89–96. https://doi.org/10.1002/hed.10179.

28. Bell EB, Cohen ER, Sargi Z, Leibowitz J. Free tissue reconstruction of the anterior skull base: a review. World J Otorhinolaryngol Head Neck Surg. 2020;6(2):132–6. https://doi.org/10.1016/j.wjorl.2020.01.004.

29. Riley CA, Tabaee A, Conley L, et al. Long-term sinonasal outcomes after endoscopic skull base surgery with nasoseptal flap reconstruction. Laryngoscope. 2019;129(5):1035–40. https://doi.org/10.1002/lary.27637.

30. Bhenswala PN, Schlosser RJ, Nguyen SA, Munawar S, Rowan NR. Sinonasal quality-of-life outcomes after endoscopic endonasal skull base surgery. Int Forum Allergy Rhinol. 2019;9(10):1105–18. https://doi.org/10.1002/alr.22398.

31. Bolk KG, Roth KA, Sharma A, Crosby DL. Patient-reported outcomes in sinonasal and skull base malignancy: an assessment of study quality and clinical relevance. Am J Rhinol Allergy. 2020;34(6):822–9. https://doi.org/10.1177/1945892420930967.
32. Little AS, Kelly D, Milligan J, et al. Prospective validation of a patient-reported nasal quality-of-life tool for endonasal skull base surgery: The Anterior Skull Base Nasal Inventory-12. J Neurosurg. 2013;119(4):1068–74. https://doi.org/10.3171/2013.3.JNS122032.
33. Patel ZM, DelGaudio JM. Olfaction following endoscopic skull base surgery. Curr Opin Otolaryngol Head Neck Surg. 2016;24(1):70–4. https://doi.org/10.1097/moo.0000000000000216.
34. Kim BY, Kang SG, Kim SW, et al. Olfactory changes after endoscopic endonasal transsphenoidal approach for skull base tumors. Laryngoscope. 2014;124(11):2470–5. https://doi.org/10.1002/lary.24674.
35. Rotenberg BW, Saunders S, Duggal N. Olfactory outcomes after endoscopic transsphenoidal pituitary surgery. Laryngoscope. 2011;121(8):1611–3. https://doi.org/10.1002/lary.21890.
36. Bedrosian JC, McCoul ED, Raithatha R, Akselrod OA, Anand VK, Schwartz TH. A prospective study of postoperative symptoms in sinonasal quality-of-life following endoscopic skull-base surgery: dissociations based on specific symptoms. Int Forum Allergy Rhinol. 2013;3(8):664–9. https://doi.org/10.1002/alr.21161.
37. Hart CK, Theodosopoulos PV, Zimmer LA. Olfactory changes after endoscopic pituitary tumor resection. Otolaryngol Head Neck Surg. 2010;142(1):95–7. https://doi.org/10.1016/j.otohns.2009.09.032.
38. Sowerby LJ, Gross M, Broad R, Wright ED. Olfactory and sinonasal outcomes in endoscopic transsphenoidal skull-base surgery. Int Forum Allergy Rhinol. 2013;3(3):217–20. https://doi.org/10.1002/alr.21103.
39. Kuwata F, Kikuchi M, Ishikawa M, et al. Long-term olfactory function outcomes after pituitary surgery by endoscopic endonasal transsphenoidal approach. Auris Nasus Larynx. 2020;47(2):227–32. https://doi.org/10.1016/j.anl.2019.07.002.
40. Li P, Luo K, Zhang Q, Wang Z. Superior turbinate management and olfactory outcome after endoscopic endonasal transsphenoidal surgery for pituitary adenoma: a propensity score-matched cohort study. Int Forum Allergy Rhinol. 2020;10(12):1276–84. https://doi.org/10.1002/alr.22694.

Chapter 32
Outcomes of Lateral Skull Base Reconstruction

Dario Ebode, Ariel Finberg, Brandon Kamrava, Ali Al Qassim, and Adrien Eshraghi

Introduction

Cerebrospinal fluid (CFS) leaks of the lateral skull base are a rare entity. Typically, tegmen dehiscence is secondary to iatrogenic injury, trauma, or chronic infection; however, an estimated 18% of dehiscence is idiopathic [1, 2]. Proposed risk factors include idiopathic intracranial hypertension, morbid obesity, and arachnoid granulations [3, 4].

Reconstruction of the lateral skull base (LSB) is mostly necessary to prevent or repair a CSF leak. Untreated CSF leaks are associated with around 20% risk of developing meningitis and an increased mortality rate [5, 6]. Besides, they are a significantly costly problem, with an estimated median cost of over $50,000 per patient in 2017 [7].

In this chapter, we will be discussing the outcomes, especially postoperative CSF leak, of the different surgical approaches to reconstruct the LSB.

First, we will present the outcomes of each approach commonly used for the reconstruction of a defect located in the LSB: the transmastoid approach (TM), the middle crania fossa (MCF) approach, the combined approach, and the petrosectomy with middle ear obliteration (MEO).

Then, we will review the different methods used to prevent a CSF leak after LSB surgery.

Finally, we will present the outcomes of the LSB reconstruction after a large resection with muscle or musculocutaneous flaps.

D. Ebode · A. Finberg · B. Kamrava · A. Al Qassim · A. Eshraghi (✉)
Department of Otolaryngology, University of Miami–Miller School of Medicine, Miami, FL, USA
e-mail: AEshraghi@med.miami.edu

Outcomes for Reconstruction of Lateral Skull Base Defects

Transmastoid Approach

Overview

The TM approach is the least morbid approach for LSB reconstruction as it does not need a craniotomy or any temporal lobe retraction.

It provides excellent exposure of the tegmen mastoideum and is required if the defect is in the posterior fossa [8].

It is generally advised for defects <1 cm, but some authors report that larger defects (<2 cm) can also be treated by this approach [8–11]. In addition, this approach allows the surgeon to treat any middle ear disorder concurrently such as a tympanic membrane perforation or a cholesteatoma.

However, certain medial defects of the tegmen tympani may require a dislocation of the ossicular chain to access, which may result in a permanent conductive hearing loss. There have been reports of improved hearing outcomes with use of reconstruction; however, these patients had preoperative pathology of the ossicular chain [12].

Outcomes

This approach generally provides reliable outcomes (Table 32.1). A recent meta-analysis from Karkas et al. reports a 6.6% rate for recurrent CSF leaks over an average follow-up of 12 months [13].

In addition, average length of stay is significantly shorter with a TM approach than a MCF approach (1.7 vs. 6.3 days) [14].

Table 32.1 Improvement of air-bone gap and postoperative CSF leak after LSB reconstruction with a trans mastoid approach among several studies

Reference	Number of patients	ABG improvement	Mean follow up (months)	Treatment failure
Sanna et al. 2009 [15]	37	ND	38.4	2.3%
Semaan et al. 2011 [12]	31	5 dB	30	0%
Oliaei et al. 2012 [16]	11	ND	13.5	0%
Kim et al. 2014 [11]	15	12 dB	15.4	7%
Perez et al. 2018 [14]	26	10 dB	23	13%
Ren et al. 2021 [8]	20	13 dB	17	10%

ABG air-bone gap, *ND* no data, treatment failure includes recurrent CSF leak, meningocele or meningoencephalocele

Theoretical complications can include epidural or subdural hematomas and meningitis. Given that the ossicular chain is sometimes dissected with this approach, there is a small but significant risk for hearing loss. Nevertheless, none of these complications have been described in the following studies.

Take Home Message

As this approach provides a high success rate with limited morbidity and a short hospitalization, some authors advocate for this approach as the primary approach for most cases. However, the management of large or multiple medial defects of the tegmen tympani can be difficult and may place patients at risk of postoperative hearing loss.

Middle Cranial Fossa Approach

Overview

The MCF approach allows for the best exposure of the middle cranial fossa floor. The exposure of the whole tegmen tympani and tegmen mastoideum facilitates the identification and treatment of multiple defects. Additionally, as the ossicular chain remains intact, there is limited risk of worsening the patient's hearing. Nevertheless, in case of dehiscence of the superior semicircular canal, this one can be damaged during the surgery and lead to a hearing loss.

The principal disadvantage of this approach is the need of a craniotomy and the retraction of the temporal lobe, which typically leads to a longer recovery period. These drawbacks can be limited by an endoscope-assisted repair via a keyhole craniotomy [17]. The dissection of the ossicular chain and the treatment of middle ear pathology is not possible with this approach and can make the management of a meningocele in contact with the ossicular chain challenging. This approach is not able to address the posterior fossa, and if there is a defect there, the surgeon may not be able to repair it with this approach alone [8].

Outcomes

The MCF approach provides excellent results with a high success rate for lateral CSF leaks (Table 32.2). Multiple studies have shown a low recurrence rate for postoperative CSF leaks, with a long-term follow-up. In addition, the treatment of the meningocele or middle ear effusion often leads to a closure of the ABG in most patients.

The craniotomy and the retraction of the temporal lobe may theoretically expose to severe complications such as subdural or epidural hematoma, meningitis, or

Table 32.2 Improvement of air-bone gap and postoperative CSF leak after LSB reconstruction with a middle cranial fossa approach among several studies

Reference	Number of patients	ABG improvement	Mean follow up (months)	Treatment failure
Leonneti et al. 2005 [19]	51	ND	59	4.2%
Gubbels et al. 2007 [21]	15	ND	13	7%
Sanna et al. 2009 [15]	37	ND	38.4	3%
Nelson et al. 2016 [20]	65	ND	19.5	7.7%
Cheng et al. 2019 [10]	47	ND	ND	7%
Brenet et al. 2019 [22]	35	ND	61	6%
Alwani et al. 2019 [6]	27	96% closed ABG	4	0%
Ren et al. 2021 [8]	8	ND	17	12.5%

ABG air-bone gap, *ND* no data, *PTA* pure tone average, treatment failure includes recurrent CSF leak, meningocele or meningoencephalocele

seizure. However, the review of the literature shows that postoperative complications are rare [18]. Leonetti et al. reported four cases of minor wound infections, Sanna et al. reported one case of extradural hematoma, and Cheng et al. reported one case of delayed facial paralysis [10, 15, 19]. However, in one series of 65 cases, approximately 33% of the patient has postoperative complications, with three patients requiring return to the operating room [20].

Take Home Message

The MCF approach is generally the preferred approach for larger or multiples defects. Despite the need of a craniotomy and a temporal retraction, postoperative complications are rare if the surgery is performed by a trained surgeon.

Combined Approach

Overview

The TM or MCF approaches can be combined if needed. This approach allows for visualization and repair of more anterior defects that cannot be reached with a TM approach alone and more posterior defects that cannot be treated with an MCF approach alone. Also, meningoencephaloceles can be dissected from both sides of the tegmen and separated from any fibrous adhesions [9].

However, the morbidity may increase given the increased operating time needed for the two procedures and additional anatomic structures encountered [22].

Outcomes

Table 32.3 shows several studies reporting excellent results.

Stevens et al. describe a high success rate (96.5%) without any major complications, and Kenning et al. had similar results overall [23, 24].

Son et al. found that a combined approach was useful in the majority of their patients for successfully repairing the leak and also improved the ABG in some patients. Worth noting however was that 5% of patients experienced permanent sensorineural hearing loss. Carlson et al. studied nearly twice the patients and didn't report any sensorineural hearing loss [18]. However, 17% had a worse pure tonal average (PTA) after the surgery. He also reported one case of postoperative seizure, one case of transient facial palsy, and one case of myocardial infarction, although it remains unclear if these patients received a combined approach or an MCF approach alone.

Table 32.3 Improvement of air-bone gap and postoperative CSF leak after LSB reconstruction with a combined approach among several studies

Reference	Number of patients	ABG improvement	Mean follow up (months)	Treatment failure
Souliere et al. 1998 [25]	6	ND	24.5	0%
Kenning et al. 2012 [24]	22	ND	10.4	4%
Carlson et al. 2013 [18]	57	ND	14.5	4%
Son et al. 2014 [9]	30	>15db	17	4–8%
Stevens et al. 2017 [23]	28	9.7 dB	25.5	3,5%

ABG air bone gap, *ND* no data, *CSF* cerebrospinal fluid, treatment failure includes recurrent CSF leak, meningocele or meningoencephalocele

Take Home Message

The combined approach shows a good success rate for LSB reconstruction for a CSF leak. However, a less invasive approach should always be considered first.

Petrosectomy with Middle Ear Obliteration

Overview

Subtotal petrosectomy with middle ear obliteration (MEO) approach is a relatively safe method of closing temporal bone defects. The goal is to obliterate all accessible pneumatized spaces in the petrous bone and close all possible fistulas. SP allows good exposure of both the middle and posterior fossa plates and has a low CSF leak recurrence rate. As this approach does not include any intracranial procedure, the risk of intracranial hematoma is low. It can be a safer approach for patients with high comorbidities or anticoagulant treatment [26].

Unfortunately, this obliteration of the petrous bone and middle ear causes maximum conductive hearing loss. In addition, the closure of the external auditory canal does not allow any clinical surveillance for cholesteatoma, and regular imaging must be performed if needed. Thus, this approach should be considered the first option mainly in patients with anacusis on the affected side with recurrent temporal bone CSF leakage.

Causes of recurrence could be excision of intracanalicular tumors, which need extensive drilling, giant vestibular schwannoma, gamma knife radiotherapy prior to surgical excision of cerebellopontine angle tumor, revision surgery, congenital, and others [27].

Outcomes

The MEO is known to be very efficient and definitive treatment for recurrent CSF leaks [15]. As this treatment is considered to be aggressive and has limited indications, only few results are described in the literature. The majority of them described excellent outcomes with a low rate of recurrent CSF leak (Table 32.4).

It should be noted this approach is often used as secondary approach, after the failure of a prior surgical treatment and that patients treated with MEO often have more comorbidities than non-MEO patients [26]. However, the post-operative CSF leak rate does not seem to be higher than other approaches.

Coker et al. was the first to suggest subtotal petrosectomy for closing persistent CSF leak. He performed it in 13 cases of CSF leak, and no postoperative recurrence was reported [28].

Magliulo et al. reported 100% control of temporal CSF leak in a study involved eight patients with different causes of recurrent CSF leak [27]. A similar result was

Table 32.4 Postoperative CSF leaks after a middle ear obliteration among several studies

Reference	Number of patients	Mean follow-up (months)	Postoperative CSF leak
Coker et al. 1986 [28]	13	ND	0%
Leoneti et al. 2005 [19]	2	59	0%
Sanna et al. 2009 [15]	55	38.4	0%
Magliulo et al. 2014 [27]	8	102	0%
Kuckowski et al. 2014 [30]	2	24	0%
Ren et al. 2021 [8]	3	16.9	0%

CSF cerebrospinal fluid, *ND* no data

reported by Kronenberg et al., who reported CSF leak in four patients treated with subtotal petrosectomy after vestibular schwannoma removal. The internal auditory canal was the usual pathway for CSF leakage as well as retrosigmoid, retrolabyrinthine, and retro- or perifacial cells [29].

Take Home Message

MEO is a reliable option to treat recurrent CSF leaks, but it should only be used on patients with non-serviceable hearing, after the failure of a prior surgical procedure or if comorbidities of the patient do not allow any other approaches.

Associated Treatments and Management of the Intracranial Hypertension

An elevated intracranial pressure (ICP) is thought to be a risk factor for spontaneous lateral and anterior skull base CSF leaks [24, 31]. In addition, the closure of a CSF leak leads to an elevation of the ICP in the postoperative period [32]. Surgeons use mainly two different techniques to manage the ICP:

- A lumbar drain can be placed to monitor and manage the ICP [24]. It is usually removed a few days after the surgery. Nelson et al. investigated the necessity of perioperative LD placement for MCF repairs of spontaneous CSF leaks. They prospectively performed 44 MCF repairs without perioperative LD placement, and 6.8% developed postoperative otorrhea. They argued that a lumber drain was not systematically needed for a successful repair of a CSF leak. Unfortunately, statistical significance and patient comorbidities were not provided; however, one can argue that LD may be placed case by case, especially in high-risk patients such as morbidly obese or those with obstructive sleep apnea. They also reported an increased length of stay and an increased estimated cost for patients with lumbar drain [20].

- Administration of acetazolamide, a carbonic anhydrase inhibitor, decreases the production of CSF by 39% and as shown efficiency in reducing the ICP [32, 33]. However, its effect on postoperative CSF leaks is yet to demonstrate clinical value.

An elevated ICP should be diagnosed as it remains a potential risk factor for a recurrent CSF leak. Currently, it remains unclear if the use of a lumbar drain or acetazolamide improve the short- or long-term outcomes for LSB reconstruction.

Conclusion

Each surgical approach shows good results with limited risk of complications. The selection of the approach should be based on the characteristic of the defect (i.e., size, number, and location of the defect(s), the patients' comorbidities (i.e., age, anticoagulant treatment, hearing, other medical conditions), and the surgeons' preference (Table 32.5).

Table 32.5 Characteristics and outcomes of each lateral skull base reconstruction approaches

Surgical approach	Advantage	Disadvantage	Indication	Relative contraindication	Recurrent CSF leak rate
TM	Less invasive Ability to access the middle ear	Risk of hearing loss	Small defects in the tegmen mastoideum Concurrent middle ear pathology Posterior fossa defects	Anterior temporal CSF leak Large or multiple defects	0–10%
MCF	Large access to the MCF floor Limited risk of damage to the ossicular chain	Extended hospitalization Inability to access the middle ear	Large or multiple defects of the LSB	Middle ear pathology Posterior fossa defect	0–12.5%
Combined	Access to largest area of skull base and middle ear	Increased morbidity	Large and complicated defects of the LSB Concurrent middle ear pathology		0–8%
MEO	Definitive treatment for recurrent CSF leaks	Complete conductive hearing loss Imaging required for cholesteatoma surveillance	Ipsilateral anacusis Recurrent lateral CSF leaks		0–9%

TM transmastoid, *MCF* middle cranial fossa approach, *MEO* petrosectomy with middle ear obliteration, *CSF* cerebrospinal fluid

Reconstruction of the Lateral Skull Base After Accessing the Cerebellopontine Angle

Retrosigmoid Approach

Overview

The retrosigmoid (RS) approach is one of the most commonly used approaches to access the cerebellopontine angle (CPA) and is often preferred by surgeons because of its indications for tumors of all sizes and ability to preserve hearing [34].

Outcomes

Similar to the other approaches, the RS approach has a significant risk of CSF leak, and there have been many studies that look at how best to perform the reconstruction. Recently, there have been new techniques on how to optimize the closure of the internal auditory canal (IAC), and now the focus is on how best to close the site of the approach [34–41]. There have been many attempted strategies to prevent CSF leaks such as dural closure, bone wax, temporalis muscle, temporalis fascia, titanium mesh, and fat grafts [41–43] (Table 32.6).

Table 32.6 Postoperative CSF leaks after a retrosigmoid approach among several studies

Reference	Number of patients	Technique used	CSF leak rate
Lebowitz et al. 1995 [39]	46	Fibrin glue to close IAC and retrosigmoid air cells	15%
Gal et al. 1999 [38]	35	Bone wax to occlude perisigmoid air cells	2.8%
Becker et al. 2003 [44]	100	Bone wax into the IAC	10%
Selesnick et al. 2004 [42]	2273	ND	10.6%
Ansari et al. 2012 [45]	1067	ND	10.3%
Fredrickson et al. 2013 [36]	79	Calcium phosphate cement cranioplasty	0%
Ling et al. 2014 [41]	58	Bone wax and fat graft for the IAC, autologous fat graft and titanium mesh	0%
Azad et al. 2016 [35]	24	Abdominal fat graft for the IAC, bone wax for air cells, additional fat graft	0%
Foster et al. 2016 [37]	672	Calcium phosphate cement cranioplasty	6%
Luryi et al. 2017 [40]	19	Calcium phosphate cement cranioplasty	0%
Hwa et al. 2021 [46]	196	Bone wax occluded air cells, and either norian Or cranios bone cement was used for the cranioplasty	18%–no cement 8%–norian cement 1%–cranios cement

IAC internal auditory canal, *CSF* cerebrospinal fluid, *ND* no data

With the exception of Lebowitz et al. and Hwa et al., all of these studies are retrospective and are not compared against a control [30, 37]. Worth noting is that Lebowitz et al. did not see a difference in CSF leak in patients that did or did not receive the fibrin glue [39].

Take Home Message

The RS approach is a reliable way to access the CPA by aiming to preserve the patient's hearing while also being the approach of choice for larger tumors of the CPA. CSF leaks are a known complication in postoperative time and must be prevented by appropriate identification of opened temporal bone cells and their obliteration during the surgery before closure of the surgical wound.

Translabyrinthine Approach

Overview

The translabyrinthine (TL) approach is mostly used to treat vestibular schwannomas. It requires the sacrifice of the vestibula, which results in temporary vertigo and a complete hearing loss, but offers a better exposure of the IAC.

Outcomes

There is a risk of developing a CSF leak after a TL approach, and the reconstruction should be done carefully.

A meta-analysis from 2004 found a CSF leak rate of 9.5%; however, this rate varies between 0.8% and 21% among other large series (Table 32.7).

The reconstruction after a TL approach classically uses an abdominal fat graft to fill the cavity. In addition, some teams use various techniques to reduce the risk of CSF leak including bone wax, titanium mesh, bone cement, or watertight periosteal closure.

The rate of CSF leak is similar after a TL or RS approach [42, 44, 45].

Table 32.7 Postoperative CSF leaks after a translabyrinthine approach among several studies

Reference	Number of patients	Technique used	CSF leak
Hoffmann et al. 1994 [47]	146	ND	21%
Arriaga et al. 2002 [48]	54	Abdominal fat graft	12.5%
	54	Hydroxyapatite cement	3.7%
Becker et al. 2003 [44]	100	Abdominal fat graft	13%
Selesnick et al. 2004 [42]	3118	ND	9.50%
Fayad et al. 2007 [49]	389	Abdominal fat graft + titanium mesh	3.3%
Merkus et al. 2010 [50]	1803	Abdominal fat graft	0.8%
Ansari et al. 2012 [45]	1623	ND	7.10%
Russel et al. 2017 [51]	275	Bone pate, bone wax, abdominal fat graft	12%
Obaid et al. 2018 [52]	129	ND	7.8%
Selleck et al. 2021 [53]	94	Abdominal fat graft+ mesh	12.8%
	38	Abdominal fat graft + periosteal closure	0%

CSF cerebrospinal fluid, *ND* no data

Take Home Message

The TL approach has a significant risk of a CSF leak. The best reconstruction technique after a TL approach is still up for debate. Most of the centers used abdominal fat; however, various surgical techniques are used including hydroxyapatite cement, titanium mesh, or periosteal closure.

Middle Cranial Fossa Approach

Overview

The MCF approach is also used for CPA surgery. Its indications have decreased in the recent years. It allows for hearing preservation but places the facial nerve between the surgeon and the acoustic neuroma, especially in case of a vestibular schwannoma from the inferior vestibular nerve.

Outcomes

CSF leaks after an MCF approach for an acoustic neuroma range from 5.7% to 12.8% in recent studies (Table 32.8). A recent meta-analysis from Ansari et al. reports a 5.3% leak rate. Of note, Scheich et al. reports two case of postoperative meningitis (1%).

Table 32.8 Postoperative CSF leaks after a trans labyrinthine approach among several studies

Reference	Number of patients	Technique used	CSF leak
Slattery et al. 2001 [54]	433	ND	5.7%
Oghalaï et al. 2003 [55]	149	ND	10%
Becker et al. 2003 [44]	100	Bone wax into the IAC	10%
Selesnick et al. 2004 [42]	573	ND	10.6%
Sameshima et al. 2010 [56]	43	ND	4.7%
Ansari et al. 2012 [45]	436	ND	5.3%
Scheich et al. 2017 [57]	203	Temporal muscle graft and bone wax	12.8%

CSF cerebrospinal fluid, *ND* no data, *IAC* internal auditory canal

Take Home Message

Although less common, the MCF approach is a great access to the CPA for small growing tumors of the IAC with good hearing. But it is not without its disadvantages. The rate of CSF leak with this approach is similar to the other approaches and range from 4.7% to 12.8%.

Locoregional and Free Flaps

Overview

After a large resection of a skull base tumor involving the temporal bone, muscle or musculocutaneous flaps are often necessary. They can offer several advantages, such as the protection of the brain and the dura, skin for closing, providing tissue volume for large reconstructions, enhancing cosmetic appearance, or providing tissue for a facial nerve reconstruction [58].

The flaps are often associated with other surgical techniques such as a reconstruction of the dura with an autologous or synthetic graft or the obliteration of the defect with abdominal fat [58]. Bone wax or hydroxyapatite can be considered for sealant of surrounding bony air cells. The elimination of dead space within the neck through use of multilayered closure and numerous tacking suture may reduce the dependent capture of CSF into the neck postoperatively if sufficient closure could not be achieved, especially in cases of malignancy requiring large resections.

A large variety of flaps can be used, including local flaps (temporalis muscle, sternocleidomastoid muscle, supraclavicular, and submental), pedicled flaps (infraclavicular, pectoralis major, latissimus dorsi, and trapezius flap), or free flaps (anterolateral thigh, radial forearm, and rectus abdominis) (Table 32.9).

Table 32.9 Postoperative CSF leaks and wound complications after a flap reconstruction of the LSB among several studies

Reference	Number of patients	Flap	Wound complication	Postoperative CSF leak
Marzo et al. 2005 [61]	8	Pedicled flap (trapezius flap)	12.5%	0%
Resto et al. 2007 [62]	8	Pedicled flap (pectoralis major)	0%	0%
Hanasono et al. 2012 [60]	27	Rotational flap (temporalis muscle)	7.4%	0%
	90	Free flap (70 ALT, 8 rectus abdominis, 12 others)	3.3%	4.4%
Patel et al. 2015 [59]	21	Rotational flap (10 SCM, 9 temporalis, 2 other)	19%	0%
	11	Pedicled flap (9 pectoralis, 1 latissimus dorsi, 1 trapezius)	36%	9%
	10	Free flap (4 ALT, 2 RFA, 2 rectus abdominis, 1 gracilis, 1 fibula)	0%	10%
Howard et al. 2016 [63]	16	Rotational flap (submental)	0%	0%
	6	Pedicled flap (latissimus dorsi)	0%	0%
	9	Free flap (anterolateral tight)	0%	0%

CSF cerebrospinal fluid, *ND* no data, *SCM* sternocleidomastoid muscle, *RFA* radial forearm, *ALT* anterolateral thigh

Outcomes

Locoregional flaps, as compared to pedicled and free flaps, often provide shorter operative times a shorter and length of stay [59, 60].

For patients who have already received radiation to the field preoperatively, which decreases the area's healing capacity, the rate of wound complications can be significantly higher with local and pedicled flaps. In these cases, free flaps, especially an anterolateral thigh flap, are good options.

Take Home Message

Large tumor resections involving the temporal bone often require a locoregional or free flap. Locoregional flaps have a shorter operating time and a shorter length of stay, but free flaps should be preferred for irradiated tissue.

Conclusion

Whether repairing an existing defect, preventing a CSF leak after an LSB surgery, or after a large oncological resection, multiple situations can require an LSB reconstruction.

Depending on the situation, various techniques are available to the surgeon. Each approach has its own advantages and disadvantages, and one should prefer the least invasive technique allowing for the successful repair of the defect.

The systematic use of associated treatments such as acetazolamide or lumbar drains is controversial, and their effectiveness needs to be further evaluated.

Overall, all approaches show strong results with rare cases of failure. This chapter serves to highlight the benefits and outcomes that can be expected from each approach used for LSB reconstruction.

References

1. Stucken EZ, Selesnick SH, Brown KD. The role of obesity in spontaneous temporal bone encephaloceles and CSF leak. Otol Neurotol. 2012;33(8):1412–7.
2. Savva A, Taylor MJ, Beatty CW. Management of cerebrospinal fluid leaks Involving the temporal bone: report on 92 patients. Laryngoscope. 2003;113(1):50–6.
3. Yew M, Dubbs B, Tong O, Nager GT, Niparko JK, Tatlipinar A, et al. Arachnoid granulations of the temporal bone: a histologic study of dural and osseous penetration. Otol Neurotol. 2011;32(4):602–9.
4. Goddard JC, Meyer T, Nguyen S, Lambert PR. New considerations in the cause of spontaneous cerebrospinal fluid otorrhea. Otol Neurotol. 2010;31(6):940–5.
5. Liao L-J, Hsu W-L, Wang C-T, Lo W-C, Lai M-S. Analysis of sentinel node biopsy combined with other diagnostic tools in staging cN0 head and neck cancer: a diagnostic meta-analysis. Head Neck. 2016;38(4):628–34.
6. Alwani M, Bandali E, Van Buren L, Yates CW, Nelson RF. Audiologic improvement following MCF approach for spontaneous cerebrospinal fluid leaks. Otol Neurotol. 2019;40(8):1026–33.
7. Chern A, Hunter JB, Bennett ML. Cost analysis of cerebrospinal fluid leaks and cerebrospinal fluid leak prevention in patients undergoing cerebellopontine angle surgery. Otol Neurotol. 2017;38(1):147–51.
8. Ren Y, Tawfik KO, Cueva RA. Audiometric outcomes following transmastoid and middle cranial fossa approaches for repair of cerebrospinal fluid otorrhea. Otol Neurotol. 2021;42(3):424–30.
9. Son HJ, Karkas A, Buchanan P, Giurintano JP, Theodosopoulos P, Pensak ML, et al. Spontaneous cerebrospinal fluid effusion of the temporal bone: repair, audiological outcomes, and obesity. Laryngoscope. 2014;124(5):1204–8.
10. Cheng E, Grande D, Leonetti J. Management of spontaneous temporal bone cerebrospinal fluid leak: a 30-year experience. Am J Otolaryngol. 2019;40(1):97–100.
11. Kim L, Wisely CE, Dodson EE. Transmastoid approach to spontaneous temporal bone cerebrospinal fluid leaks: hearing improvement and success of repair. Otolaryngol Head Neck Surg. 2014;150(3):472–8.
12. Semaan MT, Gilpin DA, Hsu DP, Wasman JK, Megerian CA. Transmastoid extradural–intracranial approach for repair of transtemporal meningoencephalocele: a review of 31 consecutive cases. Laryngoscope. 2011;121(8):1765–72.

13. Karkas A, Khneisser E. Trans-mastoid approach for cerebrospinal fluid leak repair. Curr Opin Otolaryngol Head Neck Surg. 2019;27(5):334–8.
14. Perez E, Carlton D, Alfarano M, Smouha E. Transmastoid repair of spontaneous cerebrospinal fluid leaks. J Neurol Surg B Skull Base. 2018;79(5):451–7.
15. Sanna M, Paolo F, Russo A, Falcioni M. Management of meningoencephalic herniation of the temporal bone: personal experience and literature review. Laryngoscope. 2009;119(8):1579–85.
16. Oliaei S, Mahboubi H, Djalilian HR. Transmastoid approach to temporal bone cerebrospinal fluid leaks. Am J Otolaryngol. 2012;33(5):556–61.
17. Roehm PC, Tint D, Chan N, Brewster R, Sukul V, Erkmen K. Endoscope-assisted repair of CSF otorrhea and temporal lobe encephaloceles via keyhole craniotomy. J Neurosurg. 2017;128(6):1880–4.
18. Carlson ML, Copeland WR, Driscoll CL, Link MJ, Haynes DS, Thompson RC, et al. Temporal bone encephalocele and cerebrospinal fluid fistula repair utilizing the middle cranial fossa or combined mastoid–middle cranial fossa approach: clinical article. J Neurosurg. 2013;119(5):1314–22.
19. Leonetti JP, Marzo S, Anderson D, Origitano T, Vukas DD. Spontaneous transtemporal CSF leakage: a study of 51 cases. Ear Nose Throat J. 2005;84(11):700, 702-4, 706.
20. Nelson RF, Roche JP, Gantz BJ, Hansen MR. Middle cranial fossa (MCF) approach without the use of lumbar drain for the management of spontaneous cerebral spinal fluid (CSF) leaks. Otol Neurotol. 2016;37(10):1625–9.
21. Gubbels SP, Selden NR, Delashaw JBJ, McMenomey SO. Spontaneous middle fossa encephalocele and cerebrospinal fluid leakage: diagnosis and management. Otol Neurotol. 2007;28(8):1131–9.
22. Brenet E, Dubernard X, Kleiber J-C, Bazin A, Chays A, Herman P, et al. Surgical management of spontaneous temporal bone cerebrospinal fluid leaks: results of a strategy based on defect location. A bicentric retrospective study of 44 cases. Clin Otolaryngol. 2019;44(6):1190–4.
23. Stevens SM, Crane R, Pensak ML, Samy RN. Analysis of audiometric outcomes following combined middle cranial fossa/transmastoid approaches for spontaneous cerebrospinal fluid otorrhea. Otolaryngol Head Neck Surg. 2017;156(5):924–32.
24. Kenning TJ, Willcox TO, Artz GJ, Schiffmacher P, Farrell CJ, Evans JJ. Surgical management of temporal meningoencephaloceles, cerebrospinal fluid leaks, and intracranial hypertension: treatment paradigm and outcomes. Neurosurg Focus. 2012;32(6):E6.
25. Souliere CR Jr, Langman AW. Combined mastoid/middle cranial fossa repair of temporal bone encephalocele. Skull Base. 1998;8(04):185–9.
26. Stevens SM, Crane R, Pensak ML, Samy RN. Middle ear obliteration with blind-sac closure of the external auditory canal for spontaneous CSF otorrhea. Otolaryngol Head Neck Surg. 2017;156(3):534–42.
27. Magliulo G, Iannella G, Appiani MC, Re M. Subtotal petrosectomy and cerebrospinal fluid leakage in unilateral anacusis. J Neurol Surg B Skull Base. 2014;75(6):391–6.
28. Coker NJ, Jenkins HA, Fisch U. Obliteration of the middle ear and mastoid cleft in subtotal petrosectomy: indications, technique, and results. Ann Otol Rhinol Laryngol. 1986;95(1):5–11.
29. Kronenberg J, Bendet E, Findler G, Roth Y. Cerebrospinal fluid (CSF) otorhinorrhoea following vestibular schwannoma surgery treated by extended subtotal petrosectomy with obliteration. J Laryngol Otol. 1993;107(12):1122–4.
30. Kuczkowski J, Niemczyk K, Stankiewicz C, Pilarska E, Szurowska E, Plichta Ł. Lateral petrosectomy with obliteration cavity for spontaneous cerebrospinal otorrhea in children. Am J Otolaryngol. 2014;35(5):651–4.
31. Brainard L, Chen DA, Aziz KM, Hillman TA. Association of benign intracranial hypertension and spontaneous encephalocele with cerebrospinal fluid leak. Otol Neurotol. 2012;33(9):1621–4.
32. Chaaban MR, Illing E, Riley KO, Woodworth BA. Acetazolamide for high intracranial pressure cerebrospinal fluid leaks. Int Forum Allergy Rhinol. 2013;3(9):718–21.

33. Carrion E, Hertzog JH, Medlock MD, Hauser GJ, Dalton HJ. Use of acetazolamide to decrease cerebrospinal fluid production in chronically ventilated patients with ventriculopleural shunts. Arch Dis Child. 2001;84(1):68–71.
34. Elhammady MS, Telischi FF, Morcos JJ. Retrosigmoid approach: indications, techniques, and results. Otolaryngol Clin North Am. 2012;45(2):375–97.
35. Azad T, Mendelson ZS, Wong A, Jyung RW, Liu JK. Fat graft-assisted internal auditory canal closure after retrosigmoid transmeatal resection of acoustic neuroma: technique for prevention of cerebrospinal fluid leakage. J Clin Neurosci. 2016;24:124–7.
36. Frederickson AM Jr, RFS. The utility of calcium phosphate cement in cranioplasty following retromastoid craniectomy for cranial neuralgias. Br J Neurosurg. 2013;27(6):808–11.
37. Foster KA, Shin SS, Prabhu B, Fredrickson A, Sekula RF. Calcium phosphate cement cranioplasty decreases the rate of cerebrospinal fluid leak and wound infection compared with titanium mesh cranioplasty: retrospective study of 672 patients. World Neurosurg. 2016;95:414–8.
38. Gal TJ, Bartels LJ. Use of bone wax in the prevention of cerebrospinal fluid fistula in acoustic neuroma surgery. Laryngoscope. 1999;109(1):167–9.
39. Lebowitz RA, Hoffman RA, Roland JT Jr, Cohen NL. Autologous fibrin glue in the prevention of cerebrospinal fluid leak following acoustic neuroma surgery. Am J Otol. 1995;16(2):172–4.
40. Luryi AL, Bulsara KR, Michaelides EM. Hydroxyapatite bone cement for suboccipital retrosigmoid cranioplasty: a single institution case series. Am J Otolaryngol. 2017;38(4):390–3.
41. Ling PY, Mendelson ZS, Reddy RK, Jyung RW, Liu JK. Reconstruction after retrosigmoid approaches using autologous fat graft-assisted medpor titan cranioplasty: assessment of postoperative cerebrospinal fluid leaks and headaches in 60 cases. Acta Neurochir. 2014;156(10):1879–88.
42. Selesnick SH, Liu JC, Jen A, Newman J. The incidence of cerebrospinal fluid leak after vestibular schwannoma surgery. Otol Neurotol. 2004;25(3):387–93.
43. Boghani Z, Choudhry OJ, Schmidt RF, Jyung RW, Liu JK. Reconstruction of cranial base defects using the medpor titan implant: cranioplasty applications in acoustic neuroma surgery. J Neurol Surg B Skull Base. 2013;74(S 1):A279.
44. Becker SS, Jackler RK, Pitts LH. Cerebrospinal fluid leak after acoustic neuroma surgery: a comparison of the translabyrinthine, middle fossa, and retrosigmoid approaches. Otol Neurotol. 2003;24(1):107–12.
45. Ansari SF, Terry C, Cohen-Gadol AA. Surgery for vestibular schwannomas: a systematic review of complications by approach. Neurosurg Focus. 2012;33(3):E14.
46. Hwa TP, Luu N, Henry LE, Naples JG, Kaufman AC, Brant JA, et al. Impact of reconstruction with hydroxyapatite bone cement on CSF leak rate in retrosigmoid approach to vestibular schwannoma resection: a review of 196 cases. Otol Neurotol. 2021;42:918.
47. Hoffman RA. Cerebrospinal fluid leak following acoustic neuroma removal. Laryngoscope. 1994;104(1):40–58.
48. Arriaga MA, Chen DA. Hydroxyapatite cement cranioplasty in translabyrinthine acoustic neuroma surgery. Otolaryngol Head Neck Surg. 2002;126(5):512–7.
49. Fayad JN, Schwartz MS, Slattery WH, Brackmann DE. Prevention and treatment of cerebrospinal fluid leak after translabyrinthine acoustic tumor removal. Otol Neurotol. 2007;28(3):387–90.
50. Merkus P, Taibah A, Sequino G, Sanna M. Less than 1% cerebrospinal fluid leakage in 1,803 translabyrinthine vestibular schwannoma surgery cases. Otol Neurotol. 2010;31(2):276–83.
51. Russel A, Hoffmann CP, Nguyen DT, Beurton R, Parietti-Winkler C. Can the risks of cerebrospinal fluid leak after vestibular schwannoma surgery be predicted? Otol Neurotol. 2017;38(2):248–52.
52. Obaid S, Nikolaidis I, Alzahrani M, Moumdjian R, Saliba I. Morbidity rate of the retrosigmoid versus translabyrinthine approach for vestibular schwannoma resection. J Audiol Otol. 2018;22(4):236–43.

53. Selleck AM, Hodge SE, Brown KD. Cerebrospinal fluid leak following translabyrinthine vestibular schwannoma surgery—is mesh cranioplasty necessary for prevention? Otol Neurotol. 2021;42(5):e593.
54. Slattery WHI, Francis S, House KC. Perioperative morbidity of acoustic neuroma surgery. Otol Neurotol. 2001;22(6):895–902.
55. Oghalai JS, Buxbaum JL, Pitts LH, Jackler RK. The effect of age on acoustic neuroma surgery outcomes. Otol Neurotol. 2003;24(3):473–7.
56. Sameshima T, Fukushima T, McElveen JT Jr, Friedman AH. Critical assessment of operative approaches for hearing preservation in small acoustic neuroma surgery: retrosigmoid vs middle fossa approach. Neurosurgery. 2010;67(3):640–5.
57. Scheich M, Ginzkey C, Ehrmann Muller D, Shehata Dieler W, Hagen R. Complications of the middle cranial fossa approach for acoustic neuroma removal. J Int Adv Otol. 2017;13(2):186–90.
58. Homer JJ, Lesser T, Moffat D, Slevin N, Price R, Blackburn T. Management of lateral skull base cancer: United Kingdom national multidisciplinary guidelines. J Laryngol Otol. 2016;130(S2):S119–24.
59. Patel NS, Modest MC, Brobst TD, Carlson ML, Price DL, Moore EJ, et al. Surgical management of lateral skull base defects. Laryngoscope. 2016;126(8):1911–7.
60. Hanasono MM, Silva AK, Yu P, Skoracki RJ, Sturgis EM, Gidley PW. Comprehensive management of temporal bone defects after oncologic resection. Laryngoscope. 2012;122(12):2663–9.
61. Marzo SJ, Leonetti JP, Petruzzelli GJ, Vandevender D. Closure of complex lateral skull base defects. Otol Neurotol. 2005;26(3):522–4.
62. Resto VA, McKenna MJ, Deschler DG. Pectoralis major flap in composite lateral skull base defect reconstruction. Arch Otolaryngol Head Neck Surg. 2007;133(5):490–4.
63. Howard BE, Nagel TH, Barrs DM, Donald CB, Hayden RE. Reconstruction of lateral skull base defects: a comparison of the submental flap to free and regional flaps. Otolaryngol Head Neck Surg. 2016;154(6):1014–8.

Chapter 33
Medicolegal Issues in Skull Base Reconstruction

Janet S. Choi and Joni K. Doherty

Informed Consent

Skull base reconstruction can be challenging due to complex anatomy and potential major complications. A broad range of reconstructive techniques is available for skull base defects in head and neck surgery. The method of reconstruction depends on a variety of factors including the extent and location of the defect, etiology and presence of CSF leak, patient comorbidities, desired functional and cosmetic outcomes, and previous history or future need for adjuvant therapy [1–3]. Multiple methods can be often acceptable with differential benefits and risks. Therefore, informed consent is an essential step in ensuring that patients are fully aware of the risks, benefits, and alternatives. The informed consent process comprises two major components derived from the rights that affect the patient: (1) the right to receive adequate information enabling the patient to make the best decision and (2) the patient's right to give consent [4].

Adequate information for a given skull base reconstruction surgery includes, but is not limited to, the nature of the surgery, the expected benefits, material risks and adverse effects, alternative treatments including conservative options, and the consequences of both having and not having the recommended procedures. Surgeons should provide patients information on the nature of the surgery including the details of the surgical procedure where a reasonable patient would understand [5]. The primary goal of skull base reconstructive surgeries is to repair dural defect to

J. S. Choi
Department of Otolaryngology—Head and Neck Surgery, University of Minnesota, Minneapolis, MN, USA

J. K. Doherty (✉)
Department of Otolaryngology—Head and Neck Surgery, University of Southern California, Los Angeles, CA, USA
e-mail: joni.doherty@med.usc.edu

E. C. Kuan et al. (eds.), *Skull Base Reconstruction*, https://doi.org/10.1007/978-3-031-27937-9_33

475

obtain watertight separation between the intracranial contents and the adjacent cavities. Major expected benefits of the surgery include prevention of cerebrospinal fluid (CSF) leak, pneumocephalus, and infections such as meningitis. Additionally, skull base reconstruction may provide coverage of exposed major vascular structures, provide coverage of vascularized soft tissue for better wound healing if previously irradiated, and improve cosmesis for large defects. Improvement in quality of life and functional outcomes have been reported in prior literature for patients who underwent skull base reconstruction. Gil et al. reported that the quality of life improved 6-months postoperation among patients after anterior skull base reconstruction [6, 7]. Patients who underwent reconstruction due to benign pathology had higher improvement in quality of life in comparison to patients with malignant pathology [6, 7]. The surgical approach (endoscopic vs. open approach, combined vs. open approach) did not affect quality of life among these patients [7, 8].

Major risks of skull base reconstruction surgeries include CSF leak, pneumocephalus, intracranial infections, cerebral infarct with its serious downstream effects (i.e., cognitive impairment, cranial nerve deficits, diplopia, dysphagia, and dysarthria), orbital complications, and death. A systematic review on outcomes of anterior skull base reconstruction reported that the overall reported rate of CSF leak in previous literature ranged from 0 to 14% [9]. CSF leak rate for reconstruction with free grafts at 15.6% was significantly higher than leak rate at 6.7% for vascularized reconstructions for large dural defects [10]. Complication rates of pneumocephalus and intracranial infections such as meningitis ranged from 0 to 7% and 0 to 13.5%, respectively [9]. Mortality rate from anterior skull base reconstruction ranged from 0 to 7% [9]. Thompson et al. compared reconstruction outcomes for various lateral skull base closure techniques and reported major complications to be at 8% with the most frequent being stroke at 3% [11, 12]. If locoregional or free flaps are used for reconstruction, flap-related complications including flap necrosis, partial or total flap failure, and donor site morbidities should be discussed. Flap failure rates were reported to range from 0 to 35% for locoregional flaps and from 0 to 14% for free flaps [9].

Minor risks of the skull base reconstruction surgery include wound complications (e.g., dehiscence, infection), bleeding/hematoma, temporary or permanent changes of smell and taste, chronic rhinosinusitis/mucocele, pain, numbness, swelling, and scarring. Wound complications have been reported in up to 45% of skull base reconstruction cases [9, 11]. Surgeons should discuss that patients may need prolonged hospital stay, activity restrictions, CSF diversion procedures, or a revision surgery when complications occur. Any alternative treatment options including observation, medical management, and CSF diversion procedures (e.g., EVDs, lumbar drains, shunts, and dural venous sinus stenting) should be discussed along with all surgical options. The pros and cons of all management options in context of each patient's medical condition should be highlighted.

After adequate information is provided to the patients, it is essential for surgeons to assess the patient's understanding of the information given the broad range of skull base reconstruction options. Patients then should preserve the right to consent freely without coercion. It is important to avoid providing misinformation or exaggerating the harm of not following the recommended treatment or the benefits of accepting the treatment. Efforts should be made to promote the informed consent process to be a shared decision-making process through a collaborative communication between surgeons and patients, integrating the best evidence available along with the patients' values and preferences [5].

Litigation

Skull base defects can be successfully treated in most cases with recent advancement in understanding of anatomy, etiology, and medical and surgical management options. Still, there exist cases with inadequate and inappropriate management and surgical complications that may lead to significant patient morbidity and mortality and further malpractice litigations.

According to the malpractice report published in 2019, 83% of surveyed otolaryngologists reported that they have been sued at least once during their career, listing otolaryngology as a top third highly litigated surgical specialty after general surgery and urology [13]. Ceremsak et al. reported that Rhinology was the most frequently implicated subspecialty in medical malpractice in otolaryngology comprising 28% of all cases identified between 2010 and 2019, followed by head and neck surgery comprising 17% [14]. Although no previous studies have reviewed litigation characteristics specific to the skull base defect management and reconstruction surgeries, the risk for litigation is expected to be high where management involves highly litigated subspecialties such as rhinology, head and neck surgery, neurotology, and neurosurgery. In otolaryngology, the most common procedure identified to be involved in medical malpractice litigations is endoscopic sinus surgery, which is routinely utilized in anterior skull base reconstruction [14]. Nearly half of the malpractice allegations were on improper surgical performance (49%) followed by failure to diagnose, refer, or treat (32%); medical complications (6%); unnecessary procedures/treatment (5%); and consent issue (4%) [14].

Medical malpractice is a specific subset of tort law that is defined as any act or omission by a physician during treatment of a patient that deviates from standards of care and causes an injury to the patient [15]. During evaluation, physicians should obtain a thorough history and physical exam and obtain appropriate imaging and consultation within the standards of care to minimize risks of malpractice litigations. Many malpractice claims have been identified where physicians were litigated due to a failure to timely and properly formulate appropriate differential diagnosis, failure to timely refer to consultants, and delayed diagnosis of skull base defects and tumor [16, 17]. If surgical intervention is offered, physicians must describe the recommended intervention and disclose the benefits, risks, and alternatives to obtain informed consent on the reasonable patient (what would the average patient need to know to make an informed decision) and reasonable physician standard (what would the typical physician discuss about the intervention) [16].

Surgical complications may occur despite meticulous technique and lead to a malpractice litigation. Common surgical complications cited in skull base reconstruction lawsuits include intracranial complications (e.g., CSF leak, brain injury, meningitis, hemorrhage), neurologic injuries, death, and need for additional surgery [16]. Anterior skull base reconstruction complications commonly implicated in malpractice litigations additionally include orbital injuries (blindness, diplopia), anosmia, and atrophic rhinitis. Complications commonly involved in lateral skull base reconstruction malpractice litigations include facial nerve paralysis, hearing loss, and tympanic membrane perforation [18].

A recent review of otolaryngology malpractice cases from 2010 to 2019 reported that 89% of the identified cases with available liability data were ruled in favor of the defendant otolaryngologists [14]. The rate of liability outcome in favor of physicians ranged from 47 to 89% depending on the allegation type and study period [14, 16, 18–22]. The average payment to plaintiff was $4.24 million ranging from $15,000 to $10.25 million [14]. Reviews of malpractice cases of rhinology-related cases including endoscopic sinus surgery reported that 56–62% cases were ruled in favor of the defendants [21, 23]. Lydiatt et al. reported that 23% of cases involving sinonasal diseases were ruled in favor of plaintiffs with a median judgement award of $650,000 and 15% of cases were settled with a median settlement of $575,000 [21]. A review of malpractice cases involving vestibular schwannoma often implicated in lateral skull base reconstruction reported that 56% of cases were ruled in favor of the defendants with judgment amount ranged from $400,000 to $2 million [24]. Of the malpractice claims involving facial nerve paralysis, 47% resulted in ruling favoring defendants with a mean plaintiff award of $578,000 and a mean settlement of $337,000 [20]. Previous reviews on medical malpractices cases were based on professional databases such as WestLaw and LexisNexis, which may not be comprehensive. A majority of malpractice cases are expected to be settled confidentially out of court and not documented in these databases.

Tips to Minimize Risk

Even the most skilled physicians may find themselves the subject of medical malpractice litigation. Medical malpractice claims present a significant financial, emotional, and time burden for physicians and healthcare systems [25, 26]. Previous studies in various surgical fields have demonstrated that malpractice claims can be reduced by improving physician-patient communication and physician education based on risk management and prevention strategies developed from litigation analysis [27–32].

Patient-centered communication is a vital step in establishing rapport with patients with positive impact on patient behavior, care outcomes, and satisfaction often leading to the reduction of litigation risk. Klimo et al. reported that poor physician communication and interpersonal skills, an appearance of withholding information, and an impression that the physician was rushed and uninterested in patient concerns were significantly associated with a higher risk of litigation [33]. Details on the treatment options available and why a particular option is recommended should be discussed with the patients [31]. Unrealistic patient expectations on functional or cosmetic outcomes and specific risks should be addressed before the treatment begins. Radiologic findings should be reviewed with patients with actual images when possible. Any anatomical variants noted on radiology imaging should be discussed prior to the intervention. Discussions with the patients should be thoroughly documented as the medical record is the main source of evidence and defense during malpractice litigation.

During surgery, measures should be taken to minimize complications whenever possible within the standard of care. There have been many advancements in surgical technologies in skull base reconstruction to improve technical accuracy and reduce complications. For example, intraoperative image-guided systems can assist surgeons in identifying anatomical landmarks that may have been altered by trauma, tumor invasion, or previous surgery or radiation during skull base reconstruction. Although Ramakrishnan et al. reported that the use of image guidance has not clearly been shown to decrease surgical complications or improve outcomes in a systematic review of endoscopic sinus surgeries [34, 35], image-guided surgery should be considered in skull base reconstruction for advanced diseases and revision cases if indicated. Appropriate choice of surgical approach such as endoscopic versus open in anterior skull base reconstruction is also important. Systematic reviews have shown that the complication rates were significantly lower among patients who underwent endoscopic approach for anterior skull base defect in comparison to open repair [10, 36]. The use of image guidance and surgical approach in skull base reconstruction can be based on clinical judgment and applied on a case-by-case basis. Cranial nerve monitoring should be adapted when appropriate for lateral skull base reconstruction. Previous studies have shown that the facial nerve anatomical preservation rates were significantly higher among monitored group in comparison to unmonitored group especially among patients with large skull base tumors [37, 38]. Auditory brain stem responses and electrocochleography can be recorded intraoperatively as a method of monitoring auditory functioning with limitations [39–41]. After surgery, detailed and honest operative reports including clear indications and complications that occurred during the surgery should be documented.

When complication occurs during medical care or treatment, it is always better to have a forthright conversation with the patient explaining what happened and why. Vincent et al. have reported that what patients want from their physicians following a medical error is an apology and the assurance that what happened to them will not happen to someone else [42]. Adverse patient outcomes are distressing to both physicians and patients, and physicians may be fearful and reluctant to disclose details. However, it is important to understand that not every error is the result of negligent behavior. In fact, only 1–2% of adverse events led to malpractice claims [43–45]. What is commonly considered to be below the standard of care would be the physician's failure to explain this potential complication as part of the informed consent, failure to describe the symptoms to watch for after the procedure that might indicate that a complication has occurred, failure to tell the patient that a complication did occur, and failure to recognize the complication in a timely manner [46]. Witman et al. reported that the malpractice litigation is more likely to occur among cases where physician did not disclose an error [47].

Diagnosis and management of skull base defect involves multidisciplinary team comprising primary care physician, neurologist, radiologist, pathologist, rhinologist, neurotologist, neurosurgeons, and head and neck surgeons. If an invasive intervention is recommended, it is important to form a team of skilled surgeons to provide the best practice. Most malpractice claims of surgical complications start with a key question whether the surgeon was qualified to perform the procedure. Surgeons should perform procedures within the range of their routine practice based on their training and experience. Assistant from an appropriately trained colleagues should be requested if there need skills outside of their routine scope of practice to provide the treatment or when complications occur [17, 48].

Skull base reconstruction carries significant risks inherent to the intricate anatomy and various pathology. Unexpected complications may arise from various steps of skull base defect management leading to malpractice claims. Proper evaluation, consultation, patient selection for interventions, and meticulous techniques in surgery along with the honest and open communication with patients during the entire process of evaluation and management may help avoid malpractice claims and, more importantly, provide the best patient care.

References

1. Naik AN, Lancione PJ, Parikh AS, et al. Anterior skull base reconstruction: a contemporary. 2021.
2. Moyer JS, Chepeha DB, Teknos TN. Contemporary skull base reconstruction. Curr Opin Otolaryngol Head Neck Surg. 2004;12(4):294–9.
3. Ein L, Sargi Z, Nicolli EA. Update on anterior skull base reconstruction. Curr Opin Otolaryngol Head Neck Surg. 2019;27(5):426–30.
4. Ferreres AR. Surgical ethics: principles and practice. Cham: Springer; 2019.
5. Spatz ES, Krumholz HM, Moulton BW. The new era of informed consent: getting to a reasonable-patient standard through shared decision making. JAMA. 2016;315(19):2063–4.
6. Gil Z, Abergel A, Spektor S, et al. Quality of life following surgery for anterior skull base tumors. Arch Otolaryngol Head Neck Surg. 2003;129(12):1303–9.
7. Gil Z, Abergel A, Spektor S, Khafif A, Fliss DM. Patient, caregiver, and surgeon perceptions of quality of life following anterior skull base surgery. Arch Otolaryngol Head Neck Surg. 2004;130(11):1276–81.
8. Fliss DM, Abergel A, Cavel O, Margalit N, Gil Z. Combined subcranial approaches for excision of complex anterior skull base tumors. Arch Otolaryngol Head Neck Surg. 2007;133(9):888–96.
9. Lim X, Rajagopal R, Silva P, Jeyaretna DS, Mykula R, Potter M. A systematic review on outcomes of anterior skull base reconstruction. J Plast Reconstr Aesthet Surg. 2020;73(11):1940–50.
10. Harvey RJ, Parmar P, Sacks R, Zanation AM. Endoscopic skull base reconstruction of large dural defects: a systematic review of published evidence. Laryngoscope. 2012;122(2):452–9.

11. Thompson NJ, Roche JP, Schularick NM, Chang KE, Hansen MR. Reconstruction outcomes following lateral skull base resection. Otol Neurotol. 2017;38(2):264–71.
12. Howard BE, Nagel TH, Barrs DM, Donald CB, Hayden RE. Reconstruction of lateral skull base defects: a comparison of the submental flap to free and regional flaps. Otolaryngol Head Neck Surg. 2016;154(6):1014–8.
13. Kane L. Medscape malpractice report 2019. 2019. https://www.medscape.com/slideshow/2019-malpractice-report-6012303. Accessed 20 May 2021.
14. Ceremsak J, Miller LE, Gomez ED. A review of otolaryngology malpractice cases with associated court proceedings from 2010 to 2019. Laryngoscope. 2021;131(4):E1081–5.
15. Bal BS. An introduction to medical malpractice in the United States. Clin Orthop Relat Res. 2009;467(2):339–47.
16. Patel AM, Still TE, Vaughan W. Medicolegal issues in endoscopic sinus surgery. Otolaryngol Clin North Am. 2010;43(4):905–14.
17. Sioshansi PC, Chen T, Babu SC. Malpractice in skull base surgery. In: Anderson EJ, et al., editors. Litigation in otolaryngology: minimizing liability and preventing adverse outcomes. Cham: Springer; 2021. p. 87.
18. Blake DM, Svider PF, Carniol ET, Mauro AC, Eloy JA, Jyung RW. Malpractice in otology. Otolaryngol Head Neck Surg. 2013;149(4):554–61.
19. Svider PF, Husain Q, Kovalerchik O, et al. Determining legal responsibility in otolaryngology: a review of 44 trials since 2008. Am J Otolaryngol. 2013;34(6):699–705.
20. Lydiatt DD. Medical malpractice and facial nerve paralysis. Arch Otolaryngol Head Neck Surg. 2003;129(1):50–3.
21. Lydiatt DD, Sewell RK. Medical malpractice and sinonasal disease. Otolaryngol Head Neck Surg. 2008;139(5):677–81.
22. Dawson DE, Kraus EM. Medical malpractice and rhinology. Am J Rhinol. 2007;21(5):584–90.
23. Kovalerchik O, Mady LJ, Svider PF, et al. Physician accountability in iatrogenic cerebrospinal fluid leak litigation. Int Forum Allergy Rhinol. 2013;3(9):722–5.
24. Birkenbeuel J, Vu K, Lehrich BM, et al. Medical malpractice of vestibular schwannoma: a 40-year review of the United States legal databases. Otol Neurotol. 2019;40(3):391–7.
25. Studdert DM, Mello MM, Sage WM, et al. Defensive medicine among high-risk specialist physicians in a volatile malpractice environment. JAMA. 2005;293(21):2609–17.
26. Seabury SA, Chandra A, Lakdawalla DN, Jena AB. On average, physicians spend nearly 11 percent of their 40-year careers with an open, unresolved malpractice claim. Health Aff. 2013;32(1):111–9.
27. Kern KA. Preventing the delayed diagnosis of breast cancer through medical litigation analysis. Surg Oncol Clin N Am. 1994;3(1):101–23.
28. Diercks DB, Cady B. Lawsuits for failure to diagnose breast cancer: tumor biology in causation and risk management strategies. Surg Oncol Clin N Am. 1994;3(1):125–39.
29. Levinson W. Physician-patient communication: a key to malpractice prevention. JAMA. 1994;272(20):1619–20.
30. Levinson W, Roter DL, Mullooly JP, Dull VT, Frankel RM. Physician-patient communication: the relationship with malpractice claims among primary care physicians and surgeons. JAMA. 1997;277(7):553–9.
31. Huntington B, Kuhn N. Communication gaffes: a root cause of malpractice claims. Proc (Bayl Univ Med Cent). 2003;16(2):157–61; discussion 161.
32. Svider PF, Kelly SP, Baredes S, Eloy JA. Overview of malpractice litigation in otolaryngology. In: Anderson EJ, et al., editors. Litigation in otolaryngology: minimizing liability and preventing adverse outcomes. Cham: Springer; 2021. p. 1–10.
33. Klimo GF, Daum WJ, Brinker MR, McGuire E, Elliott MN. Orthopedic medical malpractice: an attorney's perspective. Am J Orthop (Belle Mead NJ). 2000;29(2):93–7.
34. Ramakrishnan VR, Orlandi RR, Citardi MJ, Smith TL, Fried MP, Kingdom TT. The use of image-guided surgery in endoscopic sinus surgery: an evidence-based review with recommendations. Int Forum Allergy Rhinol. 2013;3(3):236–41.

35. Ramakrishnan VR, Kingdom TT. Does image-guided surgery reduce complications? Otolaryngol Clin North Am. 2015;48(5):851–9.
36. Komotar RJ, Starke RM, Raper DM, Anand VK, Schwartz TH. Endoscopic endonasal versus open repair of anterior skull base CSF leak, meningocele, and encephalocele: a systematic review of outcomes. J Neurol Surg A Cent Eur Neurosurg. 2013;74(04):239–50.
37. Acioly MA, Liebsch M, de Aguiar PH, Tatagiba M. Facial nerve monitoring during cerebellopontine angle and skull base tumor surgery: a systematic review from description to current success on function prediction. World Neurosurg. 2013;80(6):e271–300.
38. Nissen AJ, Sikand A, Curto FS, Welsh JE, Gardi J. Value of intraoperative threshold stimulus in predicting postoperative facial nerve function after acoustic tumor resection. Am J Otol. 1997;18(2):249–51.
39. Oh T, Nagasawa DT, Fong BM, et al. Intraoperative neuromonitoring techniques in the surgical management of acoustic neuromas. Neurosurg Focus. 2012;33(3):E6.
40. Kartush JM, Larouere MJ, Graham MD, Bouchard KR, Audet BV. Intraoperative cranial nerve monitoring during posterior skull base surgery. Skull Base Surg. 1991;1(2):85–92.
41. Simon MV. Neurophysiologic intraoperative monitoring of the vestibulocochlear nerve. J Clin Neurophysiol. 2011;28(6):566–81.
42. Vincent C, Phillips A, Young M. Why do people sue doctors? A study of patients and relatives taking legal action. Lancet. 1994;343(8913):1609–13.
43. Brennan TA, Leape LL, Laird NM, et al. Incidence of adverse events and negligence in hospitalized patients. Results of the harvard medical practice study I. N Engl J Med. 1991;324(6):370–6.
44. Leape LL, Brennan TA, Laird N, et al. The nature of adverse events in hospitalized patients. Results of the harvard medical practice study II. N Engl J Med. 1991;324(6):377–84.
45. Localio AR, Lawthers AG, Brennan TA, et al. Relation between malpractice claims and adverse events due to negligence: results of the harvard medical practice study III. N Engl J Med. 1991;325(4):245–51.
46. Maithel SK. Iatrogenic error and truth telling: a comparison of the United States and India. Issues Med Ethics. 1998;6(4):125–7.
47. Witman AB, Park DM, Hardin SB. How do patients want physicians to handle mistakes?: a survey of internal medicine patients in an academic setting. Arch Intern Med. 1996;156(22):2565–9.
48. Mathew R, Asimacopoulos E, Valentine P. Toward safer practice in otology: a report on 15 years of clinical negligence claims. Laryngoscope. 2011;121(10):2214–9.

Part VII
Future Applications

Chapter 34
Emerging Developments in Skull Base Reconstruction

Khodayar Goshtasbi, Bobby A. Tajudeen, Harrison W. Lin, Hamid R. Djalilian, and Edward C. Kuan

Laser Tissue Welding

Laser tissue welding (LTW) is a technology that has been studied both experimentally and clinically in mucosal and vascular repair [1], intestinal and colorectal repair [2], sealing air leaks after lung surgery [3], corneal cut closure [4], and endoscopic cranial base reconstruction [5, 6]. This technique applies laser energy (808-nm diode) to a chromophore-doped biological solder to create instant fluid-tight wound repairs with minimal foreign-body reaction [7]. Given the continuous challenges in skull base reconstruction and prevalence of postoperative CSF leaks, LTW can theoretically offer primary wound closure by endoscopic sealing of wound edges using a laser and biological solder that controls for post-repair leaks [6].

It has been more than a decade since the first endonasal LTW human experiment was published, where patients' solders persisted for up to 26 days and withstood the hydrostatic intracranial pressures [5]. Furthermore, the study reported no equipment malfunctions or patient complications, and inflammation, edema, and thermal energy were not statistically different than a control group. A subsequent animal study by the same researchers reported on a novel polysaccharide soldering gel to address the limitations of the previously used hyaluronic acid-based liquid solder, which would improve bridge tissue gaps and burst pressure, minimize gravitational displacement, and avoid intraoperative dilution from bleeding or irrigation and

K. Goshtasbi · H. W. Lin · H. R. Djalilian · E. C. Kuan (✉)
Otolaryngology-Head and Neck Surgery and Neurological Surgery, University of California, Irvine, Irvine, CA, USA
e-mail: harriswl@hs.uci.edu; hdjalili@hs.uci.edu; eckuan@hs.uci.edu

B. A. Tajudeen
Otorhinolaryngology-Head and Neck Surgery, Rush University Medical Center, Chicago, IL, USA
e-mail: bobby_tajudeen@rush.edu

E. C. Kuan et al. (eds.), *Skull Base Reconstruction*,
https://doi.org/10.1007/978-3-031-27937-9_34

successful resorption without long-term deleterious effects [6]. Since these publications, there have been no major advancements in our understanding of LTW and anterior skull base reconstruction, or potential applications to endoscopic lateral skull base reconstruction. Future studies are needed to investigate the technical feasibility and safety of this technology, especially thermal conduction around critical neurovascular structures, and further optimize the solder formulations in skull base reconstruction.

Endoscopic CNS Drug Delivery

The drug delivery of large molecule therapeutics to the central nervous system for treating neurodegenerative disorders is limited by the blood-brain barrier (BBB). Reduction of brain-derived neurotrophic factor (BDNF) levels are associated with several neurodegenerative disorders [8], which have led to various efforts for BDNF augmentation to mitigate disease progression [9]. A novel minimally invasive nasal depot (MIND) technique was recently introduced for direct trans-nasal drug delivery to the olfactory submucosal space [10]. To overcome limitations of topical intranasal drug administration, this technique suspended the drug in a gel carrier that gets endoscopically injected into the olfactory epithelium's submucosa (directly surrounding the olfactory neurons) and achieved 40% of direct intracerebroventricular delivery [10].

Another method to bypass the BBB is transmucosal drug delivery using mucosal graft techniques. Animal studies have demonstrated that the mucosal graft could transport molecules 1000x larger than what BBB directly permits (up to 500 kDa) by creating a permanent semipermeable window in the BBB using purely autologous tissues [11]. These mucosal grafts could thus bypass the BBB and deliver CNS therapeutics when engrafted over an arachnoid defect, with an efficacy similar to direct intrastriatal injections [12]. Proper human studies are warranted to investigate the utility of this technique, given human mucosal graft area-to-brain volume ratio is higher than the studied animals, and that in animal brain, diffusion to more distal regions via CSF circulation is less possible [13].

Point-of-Care CSF Detection

Prompt and accurate diagnosis of CSF leak is unfortunately challenging and far from adequate. For most clinicians, characterizing a colorless and odorless discharge such as CSF involves a high degree of clinical suspicion and may include a combination of history and physical examination, imaging, and laboratory testing. It is also common to acquire high-resolution computed tomography and magnetic resonance imaging to aid with diagnosis, which may be timely, costly, and contraindicated in selected patients, without certainty of diagnosis [14]. Moreover, signs and symptoms of CSF leak are nonspecific and may include headache, tinnitus, malaise, fever, or nasal/ear drainage, thereby risking misdiagnosis even by the most experienced of clinicians. This may also lead to a delay in diagnosis and management, leading to iatrogenic complications, antibiotic resistance, and substantial costs associated with unnecessary treatments [15–17]. The current standard of diagnosis requires sending samples to an outside laboratory and waiting 4–7 days for results, which may not be completely reliable depending on sample contamination (e.g., co-presence of blood or dilution by mucus/secretions). Despite the great need to create a reliable, fast, and user-friendly CSF detection tool, there currently exist no FDA-approved or widely used point-of-care (POC) devices available.

Current attempts to create such a POC device have aimed to quantify beta-trace protein (βTP) or beta-2 transferrin (β2TF), which are both reliable indicators of CSF [18, 19]. Development of the first rapid POC test kit has been recently published where the researchers utilized a barcode-style lateral-flow immunoassay for βTP quantification [20]. The reported test kit is composed of the lateral-flow immunoassay, collection swab, dilution buffers, disposable pipettes, and instructions, designed for an untrained user to test a solution in 20 min [20]. Future studies to continue investigating the sensitivity and specificity of the test especially when testing contaminated samples (e.g., with blood) are warranted before potential mass adoption.

Alternative targets for detection have also been explored. Dickkopf-related protein 3 (DKK3), which is a protein present in CSF and in trace amounts within serum, has been studied as a potential target for detection. Given limited renal clearance, it is less likely to generate false positives in patients with renal disease. Using immunoblotting techniques, Michaelides et al. were able to detect DKK3 in CSF with as little as 0.25 μL of volume within 10 min; conversely, no DKK3 was detected in as much as 15 μL of serum, with minimal cross-contamination by blood [21]. This technology has the potential to bypass specialized laboratory testing and prevent treatment delays for those patients with suspected CSF leak.

Another study quantified β2TF using an immunochromatographic assay testing strip via implementing sialic acid-specific lectins [22]. Specifically, immobilized lectin is implemented into deletion lines to capture sialotransferrins at the beginning of the test strip. Near the end of the strip, immobilized anti-transferrin antibodies are able to detect the remaining β2TF [22]. Despite the success of this two-stage detection system, future studies are warranted to address several limitations including the requirement for sample pre-treatment, assay time of 70 min excluding pre-treatment time, and mere testing of artificial positive and negative clinical samples. Despite the limitations of these studies, their significant achievements lay the groundwork for subsequent studies to validate POC CSF-detection devices and markedly improve skull base patient care.

Indocyanin Green in Skull Base Surgery and Reconstruction

Endoscope-integrated indocyanine green (ICG) was first introduced to skull base surgery to visually differentiate pituitary adenomas from surrounding tissues, therefore minimizing injury to surrounding structures and facilitating complete resection of the tumor [23]. Since then, this technology has evolved into various applications in skull base surgery to visualize vascular structures and confirm vascular patency and biopsy intraventricular tumors [24–27]. Near-infrared florescence imaging using second-window indocyanine green, which relies on the passive accumulation of ICG within skull base tumors such as pituitary adenoma, also has potential to serve as an adjunct to accurately localize the tumor and all the surrounding structures and thus improve surgical outcomes [28, 29]. In the fields of plastic and head and neck reconstructive surgery, there have been numerous publications on the utility of ICG to test the viability of local, pedicled, or free flaps [30–32]. For endoscopic skull base reconstruction, endoscope-integrated ICG has been recently utilized to evaluate nasoseptal flap perfusion [33, 34]. This is an important topic since there are no validated techniques to intraoperatively evaluate the vascularized flap's viability, which may be compromised pre- or peri-operatively, during endoscopic reconstruction of skull base defects.

One study tested ICG near-infrared fluorescence endoscopy on 38 patients undergoing endoscopic skull base reconstruction with nasoseptal flap [34]. When the pedicle and body of the flap both enhanced intraoperatively, all of those patients showed MRI contrast enhancement postoperatively, and there were no instances of flap necrosis. Two of the three patients with no ICG enhancement experienced flap necrosis, and of the 15 patients with either just pedicle or just body only enhancement, one experienced flap necrosis. The authors found no association between ICG enhancement and postoperative CSF leak. The study also noted an important limitation that would need to be addressed in future studies, namely, the subjective intraoperative evaluation of ICG assessment as opposed to an objective measurement such as in Hounsfield units. Another study also reported on the experience of five patients, where all the nasoseptal flaps were enhanced on intraoperative ICG evaluation, and they corresponded to appropriate postoperative healing of all flaps without complications [33]. ICG near-infrared imaging of nasoseptal flap can also be correlated with postoperative MRI flap enhancement [34].

Wound Healing Models in Skull Base Reconstruction

There are continuous scientific developments to appropriately reconstruct the skull base, prevent CSF leak, and minimize postoperative complications or need for reoperation. The reconstruction aims to form a tight dural seal that contains CSF, prevents air from passing into intracranial space, and separates the unsterile sinonasal tract from the sterile subdural space. Although appropriate dural healing is crucial to prevent CSF leaks, there remain many gaps in knowledge on the topic of healing. One study constructed a bacterial cellulose membrane as a novel dura patch, which could form an elastic, resistant, and nontoxic biogel, which accommodates collagen and growth factors [35]. Bacterial cellulose has been widely studied for wound healing in other fields because of its unique characteristics such as high water content, crystallinity, mechanical stability, and high degree of polymerization, and its biomechanics, biocompatibility, and reported fibroblastic ingrowth make it a potential candidate for dural repair [35]. Healing can also be promoted by the inflammatory response triggered by fibrin glue, which was shown to reduce rates of CSF leak via strengthening the repair and improving graft adherence [36]. It was also reported that stimulating factors (e.g., fibroblast growth factor type 2 and insulin) can further stimulate dural closure in an in vitro dural healing model [37], which can become imbedded in closure material or be applied over dural suture lines in the future. The healing effects of autologous mucosal grafts, tested in injured rabbit maxillary sinuses, were recently compared to spontaneous wound healing and showed improved cellular composition with larger areas of ciliary epithelium and lengthier/narrower cilia [38]. Notably, a new dural healing model using human cells has been introduced [39], which will continue improving upon our understanding of dural healing and closure compared to the standard animal-based healing models.

Biomechanical Models for Skull Base Reconstruction

There are several techniques to seal skull base defects and prevent CSF leaks. These include vascularized pedicled flaps (e.g., nasoseptal flap), synthetic grafts (e.g., collagen, fibrin glue), and free-graft repairs (e.g., fat, temporalis fascia) [40]. There are currently no gold-standards among these techniques, and all are commonly performed according to surgeons' preference. As such, there are active investigations regarding the biomechanical properties and strength/durability of various graft types. For instance, it was shown that burst strength of different repair techniques could be compared using a simple in vitro methodology, where authors showed the biomechanical advantage of Tisseel fibrin compared to suture, U-CLIP, and underlay/overlay techniques [41]. This is in-line with a more recent ex vivo study of six repair techniques, where Tisseel supported greater pressures than repairs without tissue sealant for large dural defects [42]. Another in vitro study tested the biomechanical properties of various soft tissue skull base repairs with reported absolute breaking strengths. They showed that the fibrin glue and pericranium combination was the strongest repair with the ability to withstand six times normal intracranial pressure, which supported the use of fibrin glue as a sealant and the use of pericranium as an alternative free graft when no other autologous grafts are available [40]. Furthermore, an ex vivo model study investigated the failure pressure of autologous mucosa/Tisseel, fat graft, and bath plug techniques on 5-mm dural defects. They showed that the bath plug technique had the highest tolerance pressure and the only one to withstand normal adult CSF pressure, while the fat graft had the highest variability and inconsistency between trials [43]. It should however be noted that such ex vivo biomechanical models are limited in the inability to assess wound healing, additive strengths of vascularized tissues, and other properties that make real-life human dural repair multifaceted.

Augmentation of dural repair with an acrylic plate under a foley catheter for diffuse support was recently tested in an ex vivo model. This resulted in tolerating the greatest amount of intracranial pressure (and the only one withstanding the upper limits of normal adult pressure) compared to other tested repairs (mucosa with fibrin glue with or without foley catheter) [44]. Some studies have utilized a pressure testing apparatus to test the biomechanical characteristics of various repairs [36]. Studies in live models are needed to replicate these findings while accounting for the effects of wound healing, blood coagulation, changing temperature, and pedicled flap repair on the fibrin sealant. The novel use of titanium clips compared to tissue glue was studied in an ex vivo porcine biomechanical model, showing that tissue glue (collagen matrix graft with polyethylene glycol glue) had the highest and novel titanium clips had the lowest failure pressures [45]. Despite this finding, there is certainly a continued need for invention of novel material with the highest biomechanical viability and endurance.

Training Through Simulations and 3D Printed Models

Technological developments in the past decade are offering novel opportunities to improve training in skull base surgery and reconstruction, including surgical simulations and three-dimentional (3D)-printed models. In addition to allowing extra practice in a safe environment, this can allow trainees to experience rare conditions that are otherwise not encountered often during training. For instance, given internal carotid artery (ICA) injury and its management is rarely encountered during training [46], there were recent efforts to develop cadaveric stimulation models of ICA injury for residents and attendings. These efforts showed significant improvement in performance and confidence after participating in the brief and low-cost simulation [47, 48]. Similarly, a perfusion-based human cadaveric model was developed for simulation of dural venous sinus injury and repair, which was beneficial in improving management skills of the participating residents [49]. Perfusion-based human cadaveric models were also utilized to simulate CSF leak repair, which led to an increase in knowledge and confidence of the participants [50].

Compared to cadaveric models, virtual reality (VR) models allow for artificial incorporation of anatomical variations, rare scenarios, and repeated attempts at various tasks [51]. In lateral skull base surgery education, one study developed an interactive stimulation that combined a 3D operative perspective from the lead surgeon with VR models of the temporal bone that could be manipulated [52]. An anatomy-specific VR surgical rehearsal for cortical mastoidectomy with facial recess was also developed, which resulted in significant increase in confidence and performance of the training participants [53]. VR haptic simulators have also been introduced to the field of anterior skull base surgery to provide a realistic training environment [54]. The incorporation of these technologies may prove promising in the training of skull base reconstruction in the future.

The development of 3D-printed models has also optimized teaching and improved trainee's understanding and subsequent performance. The applications of 3D technology and their incorporation into surgical training are increasing because of their cost, availability, lack of regulatory requirements, and ability to customize and create rare variations [55]. Three-dimensional models have been developed to simulate surgery for complex intracranial lesions [56], cranial nerve management [57], endoscopic anterior skull base simulation [55], and lateral skull base training [58]. Lastly, these technologies can provide both educational opportunities as well as novel approaches for treatment and reconstruction of skull base lesions. One study described a challenging case of a petrous apex cyst through a subcochlear surgical corroider, where the combination of VR, 3D-printed model, and navigation enabled a safe transcanal endoscopic approach [59].

References

1. Mistry YA, Natarajan SS, Ahuja SA. Evaluation of laser tissue welding and laser-tissue soldering for mucosal and vascular repair. Ann Maxillofac Surg. 2018;8(1):35–41.
2. Huang H-C, Walker CR, Nanda A, Rege K. Laser welding of ruptured intestinal tissue using plasmonic polypeptide nanocomposite solders. ACS Nano. 2013;7(4):2988–98.
3. Schiavon M, Marulli G, Zuin A, Lunardi F, Villoresi P, Bonora S, et al. Experimental evaluation of a new system for laser tissue welding applied on damaged lungs. Interact Cardiovasc Thorac Surg. 2013;16(5):577–82.
4. Tal K, Strassmann E, Loya N, Ravid A, Kariv N, Weinberger D, et al. Corneal cut closure using temperature-controlled CO2 laser soldering system. Lasers Med Sci. 2015;30(4):1367–71.
5. Bleier BS, Cohen NA, Chiu AG, O'Malley BWJ, Doghramji L, Palmer JN. Endonasal laser tissue welding: first human experience. Am J Rhinol Allergy. 2010;24(3):244–6.
6. Bleier BS, Palmer JN, Cohen NA. Evaluation of a polysaccharide gel for laser-assisted skull base repair. Am J Rhinol Allergy. 2013;27(2):148–50.
7. Meier JC, Bleier BS. Novel techniques and the future of skull base reconstruction. Adv Otorhinolaryngol. 2013;74:174–83.
8. Zuccato C, Cattaneo E. Brain-derived neurotrophic factor in neurodegenerative diseases. Nat Rev Neurol. 2009;5(6):311–22.
9. Sampaio TB, Savall AS, Gutierrez MEZ, Pinton S. Neurotrophic factors in Alzheimer's and Parkinson's diseases: implications for pathogenesis and therapy. Neural Regen Res. 2017;12(4):549–57.
10. Padmakumar S, Jones G, Pawar G, Khorkova O, Hsiao J, Kim J, et al. Minimally invasive nasal depot (MIND) technique for direct BDNF AntagoNAT delivery to the brain. J Control Release. 2021;331:176–86.
11. Bleier BS, Kohman RE, Feldman RE, Ramanlal S, Han X. Permeabilization of the blood-brain barrier via mucosal engrafting: implications for drug delivery to the brain. PloS One. 2013;8(4):e61694.
12. Bleier BS, Kohman RE, Guerra K, Nocera AL, Ramanlal S, Kocharyan AH, et al. Heterotopic mucosal grafting enables the delivery of therapeutic neuropeptides across the blood brain barrier. Neurosurgery. 2016;78(3):448–57; discussion 457.

13. Marianecci C, Rinaldi F, Hanieh PN, Di Marzio L, Paolino D, Carafa M. Drug delivery in overcoming the blood-brain barrier: role of nasal mucosal grafting. Drug Des Devel Ther. 2017;11:325–35.
14. Reddy M, Baugnon K. Imaging of cerebrospinal fluid rhinorrhea and otorrhea. Radiol Clin North Am. 2017;55(1):167–87.
15. Ramakrishnan VR, Kingdom TT, Nayak JV, Hwang PH, Orlandi RR. Nationwide incidence of major complications in endoscopic sinus surgery. Int Forum Allergy Rhinol. 2012;2(1):34–9.
16. van de Beek D, Drake JM, Tunkel AR. Nosocomial bacterial meningitis. N Engl J Med. 2010;362(2):146–54.
17. Villwock JA, Villwock MR, Deshaies EM, Goyal P. Clinical and economic impact of time from admission for CSF Rhinorrhea to surgical repair. Laryngoscope. 2019;129(3):539–43.
18. Bachmann-Harildstad G. Diagnostic values of beta-2 transferrin and beta-trace protein as markers for cerebrospinal fluid fistula. Rhinology. 2008;46(2):82.
19. Mantur M, Łukaszewicz-Zając M, Mroczko B, Kułakowska A, Ganslandt O, Kemona H, et al. Cerebrospinal fluid leakage--reliable diagnostic methods. Clin Chim Acta. 2011;412(11–12):837–40.
20. Bradbury DW, Kita AE, Hirota K, St John MA, Kamei DT. Rapid diagnostic test kit for point-of-care cerebrospinal fluid leak detection. SLAS Technol. 2020;25(1):67–74.
21. Michaelides EM, Kuang H, Pieribone VA. Dickkopf-related protein 3 as a sensitive and specific marker for cerebrospinal fluid leaks. Otol Neurotol. 2016;37(3):299–303.
22. Oh J, Kwon S-J, Dordick JS, Sonstein WJ, Linhardt RJ, Kim M-G. Determination of cerebrospinal fluid leakage by selective deletion of transferrin glycoform using an immunochromatographic assay. Theranostics. 2019;9(14):4182–91.
23. Litvack ZN, Zada G, Laws ERJ. Indocyanine green fluorescence endoscopy for visual differentiation of pituitary tumor from surrounding structures. J Neurosurg. 2012;116(5):935–41.
24. Tsuzuki S, Aihara Y, Eguchi S, Amano K, Kawamata T, Okada Y. Application of indocyanine green (ICG) fluorescence for endoscopic biopsy of intraventricular tumors. Childs Nerv Syst. 2014;30(4):723–6.
25. Cho A, Cho SS, Buch VP, Buch LY, Lee JYK. Second window Indocyanine green (SWIG) near infrared fluorescent transventricular biopsy of pineal tumor. World Neurosurg. 2020;134:196–200.
26. Mielke D, Malinova V, Rohde V. Comparison of intraoperative microscopic and endoscopic ICG angiography in aneurysm surgery. Neurosurgery. 2014;10(Suppl 3):418–25.
27. Acerbi F, Vetrano IG, Sattin T, de Laurentis C, Bosio L, Rossini Z, et al. The role of indocyanine green videoangiography with FLOW 800 analysis for the surgical management of central nervous system tumors: an update. Neurosurg Focus. 2018;44(6):E6.
28. Cho SS, Buch VP, Teng CW, De Ravin E, Lee JYK. Near-infrared fluorescence with second-window indocyanine green as an adjunct to localize the pituitary stalk during skull base surgery. World Neurosurg. 2020;136:326.
29. Cho SS, Lee JYK. Intraoperative fluorescent visualization of pituitary adenomas. Neurosurg Clin N Am. 2019;30(4):401–12.
30. Hitier M, Cracowski J-L, Hamou C, Righini C, Bettega G. Indocyanine green fluorescence angiography for free flap monitoring: a pilot study. J Craniomaxillofac Surg. 2016;44(11):1833–41.
31. Yano T, Okazaki M, Tanaka K, Tsunoda A, Aoyagi M, Kishimoto S. Use of intraoperative fluorescent indocyanine green angiography for real-time vascular evaluation of pericranial flaps. Ann Plast Surg. 2016;76(2):198–204.
32. Yeoh MS, Kim DD, Ghali GE. Fluorescence angiography in the assessment of flap perfusion and vitality. Oral Maxillofac Surg Clin North Am. 2013;25(1):61–6, vi.
33. Kerr EE, Jamshidi A, Carrau RL, Campbell RG, Filho LFD, Otto BA, et al. Indocyanine green fluorescence to evaluate nasoseptal flap viability in endoscopic endonasal cranial base surgery. J Neurol Surg B Skull Base. 2017;78(5):408–12.

34. Geltzeiler M, Nakassa ACI, Turner M, Setty P, Zenonos G, Hebert A, et al. Evaluation of intranasal flap perfusion by intraoperative indocyanine green fluorescence angiography. Oper Neurosurg (Hagerstown). 2018;15(6):672–6.
35. Hosemann W, Goede U, Sauer M. Wound healing of mucosal autografts for frontal cerebrospinal fluid leaks—clinical and experimental investigations. Rhinology. 1999;37(3):108–12.
36. de Almeida JR, Ghotme K, Leong I, Drake J, James AL, Witterick IJ. A new porcine skull base model: fibrin glue improves strength of cerebrospinal fluid leak repairs. Otolaryngol Head Neck Surg. 2009;141(2):184–9.
37. Goldschmidt E, Ielpi M, Loresi M, D'adamo M, Giunta D, Carrizo A, et al. Assessing the role of selected growth factors and cytostatic agents in an in vitro model of human dura mater healing. Neurol Res. 2014;36(12):1040–6.
38. Topdag M, Kara A, Konuk E, Demir N, Ozturk M, Calıskan S, et al. The healing effects of autologous mucosal grafts in experimentally injured rabbit maxillary sinuses. Clin Exp Otorhinolaryngol. 2016;9(1):44–50.
39. Goldschmidt E, Hem S, Ajler P, Ielpi M, Loresi M, Giunta D, et al. A new model for dura mater healing: human dural fibroblast culture. Neurol Res. 2013;35(3):300–7.
40. Fandiño M, Macdonald K, Singh D, Whyne C, Witterick I. Determining the best graft-sealant combination for skull base repair using a soft tissue in vitro porcine model. Int Forum Allergy Rhinol. 2013;3(3):212–6.
41. de Almeida JR, Morris A, Whyne CM, James AL, Witterick IJ. Testing biomechanical strength of in vitro cerebrospinal fluid leak repairs. J Otolaryngol Head Neck Surg. 2009;38(1):106–11.
42. Lin RP, Weitzel EK, Chen PG, McMains KC, Chang DR, Braxton EE, et al. Failure pressures after repairs of 2-cm × 2.5-cm rhinologic dural defects in a porcine ex vivo model. Int Forum Allergy Rhinol. 2016;6(10):1034–9.
43. Lin RP, Weitzel EK, Chen PG, McMains KC, Majors J, Bunegin L. Failure pressures of three rhinologic dural repairs in a porcine ex vivo model. Int Forum Allergy Rhinol. 2015;5(7):633–6.
44. Chen PG, Clampitt MR, Chorath KT, Lin RP, Weitzel EK, McMains KC, et al. Augmentation of dural defect repairs strength with an acrylic plate in a porcine ex vivo model. Am J Rhinol Allergy. 2019;33(6):757–62.
45. Chorath K, Krysinski M, Bunegin L, Majors J, Weitzel EK, McMains KC, et al. Failure pressures of dural repairs in a porcine ex vivo model: novel use of titanium clips versus tissue glue. Allergy Rhinol (Providence). 2019;10:2152656719879677.
46. Rowan NR, Turner MT, Valappil B, Fernandez-Miranda JC, Wang EW, Gardner PA, et al. Injury of the carotid artery during endoscopic endonasal surgery: surveys of skull base surgeons. J Neurol Surg B Skull Base. 2018;79(3):302–8.
47. Donoho DA, Pangal DJ, Kugener G, Rutkowski M, Micko A, Shahrestani S, et al. Improved surgeon performance following cadaveric simulation of internal carotid artery injury during endoscopic endonasal surgery: training outcomes of a nationwide prospective educational intervention. J Neurosurg. 2021:1–9.
48. Donoho DA, Johnson CE, Hur KT, Buchanan IA, Fredrickson VL, Minneti M, et al. Costs and training results of an objectively validated cadaveric perfusion-based internal carotid artery injury simulation during endoscopic skull base surgery. Int Forum Allergy Rhinol. 2019;9(7):787–94.
49. Strickland BA, Ravina K, Kammen A, Chang S, Rutkowski M, Donoho DA, et al. The use of a novel perfusion-based human cadaveric model for simulation of dural venous sinus injury and repair. Oper Neurosurg (Hagerstown). 2020;19(3):E269–74.
50. Christian EA, Bakhsheshian J, Strickland BA, Fredrickson VL, Buchanan IA, Pham MH, et al. Perfusion-based human cadaveric specimen as a simulation training model in repairing cerebrospinal fluid leaks during endoscopic endonasal skull base surgery. J Neurosurg. 2018;129(3):792–6.
51. Lavigne P, Yang N. Training and surgical simulation in skull base surgery: a systematic review. Curr Otorhinolaryngol Rep. 2020;8(2):154–9.

52. Barber SR, Jain S, Mooney MA, Almefty KK, Lawton MT, Son Y-J, et al. Combining stereoscopic video and virtual reality simulation to maximize education in lateral skull base surgery. Otolaryngol Head Neck Surg. 2020;162(6):922–5.
53. Locketz GD, Lui JT, Chan S, Salisbury K, Dort JC, Youngblood P, et al. Anatomy-specific virtual reality simulation in temporal bone dissection: perceived utility and impact on surgeon confidence. Otolaryngol Head Neck Surg. 2017;156(6):1142–9.
54. Kim DH, Kim HM, Park J-S, Kim SW. Virtual reality haptic simulator for endoscopic sinus and skull base surgeries. J Craniofac Surg. 2020;31(6):1811–4.
55. Low CM, Morris JM, Price DL, Matsumoto JS, Stokken JK, O'Brien EK, et al. Three-dimensional printing: current use in rhinology and endoscopic skull base surgery. Am J Rhinol Allergy. 2019;33(6):770–81.
56. Lan Q, Zhu Q, Xu L, Xu T. Application of 3D-printed craniocerebral model in simulated surgery for complex intracranial lesions. World Neurosurg. 2020;134:e761–70.
57. Lin J, Zhou Z, Guan J, Zhu Y, Liu Y, Yang Z, et al. Using three-dimensional printing to create individualized cranial nerve models for skull base tumor surgery. World Neurosurg. 2018;120:e142–52.
58. Mooney MA, Cavallo C, Zhou JJ, Bohl MA, Belykh E, Gandhi S, et al. Three-dimensional printed models for lateral skull base surgical training: anatomy and simulation of the transtemporal approaches. Oper Neurosurg (Hagerstown). 2020;18(2):193–201.
59. Barber SR, Wong K, Kanumuri V, Kiringoda R, Kempfle J, Remenschneider AK, et al. Augmented reality, surgical navigation, and 3D printing for transcanal endoscopic approach to the petrous apex. OTO Open. 2018;2(4):2473974X18804492.

Index